**This book is to be returned on or before
the last date stamped below.**

RUSKIN, Asa P.

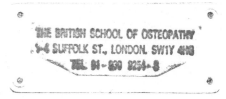
# CURRENT THERAPY IN PHYSIATRY

## Physical Medicine and Rehabilitation

*Edited by*

## ASA P. RUSKIN, M.D., F.A.C.P.

*Director, Department of Rehabilitation Medicine,*
*Kingsbrook Jewish Medical Center, Brooklyn, New York;*
*Associate Clinical Professor, Rehabilitation Medicine,*
*Albert Einstein College of Medicine, Bronx, New York*

## W. B. SAUNDERS COMPANY

*Philadelphia /London /Toronto /Mexico City /Rio de Janeiro /Sydney /Tokyo*

W. B. Saunders Company:   West Washington Square
Philadelphia, PA 19105

1 St. Anne's Road
Eastbourne, East Sussex BN 21 3UN, England

1 Goldthorne Avenue
Toronto, Ontario M8Z 5T9, Canada

Apartado 26370—Cedro 512
Mexico 4, D.F., Mexico

Rua Coronel Cabrita, 8
Sao Cristovao Caixa Postal 21176
Rio de Janeiro, Brazil

9 Waltham Street
Artarmon, N.S.W. 2064, Australia

Ichibancho, Central Bldg., 22–1 Ichibancho
Chiyoda-Ku, Tokyo 102, Japan

**Library of Congress Cataloging in Publication Data**

Main entry under title:

Current therapy in physiatry.

   1. Physical therapy.   2. Physically handicapped—
Rehabilitation.   I. Ruskin, Asa P.   [DNLM:
1. Rehabilitation.   2. Physical therapy.   WB 460 C976]
RM700.C87   1984      615.8'2            82-19138
ISBN 0-7216-7853-X

Current Therapy in Physiatry                     ISBN   0-7216-7853-X

Last digit is the print number:     9   8   7   6   5   4   3   2

# DEDICATIONS

- In memory of my parents, Simon and Frances, for whom books were everything.

- In memorium to our friend and collaborator, Dr. Arthur Abramson.

# THANKS

- For my early clinical training, to my professors at the Faculté de Médecine de Paris, and especially Monsieur le Professeur Henri Baruk, in whose service humanism was paramount.

- To my mentors who first introduced me to the specialty of Physical Medicine and Rehabilitation, Dr. Joseph Rogoff and Dr. Jerome Tobis.

- To my wife Francine, whose sacrifices advanced my career at great cost to her own.

- A special thanks to my secretary, the indispensable Marge Stone.

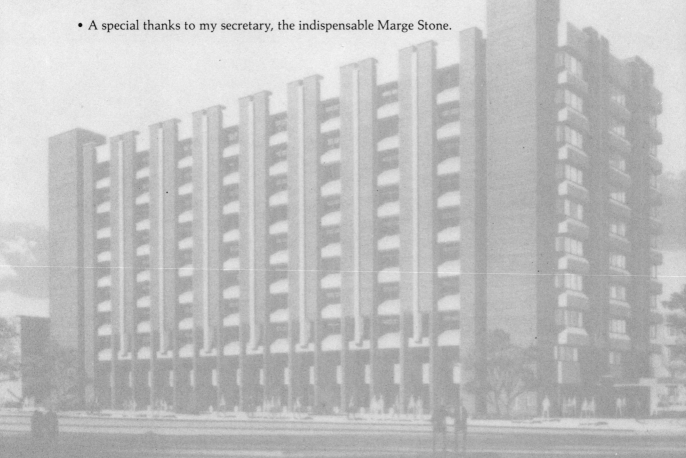

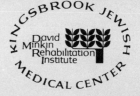

KINGSBROOK JEWISH MEDICAL CENTER

David Minkin Rehabilitation Institute

# CONTRIBUTORS

ARTHUR S. ABRAMSON, M.D. (deceased 11/3/82)

Professor and Chairman, Department of Rehabilitation Medicine, Albert Einstein College of Medicine, Bronx, N.Y.

AUGUSTA ALBA, M.D.

Clinical Associate Professor, New York University School of Medicine; Deputy Director, Department of Rehabilitation Medicine, Goldwater Memorial Hospital, New York University Medical Center, Roosevelt Island, New York, N.Y.

JUSTIN ALEXANDER, PH.D.

Associate Professor, Department of Rehabilitation Medicine, Albert Einstein College of Medicine, Bronx; Professor and Chairman, Division of Physical Therapy, Ithaca College, Ithaca; Director, Physical Therapy, Bronx Municipal Hospital Center-Albert Einstein College of Medicine, Bronx, N.Y.

THOMAS L. ASHCOM, JR., O.T.R., C.R.C.

Director, Occupational Therapy/Vocational Services, Magee Rehabilitation Hospital, Philadelphia, PA.

JOHN V. BASMAJIAN, M.D., F.A.C.A., F.R.C.P. (C.)

Professor of Medicine and Director of Rehabilitation Programs, McMaster University School of Medicine; Director, Chedoke Rehabilitation Centre, Chedoke-McMaster Hospitals, Hamilton, Ontario, Canada.

S. ELAINE BENNETHUM, M.S., O.T.R., R.P.T.

Clinical Supervisor of Occupational Therapy, Goldwater Memorial Hospital, New York University Medical Center, Roosevelt Island, New York, N.Y.

NANCY A. BROOKS, M.A.

Assistant Professor, Sociology, Wichita State University, Wichita, KA.

LORRAINE E. BUCHANAN, R.N., M.S.N.

Project Coordinator, Regional Spinal Cord Injury Center of Delaware Valley, Thomas Jefferson University, Philadelphia, PA.

RENÉ CAILLIET, M.D.

Chairman and Professor, Department of Rehabilitation Medicine, University of Southern California, Los Angeles; Director, Department of Rehabilitation Medicine, Santa Monica Hospital Medical Center, Santa Monica, CA.

DIANA D. CARDENAS, M.D.

Assistant Professor, Department of Rehabilitation Medicine, University of Washington; Director, Outpatient Rehabilitation Services, University Hospital; Attending Physician, University Hospital, Harborview Medical Center, Children's Orthopedic Hospital and VA Hospital, Seattle, WA.

MICHAEL CHAIKEN, M.S.

Assistant Professor, Long Island University; Instructor, City University of New York; Chief of Recreation Therapy, Kingsbrook Jewish Medical Center, Brooklyn, N.Y.

R. CHAWLA, O.T.R.

Assistant Lecturer, Rehabilitation Medicine, New York Medical College, Valhalla; Chief, Occupational Therapy, Metropolitan Hospital, New York, N.Y.

SANDRA M. COHEN, M.A., R.P.T.

Formerly Physical Therapist, Kingsbrook Jewish Medical Center, Brooklyn, N.Y.

VICTOR CUMMINGS, M.D.

Eleanor Coghlin Chairman and Professor of Rehabilitation Medicine, Medical College of Ohio; Director of Rehabilitation Medicine, Coghlin Memorial Rehabilitation Pavillion and Medical College of Ohio Hospital, Toledo, OH.

ROGER DAVIS, B.S.

Recreational Therapist, Kingsbrook Jewish Medical Center, Brooklyn, N.Y.

J. ROBIN DEANDRADE, M.D.

Professor, Department of Orthopedics, Professor, Department of Rehabilitation Medicine, Chairman Emeritus, Department of Rehabilitation Medicine, Emory University School of Medicine; Chief of Orthopaedic Service, VA Medical Center; Attending Orthopaedic Surgeon, Emory University Hospital, Grady Memorial Hospital, Egleston Children's Hospital, Atlanta, GA.

EDWARD F. DELAGI, M.D.

Professor Emeritus, Department of Rehabilitation Medicine, Albert Einstein College of Medicine; Attending Physician, Bronx Municipal Hospital Center and the Hospital of Albert Einstein College of Medicine, Bronx, N.Y.

JAMES T. DEMOPOULOS, M.D.

Professor and Vice Chairman, Department of Rehabilitation Medicine, Mt. Sinai School of Medicine, City University of New York; Director, Department of Rehabilitation Medicine, Beth Israel Medical Center, New York, N.Y.

JOHN F. DITUNNO, JR., M.D.

Professor and Chairman of Rehabilitation Medicine, Jefferson Medical College; Chairman, Department of Rehabilitation Medicine, Thomas Jefferson University Hospital; Project Director, Regional Spinal Cord Injury Center of Delaware Valley, Thomas Jefferson University Hospital, Philadelphia, PA.

KEVIN EARLS, M.S., O.T.R.

Staff Therapist, Kingsbrook Jewish Medical Center, Brooklyn, N.Y.

ALICE L. EASON, M.P.A., R.P.T.

Chief, Physical Therapy Service, Goldwater Memorial Hospital, New York University Medical Center, Roosevelt Island, New York, N.Y.

BARBARA EISNER, M.P.S.

Recreational Therapist, Kingsbrook Jewish Medical Center, Brooklyn, N.Y.

ANDREW A. FISCHER, M.D., PH.D.

Associate Professor of Physical Medicine and Rehabilitation, Mt. Sinai School of Medicine, New York; Chief, Rehabilitation Medicine Service, VA Medical Center, Bronx; Director, Pain Diagnostic and Rehabilitation Center of Long Island, Great Neck, N.Y.

ROBERT M. FRAZIER, M.A.

Director of Recreation Therapy, Cobble Hill Nursing Home, Brooklyn, N.Y.

SUSAN O. GANS, M.S., O.T.R.

Chief, Occupational Therapy, Department of Rehabilitation Medicine, Albert Einstein College of Medicine, Bronx Municipal Hospital Center-Jacobi Hospital, Bronx, N.Y.

ROBERT L. HEINEMAN, L.P.T.

Formerly Affiliated with the Department of Rehabilitation Medicine, Thomas Jefferson University Hospital, Philadelphia, PA.

J. P. HELD

Professeur, Faculté de Médecine, Paris Ouest; Directeur, Clinique de Reeducation Motrice, Hospital Raymond Poincaré, Paris, France

GAIL M. HERRING, M.S.W., A.C.S.W.

Chief, Social Service, Goldwater Memorial Hospital, New York University Medical Center, Roosevelt Island, New York, N.Y.

CATHERINE HINTERBUCHNER, M.D.

Professor and Chairman of Rehabilitation Medicine, New York Medical College; Chief and Attending Physician of Rehabilitation Medicine, Metropolitan Hospital Center, New York; Attending Physician in Rehabilitation Medicine, Westchester County Medical Center, Valhalla, N.Y.

JUDITH HIRSCHWALD, M.S.W.

Patient Systems Coordinator, Regional Spinal Cord Injury Center of Delaware Valley, Thomas Jefferson University Hospital; Director of Social Services, Magee Rehabilitation Hospital; Lecturer, University of Pennsylvania School of Social Work, Philadelphia, PA.

LEE S. GOLDSMITH, M.D., L.L.B., F.C.L.M.

Adjunct Associate Professor of Law, Fordham Law School; Partner, Goldsmith and Tabak, New York, N.Y.

MASAYOSHI ITOH, M.D., M.P.H.

Associate Professor of Clinical Rehabilitation Medicine, New York University School of Medicine; Associate Director, Department of Rehabilitation Medicine, Goldwater Memorial Hospital, New York University Medical Center, Roosevelt Island, New York, N.Y.

STANLEY R. JACOBS, M.D.

Assistant Professor, Rehabilitation Medicine, Jefferson Medical College; Director, Consultation Service, Department of Rehabilitation Medicine, Thomas Jefferson University Hospital; Head, Division of Rehabilitation Medicine, Department of Medicine, Mt. Sinai-Daroff Medical Center, Philadelphia, PA.

KAREN JOELSON, M.A., C.C.C.

Formerly Speech Pathologist, Kingsbrook Jewish Medical Center, Brooklyn, N.Y.

LAWRENCE I. KAPLAN, M.D.

Clinical Professor of Rehabilitation Medicine, Mt. Sinai School of Medicine; Director, Department of Rehabilitation Medicine, Mt. Sinai Services, City Hospital Center, Elmhurst; Attending Physician, Mt. Sinai Medical Center, New York, N.Y.

SHANTI S. KARWAL, M.D.

Assistant Attending, Department of Rehabilitation Medicine; Director, Work Physiology Laboratory, Kingsbrook Jewish Medical Center, Brooklyn, N.Y.

ALI A. KHALILI, M.D.

Associate Professor, Department of Rehabilitation Medicine, Northwestern University, McGaw Medical Center, Chicago; Director and Chairman, Department of Rehabilitation Medicine, Grant Hospital of Chicago; Consulting Physiatrist, Rehabilitation Institute of Chicago; Consulting Physiatrist, Memorial Hospital of DuPage County, Elmhurst, IL.

HANS KRAUS, M.D.

Associate Professor of Rehabilitation Medicine, New York University College of Medicine, New York, N.Y.

NANCY G. KUTNER, PH.D.

Assistant Professor (Medical Sociologist), Department of Rehabilitation Medicine, Emory University School of Medicine, Atlanta, GA.

JANET G. LAMANTIA, R.N., M.A.

Clinical Coordinator, Regional Spinal Cord Injury Center of Delaware Valley, Thomas Jefferson University Hospital; Clinical Coordinator, Spinal Cord Injury Follow-Up Program, Magee Rehabilitation Hospital, Philadelphia, PA.

MATHEW H. M. LEE, M.D., M.P.H., F.A.C.P.

Professor of Clinical Rehabilitation Medicine, Clinical Professor of Behavioral Sciences and Community Health, Clinical Professor of Oral and Maxillofacial Surgery, College of Dentistry, New York University; Director, Department of Rehabilitation Medicine, Goldwater Memorial Hospital, New York University Medical Center, Roosevelt Island, New York, N.Y.

KURT G. LEICHTENTRITT, M.D.

Consultant in Rehabilitation Medicine, Albert Einstein College of Medicine; Director of Rehabilitation Medicine, Pelham Bay General Hospital; Medical Director, Astor Gardens Nursing Home; Emeritus Associate Attending at Montefiore Hospital and Medical Center; Associate Attending, Bronx Municipal Hospital; Consultant, Westchester Square Hospital; Consultant, St. Barnabas Hospital, Bronx, N.Y.

MICHAEL H. LEVINE, M.S.

Recreation Leader, Kingsbrook Jewish Medical Center, Brooklyn, N.Y.

W. T. LIBERSON, M.D.

Department of Rehabilitation Medicine, Brooklyn Hospital, Brooklyn, N.Y.

MELANIA M. LIBERTO, M.S.

Staff Psychologist, Magee Rehabilitation Hospital, Philadelphia, PA.

LESLIE LINVILLE, M.S., O.T.R.

Occupational Therapist, Kingsbrook Jewish Medical Center, Brooklyn, N.Y.

HEINZ I. LIPPMANN, M.D., F.A.C.P., F.A.C.A.

Professor Emeritus of Rehabilitation Medicine, Albert Einstein College of Medicine; Chief, Peripheral Vascular Clinic, Bronx Municipal Hospital Center (AECOM); Consultant in Peripheral Vascular Diseases, Englewood Hospital, Englewood; Consultant, Physical Medicine and Rehabilitation, East Orange VA Hospital, East Orange; Director, Rehabilitation Medicine, Barnert Memorial Hospital, Paterson, N.J.; Director, Physical Medicine and Rehabilitation, Workmen's Circle Home and Infirmary for the Aged, Bronx, N.Y.

KAREN LUCAS, B.S.

Counselor, Office of Vocational Rehabilitation. Stationed at Department of Rehabilitation Medicine, Thomas Jefferson University Hospital, Philadelphia, PA.

CHRISTOPHER MACDONALD, M.S.

Senior Psychologist, Goldwater Memorial Hospital, New York University Medical Center, Roosevelt Island, New York, N.Y.

CAROL MANLY, M.A., C.C.C.

Assistant Chief, Speech Pathology and Audiology Service, Goldwater Memorial Hospital, New York University Medical Center, Roosevelt Island, New York, N.Y.

CARL H. MARQUETTE, PH.D.

Clinical Assistant Professor, Rehabilitation Medicine, Clinical Assistant Professor, Psychiatry and Human Behavior, Jefferson Medical College; Chief, Psychology Section, Department of Rehabilitation Medicine, Thomas Jefferson University Hospital; Director, Department of Psychology, Magee Rehabilitation Hospital, Philadelphia, PA.

DEBORAH MCMURDO, O.T.R.

Formerly affiliated with the Department of Rehabilitation Medicine, Thomas Jefferson University Hospital, Philadelphia, PA.

MARGO S. MEISSNER, M.A., R.P.T.

Formerly Physical Therapist, Kingsbrook Jewish Medical Center, Brooklyn, N.Y.

MADELYN MELTZER, M.A., O.T.R.

Senior Occupational Therapist, Kingsbrook Jewish Medical Center, Brooklyn, N.Y.

GAIL MILLER, B.S., L.P.T.

Director of Physical Therapy Department, Magee Rehabilitation Hospital, Philadelphia, PA.

MICHAEL MITTELMANN, M.D.

Medical Director, Claim Department, Commercial Insurance Division, Ætna Life & Casualty, Hartford, Connecticut; Chairman-Elect, Insurance Rehabilitation Study Group; Chairman, Rehabilitation Subcommittee (of the Disability Insurance Committee), Health Insurance Association of America; Member; Rehabilitation Practices Committee of American Congress of Rehabilitation Medicine.

P. MUKKAMALA, M.D.

Assistant Professor of Community Medicine, West Virginia University Medical School; Medical Director, West Virginia Rehabilitation Center, Institute, W.V.

ROSEMARY MURRAY, M.A., R.N.

Director, Mt. Sinai Hospital School of Continuing Education in Nursing, New York, N.Y.

FRANK NASO, M.D.

Professor, Rehabilitation Medicine, Assistant Professor, Medicine, Jefferson Medical College; Director, Rehabilitation Unit, Department of Rehabilitation Medicine, Thomas Jefferson University Hospital, Philadelphia, PA.

ALICE MERTZ NOLAN, R.N., M.A.

Head Nurse, Elmhurst Hospital Center, Rehabilitation Medicine, Queens, N.Y.

JUDITH M. PERINCHIEF, O.T.R.

Assistant Director of Occupational Therapy, Magee Rehabilitation Hospital; Adjunct Instructor, College of Allied Health Professions and Clinical Instructor for Occupational Therapy Field Work, Temple University, Philadelphia, PA.

ALDO O. PEROTTO, M.D.

Associate Professor, Department of Rehabilitation Medicine, Albert Einstein College of Medicine; Attending Physician, Bronx Municipal Hospital Center and the Hospital of Albert Einstein College of Medicine, Bronx, N.Y.

DOROTHY PEZENIK, O.T.R.

Senior Occupational Therapist, Goldwater Memorial Hospital, New York University Medical Center, Roosevelt Island, New York, N.Y.

LOU ANN PILKINGTON, PH.D.

Formerly Chief, Pulmonary Laboratory, Goldwater Memorial Hospital, New York University Medical Center, Roosevelt Island, New York, N.Y.

HORACIO PINEDA, M.D.

Clinical Assistant Professor of Rehabilitation Medicine, Department of Physical Medicine and Rehabilitation, New York University; Attending Physiatrist, Institute of Rehabilitation Medicine, New York University, New York, N.Y.

JANIS QUINN, L.P.T.

Formerly affiliated with the Department of Rehabilitation Medicine, Thomas Jefferson University Hospital, Philadelphia, PA.

MARGARET REDDY, R.N., M.A.

Assistant Director of Nursing, Neurosensory Care Program, Thomas Jefferson University Hospital, Philadelphia, PA.

JOHN B. REDFORD, M.D.

Professor and Chairman, Department of Rehabilitation Medicine, University of Kansas College of Health Sciences and Hospital, Kansas City, KA.; Consulting Physiatrist, VA Medical Center, Kansas City, MO.

JAY D ROBERTS, M.D.

Director, Rehabilitation Medicine, Chico Community Hospital, Chico, CA.

MATEI S. ROUSSAN, M.D.

Professor of Rehabilitation Medicine, Albert Einstein College of Medicine; Attending Physiatrist, Bronx Municipal Hospital Center, Hospital of the Albert Einstein College of Medicine, Montefiore Hospital and Medical Center, Bronx, N.Y.

ETTA RYBSTEIN-BLINCHIK, PH.D.

Senior Psychologist, Department of Rehabilitation Medicine, Goldwater Memorial Hospital, New York University Medical Center, Roosevelt Island, New York, N.Y.

JOYCE S. SABARI, M.A., O.T.R.

Teaching Fellow, Department of Occupational Therapy, New York University Medical Center, New York, N.Y.

HERSCH SACHS, M.D.

Coordinator, Rehabilitation Medicine in Pediatrics, Kingsbrook Jewish Medical Center, Brooklyn, N.Y.

JOJI SAKUMA, M.D.

Clinical Associate Professor of Rehabilitation Medicine, New York Medical College; Attending Physician, Metropolitan Hospital Center, New York, N.Y.

PHOEBE SATUREN, M.D.

Professor of Clinical Rehabilitation Medicine, New York Medical College; Chief, Children's Rehabilitation, Attending Physician, Metropolitan Hospital, New York, and Westchester County Medical Center, Valhalla, N.Y.

DORIS SCHANZER, O.T.R.

Senior Occupational Therapist, Goldwater Memorial Hospital, New York University Medical Center, Roosevelt Island, New York, N.Y.

VOJIN N. SMODLAKA, M.D., SC.D.

Clinical Professor of Rehabilitation Medicine, State University of New York College of Medicine; Adjunct Professor of Sports Medicine, Long Island University; Attending Physician, Methodist Hospital, Brooklyn, City Hospital at Elmhurst, Kingsbrook Jewish Medical Center, Kings County Hospital, St. Vincent's Medical Center of Richmond, N.Y.

DORA A. SORELL, M.D.

Professor of Clinical Rehabilitation Medicine, New York Medical College; Attending Physician and Associate Director, Department of Rehabilitation Medicine, Westchester County Medical Center, Valhalla, N.Y.

LINDA SNYDER, R.P.T., M.A.

Senior Physical Therapist, Goldwater Memorial Hospital, New York University Medical Center, Roosevelt Island, New York; Physical Therapist, James Rudel HIP Center, Bronx, N.Y.

WILLIAM E. STAAS, JR., M.D.

President and Medical Director, Magee Rehabilitation Hospital; Clinical Professor of Rehabilitation Medicine, Jefferson Medical College, Thomas Jefferson University, Philadelphia, PA.

DANIEL C. SULLIVAN, M.S., C.R.C.

Adjunct Assistant Professor, Therapeutic Recreation, Temple University; Patient Systems Coordinator, Spinal Cord Injury Center of Delaware Valley, Thomas Jefferson University Hospital; Program Director, Delaware Valley Project With Industry, Magee Rehabilitation Hospital, Philadelphia, PA.

PAULINE P. TAN, B.S. Phar., B.S. Educ., B.S. O.T., O.T.R.

Chief Occupational Therapist, Kingsbrook Jewish Medical Center, Brooklyn, N.Y.

HELENE TORNICK-BRUCH, O.T.R.

Senior Occupational Therapist, Kingsbrook Jewish Medical Center, Brooklyn, N.Y.

CARMEL A. TUTHS, R.N., M.A.

Discharge Planning Coordinator and Chief, Public Health Nursing Service, Goldwater Memorial Hospital, New York University Medical Center, Roosevelt Island, New York, N.Y.

JUDITH WASSERMAN, B.S., O.T.R.

Chief, Occupational Therapist, Goldwater Memorial Hospital, New York University Medical Center, Roosevelt Island, New York, N.Y.

RUTH K. WESTHEIMER, ED.D.

Adjunct Associate Professor, New York Hospital, Cornell University; New York Hospital Cornell University, Human Sexuality Program, Belleview Hospital, New York, N.Y.

AMY WOLFSON, M.S., O.T.R.

Senior Occupational Therapist, Kingsbrook Jewish Medical Center, Brooklyn, N.Y.

# CONTENTS

## Section IV  SYSTEMIC DISORDERS

## Section V  SPINAL CORD

## Section VI  PEDIATRIC HABILITATION

## Section VII  PSYCHOSOCIAL ASPECTS

# Introduction

Modern medical science has made dramatic progress in prolonging life by overcoming disease and the effects of injury. The often-unappreciated corollary has been a geometric rise in the number of persons suffering chronic disease and disability. At the present time it is estimated that over 50 per cent of the population is suffering one or more chronic diseases and that a full 70 per cent of the population will be disabled at some point in life.

Prior to the advent of antibiotics in the 1940s, spinal cord injury meant death within a few weeks or months and no thought of rehabilitation was feasible. In the 1970s casualties of our civilian life style were creating more than 10,000 new cases of spinal cord injury per year with an almost-normal life expectancy such that at the present time the number of spinal cord–injured wheelchair-bound individuals in the United States approaches 500,000. In similar fashion, victims of all manner of disease and disability are not only living for much longer periods but are rightfully demanding a higher quality of life and full participation in society.

Parallel to the rapidly expanding needs of these individuals, a medical specialty has developed whose primary interest is the restoration of function to those suffering physical disability regardless of cause.

Because of the staggeringly large numbers of individuals involved, it is necessary for all physicians and health practitioners, whatever their specialty, to have more than a perfunctory knowledge of developments in this field.

It is the primary purpose of this book to present in adequate depth some of the major areas of physiatric concern. All the physicians who have made clinical contributions to this book are physiatrists who have undergone the same basic training in physical medicine and rehabilitation (see Chap. 33 on physiatry), although their areas of special interest vary widely. Each chapter is designed to provide useful and practical information that can be applied in the day-to-day practice of all primary care physicians and a large number of specialists.

An immediately apparent difference between this and the usual medical textbook is the presence of contributions by nonphysicians. The provision of holistic health care that considers all aspects of the patient's problem in an integrated fashion has outgrown the possibility of a single individual, the physician, being thoroughly competent in all aspects, or having the time to provide all of the required services. However, it is imperative in this era of growing specialization that the physician have a thorough understanding of the services that can be provided by other health professionals and that the physician recognize the full extent and quality of these services as well as their boundaries and limitations. In those regions in which access to allied health professionals is limited, it behooves physicians to acquire personal knowledge so that they may advise the patient and family more adequately. Very few physicians have read textbooks designed for nurses or therapists. However, there is a wealth of information in the allied health professional contributions that the physician will find useful in daily practice and overall supervision of the patient's care (see Chap. 32).

All too many physicians simply refer a patient to a dealer to purchase a wheelchair without recognizing the multitude of variations that make it a specific prescription item. Likewise, too few of us think to prescribe specific leisure activities for a disabled patient or can advise on such basic questions as how a stroke patient may be taught to dress himself.

Several chapters in the book overlap and provide different perspectives and techniques for approaching the same problem. This is especially true in the chapters concerning the treatment of pain as well as some of the other sections. This only underlines the basic truth that for most problems there is no one correct answer, and in the treatment of any individual patient one may wish to combine and modify a variety of different approaches.

The last section of the book will also be noted as

a departure from a standard medical text, providing as it does chapters by a sociologist, a physician executive in the insurance industry, and a physician attorney, as well as an educator. Comprehensive care of patients with disability requires that the physician be familiar in these many areas that profoundly affect the patient's life. In these chapters, as in the others, special attention was paid to presenting information that will be both practical and useful in daily medical practice with references and indications for those who wish to delve deeper in these important subjects.

# Section I

# STROKE

# 1
# Stroke

## Understanding Stroke and its Treatment
*by Asa Ruskin, M.D.*

In order to appreciate what happens to the person who has sustained brain damage from a cerebrovascular accident (CVA), it is first necessary to conceptualize the dynamic functioning of the brain. For most of us this means discarding the simple schematic diagrams and functional maps that were the standard in neuroanatomical teaching for almost a hundred years. The nineteenth century anatomist treated the brain in much the same way as any other organ and described various readily apparent subdivisions (lobes, medulla, pons, ganglia). The early neurophysiologists attempted to ascribe function to these identifiable segments. The late nineteenth and early twentieth century saw a great deal of neurophysiological research, much of it dubious and not reproducible, carried out primarily on lower mammals and occasionally on primates. Much of this work would not have passed muster by today's standards because of the workers' inadequate understanding of the effects of electrical stimulation and failure to take into account a host of unforeseen variables such as intensity of stimulation, degree of anesthesia, lack of reproducibility, lack of identification of areas stimulated, and failure to appreciate the importance of time intervals for recuperation, regeneration, and degeneration.

One of these early concepts that is still perpetuated in many textbooks was the famous cortical map illustrating many numbered areas of the brain as having specific and discrete functions, separate and distinct from other portions of the brain, in identifiable positions. It is frequently not recalled that the various research projects producing cortical maps did not agree in their findings and, even worse, that studies done on lower primates were simply transposed over the picture of a human brain and considered to have been "homologized for man."

This schematic and mechanistic view of the brain produced in many clinicians' minds what might be called the "apple pie" concept of brain damage. In this way of thinking, occlusion of a specific artery results in damage that might be likened to removing a slice of pie from an otherwise intact brain with the clinical picture dependent on the functions subserved by that particular slice of the brain "pie." Thus in the classical context an infarction involving the right precentral motor area would produce a left hemiplegia, and if it involved the postcentral region, a left hemianesthesia would be added. In like fashion, effects on different regions would produce the other classical stroke syndromes, different ones being described for each cerebral circulatory region.

While we are still far from total understanding of the workings of the human brain, a more modern dynamic and holistic picture has evolved over the

Photographs for this chapter by Herbert A. Fischler, M.A., R.B.P., F.R.M.S., Chief of AudioVisual Resources, Kingsbrook Jewish Medical Center, Brooklyn, N.Y.

last three or four decades, pari pasu with the development of the electronic era and concepts of the computer age.

## THE NEURON

Basic to a holistic concept of the brain is understanding its smallest structural element, the neuron. The primary cell of the nervous system, as shown in Figure 1–1, consists of a cell body with a highly arborized dendritic tree, giving rise to a single axon whose length can vary from microscopic dimensions to a few feet in length.

Scattered all over the dendritic tree and the cell body are a vast number of terminal buttons from the axons of other cells carrying information that may be either excitatory or inhibitory. The numbers of these inputs can range from an average of 10,000 for a single cerebral cortical cell to over a 100,000 per cell in the cerebellum. The single neuron is only capable of choosing between firing or not firing. That "simple" decision can depend on the analysis of many thousands of inputs, further complicated by the fact that the excitatory and inhibitory inputs can be immeshed in internal feedback loops and highly complex intertwining of incoming messages such that there might be excitatory endings terminating on incoming inhibitory endings in an infinite variety of permutations and combinations. With this in mind, we begin to see that no single cell of the nervous system functions independently of a vast array of information, making that "simple" decision to fire highly sophisticated indeed. The largest amount of the central nervous system white matter is utilized, not by direct pathways as was previously thought, but by internuncial neurons participating in feedback and feedforward types of communication. Thus all the cells are interrelated in a highly integrated whole, and the two sides of the central nervous system are united at every level of the neuraxis.

With a human brain containing over one billion such cells, we can begin to appreciate the organizational substrata of human thought and behavior. The simplest of activities such as picking up an apple from a bowl requires the participation of the whole of the central nervous system as well as the entire musculoskeletal system. The apple must be seen and observed. It must be recognized and remembered, and the desire to pick it up formulated. Movement of the eyes, including adaptation to light and distance, must precede coordinated movement of the head and neck followed by integrated realignment of the center of gravity and the musculoskeletal system, allowing the hand to reach forward and in a coordinated and smooth fashion grasp the apple with the appropriate strength to lift it, and neither drop nor crush it. It is of utmost importance to emphasize that this simple activity requires the participation of both sides of the nervous system and the integrated function of both halves of the body. When damage occurs in any portion of the brain, not only are those functions that might be the primary concern of that region disturbed, the entire brain suffers from the loss of communication with that injured portion. This communication, it must be remembered, is a "two-way street." Therefore, the remaining "normal" portions of the brain are not only deprived of input from the damaged area, but they are also subject to abnormal messages and misinformation generated as a result of the lesion.

From this basic understanding of the neuron, it

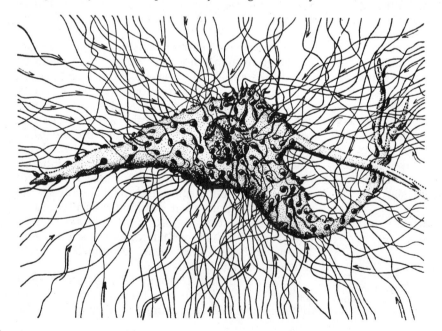

**Figure 1–1.** Mononeuron body and dendrites with representative synaptic terminals of axons of other neurons transmitting excitatory or inhibitory impulses. Many excitatory impulses must arrive at the motoneuron nearly simultaneously to exceed the excitatory threshold and generate an impulse transmitted over the axon. (From How Cells Communicate, by B. Katz. Scientific American 205:209–220. Copyright © 1961 by Scientific American, Inc. All rights reserved.)

is easy to recognize that there is no such thing as a simple stroke with hemiplegia. The victim of the stroke will have significant difficulties with both sides of the body and these difficulties will extend in some degree to all functions of the brain. Motor function will be impaired on both sides. Balance and coordination will not be the same. Sensory perception and spatial orientation will be impaired with far-reaching and often disastrous effects. Memory, cognition, and behavior will all be altered, often presenting the most formidable challenges to rehabilitation.

## PHYSIOLOGICAL BASIS FOR REHABILITATION TECHNIQUES

Two major principles underlie the modern concepts of plasticity in the central nervous system on which a great number of rehabilitative techniques are based.

The first of these is the polysensory function of the neuron.[1] No longer can we think in terms of the classical giant cell of Betz with its purely motor function initiating voluntary motor action via a discrete "pyramidal tract" to the anterior horn cell. We must now think in terms of a polysensory neuron receiving inputs from the visual system, the auditory system, the vestibular system, the proprioceptive systems, and the exteroceptive systems. We must remember that via the abundant interhemispheric cross connections, each of these sensory inputs is arriving at each cell from both sides of the brain, enabling the brain to enjoy stereooptics, stereophonics, stereo-orientation, and stereognosis of both internal and external stimuli. Thus if cells are deprived on one category of input, they are capable of compensation via other inputs. These polysensory neurons or pools of neurons are also capable of memory storage with the degree of complexity that allows for human thought and learning.

The second basic principle arises from the hierarchical structure of the nervous system as it slowly developed up the evolutionary ladder, culminating in the human (and perhaps cetaceous) brain.

We tend to think of finely tuned motor skills and dexterity as the cortical prerogative of the higher primates and man. However, one has only to think of the sea gull swooping down to pluck a fish from the water to admire the finesse of observation and action that can be accomplished almost entirely by the basal ganglia in birds. In cats and dogs, we know that if we remove the cerebral cortex from one hemisphere, almost no motor impairment is detected, although the animal has contralateral hemianopia. In decorticate cats, if the basal ganglia and thalami are undisturbed, the animal can walk, sit, or stand in a fairly normal fashion. However, if the midbrain has been sectioned, the cat develops decerebrate rigidity. In monkeys the cerebral cortex plays a much more important role; removal of the "precentral motor cortex," or all of the cortex from one hemisphere, will produce a severe or total contralateral paralysis. After a period of time, however, movement will begin to return and the monkey will regain significant function in the lower extremities and some function of the upper extremities.[2-7] It has also been shown that each cerebral cortex provides a significant degree of ipsilateral innervation and further that the ipsilateral innervation is more extensive in the lower extremities than in the upper.

The hierarchical structure flowing from these and many other types of experiments allows one to subdivide the central nervous system along phylogenetic lines (Fig. 1–2), separating the archi, or reptilian brain, which develops first and on which was successively and progressively superimposed the older and the newly evolved systems. The ontogenetic development of the brain follows to some extent the evolutionary development of the species in that the central core, or autonomic and ventricular systems and the archi cerebellovestibular system, is the first to mature, with the newer cortical (neo) system not fully matured until some years after birth. It is these subcortical systems that provide the organizational substrata for the vast multitude of reflex activities that permit highly complex bilaterally integrated sensory and motor functions to take place without impinging on cortical or conscious awareness. It is through the judicious and manageable use of these reflexes, both inhibitory and facilitatory, that much useful function can be reacquired by the brain-damaged person and even-

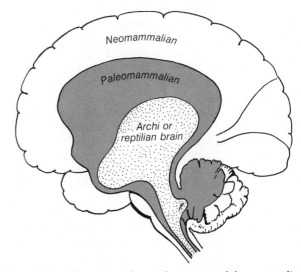

**Figure 1–2.** The archi, paleo, and neo parts of the mammalian central nervous system.

tually brought under the conscious control of the ipsilateral and remaining contralateral portions of the brain.

## TREATMENT OF STROKE

Although there has been a recent long-term downward trend, cerebral vascular disease is still the third most common cause of death in the United States.[9] Results of the recent Harvard Cooperative Stroke Registry, in which 694 patients were studied, revealed a diagnosis of thrombosis in 53 per cent, cerebral embolism in 31 per cent, and intracerebral hematoma in 10 per cent, with subarachnoid hemorrhage accounting for 6 per cent.[10] As a higher percentage of intracerebral hemorrhage and many cases of emboli are associated with coma at onset, in which the mortality rate is 86 per cent,[11] the vast majority of patients seen in a rehabilitation center are those who have suffered cerebral vascular thrombosis of arteriosclerotic origin or minor cerebral embolism. It is these patients, principally from the former category, with which this chapter is primarily concerned.

Specific treatment of the stroke itself may be divided into medical and surgical approaches. In a clinical and statistical comparison of different treatments in 300 patients[11] it was concluded that, in ischemic stroke, use of antiedema agents, including dexamethasone, hypertonic mannitol, and vasodilating ergot alkaloids (Hydergine), did not prove more helpful than the usual supportive care measures. However, we would seriously consider using these medications in the early treatment of patients manifesting moderate to severe alteration in level of consciousness, obtundation, or coma.

The majority of ischemic stroke patients seen for rehabilitation are those who have had brief or no loss of consciousness and who have been receiving general medical care or nursing home care. These patients, because of cognitive and behavioral changes, often have been allowed to become partially dehydrated. This is often combined with a tendency to hypercoagulability, a generalized decrease in patency of cerebral levels due to arteriosclerosis and frequently a reduced cardiac output from associated arteriosclerotic heart disease, decreased activity, and bed rest. In these patients the overall effect can be a significant increase in neurological deficit, confusion, and a decreased level of consciousness. These patients can often show a dramatic improvement with adequate intravenous fluid supplements, restoration of electrolyte balance, and nutritive supplement. In our experience the use of oral papaverine in adequate dosage, 200 mg t.i.d., or the equivalent intravenously, has a vasodilating effect that seems helpful. Also on occasion intermittent inhalation of carbogen (oxygen 95 per cent, carbon dioxide 5 per cent), given for 10 minutes per hour by simple mask or nasal catheter, may prove beneficial. The two last-named modalities have also proven quite helpful as adjunctive treatments for frequent transient ischemic attacks (TIAs).

Use of anticoagulant agents in the patient with completed stroke has for the most part been discontinued because of the high incidence of hemorrhagic complications.

Transient ischemic attacks affected 26 per cent of all patients in the Harvard Registry, and 24 per cent had a history of previous stroke. One of the most exciting additions to the medical armamentarium for this condition is the use of aspirin, 325 mg once a day. A study of 585 patients[12] showed that its use reduced the risk of TIAs by 19 per cent and the risk of stroke or death by 31 per cent. The results are even more positive when the statistics are limited to men, in whom a 48 per cent reduction in stroke or death was reported. Aspirin and other platelet-antiaggregating agents are rapidly becoming the treatment of choice in these instances, having a much lower incidence of complications than anticoagulant therapy.[13] At the present time anticoagulants should probably be restricted to carefully selected patients suffering cerebral emboli of cardiac or other origin.[14]

Treatment of underlying medical problems is naturally a priority concern. Cerebral vascular ischemia or hemorrhage may be a complication in many specific diseases. These include such entities as sickle cell anemia, collagen diseases with arteritis, lymphomas, and blood dyscrasias. Specific treatment of these entities is beyond the scope of this work; however, because of their extreme frequency, we must pay special attention to treatment of underlying diabetes mellitus and the diagnosis and treatment of associated cardiovascular disease. Myocardial infarction is a frequent precipitating factor in the etiology of cerebral ischemia brought about by sudden drop in blood pressure in an individual predisposed by reason of arteriosclerotic cerebrovascular and carotid stenosis. Often the myocardial incident is minor and may be overlooked because of the dramatic magnitude of the cerebral symptoms and the patient's inability to give an adequate history of the moments preceding onset (see Chapter 18).

It is also important to rule out associated neurological conditions and make a neurological differential diagnosis. One neurological condition that frequently accompanies stroke is Parkinson's syndrome, which may be related to the cerebral vascular disease itself or to the high incidence of both conditions in the same age group. As manifestations of this syndrome can be masked by the cerebral vascular neurological deficit, it is of utmost importance to examine the intact side carefully for evidence of cogwheel phenomenon and to be particularly alert for the condition in patients having a history of bilateral cerebral vascular episodes or manifesting a classical pseudobulbar palsy.

Surgical treatment must be limited to a very carefully selected group of patients; its success depends on the availability of a highly sophisticated and practiced neurosurgical team capable of achieving optimal results. The clinical outcome of 40 patients with ischemia or infarction of the internal carotid artery who underwent anastomosis of the temporal to the middle cerebral artery[15] showed a striking reduction in the number of recurrent TIAs. Of this group of 34 patients, in whom the median age was 56, more than half who had had focal neurological deficits before the operation improved postoperatively. However, none of these patients had had severe motor deficit. The more widely utilized carotid endarterectomy has also been associated with favorable results with highly selected groups of patients.

It must be remembered that cerebral angiography has significant hazards when undertaken in patients with arteriosclerotic vascular disease. In one study, an incidence of cerebral complications exceeding 12 per cent has been reported, in which 5 to 6 per cent suffered permanent neurological deficit.[16] We do not think that cerebral angiography is warranted except for those patients in whom vascular surgery is a serious consideration, or in whom the neurological diagnosis is obscure after all other noninvasive diagnostic procedures, including computerized axial tomography, have been done and in whom the possibility of a surgically correctable condition is considered.

Treatment of spasticity is an overriding concern throughout the management of the brain-damaged patient. Various techniques and considerations are discussed in depth elsewhere in this work. A few medications have proven to be useful adjuncts for this purpose. Several have been introduced with much fanfare and later found to have limited clinical application. Among the medications that we currently employ, oral baclofen has proven helpful, starting with 10 mg once a day and increasing slowly to a maximum of 20 mg t.i.d. As with all conditions, some patients will respond more readily to one drug than another, and failure to have significant improvement with one does not prejudge the outcome that might be achieved with a different product.

It must be emphasized that drug treatment alone is rarely, if ever, sufficient and must always be combined with appropriate physical therapy, occupational therapy, and correct rehabilitation nursing techniques, as well as selected nerve block and surgical approaches when needed (see Chapter 24). It should be remembered that a certain degree of spasticity in the lower extremity can be functionally useful, allowing the hemiplegic patient to stand and walk without the need for bracing at the knee. If the response to antispastic medication is too good, the patient may lose some of the functionally useful spasticity and his overall level of achievement can be reduced rather than augmented.

Valium has been widely used to reduce spasticity and can be helpful in selected cases. Drawbacks are a tendency of this drug to produce somnolence at higher doses and a propensity to increase the degree of depression that these patients frequently manifest. It can be most useful in those patients for whom spasticity is a particular problem at night and can be given for this purpose in a single evening dose.

Spasticity as well as other neurological manifestations of reduced higher cortical control, such as tremor and ataxia, are often aggravated by the patient's anxiety. In cases in which this seems to be a factor, use of simple antianxiety medication such as phenobarbitol can be most helpful.

Different medications have been brought out for spasticity, and we have occasionally used Dantrium, among others. In all instances, the same precautions indicated for baclofen should be kept in mind, and the clinician should familiarize himself with the side effects and precautions to be observed for each.

## COGNITIVE AND BEHAVIORAL CHANGES

Neurological texts describe a large number of specific syndromes associated with lesions in precise areas of the brain. These can give rise to purportedly limited cognitive dysfunction such as the inability to recognize one's fingers and to do simple arithmetic (Gerstmann's syndrome), the inability to recognize faces (prosopagnosia), streets, or places, inability to read while maintaining other language skills (alexia), isolated inability to read music for a musician (amusia), various deficits in precise language function with maintenance of other functions, and assorted other fascinating syndromes for which the reader is referred to standard neurological works. Much has been made of describing specific defects related to occlusion of particular arteries or regions. These studies have for the most part been done by observations on patients with discrete tumors or small isolated infarctions as well as those undergoing neurosurgical procedures. While these eponymous syndromes have considerable theoretical and academic interest, their clinical value is more restrained.

While the brain certainly has been shown to have various localized areas involved with relatively specific functions, I have emphasized the high degree of integration and interdependence of all its areas as the reason why any lesion, no matter how small, will become manifested to a greater or lesser degree by creation of a disturbance in the cognitive integrity of the whole.

The major function of the white matter is to ensure transmission between neurons, which provides for integration of functions of the various parts. It is disturbances of this integrating ability that cause the most profound changes in cognitive function by impairing perceptual awareness of the multiple sensory inputs—visual, auditory, tactile, and somesthetic—as well as impairing the integration of these inputs with appropriate motor responses. It must be remembered that in the clinical setting the average stroke patient usually has diffuse cerebrovascular disease, perhaps previous episodes of stroke or transient cerebral ischemia, and frequently other conditions resulting in impaired cerebral circulation, such as decreased cardiac output, hypercoagulability, and anemia, as well as the effects of aging itself. Therefore, from a practical standpoint, we must consider that while there might be one major area of infarction precipitating the hemiplegia that brought the patient to medical attention, there will be areas of impaired function located diffusely throughout one or both hemispheres.

Studies revealing major asymmetric functions of the two hemispheres that were done in the 1960s revealed that the left hemisphere not only is predominant in localization of language function but also appears to be important for all types of mathematical and analytical thinking of the deductive type. The right hemisphere is more involved with spacial orientation, body image, and inductive modes of reasoning. However, in approaching the rehabilitation of a stroke patient with a major lesion in one or the other hemisphere, we must remember that normal thinking and carrying out of activities requires integrated function of both these hemispheres, neither of which is really dominant over the other. For example, a professional writer who has sustained damage to the right hemisphere with "conserved" language function might well still be able to communicate for routine daily activity and be able to write simple material, but his syntax will probably suffer and the ability to write creatively will be significantly impaired, as will other cognitive functioning to be described.

## DENIAL AND HEMI-INATTENTION

Probably because of inability to analyze and integrate incoming sensory matter due to the disruptive brain lesion, as well as perhaps the internal production of abnormal signals, a very high percentage of stroke patients have a form of denial of illness (anasognosia) as well as a lateralized denial of one half of their own body and the environment

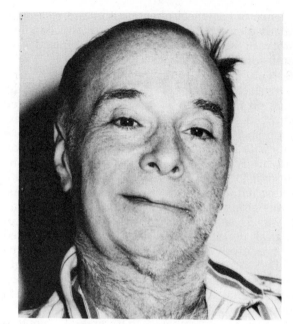

**Figure 1–3.** Failure to shave or comb hemiplegic side.

on that side. This produces a hemi-inattention. It is fundamental to realize that with this and the other cognitive disturbances the patient is totally unaware of the existence of these deficits and therefore will not complain of them. It is the examiner who

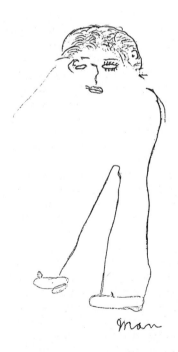

Draw a Man or a Lady

man

**Figure 1–4.**

must elicit the information by direct questioning, testing, and observation.

If patients are able to communicate in the early phase after the stroke, they are quite likely to deny any dysfunction and will explain that they are in the hospital "because my doctor sent me in," "because of my arthritis," and in some instances they will be unaware that they are in a hospital. A patient with left hemiplegia, for example, when requested to raise the right arm, might do so quite readily. Then when asked to raise the left arm, he might respond "I just did," or he might raise the left arm by grasping it with the right hand and elevating it. When further questioned, he might report that it had moved perfectly well. Another patient complained that a man in the next bed bothered her by keeping his hand on her breast, totally unaware that the hand she referred to was her own on the hemiplegic side.

As the patient improves, this gross denial of illness usually recedes, but the hemi-inattention and apraxic problems persist. These patients have considerable difficulty in spacial orientation. They are unable to localize stimuli, their own limbs, and objects in space. They may totally disregard stimuli coming from the involved side, even though they can hear, see, or feel those stimuli and are aware that they are occurring, occasionally localizing the stimulus and responding as though it were on the intact side. It is not uncommon to see patients, with hemiplegia wash, shave, comb, and dress only one side of the body, being totally unaware that they have neglected these grooming tasks for the other side, even though they are physically capable. Even after being presented with a mirror, the patient might not realize the omission (Fig. 1–3). In specific test situations, when asked to draw figures, patients will neglect or improperly construct one side of the figure, even though there may be no visual defect or the entire test is placed in their intact visual field (Fig. 1–4). This is especially dramatic when done by a person with artistic ability (Figs. 1–5 and 6).

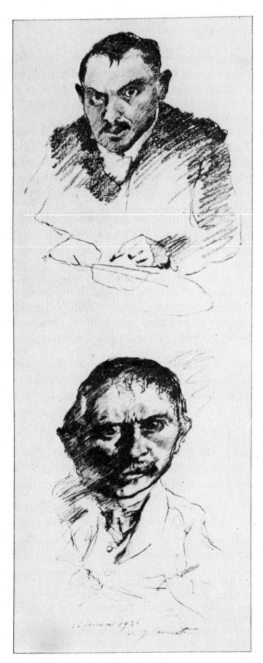

**Figure 1–5.** Self-portrait by artist before and after a stroke.

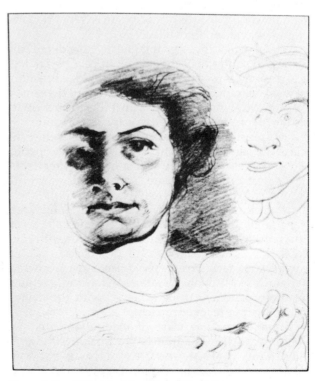

**Figure 1–6.** Self-portrait by artist after stroke.

It can readily be appreciated that in view of these impairments in perception and cognitive function, retraining a patient in the "simple" acts of daily living is not an easy undertaking. It is usually not understood by the family and lay people, often including hospital administrators, that the skills of a highly trained occupational therapist are necessary to teach a patient to put on his shirt when he has lost the concept of what the sleeve is to the shirt and the ability to localize his arm and the clothing in space and visualize the act of dressing. The same holds true for all other aspects of rehabilitation.

### DEPRESSION AND BEHAVIORAL ADJUSTMENTS

As a result of the sensory alterations and deprivations of which the patients are themselves totally unaware, behavioral changes are inevitable. The patient knows that he is unable to put on his shirt but does not understand why. Likewise he might recognize that he is unable to communicate properly, again without understanding the reason for this. The patient, as a result of repeated failures, tends to become withdrawn and "depressed." This is frequently made worse by the well-meaning family member or friend who mistakenly "encourages" him with statements such as, "Come on, John, you can do it if you only try harder."

The patient who is likely to misconstrue and poorly interpret sensory input and communications will also tend to "explain" these misinterpretations by projecting unwarranted accusations on members of the family and on the health professionals caring for him, leading to a type of paranoid behavior and hostility.

While some investigators have considered the depressed attitude of the patient to be a psychological response to or grieving for the lost function, several significant differences between depressed stroke patients and those with other forms of reactive depression make this explanation unlikely. The depressed stroke patient does not manifest the classical signs of insomnia and loss of appetite. These patients do not manifest a general tendency to neglect of personal care, and they do not ordinarily respond to a psychotherapeutic approach. Furthermore, the tricyclic and similar antidepressant medications do not produce significant amelioration. In view of these inconsistencies with classical depressive neurosis and psychosis, I would suggest the term *organic pseudodepression* to characterize this condition. Treatment and improvement of these patients can be achieved with the overall rehabilitation team approach.

Examples of one class of medications that we have found useful adjuncts are Ritalin, 10 mg orally, b.i.d. at 8 A.M. and 2 P.M. (avoiding an evening dose that might disturb sleep) or Dexedrine, 2 to 5 mg orally at similar times or in a long-acting spansule form, 10 to 15 mg once daily in the morning. I believe that these medications are helpful not only for their mood-elevating characteristic but also their ability to enhance the patient's attention span and thereby perhaps improve his interpretation of stimuli. These drugs are known for producing cortical excitation and in minimally brain-damaged children help to compensate in some measure for loss of cortical inhibitory function on lower centers.

## PRINCIPLES OF MOTOR REHABILITATION

Damage to the cerebral cortex and integrative circuits typically produces a hemiplegia with spasticity in which the so-called "antigravity" muscles predominate over their antagonists. This causes in the lower extremity an extension of the leg with external rotation as well as inversion and plantar flexion of the foot. There is also tendency to traction or hiking of the pelvis. In the upper extremity, a depression of the shoulder is present combined with internal rotation and flexion at the elbow, together with flexion of the wrist and fingers. This reflex spasticity is rapidly complicated by soft tissue contracture that tends to freeze the extremities in this abnormal posture.

Much of the rehabilitation effort by the team, using the techniques of physical therapy, occupational therapy, and rehabilitation nursing, is directed at correcting this postural deformation. This is done with techniques that encourage inhibitory reflexes in those muscle groups that are contracted while stimulating facilitatory reflex contraction of the opposing muscles, as well as various techniques to prevent or reduce the concomitant soft tissue contractures. It is important that the fight against the hemiplegic posture be carried out on a 24-hour basis, not only by the intermittent therapy sessions but by correct posturing and positioning of the patient when in bed or when sitting in a chair. The physiatrist must ensure that all the personnel of the rehabilitation center are aware of and practicing these techniques correctly. The practitioner must educate the patient's family to do likewise when treatment is given at home.

## REFERENCES

1. Moore, J. C.: Neuroanatomical considerations relating to recovery of function following brain lesions. *In* Bach y Rita, P. (ed.): Recovery of Function: Theoretical Consideration for Brain Injury Rehabilitation. Baltimore, University Park Press, 1980.
2. Bard, P.: Studies on the cerebral cortex. I. Localized control of placing and hopping reactions in the cat and their normal management by small cortical remnants. Arch. Neurol. Psychiatr. 30:40, 1933.

3. Bard, P.: Medical Physiology, 10th ed. St. Louis, C. V. Mosby Co., 1956.
4. Bard, P. and Macht, M. B.: The behavior of chronically decerebrate cats. *In* Wolstenholme, G. E. and O'Connor, C. M. (eds.): Neurological Basic of Behavior. London, J. & A. Churchill, Ltd., 1958.
5. Bard, P. and Rioch, D. M.: A study of four cats deprived of neocortex and additional portions of the forebrain. Bull. Johns Hopkins Hosp. 60:73–147, 1937.
6. Bazett, H. C. and Penfield, W. G.: A study of the Sherrington decerebrate animal in the chronic as well as the acute condition. Brain 45:185–265, 1922.
7. Travis, A. M. and Woolsey, C. N.: Motor performance of monkeys after bilateral partial and total cerebral decortications. Am. J. Phys. Med. 35:273–310, 1956.
8. Bucy, P. C. and Fulton, J. F.: Ipsilateral representation in the motor and pre-motor cortex of the monkey. Brain 56:318–382, 1933.
9. Soltero, I. et al.: Trends in mortality from cerebrovascular diseases in the United States, 1960–1975. Stroke 9:549–558, 1978.
10. Mohr, J. P. et al.: The Harvard Cooperative Stroke Registry: A prospective registry. Neurology 28:754–762, 1978.
11. Santambrogio, S. et al.: Is there a real treatment for stroke? Clinical and statistical comparison of different treatments in 300 patients. Stroke 9:130–132, 1978.
12. Barnett, H. J. M. et al.: Randomized trial of aspirin and sulfinpyrazone in threatened stroke. N. Engl. J. Med. 299:53–59, 1978.
13. Silverstein, A.: Neurologic complications of anticoagulation therapy: A neurologist's review. Arch. Intern. Med. 139:217–220, 1979.
14. Milliken, C. H. and McDowell, F. H.: Treatment of transient ischemia Attacks. Stroke 9:299–308, 1978.
15. Lee, M. C. et al.: Superficial temporal to middle cerebral artery anastomosis: Clinical outcome in patients with ischemia or infarction in internal carotid artery distribution. Arch. Neurol. 36:1–4, 1979.
16. Faught, E. et al.: Cerebral complications of angiography for transient ischemia and stroke: Prediction of risk. Neurology, 29:4–15, January, 1979.

# Physical Therapy

*by Sandra M. Cohen, M.A., R.P.T. and Margo S. Meissner, M.A., R.P.T.*

Physical therapy should be initiated as soon as possible following onset of stroke. This may occur even before the patient's condition is stable. Treatment procedures and goals vary according to the status of the patient.

Initially the purpose of physical therapy is to maintain range of motion, prevent contractures and edema, and improve the emotional outlook of the patient for physical rehabilitation. As the patient improves, the emphasis of physical therapy varies according to this improvement. The stroke patient may pass through particular stages of recovery or perhaps remain at one stage indefinitely. These stages of recovery define the state of muscle control and functional ability available. Recovery of the involved upper and lower extremity may progress at different speeds. Upper extremity function usually lags behind the involved lower extremity. The physical therapist must first assess the stage of recovery for selection of the most appropriate techniques of treatment. Throughout the physical therapy program, this assessment continues to determine progress and effectiveness of treatment. Techniques of treatment are altered according to progress.

Constant communication among the physical therapist, physician, and other team members is most advantageous for a coordinated approach to treatment. This becomes especially important for proper discharge planning. The team should set long-term goals to make reasonable and realistic plans for the patient.

Methods of treatment vary according to the orientation of the therapist, but the goals of treatment are basically the same.

Following onset of stroke, there is no voluntary movement of the affected limbs. The involved extremities are flaccid; little or no muscular resistance can be elicited upon passive movement. The hemiplegic side is nonfunctional. The patient is unable to sustain sitting without external support, and assistance is required for all positional changes and transfer activities. At this stage the functional prognosis is adequate sitting balance, safe transfers, bed mobility, and brief standing. Ambulation is a possibility achieved with difficulty. This would entail the use of a long leg brace, shoe lift, quadruped (quad) cane and, most likely, assistance. The patient ambulates with a stiff knee, calling for high energy consumption.

As the patient recovers, spasticity develops. Any attempt at voluntary movement will result in a weak synergistic muscle activation pattern that may not produce an actual limb movement. Great effort made by the uninvolved side may lead to associated movements in the hemiplegic limbs. Eventually spasticity becomes more marked. Voluntary attempts at movement result in a more defined synergistic pattern (Fig. 1–7). Synergy as defined by Brunnstrom is the action of a group of muscles that work together as a unit; it is of primitive and automatic nature, and is present on a spinal cord level. Flexor and extensor synergies exist in both upper and lower extremities and are dominated by

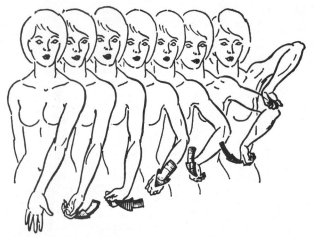

**Figure 1–7.** Pattern of upper extremity synergic reflex flexion resulting in flexion, abduction, internal rotation of the shoulder, flexion of the elbow, pronation of the forearm, and flexion of the wrist and fingers. (From Buerger, A. A. and Tobis, J. S.: Neurophysiologic Aspects of Rehabilitation Medicine. Springfield, Charles C Thomas, 1974.)

particular muscle groups. Flexion usually predominates in the upper extremity and extension predominates in the lower extremity. In the upper extremity elbow flexion is the strongest flexor component. Shoulder adduction and forearm pronation are the strongest extensor components.

In the lower extremity, hip flexion appears to be the strongest flexion component and knee extension, hip adduction and ankle plantar flexion are all strong extension components. Knee extension usually predominates (Fig. 1–8).

Synergistic patterns of movements can be incorporated into the gait pattern. As a result, the pattern of ambulation is relatively improved. A long leg brace is no longer required, making gait more functional and less energy-consuming. Spasticity of the lower extremity may be supportive for function unless dominance of certain synergy components interferes with movement. The upper extremity is not functional when dominated by synergistic movements. At this stage of recovery the patient should become independent in transfer activities, bed mobility, and possibly ambulation with assistive devices.

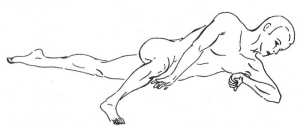

**Figure 1–8.** Maximal pattern of reciprocal reflex synergies. (From Buerger, A. A. and Tobis, J. S.: Neurophysiologic Aspects of Rehabilitation Medicine. Springfield, Charles C Thomas, 1974.)

As spasticity decreases, movements that deviate from the basic limb synergy become available. The functional capability of the patient continues to improve. The upper extremity can be employed for supportive purposes. Ambulation not only becomes independent but also assumes a more normal gait pattern, requiring less aid from assistive devices.

When spasticity is at a minimum and movement is relatively independent of the basic limb synergies (isolated movement), the patient should achieve independence in ambulation and activities of daily living without assistance or orthotic device. Both upper and lower extremity are functional, but coordination and power may not be within normal limits. Gait and movements of the involved extremities are performed slower and with less acuity than in the uninvolved limbs. Total recovery implies that spasticity is no longer demonstrated by passive limb movement. No deficit in motor control can be defined. Movements are finely coordinated with normal power and control. Full function is restored. Gait assumes a more normal pattern with equal stride, symmetry of weight bearing, and normal cadence.

An understanding of the typical stages of recovery provides good guidelines for evaluation and establishment of treatment goals. The appropriate treatment plan is designed according to the findings of the hemiplegic evaluation.

## TREATMENT

As stated earlier, following onset of stroke, the involved extremities are flaccid. The goals of treatment are to maintain range of motion, prevent contractures, and improve bed mobility, sitting balance, and transfer activities. Physical therapy treatment consists of passive range of motion and facilitation techniques to the flaccid limbs, active range of motion to the uninvolved extremities, mat activities (rolling), sitting balance, and transfer activities. Facilitation techniques could include icing, brushing, reflex positioning, vibration, and quick stretch. Bed positioning involves use of pillows to prevent hip external rotation and for upper extremity elevation to prevent edema. This is described in more detail in Chapter 3. If the patient shows no progress beyond this stage of recovery, ambulation may be initiated. This requires the use of a long leg brace, hemiwalker, or quadruped cane, shoe lift on the uninvolved side, and probably supervision. The shoe lift allows the hemiplegic's leg to clear the floor more easily.

As spasticity and synergy appear, the goals include promotion of active voluntary movement independent of synergy, improvement in standing balance, and achievement of trunk stability. Treat-

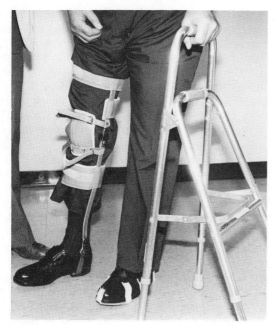

**Figure 1–9.** Note long leg brace on hemiparetic side and shoe lift under opposite foot.

ment continues as before, including active assistive exercise to the involved extremities and mat activities such as quadruped "walking" on knees and elbows. Standing activities without knee support may be initiated.

As spasticity and synergistic movement patterns become strong, the goals of physical therapy include improved active voluntary movement independent of synergy, relaxation of spasticity, and independent ambulation with quadruped cane and short leg brace.

Treatment includes active and active-assistive exercise to strengthen the poorly controlled muscle groups and relaxation techniques (such as rotational movements and positioning) to decrease spasticity. Progressive ambulation continues, including ambulation on steps and inclines.

With the development of isolated voluntary movement (independent of synergy) the goals of physical therapy include improved control and power of these movements and the functional gait pattern. The emphasis of gait training is knee stability in stance (avoiding hyperextension), hip and knee flexion during swing phase, equalization of stride, and weight shifting. Treatment includes active, resistive, and isokinetic exercise, and balance and gait training with a short leg brace and standard cane on all surfaces, steps, and inclines.

When spasticity is at a minimum and strong voluntary isolated movement exists, the physical therapy goals are to improve the power and coordination of fine motor movements and ambulation. At this stage the patient is independent in ambulation and activities of daily living without orthotic or am-

bulatory aid. Gait has a good symmetrical appearance. Treatment includes progressive isokinetic and resistive exercise, with speed and coordination emphasized. Emphasis of gait training is on speed, coordination, and endurance. This is the final stage of recovery.

## ASSISTIVE DEVICES FOR AMBULATION TRAINING

Standing balance and pre-gait activities can be initiated in the parallel bars, which provide maximum external stability and a secure environment for the patient. Once static standing balance is achieved by maintaining the center of gravity over the base of support, dynamic standing activities are begun. These activities include shifting of weight from side to side, lifting one leg while supporting body weight with the other, and placing one foot in front of the other with shifting of weight forward and back. The parallel bar is held with the uninvolved hand to assist balance and, if necessary, to bear weight; this will decrease the forces on the hemiplegic leg during stance. The parallel bars provide more stability than other assistive devices because the patient can push or pull on them. Any other device that is not secured to the floor can provide stability only with a compressive force.

Once dynamic balance is established in the parallel bars and lower extremity stability is sufficient for ambulation, either by intrinsic muscle stability alone or with extrinsic stability provided by splints or braces, the patient can progress to ambulation outside the parallel bars using a hemiwalker or a cane if he cannot ambulate unassisted.

The hemiwalker is indicated for patients who require maximal assistance for balance, particularly during stance phase on the involved lower extremity. It is designed to bear weight through a centered handle so it can be controlled with one upper extremity. The disadvantages of being dependent on a walker are that it is a large, awkward piece of equipment to use in small or crowded areas, and the patient is unable to use it to assist in stair climbing.

Canes are indicated for patients who require moderate to minimal assistance for balance. The cane should be held in the hand opposite to the affected lower extremity to provide a wider base of support when weight is placed on the affected leg. Every cane should have a good suction tip, which should be checked frequently for wear. There are three basic cane types available: quadruped (quad) cane, orthocane, and standard cane.

The quad cane provides a wider base of support during weight bearing and is considered to provide the maximum support. It is available with either a wide base (9 by 13 inches) or a narrow base (5 by 7 inches). This cane is selected for the patient who requires moderate assistance for balance. The base is small enough to fit on a standard-size step, so it can be used to assist in stair climbing. The disadvantage is that it is awkward to use in a narrow or crowded area; passersby may accidentally kick the cane or trip over it because of the wide position of the prongs.

An orthocane or a standard cane are considered for those patients who require only minimal assistance for balance. The orthocane provides for better balance and control because the upright angulation of the cane allows the patient's weight to be placed over the center of the cane. The grip surface is flattened to enhance comfort. The standard crook-top cane is inexpensive, but the weight-bearing line does not fall directly down the shaft of the cane. If the circumference of the handle is too small or too large, the patient may have difficulty gripping it.

All canes and walkers should be measured to the proper length to provide maximum safety and effectiveness. Having a cane or walker of proper height should enable the patient to stand with his elbows slightly flexed (approximately 20 degrees to 30 degrees) while gripping the device. The cane should be measured with the tip four inches in front and four inches to the side of the foot.

## COMPLICATIONS

Special consideration should be given to certain common complications of the hemiplegic patient that can affect the functional training program. Following is a discussion of the most common of these complications and how they are managed within the physical therapy program.

### SHOULDER-HAND SYNDROME

The pain associated with this syndrome* interferes significantly with the rehabilitation program. If the pain persists, the potentially functional arm may become nonfunctional, with fixed contractures at the shoulder and wrist. Proper support for the shoulder, appropriate bed positioning, and passive range of motion to prevent contractures will aid in the prevention of shoulder-hand syndrome. If it should develop, therapeutic techniques should be administered to decrease the pain and swelling and increase the range of motion. Adequate treatment cannot be based on any one specific therapeutic agent. Of primary importance are passive range of motion or active-assistive range of motion exercises for the involved extremity within the lim-

---

*See Chapter 2 for further discussion.

its of the patient's pain tolerance. These exercises should be gently administered, for if excessive pain is incurred during treatment, the patient will tend to resist further passive range of motion in anticipation of pain.

Application of a hot pack or a cold pack to the shoulder and wrist prior to passive range of motion exercises may improve pain tolerance and allow increased passive range of movement. Patients with residual active motion are encouraged to use this to pain tolerance. Suggested treatment devices include a hemiplegic sling to support the shoulder and hand and an overhead sling for reduction of edema in the hand. If massive edema of the hand is present, Jobst air compression can be used daily to assist in edema reduction.

Connective tissue massage (CTM) has been shown to be an effective means to relieve the pain involved with shoulder-hand syndrome. It is a specialized massage technique performed by the physical therapist to stimulate the mast cells to release a histamine-like substance, which acts on the autonomic nervous system. The means by which this technique succeeds in treatment of shoulder-hand syndrome has not been clarified, although counterirritation may be involved. It is possible that the slight traumatic effect of this form of massage could stimulate the release of enkephalin in the central nervous system, which would result in relief of pain.

Other modalities have been useful in the treatment of this syndrome. Pulsed ultrasound applied to the stellate ganglion on the affected side is suggested by Goodman.[2] The addition of transcutaneous electric nerve stimulation (TENS) may provide increased pain relief.

### GLENOHUMERAL SUBLUXATION

Activation of the muscles surrounding the shoulder joint is needed not only for upper limb functioning but also to prevent subluxation of the shoulder joint. Thus the flaccid hemiplegic is particularly susceptible to glenohumeral subluxation. Allowing the weight of the flaccid upper limb to dangle unsupported promotes overstretching of the shoulder joint capsule and the supportive ligamentous structures, which can cause pain and joint instability. With a hemiplegic arm sling properly worn or use of a lap board for seated activities, glenohumeral separation will be avoided. However, this does not help to stimulate activity of the muscles that is needed to protect the joint.

Facilitation techniques to promote muscle activity should be concentrated on the shoulder musculature. Activity of the supraspinatus muscle is particularly important for the prevention of subluxation of the shoulder joint. When the patient is supine, the recommended bed posture avoids abduction of the humerus with respect to the scapula as it deprives the shoulder joint of the stabilizing action of the lower portion of the glenoid fossa on the humeral head and slackens the superior portion of the capsule, thus predisposing to a downward subluxation of the humeral head. In handling the patient, traction on the affected arm is avoided. The patient is instructed to support the affected arm with the uninvolved arm when changing bed positions.

## EDEMA

The flaccid hemiplegic hand and foot are prone to edema. With the onset of edema, range of motion is decreased secondary to the swelling and often pain is elicited, possibly because of compression of internal structures. The primary treatment should be that of prevention. Since muscle activity is absent, muscle pumping is also absent and dependent edema must be prevented. This can be accomplished simply by proper positioning. The limb can be supported with pillows, a lapboard, or a sling. It should be elevated intermittently with the wheelchair foot rest when the patient is seated for long periods of time. Bed posture is also important. The patient should not lie on the affected arm or leg. When the patient is sidelying on the involved side, care should be taken to properly position the extremities.

If edema does exist, certain therapeutic procedures and modalities are useful to decrease it. Certainly, limb elevation is the position of choice. If some active movements are present in the involved extremity, exercises in the elevated position are performed. A Jobst air compression bag applied to the extremity may produce rapid beneficial results. With the limb elevated, electrical stimulation, using an alternating reciprocal type of current applied to the wrist and finger flexors and extensors or the ankle dorsiflexors and plantar flexors, has been a useful modality. Centripetal massage to the hand or foot with the limb elevated will also help decrease edema.

# Occupational Therapy

by Kevin Earls, M.S., O.T.R., Leslie Linville, M.S., O.T.R., Madelyn Meltzer, M.A., O.T.R., Helene Tornick-Bruch, O.T.R., and Amy Wolfson, M.S., O.T.R.

## WHAT IS OCCUPATIONAL THERAPY?

Occupational therapy can be described as the art and the science of channelling an individual's effort in specially selected activities that have been designed to restore and enhance his performance. Occupational therapy facilitates the learning of a wide variety of skills and functions that are essential to well-developed human adaptation. The target of these skills is an attempt to correct or diminish pathology and to promote the maintenance of health. Occupational therapy focuses on the individual's ability to complete satisfactorily essential roles and tasks needed for productive living. These roles provide for the individual a sense of mastery of himself and his environment.

Occupational therapy utilizes medical and social perspectives to examine the unique nature of the individual and *how he relates to his environment*. The role of the occupational therapist is to help the individual develop and maintain the highest level of biological, social, and psychological functioning. The aim of the occupational therapist's intervention is the alleviation of dysfunction and the development of maximum functional independence in all aspects of living.

## HISTORICAL PERSPECTIVE

The philosophical basis of occupational therapy, the utilization of goal-directed, purposeful activity as a therapeutic process, came about shortly before the beginning of the twentieth century. The cornerstone of the philosophy is that an individual through motivation can use his hands and abilities to influence the state of his own health and function. The individual's involvement in "occupation" bears a striking and direct relation to his state of health. The concept of occupation is defined as a goal-directed activity that the individual deems meaningful and therefore provides feedback concerning value, ability, and an interrelatedness to others. The occupational performance consists of cognitive, biological, emotional, and social components. Each of these components could be examined separately. However, in the light of occupational therapy, they are viewed in terms of their interrelatedness.

The growth of the field was rapidly accelerated by a need that arose from the entrance of the United States into World War I. At that time the nation was faced with large numbers of men in need of rehabilitative therapy. The army moved into action and established two groups of rehabilitation specialists, called reconstruction aides. These two groups were occupational and physical therapists.

After the war the field of occupational therapy continued to grow at a somewhat steady pace. This pace was once again rapidly accelerated when the United States entered the Second World War. Because of the critical need for personnel in the armed forces as well as in key industries, there was a need for maximum utilization of manpower. Thousands of occupational therapists were needed; new techniques for more rapid rehabilitation were developed in order that men could be physically and mentally fit for service or work.

Since the end of the war the field of occupational therapy has continued to grow—keeping abreast of advances in medical and technical sciences and involving itself in physical dysfunction, chronic disease conditions, and mental health.

## THE OCCUPATIONAL THERAPY PROCESS

The process by which the therapeutic goals are accomplished require:

1. Collection of data
2. Identification of problems
3. The knowledge of various options, interventions, and methods of treatment
4. The developmental level or stage of the individual
5. The interests, abilities, and preferences of the individual.

After the appropriate data have been compiled, the specific problem areas are clearly defined. At this point decisions can be made regarding available programs and methods of treatment of the specific problem areas, and these decisions can be implemented for the resolution of the problems. The process involves inductive reasoning to derive conclusions on the basis of data that have been collected and also deductive reasoning to make inferences from general principles that have been learned. Whether the process is based on inductive or deductive reasoning, occupational therapy is a problem-solving intervention approach.

## TREATMENT PLANNING

Once data have been collected, problems identified, and a therapeutic approach chosen, the next area of concern is treatment. An assessment is made of the individual's capabilities in order to establish a baseline of function. A treatment plan is then formulated, with the goals of the patient kept in mind. The plan works in conjunction with the treatment of other rehabilitation team members. The plan is directed toward eliminating or diminishing disability through a variety of techniques and utilizing goal-directed activity designed to focus on the individual's capabilities in all aspects of functioning. The activities utilized in the treatment program include:

1. Exercises that can be translated into purposeful activity
2. Self-care activities
3. Cognitive and perceptual activities
4. Expressive and creative activities

Occupational therapy also makes use of prevocational, vocational, educational, and leisure time activities.

Simulated or actual self-care and work-related tasks are often a major part of the treatment program. Patients may be instructed in the areas of work simplification, energy conservation, and joint or limb protection as part of the total treatment program. There is a regular reassessment of capabilities and progress in order to document gains made, to avoid secondary problems, and to reestablish goals. Preventive measures are employed, such as static and dynamic splinting, and also proper positioning of the individual in order to eliminate contractures, deformities, skin breakdown, and other secondary problems.

## FAMILY INVOLVEMENT

The individual's family is a very important part of the occupational therapy treatment process. The family should be included in the total rehabilitation process. This is often a crucial point for a successful and effective transition of the individual from the hospital to the home and community. The family should receive both instruction concerning the individual's condition (including his disabilities *and abilities*) and counseling so that their roles are clear in aiding him to attain his maximum potential. Visits by a member of the rehabilitation team to the home of the disabled person early in treatment is highly beneficial so that a greater knowledge of home environment, physical layout, and potential architectual problems can be included in the treatment program. It is important that the individual be properly prepared by training and adaptive equipment for a successful transition from the hospital or rehabilitation center to his home environment.

## EVALUATION AND TREATMENT PLAN

The first step in the occupational therapy approach to stroke rehabilitation involves a thorough evaluation of the patient's status, and establishment of a treatment plan followed by the implementation of the treatment approach.

The following sections will present each area of consideration for evaluation as well as the indicated treatment approach.

The sections are in the following order:

1. Behavioral function and social status
2. Communication
3. Perception
4. Sensation
5. Hemianopsia
6. Postural control
7. Upper extremity function
8. Activities of daily living
   A. Feeding
   B. Dressing
   C. Grooming and Hygiene
   D. Transfers
   E. Locomotion and mobility
   F. Homemaking
   G. Home evaluation

### BEHAVIORAL FUNCTION AND SOCIAL STATUS

A patient's rehabilitation is strongly dependent upon his cognitive and psychosocial status. Some areas that should be considered are state of alertness, orientation, attention span, distractability, concentration span, memory, judgment, impulsivity, mood (depression, anger, and so forth), self-image, and motivation. Most aspects of occupational therapy require the active participation of the patient. The extent to which the patient is not alert, cannot attend to or concentrate on the task, does not understand or remember the instructions, or is not motivated will severely affect his ability to participate in a meaningful way. Often it is inappropriate to begin treatment on the upper extremity, postural control, or perception, or training in basic tasks, until a reasonable level of cognitive and psychological functioning has been obtained.

The evaluation of these functions can be accomplished through interviews with the patient and observations made during various activities. Interviews with the patient's family are often helpful because the patient may exhibit different emotions and behavioral patterns with them.

Premorbid cognitive status, psychological status,

value systems, life style, (including occupation, leisure interests, and number of people living with the patient and their relationship), and interpersonal relationships will significantly affect the patient's attitudes toward and participation in the rehabilitation process. These too can be assessed through interviews with the patient and family. Premorbid status is important because the patient enters the rehabilitation situation with certain expectations of what he should or would like to accomplish. These expectations can help or hinder the rehabilitation process. If the patient has always enjoyed being an independent person, he may be motivated toward being independent again. On the other hand, if he had been independent out of necessity only, he may take this opportunity to be dependent without social stigma. If the patient had a job that he feels he will be able to return to, and would like to return to, he may be more motivated than one who welcomes an excuse not to return to work, or who, realizing he can never do the same job, feels that he has no reason to recover. If the patient has healthy close interpersonal relationships, he may feel a sense of security and acceptance that help him adjust to disability. If his relationships were less than healthy he may feel rejected, or may use the disability in a manipulative way.

Throughout the rehabilitation process, the patient's cognitive and psychosocial status should be reassessed. There should be changes associated with decrease in edema of the brain, psychological adjustment to hospitalization and disability, and adjustment of family members to the patient's illness. These changes may be positive or negative—there is not necessarily a continuous positive sequence. For instance, a patient may appear to be adjusting well and suddenly become depressed when discharge from the hospital is becoming imminent.

If the patient is being treated in a hospital setting, the therapist should always be aware of what the patient's discharge plans are. If the patient is being seen on an outpatient basis, his present life style must be considered. Rehabilitation goals will differ for a patient who will be living in a skilled nursing facility, health-related facility, home with family members who can be of assistance, or home alone. If there are family members who will be involved with the patient, they should be kept aware of the patient's status and prognosis, should be encouraged to attend therapy sessions if they are not distractive, and should be trained in how to deal with the patient. Family members often have unrealistic conceptions about the patient's abilities or limitations and this can cause strained interactions. It can also cause a patient to be placed in a nursing home when it is not necessary. If family members are kept abreast of the patient's status, they can be more realistic in their expectations and plans.

## COMMUNICATION

Communication problems that are common in stroke patients are aphasia (expressive, receptive, global), agraphia, alexia, and dysarthria. The speech pathologist ordinarily evaluates and treats the patient for these deficits. The person providing occupational therapy services must be aware of communication problems because they will affect treatment (e.g., if the patient does not understand instructions), and because the therapist will be involved in training the patient to compensate for communication deficits. Patients who are aphasic are often hemiplegic on the dominant side. They may therefore require training in change of dominance so that communication through writing is possible. They may also be trained in one-handed typing. If the patient does not have the necessary motor control, cognition, and perception for writing or typing, he may require a communication board. A communication board (Fig. 1–10) has words or pictures or both denoting objects, people, and feelings. The patient can point to what he wants to express. The alphabet can also be present on the board so that the patient's communication is not restricted (see speech therapy section, p. 48).

## PERCEPTION

### General Considerations for Evaluation of Perceptual Functioning

Careful evaluation of perceptual deficits can assist in locating a lesion, since specific brain sites are responsible for specific perceptual functions. Table 1–1 contains a list of commonly seen perceptual problems and their associated lesion sites.

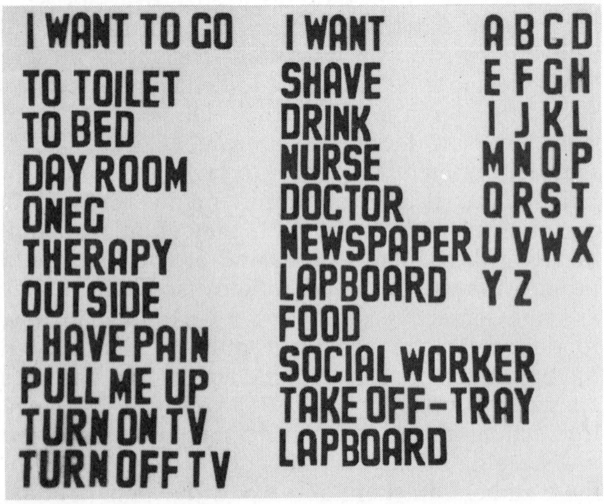

Although there are several standardized perceptual tests for children, there are few for adult populations. The tests that are administered therefore require subjective judgments by the evaluator. Careful observations of the way in which a patient performs a task are as important as the actual task performance. Problems such as short attention span, distractability, impulsivity, and so forth may be noticed. A person with a right hemispheric lesion would be more likely to be impulsive, whereas a person with left hemispheric damage would be more likely to check his work and make corrections. Other aspects, such as a person's tendency to verbalize or analyze, should be noticed. This may indicate that a person with right hemispheric damage is calling upon the left hemisphere to compensate.

The reader may notice that, later in this section when suggestions are given for specific evaluation methods, the same modality is suggested for use in testing several different functions. It is the way in which the test is administered and the observations of the patient's performance that allow the skilled evaluator to determine where the problem lies.

When administering perceptual tests the evaluator must consider prerequisite functions for each skill as well as possible interferences with the evaluation itself. The evaluator must be certain that the patient possesses the necessary sensory and motor functions, cognitive functions, and language ability required for a specific task. The evaluator must also be aware of how perceptual skills interact with one another. For instance a patient may perform poorly on a figure-ground test, but the problem may be in form constancy and not in figure-ground. Therefore, the sequence of testing is important.

It is extremely difficult, if not impossible, to find a test that purely assesses one specific perceptual skill. It is therefore necessary to observe closely and to administer several tests until the true problem is found.

The evaluator must also try to find tests that do not allow for compensation. For instance, when color perception is being tested, objects that match up in shape as well as color should not be used.

### General Considerations for Treatment of Perceptual Deficits

When treating a patient for perceptual deficits, many considerations are similar to those for evaluating. These include prerequisite functions, possible interferences, and interrelationships between various perceptual functions, compensation, life experiences, and individual psychological differences. The general approach as well as the specific task used in treating any patient will depend on all of these considerations.

**I WANT TO GO**
**TO TOILET**
**TO BED**
**DAY ROOM**
**ONEG**
**THERAPY**
**OUTSIDE**
**I HAVE PAIN**
**PULL ME UP**
**TURN ON TV**
**TURN OFF TV**

**I WANT**
**SHAVE**
**DRINK**
**NURSE**
**DOCTOR**
**NEWSPAPER**
**LAPBOARD**
**FOOD**
**SOCIAL WORKER**
**TAKE OFF-TRAY**
**LAPBOARD**

**A B C D**
**E F G H**
**I J K L**
**M N O P**
**Q R S T**
**U V W X**
**Y Z**

**Figure 1–10.** Communication board.

**TABLE 1–1.** PERCEPTUAL PROBLEMS AND ASSOCIATED LESION SITES

| | BRAIN SITE | | EXAMPLES OF FUNCTIONS |
|---|---|---|---|
| PERCEPTUAL FUNCTION | Hemisphere | Lobe | THAT MAY BE AFFECTED |
| Stereognosis | Either | Parietal | Finding objects in one's pocket |
| Body scheme | Left | Parietal | Dressing |
| Finger agnosia | Left | Parietal | Activities require fine coordination (buttoning) |
| Constructional apraxia | Either | Occipitoparietal | Dressing |
| Motor apraxia | Either | Frontal | Ability to learn new tasks or to carry out previously known tasks with a complex sequence |
| Ideomotor apraxia | Left | Parietal | |
| Ideational apraxia | Left or diffuse | Brain damage | Ability to carry out any meaningful activity |
| Laterality | Either | Parietal | Dressing |
| Form constancy | Right | Parietal | May mistake one object for another, such as a sock for a glove |
| Position in space | Right | Parietal | Dressing |
| Figure-ground | Right or large lesion or many small lesions anywhere in brain | Parietal | Ability to find objects in the environment |
| Spacial relations | Right | Parietal | Transfers, dressing |
| Depth and distance perception | Either | Parietal | Transfers, climbing stairs |
| Visual part-whole perception | Left | Occipitoparietal | Reading |
| Unilateral neglect | Right | Parietal | Dressing, shaving, bathing |
| Denial | Right | Parietal | Transfers, dressing |

There are three major categories of treatment approaches used for adult populations: *transfer of training*, *splinter skill learning*, and *compensation*. Transfer of training is used when the administrant believes that increased experience with carefully chosen perceptual tasks will improve the patient's abilities in that perceptual area, and that there will be carryover into the patient's daily life. A patient who, for example, is unable to dress himself because of poor spatial concepts may be asked to connect dots following a certain pattern. This is believed to improve spatial concepts and eventually the patient should be able to dress unaided without any specific dressing training.

Splinter skills are taught when the administrant believes that the patient's general perceptual functioning cannot be improved, but that he can learn to perform specific tasks, usually through repetition. In this case, the aforementioned patient would be given intensive dressing training. He may eventually learn to dress himself but will still not to able to perform other tasks requiring spacial concepts.

Compensation is also used when the administrant believes that the patient's general perceptual functioning cannot be improved. It is often done in association with splinter skill teaching (for instance, giving the patient cues to remember, such as the back of a shirt is where the tag is). It is also used in a more general way, such as making the patient aware of his deficits and training him to search out his own cues in any given situation.

Perceptual evaluation and treatment leave much room for the administrant's creative thinking. Each patient responds differently to any means of evaluation and treatment. Some patients find typical perceptual tasks degrading or threatening, and an alternate means must be found. Some patients will perform poorly on a typical test but will perform well on functional tasks requiring similar perceptual skills. A person's life experiences are important considerations. For instance, a former seamstress may perform poorly on a stereognosis evaluation until she is presented with a spool of thread.

In the following paragraphs, suggestions for evaluating and treating various perceptual dysfunctions are presented. It is emphasized that an understanding of the underlying neurophysiology, as well as the functional aspects of perception, is of extreme importance in administering, interpreting, and adapting these techniques.

## Perceptual Dysfunctions

### Stereognosis

*Evaluations:* With vision occluded, place familiar objects and forms in the patient's hand and have the patient indicate which object or form he feels.

*Treatment:* (1) Provide tactile stimulation to the affected arm. (2) Have the patient manipulate various objects first with vision and then with vision occluded. Provide cognitive cues.

### Body Scheme

*Evaluations:* (1) Have the patient point to various body parts. (2) Have the patient draw a person. (3) Have the patient put together a puzzle of a person.

*Treatment:* (1) Sensory input to body parts. Have the patient name the body part as it is stimulated. Have the patient stimulate his own body parts while naming them. (2) Have the patient point to your body parts first and then his. (3) Have the patient point to the body parts of a picture of a person. (4) Have the patient construct a puzzle of a person.

### Finger Agnosia

*Evaluations:* (1) Touch the patient's fingers, one at a time, and have the patient name or point to a picture of the same finger. Do this while the patient is watching, or with vision occluded. (2) Have the patient move a finger that you name.

*Treatment:* Provide increased tactile stimulation to the affected fingers.

### Constructional Apraxia

*Evaluations:* (1) Have the patient copy drawings of a house, a flower, and so forth. (2) Have the patient copy a construction built with one-inch cubes.

*Treatment:* Have the patient copy simple drawings and constructions. Start off by giving several cues. Grade the activities by giving fewer cues and more complex tasks.

### Motor, Ideomotor, and Ideational Apraxias

*Evaluations:* The Goodglass test for apraxia consists of a series of commands. The patient is asked to pretend to perform a task; if the patient cannot do this, he is asked to imitate the therapist doing it. If he still cannot do it, he is asked to actually carry out the task, if appropriate.

*Treatment:* Splinter skills are taught through very structured learning processes and much repetition.

### Laterality

*Evaluations:* (1) Ask the patient to point to right and left. (2) Ask the patient to point to right and left parts of his body (body image must be known to be intact).

*Treatment:* (1) Provide extra sensory input to one side of the body. (2) Verbalize right and left when giving instructions. (3) Have the patient verbalize right and left while performing tasks. (4) For compensation, provide cues to help the patient recognize right and left on specific objects and on his body.

### Form Constancy

*Evaluations:* (1) In the Frostig Form Constancy test, the patient is presented with several shape drawings and asked to trace all the squares and circles. (2) Form boards are used, in which the patient is asked to place forms in their appropriate spaces.

*Treatment:* Have the patient match similar shapes, forms, and objects. Grade this activity as the patient progresses.

### Position in Space

*Evaluations:* (1) Present the patient with one stimulus picture or object and several others, one of which is identical to the stimulus and all others of which are identical except for a rotational transformation. The patient must match the stimulus with its identical replica. The Frostig Position-in-Space tests includes this task.

*Treatment:* Have the patient manipulate objects, changing their position according to specific commands.

### Figure-Ground

*Evaluations:* (1) Have the patient trace over, name, or point to a specified shape or form that is imbedded in a picture. Ayres and Frostig have developed tests of this kind. (2) Ask the patient to find objects in his environment.

*Treatment:* Ask the patient to perform tasks similar to the evaluations, starting with obvious differentiations between figure and ground, and make these differentiations more discrete as the patient progresses.

### Spatial Relations

*Evaluations:* (1) Have the patient connect a group of dots to match a stimulus drawing. The Frostig Spacial Relations test includes this. (2) Have the patient build one-inch cubes to match a stimulus drawing.

*Treatment:* (1) Have the patient place objects in various relationships to each other and to himself. ("Place the block in front of you.") (2) These evaluation techniques can also be used for training purposes.

### Depth and Distance Perception

*Evaluations:* (1) Ask the patient to grasp an object from various distances and planes. (2) Ask the patient to place an object inside a box.

*Treatment:* Have the patient perform functional activities that require depth and distance perception. Provide cognitive cues.

### Visual Part-Whole Perception

*Evaluations:* (1) Have the patient copy a drawing or cube design. Observe both the finished product and the patient's approach to determine his appreciation of the relationship between the parts and the whole. (2) Present the patient with several pictures and ask him to sequence them to tell a story.

*Treatment:* These evaluations can also be used as treatments. Grade the activity from simple to complex (in terms of part-whole relationships) and provide cognitive cues.

### Unilateral Neglect

*Evaluations:* (1) Have the patient draw a picture of a person, a house, a clock. (2) Have the patient copy a drawing. (3) Have the patient cross out all of a specified letter on a page of random letters.

*Treatment:* (1) Position yourself on the patient's neglected side. (2) Position objects being worked with on the patient's neglected side. (3) Provide sensory stimulation to the neglected area. (4) Teach compensation for specific tasks such as searching for the beginning of a line with finger and eyes when reading.

### Denial

*Evaluations:* (1) Ask the patient questions about his condition. (2) Ask the patient questions about his functional abilities. (3) Observe the patient performing tasks. He may appear impulsive because he is acting as if he has no disability.

*Treatment:* Reinforce cognitive awareness of the disability.

## SENSATION

The presence of sensation, including both tactile and proprioceptive awareness, is an essential factor in determining whether or not coordinated motor function will be a reality for a stroke patient. Without sensory function, motor function is greatly impaired. The patient must learn to use vision to compensate for the loss, but this may not be entirely satisfactory. Full potential of available motor function may never be realized. Therefore, a sensory evaluation is an important assessment tool in determining the occupational therapist's treatment plan and goals for the hemiplegic patient. A complete sensory evaluation should involve the following modalities: light touch, pressure, temperature, pain, proprioception (position sense), and kinesthesia (movement sense). (Stereognosis is covered in the perception section.)

### Evaluation Procedure

Make sure the patient understands the procedure of each test. Use either demonstration or verbal instructions, depending upon which is more successful with the individual stroke patient. Test the uninvolved side so that the patient understands what the normal response feels like. Occlude vision by using a blindfold, shield, or by ask-ing the patient to close his eyes. Vary the timing and the location of the sensory stimulation. Occasionally, to test responses, ask the patient if he felt a stimulation that in fact was not provided. Record responses as *intact*–a quick, accurate response, *impaired*–incorrect or delayed response or ability to identify stimulus but not to localize it, or *absent*–no response to stimulus.

*Light touch*–Use a fine brush or cotton to lightly touch skin. If the patient indicates he felt stimulus, have him localize it by pointing to the spot with the uninvolved hand.

*Pressure*–Use a blunt object such as the eraser head of a pencil or the head of a straight pin. Again, ask for localization if the stimulus is felt.

*Pain*–Use a straight pin; alternate the sharp end with the opposite end and ask if the stimulus is sharp or dull. Ask for localization.

*Temperature*–Fill capped test tubes, one with hot water and the other with cold. Ask the patient to identify hot or cold stimulus and its location.

*Proprioception*–Place the involved upper or lower extremity into various positions and ask patient to imitate the same positioning at each joint using the uninvolved opposite body part. The therapist should hold the body part laterally at bony prominences. Perform test first with the patient watching, then with his vision occluded, to ensure understanding of the procedure.

*Kinesthesia*–Move involved extremity up or down at the joint, holding at bony prominences. Test small as well as large joints. Ask the patient whether the body part was moved up or down.

### Treatment for Sensory Loss

Treatment is directed primarily toward compensation to avoid injury and to improve motor performance. The patient must be made aware of the extent of the sensory deficit, and safety factors should be continually reinforced. If the loss is severe, the patient must be trained to check constantly on the position of the upper and lower limbs using vision. Otherwise, a patient with severe sensory loss may be seen propelling his wheelchair with the fingers of his involved hand caught in the spokes and his involved leg twisted underneath the chair.

If the hemiplegic patient is a smoker, he should be cautioned about the use of matches and cigarettes or cigars; both are potentially dangerous for someone with sensory loss. Protective clothing should be worn when the patient is outdoors in cold weather. During bathing, safety precautions must be stressed. The uninvolved upper extremity should be used to test water temperature, or a commercially available bath thermometer can be used. Kitchen activities are another source of potential danger, with the use of a gas or electric stove and knives as well as hot water. The hemiplegic patient with sensory loss who wishes to return to the role of homemaker should be evaluated for the ability to perform simple homemaking tasks safely, such as preparing a cup of coffee (see p. 42). The patient should demonstrate good judgment, an awareness of the sensory loss, and an ability to compensate visually for the loss before further training in kitchen activities commences.

### HEMIANOPSIA

Hemianopsia is a common visual deficit in hemiplegic patients. It involves the loss of vision for part of the visual field in one or both eyes. Homonymous hemianopsia is the loss of vision in the right visual field or left visual field of both eyes. Combined with sensory loss, hemianopsia can lead to a total neglect of the involved side (see p. 10). (However, the patient may have unilateral neglect without any visual or sensory loss.)

### *Evaluation Procedure*

1. Sit directly in front of the patient and have him look straight ahead at your nose. Hold similar pencils, one in each hand, at ear level of the patient. Slowly bring both pencils straight forward and ask the patient to indicate when he sees each pencil. If it appears that a deficit exists, retest to confirm results. Hold only one pencil on the side with possible visual loss and again ask the patient to indicate when he sees it.

2. With the patient seated at a table or using a wheelchair lapboard, place a sheet of unlined paper directly in front of him. Draw a horizontal line on the paper and ask the patient to divide this line exactly in half. A significant error to either the right or left of mid-line indicates visual field deficit.

### *Treatment*

Compensation is the primary treatment technique for hemianopsia. First, however, the patient should be made aware of his deficit, because many patients do not realize that they have a visual field loss. This can be done by asking the patient to perform activities that require his participation in both the right and left side of his visual field. Feeding is an excellent activity to use. The tray can be set up with coffee on one side and milk and sugar on the other, as an example.

Once the patient comprehends the extent of his visual impairment, he must be taught to turn his head to compensate for the loss. This training can be incorporated into his activities of daily living treatment.

The therapist can also provide activities chosen specifically for hemianopsia compensation. Cancellation of letters is a possible activity. On an unlined piece of paper held lengthwise, type a horizontal line of various letters, making sure to include several of one letter, for example, "A". Seat the patient at a table and place the paper directly in front of him. Then ask the patient to cancel out all the "A's." If he disregards the left or right side of the paper, remind him to turn his head to see entire width of paper.

Copying pegboard designs is another activity to use. Arrange a design on a pegboard, covering both the left and right side of the board. With the patient seated at a table, place the pegboard directly in front of him. Have him copy the design onto another pegboard. The pegs can be placed on the side with field loss to reinforce the need for the patient to turn his head.

### POSTURAL CONTROL

In the stroke patient, the most common factors that interfere with normal postural control are:

1. Disturbances of sensation on the affected side (including hemianopsia)
2. Disturbances of perception
3. Spasticity
4. Release of dominant reflexes from cortical control.

This section concentrates on the release of reflexes from cortical control. The release of these dominant reflexes causes the patient an upset of postural control and makes it difficult for him to command his neuromuscular system. Therefore, the goal of treatment is to re-establish cortical control over these dominant reflexes. In the developing infant, most movements are primitive and reflex-dominated. As he progresses through motor development, these reflexes become cortically controlled and the infant then has more controlled voluntary movements. The stroke patient must go through the same progression, with the goal of inhibition of the dominant reflexes at each stage of development.

Prior to cortical control of these reflexes it is necessary to re-establish righting and equilibrium reactions that are necessary for cortical control to be effective. These equilibrium reactions must be established at each level of development in order to attain the final goal: controlled movement.

Equilibrium responses allow the patient to regain his balance when his center of gravity is shifted by an outside force, either by reaching out with his foot or hand or stepping to the side. When these responses have been elicited, the patient is ready for effective controlled movement.

Postural control is generally evaluated in occupational therapy in three positions: supine, sitting, and standing.

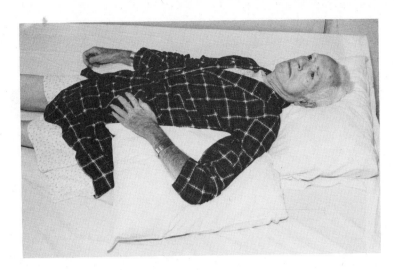

**Figure 1–11.** Correct positioning of affected (L) upper extremity is supine position.

## Supine Evaluation and Treatment

The patient is being tested in his ability to roll from supine to his side. The grading of control generally used is: (1) independence, patient needs no assistance; (2) minimal assistance; (3) moderate assistance; (4) maximal assistance; (5) dependence, patient needs total assistance from a second person.

### Correct Positioning of Patient in Bed
(Figs. 1–11–13)

In the supine position, the affected shoulder should be in protraction and external rotation and held in place by a pillow. The elbow and wrist should be in extension.

It is of great importance that the patient be positioned correctly in bed to prevent an increase of unwanted tone. In all three positions, supine, on the affected side, and on the sound side, the affected arm must be placed in protraction and external rotation, and the elbow and wrist in extension. The affected hip must be in protraction and flexion, and the knee in flexion as well (see Chapter 3 for nursing details).

These positions can be maintained by a pillow. During therapy sessions, when a rest period is required, these are the positions to revert to.

### Rolling

Rolling to the affected side is generally the easier way. The patient clasps his hands over his head and rolls to the affected side. He can lift his sound leg over his affected leg.

*Rolling to the sound side* may be more difficult initially because of the trunk rotation involved. The patient starts in the same position but may need assistance at the shoulder and pelvis to turn. The patient should attempt both directions and should be trained to maintain his balance lying on either side. In both cases, the involved arm should be brought well forward in protraction, which will happen if the hands remain clasped as the patient turns.

In *rolling to sitting*, the patient continues the roll to the affected side and is assisted to prop his elbow. Again, he must be stabilized in this position before he can assume sitting. This position will

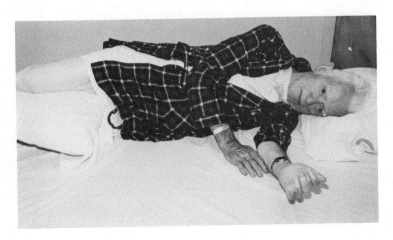

**Figure 1–12.** Correct positioning of affected extremities (L upper and lower) when sidelying on affected side.

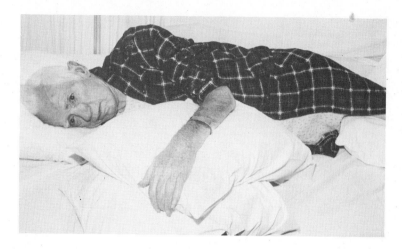

**Figure 1–13.** Correct position of affected extremities (upper and lower) in sidelying on sound side.

also give good approximation of the affected shoulder. From this position the patient can at first be helped into sitting with his sound hand, and eventually he should be able to do this independently. At this point, the patient is ready to be trained in sitting balance.

### Sitting Balance

*Static sitting balance* is defined as the ability to maintain erect, unsupported sitting without changing the center of gravity. *Dynamic sitting balance* occurs when the center of gravity is changed (by having the patient transfer his weight from one side to the other or having him reach out for an object).

Sitting balance is generally graded as follows: Poor, unable to maintain unsupported sitting; Fair, able to maintain sitting without resistance applied; Good, maintains balance with resistance. Good sitting balance is an important prerequisite for the beginning of activities of daily living training. Many stroke patients tend to lean toward the affected side when unsupported in sitting; this signifies poor sitting balance. Three techniques can be used to prevent poor sitting posture while the patient is in a chair or a wheelchair. (1) A seat belt in a wheelchair should be used to keep patient from sliding forward. (2) A lapboard (see Fig. 1–19) can be used to support the affected upper extremity and prevent the patient from slumping forward. (3) A wedged cushion can be used to keep the knees raised higher than the hips to prevent slumping forward (Fig. 1–14).

EQUILIBRIUM REACTIONS. To elicit *equilibrium reactions* in sitting, the patient is asked to sit straight in a chair with feet parallel and flat on the floor and knees apart and flexed to 90 degrees. The patient's arms should be crossed in front of him, with the sound hand supporting the affected elbow. When the patient is stabilized in this position, resistance (manual) is given to disturb balance and evoke equilibrium responses. The resistance given should be enough so that the patient can tolerate it

without production of an increase in abnormal tone. The primary areas for resistance as established by Bobath are the back of the head, shoulder girdle, and pelvic girdle (used more in standing balance training).

It is important to start slowly and gently to encourage the patient's confidence, and then increase pressure as tolerance increases. The commands given to the patient must be short and to the point. The patient should not know in which direction he is to be pushed, so that his responses will not become automatic. These principles on eliciting equilibrium reactions should be applied at each stage of progression from sitting to standing balance.

TRUNK BENDING. The patient assumes the same position as just described and bends forward at the waist and returns to a sitting position. He then

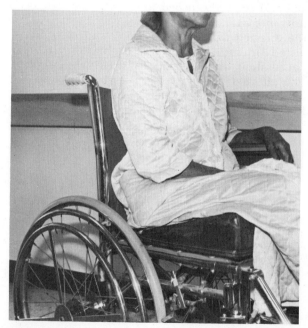

**Figure 1–14.** Wedge cushion helps prevent the patient from slumping forward.

does the same to each side. At first the patient may need assistance with this. Eventually the patient should control this movement himself.

TRUNK ROTATION. The same position is used in sitting as described. The patient rotates his trunk, bringing his arms to one side while looking straight ahead and then to the other side. The rotation should start slowly and eventually the range should be increased. For maximal rotation, the patient should be encouraged to look over his right shoulder as he swings his arms to the left and vice versa.

OTHER EXERCISES. Sitting with elbows flexed and on knees, hands clasped, the patient leans forward to increase approximation of shoulders to elbows.

Hands clasped, elbows extended, the patient leans forward to touch the floor with his hands. The patient then touches alternate legs. This exercise is good for trunk rotation.

Weight transfers should be done to each side by the patient placing his shoulders in external rotation with palms on his chair. The patient transfers his weight to each side and lifts the buttock off the chair.

For "walking" in a sitting position, the patient moves a few steps forward, alternating hips, and then backward. This is the first step in training for transfers.

### Standing Balance

EVALUATION. For static standing, the patient should be able to maintain unsupported standing without shifting the center of gravity. For dynamic standing, the patient should be able to maintain standing when the center of gravity is changed. The progression used for standing balance is: Poor, unable to maintain standing; Fair, able to maintain standing without support; and Good, able to maintain standing with resistance.

TREATMENT. Before controlled standing and ambulation can be achieved, it is necessary for the patient to go through a progression of exercises starting from prone lying on forearms. It is important that the patient be stabilized and equilibrium responses be elicited at each level of progression. These exercises are best done on a foam floor mat, which provides a slightly unstable base of support and will increase equilibrium responses. With patients who show good improvement, a tilt table may be used to provide an even more unstable base of support. A mirror is helpful as it provides the patient with visual cues about his posture and gives feedback as to whether or not he is properly maintaining his balance.

The progression of exercises from prone to standing is as follows: (1) exercises in quadruped, (2) exercises in kneeling, and (3) exercises in standing.

### Exercises in Quadruped

The patient is pronelying with forearm support: (1) Forearms parallel and facing forward. (2) Elbows flexed and directly below shoulders. (3) Knees flexed, ankles dorsiflexed (held in place with a pillow).

KNEELING WITH FOREARM SUPPORT. The patient should be flexed to 90 degrees at shoulders, elbows, hips, and knees, and weight should be well-balanced over forearms.

KNEELING ON HANDS. The shoulders should be in external rotation, elbows extended, hands flat on the floor with fingers in abduction.

1. The patient may at first need assistance to attain each position, but it is important that he eventually be able to get into them independently.

2. The patient must be stabilized in the position.

3. Manual resistance is given at key points to elicit equilibrium responses.

4. Weight transference should be done from the sound to the affected side. A mirror can be used, and as the patient transfers his weight over the affected side, he reaches toward the mirror with his sound hand. (Crossing the midline is also good for perceptual training.)

5. Rocking back and forth on forearms and knees and then hands and knees, as well as laterally, should be practiced. This is an important prerequisite for the reciprocal movements necessary for walking.

6. Crawling should be done.

EXERCISES IN KNEELING. The patient's hand should be clasped and raised forward, elbows extended.

1. The patient should be stabilized in this position.

2. Weight shifting from one knee to the other should be done.

3. Knee walking should be done.

4. Balancing over alternate knees should be done: each leg is alternated, brought forward, and flexed to 90 degrees while the other leg remains in kneeling. The patient should be stabilized in this position and then equilibrium responses should be elicited.

STABILIZED STANDING

1. The head must be in a good position so that the rest of the trunk alignment will follow.

2. The feet must be parallel and flat on the floor (not on the toes).

3. The pelvis should be in protraction.

4. Knee should be in extension (but *not* hyperextended).

5. The affected upper extremity must be in a good position (external rotation, extension at elbow and wrist, thumb abducted).

EXERCISES IN STANDING

The weight is shifted first on to the affected foot, then the sound foot.

2. The weight is shifted with the sound foot one step forward. Then this is alternated, and the affected foot is forward.

3. Equilibrium responses should be elicited by giving resistance at shoulders or hips, sufficient for patient to have to step aside with his foot or reach his foot out to stabilize himself. When equilibrium responses are automatic in standing, the patient is ready for controlled walking.

It must be remembered that equilibrium responses must be elicited at each level of development for controlled movement at any stage to be effective.

## THE HEMIPLEGIC UPPER EXTREMITY

Evaluation of the patient with a hemiplegic upper extremity is often performed based on Brunnstrom's stages of recovery. A comprehensive evaluation should include: (1) primitive abnormal postural reflexes and associated reactions present and their effect on the patient's tone and motions of the trunk and extremities, (2) the presenting stages of recovery and level of voluntary control, and (3) proprioceptive disturbances.

The evaluation is performed with the patient in supine, sitting, and if possible standing positions, starting proximally and proceeding through isolated finger and thumb movements. Range of motion of the upper extremity is tested actively to determine the amount of volitional movement. For example, the patient may be asked to perform a task such as reaching for an object on the table or from the examiner's hand, or he may be asked to touch a part of his own body such as the mouth or head. The therapist then observes motions occurring at the shoulder, elbow, wrist, and fingers and observes for signs of synergistic patterns.

Grading for the stages of recovery of the upper extremity is recorded in terms of functional ranges rather than in degrees: full, three fourths, one half, one fourth, or one eighth ranges of motion at each joint. Stage VI includes a more detailed evaluation of isolated movements and coordination of the upper extremity with special attention to fine movements of the wrist and fingers, including grasp patterns. Range of motion is also tested passively to examine for existing subluxation and for limitations caused by spasticity and/or pain commonly found in the extensors, adductors, internal rotators and horizontal adductors of the shoulder; forearm pronators; and elbow, wrist, and finger flexors.

The extremity is observed at rest for signs of spasticity, edema, or neglect.

The use of spontaneous movements is also recorded; this may be a valuable function to be utilized later in treatment.

If the patient is capable of functional movements but cannot *initiate* movement volitionally and there are no sensory deficits, he may be considered to be apraxic. For the evaluation the therapist can demonstrate the movement required using passive range of motion to the involved or uninvolved extremity, providing somatosensory and visual feedback to cue. This technique is also helpful to the confused or aphasic patient when verbal, written, or gestured communication is not comprehended.

Evaluation of the unaffected upper extremity is included to determine whether there is any decrease of function and to provide comparative information in formulating a level of expectation of function for the involved extremity. If the patient is in a more advanced stage of recovery (Brunnstrom's stages V to VI), evaluation of both upper extremities is assessed in a bilateral task requiring coordination and integration of both sides of the body. Such a task would be donning and doffing a shirt or blouse.

### Treatment

The first objective is maintenance of range of motion. Second in importance is prevention of deformities and correction of them if they do occur. A third objective is to train the patient to improve his performance in specific skills such as activities of daily living, self-care, and work and leisure activities with the *unaffected* upper extremity if the dominant extremity is affected. It is usual that most patients will not regain full function of the involved extremity, especially for skilled activities. A fourth objective is to train the patient to utilize adaptive equipment needed. A fifth objective is to retrain the affected upper extremity to its maximal level.

### Maintenance of Range of Motion

When the upper extremity is flaccid (corresponding to Brunnstrom's stage I of recovery), at least once daily the extremity should be taken through full range of motion at each joint to maintain joint freedom in the event that voluntary movement is recovered and to prevent deformity when there is no recovery. The therapist should support joints that are not being ranged. The patient may be taught to perform self-ranging exercises. Performing these exercises in supine is suggested if the patient has difficulty in moving the arm in the sitting position. As more voluntary movements develop in subsequent stages of recovery, the patient may perform range of motion more actively, with the therapist (or family) assisting to complete the full range. Care should be taken to avoid forcing the arm into ranges of pain. With an increase in spas-

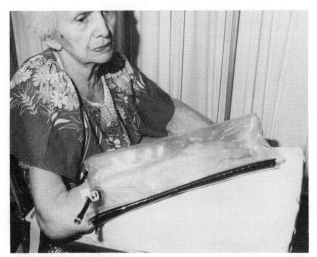

**Figure 1–15.** The Jobst air splint is used to reduce edema of the affected extremity.

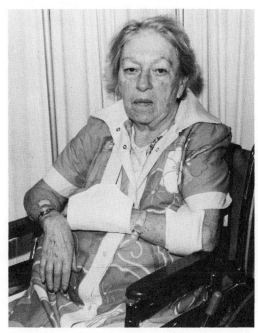

**Figure 1–16.** Hemi-sling.

ticity, movement in range of motion may become difficult for the patient (and therapist) to achieve. Some methods used for decreasing spasticity or normalizing tone include:

1. Range of motion with influence of gravity eliminated, as with the patient in supine position.

2. Slow rolling or rocking of trunk.

3. Slow, rhythmic movements with prolonged joint compression of affected extremity.

4. Joint compression with light pressure.

5. Direct facilitation to antagonist muscle or muscle group.

6. Use of moist heat to affected extremity.

7. Use of neutral heat (extremity wrapped in turkish towel 10 to 20 minutes).

8. Use of Jobst air splint (also used about 10 to 20 minutes to reduce edema) (Fig. 1–15).

9. Biofeedback to specific muscles or muscle groups.

Once spasticity is reduced, greater ranges of passive and active motion may be achieved.

### Prevention and Correction of Deformities

#### SHOULDER

For the shoulder, correct positioning of the involved extremity is employed to prevent subluxation at the gleniod-humeral joint and to assist in pushing the head of the humerus back into the glenoid fossa if there is subluxation. Relief of pain may also be achieved. This may be accomplished by positioning with use of several mechanical methods.

1. Providing the patient with the *hemi-sling* (Fig. 1–16) is controversial because of restriction of movement and possible anterior displacement of the humeral head in the fixed adducted position

with prolonged use. The sling does provide support to the flaccid extremity while the patient is standing to transfer or ambulating.

2. The *Bobath sling* (Fig. 1–17) gives proximal stabilization but is less supportive distally.

3. *Pillow(s) in the patient's lap* (Fig. 1–18) supporting the elbow and hand with the arm moderately elevated can prevent edema.

4. A *lap board* (Fig. 1–19) with or without padded elevated foam wedge can be used as an arm support. This may also be adapted to keep the hand in

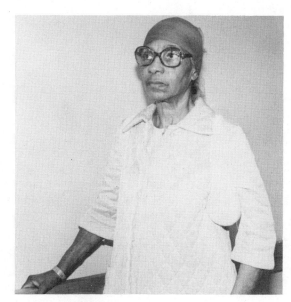

**Figure 1–17.** The Bobath sling.

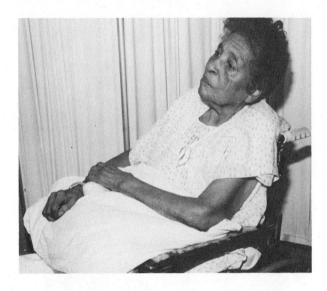

**Figure 1–18.** Pillow in lap is used to support elbow and hand.

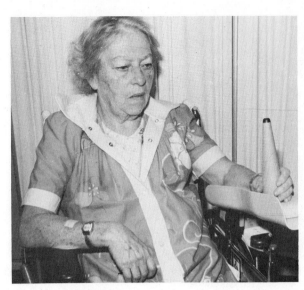

**Figure 1–19.** Lap-board can be adapted with or without padded wedge foam and/or hand roll.

a functional position—a foam roll may be placed in the hand, or the hand in neutral position can be kept in place with a padded dowel.

5. *Trough arm supports* (Fig. 1–20) may be adapted with a foam hand roll.

Other supportive devices that may be used when there is more tone present are:

6. A *latex tubing sling* (Fig. 1–21) is less supportive distally but provides stimulation (quick stretches) to the rotator cuff muscles and elbow extensors from the bounce of the tubing.

7. A *mobile suspension sling* (Fig. 1–22) is hung, or an *L-shaped metal bar* is attached, to the back of the

wheelchair. The hemiplegic extremity is supported on an adjustable sling. In addition to providing proximal support and relief of pain and reducing edema, the sling allows active movement. Stoppers may be used initially to prevent the possibility of further subluxation by the horizontal swing of the sling. (A rubber tip placed on the end of the metal bar is suggested as a safety precaution.)

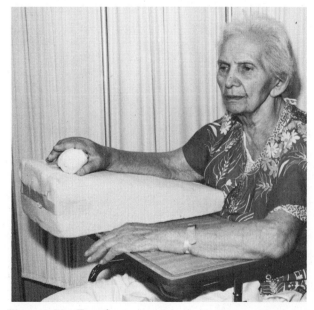

**Figure 1–20.** Trough arm support.

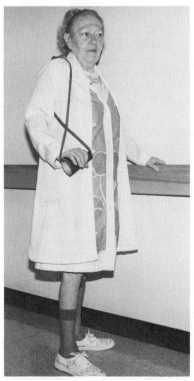

**Figure 1–21.** Latex tubing sling.

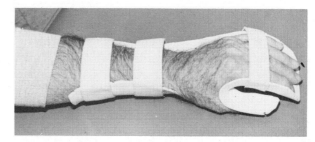

**Figure 1–23.** Static forearm hand splint or resting splint.

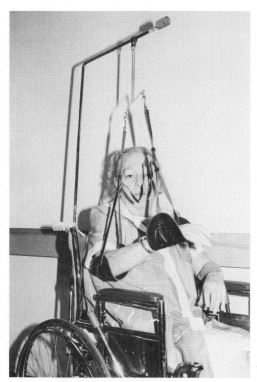

**Figure 1–22.** Mobile suspension sling.

### FOREARM AND HAND

Every effort should be made to prevent edema of the hand while the patient is in the bed and in the wheelchair. A *static forearm hand splint* (Fig. 1–23) or *volar cock-up hand splint* may be used to maintain the hand in functional position and to prevent deformities or contractures from impending spasticity. Initially to be used as a resting splint during most of the day and night with relief for daily exercise and hygiene, in later stages of recovery this may be used only as a night splint. When the patient gains wrist and finger control, use of the splint is reevaluated. In bed or in the wheelchair, the splinted extremity may be elevated distally to prevent edema or assist in reducing it.

Splinting may be contraindicated when there is an increase in flexor spasticity. Dorsal splinting may be tried to facilitate extensors of the hand and wrist for alleviating sensory stimulation to the flexor surface. Splints may be fabricated from various materials (Orthoplast and Aquaplast) available commercially or may be purchased prefabricated.

The patient should be trained to improve his performance in activities of daily living. Self-care skills should be taught, and work and leisure activities with the unaffected extremity should be encouraged. Further training should involve use of adaptive equipment. The patient should be trained to use the affected extremity to its maximal level.

Since the course of recovery in the extremity usually goes proximal to distal in early treatment, particular attention is given to the shoulder to strengthen the shoulder girdle musculature for maximal stability of the glenoid-humeral joint. Once proximal stabilization is achieved, the ability to use the involved extremity for most functional activities requiring movements away from the body is greatly increased, especially when distal recovery follows.

### Retraining and Strengthening

Retraining and strengthening may be achieved with neurophysiological techniques. A variety of treatment approaches are practiced. Each therapist should develop and adjust an approach as required by the patient's individual responses. The traditional neurophysiological approaches that are used are techniques developed by pioneers in the field. Bobath's basic principle focuses on facilitation of normal movement patterns and inhibition of compensatory movements and abnormal movement patterns in order for the patient eventually to initiate these normal movements independently. The theory of Brunnstrom utilizes the sequential appearance of flexion and extension mass movement patterns to progress to normalized integrated functional movements. Rood encouraged the use of somatosensory stimulation of trunk and limbs to elicit motor responses in the respective body segments. The Voss-Kabat-Knott approach focuses on proprioceptive input for facilitation of synergistic

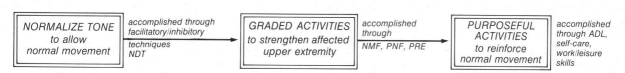

**Figure 1–24.**

muscle responses of stabilizers and prime movers used normally in various movement patterns. Each method is concerned with normalizing tone through inhibiting and/or relaxing and facilitating and/or stimulating motor activity, and increasing voluntary motion, coordination, strength, and endurance. Each method is approached on a neurophysiological basis with an understanding of the sequence of normal human motor development. Because early motor development is greatly influenced by reflex activity, these reflex mechanisms are considered to facilitate or inhibit voluntary effort.

All of the methods employ concepts of motor learning by using repetition of normal movement of past skilled performances stored in patients' long-term memory (engrams). This contributes to an increase in sensory awareness, motor planning, and subconscious sensorimotor integration. These benefits may be accomplished through frequency of stimulation for reinforcement of sensory input, verbal and visual cueing, and the integration of the body and its segments.

The development of coordinated movements is the goal of most therapeutic exercises. Development of compensatory movements or secondary neural pathways should be facilitated *only* after function in the affected extremity has been developed to its fullest. This may enable the patient to use the affected extremity assistively if not functionally. Handling and close personal interaction with the patient's conscious participation is necessary in order for the patient to "learn" muscular control and is vital for the success of these approaches.

Other devices for retraining and strengthening are progressive-resistive exercises (described by DeLorme), graded activities, and biofeedback. Also helpful are unilateral activities that not only increase strength and dexterity in the uninvolved extremity but also have resistive effects on the involved extremity. Examples are craft activities (copper tooling, rug hooking), ball playing, card playing (with slotted rack to hold cards), and writing, drawing, and painting. Graded hand grippers are helpful, as are activities of daily living, self-care, and homemaking.

Mat activities can be of benefit—for example, following the neurodevelopmental progression: rolling to side and rolling to sitting position (see section on postural control).

A ball bearing skateboard (Fig. 1–25) on a table at a comfortable height can be used for the affected extremity. The patient is seated sideways at the table. An Ace bandage may be used to secure the forearm if needed. The therapist assists in moving the arm more easily if such assistance is required. Movements achieved are horizontal adduction and abduction, scapular protraction and retraction, and

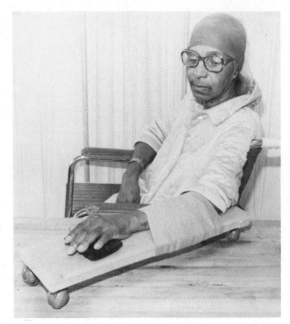

Figure 1–25. Skateboard.

elbow flexion and extension. The patient may progress to active movements; activity may be graded with added weights.

A counterbalance sling or overhead sling (Fig. 1–26) can be used to facilitate movement and in conjunction with any activity that requires the use of the involved extremity when elimination of gravity is desired. It may also be used to resist movement by adding weights.

Wand or broomstick exercises (self-assisted, active assistive) with an Ace bandage or hand mitt on the involved hand are used to aid grasp. Movements obtained are shoulder flexion and extension, horizontal adduction and abduction, elbow extension, and flexion and wrist extension. The flaccid extremity may need to be supported with the overhead sling. This activity may be graded by approximation of both hands, with the activity becoming more difficult when they are further apart. Repetitions are done slowly and rhythmically. A climbing board may be used to modify this activity. Both may be graded with sandbag weights.

Bilateral sanding is used initially with the affected hand supported with a mitt or an Ace bandage if grasp is not present; the purpose is to achieve scapular protraction and retraction, elbow flexion and extension, and wrist and finger flexion. Again, the overhead sling may be used. The activity is graded by adding weights and adjusting the incline of the board. Bilateral self-care activities include dressing, transfers, feeding, hygiene, cooking, and household chores. Bilateral gross motor activities include ball playing, shuffleboard, turkish knotting, or macramé. All these activities can be adapted to the goal desired and upgraded (soft to hard ball, large to small ball). Shuffleboard discs can be weighted. The height and position of the turkish knot and macramé frames can be adjusted. And as distal movement returns, bilateral fine motor activities to develop efficiency and precision in various grasp patterns and individual finger movements are begun. This includes crafts, writing with the involved hand (if dominant), turning pages, picking up small objects, manipulating objects, stacking, and activities with Theraplast (resistive putty). Self-care activities in this category include using feeding utensils, fastening clothing, shaving, brushing hair and teeth, and preparing meals. Also in this category are typing and playing of musical instruments, which also assist in developing rhythmic movement.

A patient may skip stages of recovery or recovery may plateau at any stage. The occupational therapist will modify his treatment approach and goals as the patient shows or does not show progress in using the affected extremity. The family should be encouraged to stay abreast of the patient's progress not only to adapt the treatment program in the home but, more importantly, to be able to set goals that demonstrate an understanding of the patient's abilities and limitations.

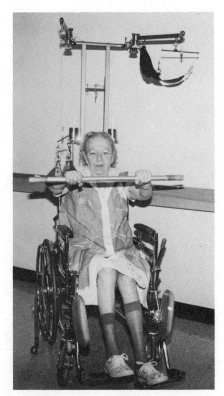

**Figure 1–26.** Counterbalance sling or overhead sling.

## ACTIVITIES OF DAILY LIVING: SELF-CARE ACTIVITIES

These are the ability to feed oneself, dressing activities, grooming and hygiene tasks, transfer, and locomotion with assistive walking device or wheelchair. Self-care activity training should be initiated as soon as the patient's medical status allows it to help alleviate the depression that adult stroke patients feel upon becoming dependent upon others for their needs. Although at first it may be easier and quicker to do these things for the patient, if the patient does not learn to care for himself he will *remain* dependent, and in the long run more time will have to be spent assisting him.

Factors influencing treatment are hemiplegia (flaccidity or spasticity), sensory loss, loss of postural control, perceptual problems, apraxia, secondary medical problems (cardiac conditions, arthritis), mentation problems (confusion, memory loss, poor judgment) and poor endurance.

It is important to understand exactly what the treatment procedure is so that it can be explained in the clearest and most concise terms to the patient. He should have a clear understanding of what is expected of him. Verbal instructions may need to be repeated frequently, especially for those patients with memory loss, and should be the same each time.

A patient with sensory loss must be taught to protect himself from injury (use visual cueing). Patients with loss of postural control must be given adequate physical support, such as a lapboard.

Articles of clothing as assistive devices should be placed within easy reach of the patient to increase his independence. Assistive equipment should be given to a patient only when absolutely necessary.

A patient's abilities must be assessed and a decision should be made as to which activities are best done in bed, in a chair or wheelchair, or in standing position. It is therefore important to coordinate activities of daily living training with the other treatment the patient is receiving (as his sitting balance improves more work can be done on transfer or dressing training).

The patient must be given adequate time for the relearning of these activities. This is particularly true of those patients with memory loss, perceptual difficulties, and those who have had to change hand dominance. If a patient is frustrated with one area of activities of daily living, another one should be tried. The first one can be returned to when the patient exhibits an increase in function. The therapist should listen to the patient's own suggestions as to the best way to accomplish an activity.

It is important to be aware of safety precautions and to remember that although a patient may appear independent in an activity, he may require supervision or guarding.

The therapist should encourage the patient to do as much for himself as possible. Grading of progression in activities of daily living training is: (1) total dependence, (2) need for assistance, (3) need for supervision, and (4) independence with or without assistive devices. The long-term goal of activities of daily living training is to have the patient achieve maximal independence in self-care. In those areas in which he has difficulty, family members should be taught procedures that will be most comfortable and safe for the patient and easiest for them.

## Dressing

For an evaluation the patient may be asked to begin with simple undressing and dressing with hospital clothing (gown, bathrobe, slippers). Evaluation may be done in supine, sitting, and/or standing positions, unilaterally or bilaterally. On a higher level, the family may be asked to bring in the patient's street clothes. His ability to dress and undress is evaluated.

The patient's status in postural control is an important consideration in determining the level of evaluation and treatment approach to be used in training of dressing activities. The patient's medical, cognitive, and perceptual status, the level of recovery of the affected upper and lower extremity, and the sensory status are other important factors affecting evaluation and treatment and the patient's ability and performance in dressing activities.

Training is also approached with the patient in supine, sitting, and/or standing positions. For instance, a patient with poor sitting balance may need to begin training sitting in a wheelchair or armchair and eventually progress to sitting without external support with his feet flat on the floor. In addition, dressing activities are taught according to the extent of recovery of the affected upper and lower extremity. For the patient with flaccid upper and lower extremities, unilateral training is taught. When the upper or lower extremity or both are flaccid, one-handed training is facilitated because the flaccid limbs can glide through the garment.

In the patient with spastic upper and lower extremities, unilateral training is begun. The spastic upper and lower extremity are more difficult to manage in one-handed dressing training. Relaxation techniques may be required to perform the task.

Minimal to moderate voluntary control of movements in bilateral training is taught. The patient is encouraged to use the affected upper extremity and a lower extremity assistively to accomplish dressing. Training progresses from unilateral to the patient's normal bilateral techniques when possible.

Since most patients do not regain full use of the involved upper extremity, emphasis is placed on *one-handed* training, especially when the patient must change dominance. Therefore, one-handed dressing techniques are described in the following section.

### One-Handed Dressing Techniques

All articles of clothing should be placed within easy reach of the patient. Reachers (commercially available) may be used to secure clothing and also to assist in dressing.

#### Front-Opening and Closing Garment

The garment (shirt or blouse, robe, jacket, dress) is put on the affected upper extremity first. Patients demonstrating impaired sitting balance should be watched closely to prevent falling. If sitting balance is not sufficient without external support the patient can perform this activity in a wheelchair or armchair rather than sitting in bed.

1. The garment is arranged flat on the patient's lap with the tag side up. The collar is placed toward the chest.
2. With the sound upper extremity, the patient arranges the hole of the sleeve close to the affected hand.
3. The sound upper extremity places the affected upper extremity into the sleeve, pushing the sleeve past the elbow and onto the shoulder.
4. With the sound upper extremity, the patient takes hold of the collar and swings the garment over to the sound shoulder.

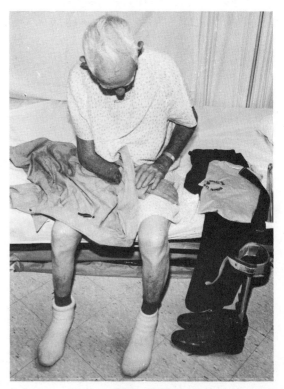

**Figure 1–27.**

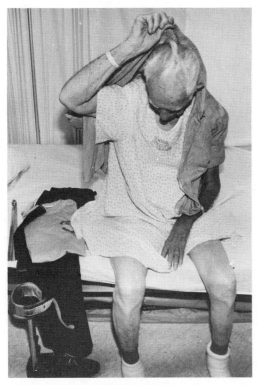

Figure 1–28.

5. The sound upper extremity is inserted in an upward outward direction into the sleeve.
6. The garment is fastened.

*Equipment:* A button hook (see p. 241) may assist in fastening smaller buttons.

The garment is removed by slipping it off the shoulder of the sound side first with a shrugging motion. The patient is asked to lean forward so that the garment is sure to be free in the back.

*Hints*

1. The sleeve of the garment on the sound side may be fastened before donning the garment. Elastic thread may be used to secure the cuff button if the cuff is too tight.
2. Teeth may be used to unfasten the sleeve of the sound side.
3. Loose-fitting garments (a size larger) are preferred.
4. Short sleeves are preferred.
5. Larger buttons or snaps are easier to fasten.

**Overhead Garment**

These are T-shirts, dresses, sweaters; start with the affected upper extremity first.

1. The garment is arranged on the patient's lap tag side down.
2. The sound upper extremity assists in putting the affected upper extremity through the body of the garment into the sleeve (or the sound upper extremity can assist the affected upper extremity into the sleeve by pulling the affected upper extremity through, from the outside of the sleeve).

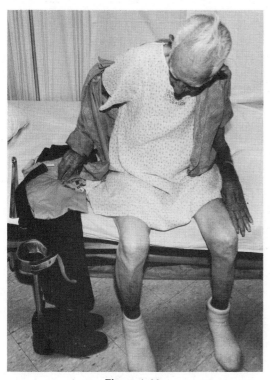

Figure 1–29.

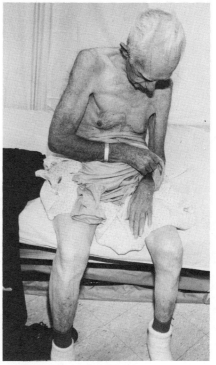

Figure 1–30.

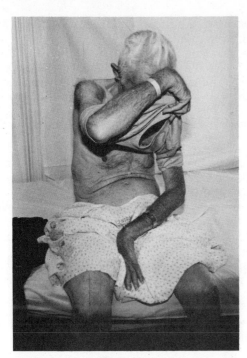

**Figure 1–31.**

*Hints:* Larger sizes are recommended. The garment is removed by reaching to the back and collar and pulling the garment overhead.

### Trousers

#### In Supine

The garment is put on affected lower extremity first, with the patient in supine position.

1. With the affected lower extremity crossed over and supported by the raised and bent sound lower extremity, the pant leg is slipped over the affected lower extremity. (The bed is tilted up at the head or the upper trunk is raised by pillows.)
2. By lowering the sound leg or by using the sound upper extremity, the patient uncrosses the affected lower extremity. The sound lower extremity is then inserted into the pant leg.
3. The buttocks are raised off the bed using the sound lower extremity bent and raised to push up. The pants are pulled over the hips and fastened. (If the patient is unable to raise his hips by this method, he can work the pants up over the hips by rolling from side to side.)

*Hints:* A loop or ring on the zipper pull may assist in fastening trousers. Belt loops may assist in pulling up pants.

3. The patient pushes the sleeve over the elbow.
4. The sound upper extremity is inserted into the sleeve.
5. The patient grabs the back of the garment and collar and lifts the garment overhead; the head is inserted.
6. The patient reaches to the back to straighten the garment.

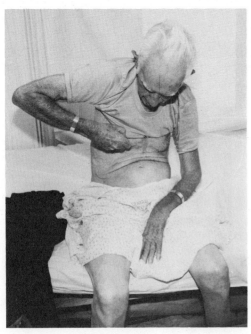

**Figure 1–32.**

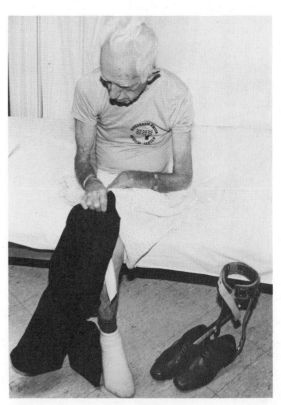

**Figure 1–33.**

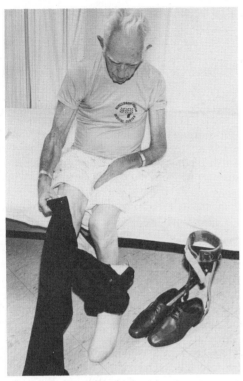

**Figure 1–34.**

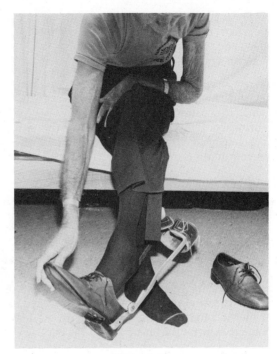

**Figure 1–35.**

### IN SITTING AND STANDING

1. Pants may be donned in a sitting position once the patient has gained trunk control. The affected lower extremity is crossed over the sound lower extremity and brought up toward the midline of the body. The pant leg is slipped over the affected lower extremity and the leg is eased down.
2. The sound lower extremity is inserted into the pant leg. (The patient may stand to fasten the trousers if the trunk control is sufficient.)

*Hint:* Suspenders fastened onto the trousers before they are donned may assist the patient in holding the pants up while he is standing.

*Equipment:* A reacher or dressing stick may be used to secure pant legs. The garment is removed on the sound side first—the patient reverses the steps.

### Short Leg Brace (With Shoe)

*Equipment:* Long-handled shoehorn and footstool.

1. All Velcro straps are opened.
2. The tongue of the shoe is folded up and back.
3. The affected lower extremity may be crossed over the sound leg and brought up to the midline of the body or brought closer by using a footstool.
4. The brace is placed behind the affected lower extremity by holding calf bar to maneuver.

Toes are inserted into the shoe of the brace sideways at first.

5. The brace is maneuvered so that toes and foot are aligned in the shoe. If the shoe is a size larger, the heel will slip into the back of the shoe when the patient pulls upward and back on the calf bar. A shoehorn at the heel or pres-

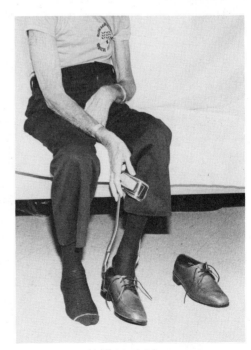

**Figure 1–36.**

sure on the affected knee (using the sound upper extremity) will assist the foot to slip into the shoe.

6. Velcro straps are fastened.

The brace is removed by the patient opening the straps and pushing down and forward on the calf bar with the sound upper extremity. The toes of the sound foot placed on the heel of the shoe of the brace to pull down the shoe heel may also assist in removing the brace.

### Long Leg Brace (With Shoe)

Most patients do not become proficient enough to don and doff a long leg brace without assistance.

### Shoes

Shoes may be donned by the same method as for trousers, step 1 in supine, substituting the shoe for trousers. The shoe is held at the heel, and steps 1 and 2 for trousers in sitting position are used. Another method that may be used is mentioned in the section on donning a short leg brace (steps 3 and 5).

*Equipment:* Long-handled shoehorn, and footstool.

*Hints*

1. Use of Velcro closures, slip-in shoes, and elastic shoe laces eliminates tying laces.
2. Some patients may be dextrous enough to be able to tie a bow with one hand. A method used without tying is:
   (a) Using sound upper extremity, ends of laces are placed through the last hole (nearest to ankle) to form loops.
   (b) The ends of the laces are put through opposite loops.

(c) The ends are pulled in opposite directions one side at a time until the loops are gone. The ends of lace will be secured under the loops.

(d) Lace ends are tucked into sides of shoe.

### Socks

The same method is used as for trousers step 1 for supine and steps 1 and 2 for sitting, substituting a sock for the trousers. The patient may widen the mouth of the sock by inserting the sound hand into the mouth of the sock and spreading the fingers.

*Equipment:* A dressing stick (see p. 240) may be used to assist in holding the mouth of the sock open.

### Brassiere (see Chapter 13)

1. Working at waist level using the sound upper extremity, the patient tucks one side of the back strap of the bra into the panties or slacks. The other side of the back strap is brought around to the front.
2. Hooks are fastened (Velcro closures are helpful).
3. The bra is reversed to the correct position. (Powder may assist in turning the bra to the front.)
4. The shoulder strap of the affected side is placed over the affected elbow toward the shoulder. (Elastic straps are easier to manage.)
5. The sound upper extremity is placed through the other shoulder strap.
6. Straps are put onto both shoulders.
7. The patient leans forward to adjust.

*Hints:* Use of a larger back size of bra is recommended (i.e., from 34B to 36B). An elastic strap at-

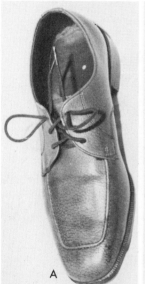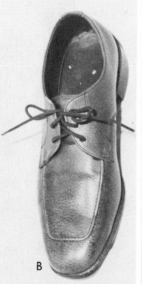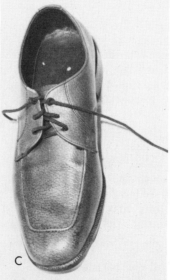

Figure 1–37.

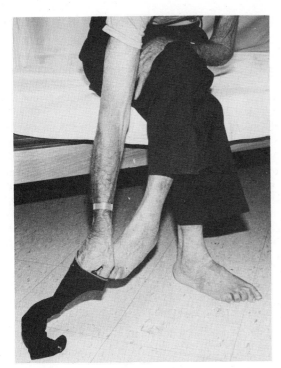

Figure 1–38.

tached to the back strap will allow extra room. Front-fastening bras may be helpful.

### Hemi-Sling

1. The hand part of the sling is placed in front, resting over the sound shoulder.
2. With the sound upper extremity the patient reaches and pulls the elbow part of the sling under and through the axillary areas of the affected upper extremity.
3. With the sound upper extremity the patient pulls the affected upper extremity through the elbow cuff and rests the elbow into the cuff.
4. Step 3 is repeated with the hand part of the sling.
5. The patient adjusts the height to comfort and sees that the affected shoulder is secure.

## HYGIENE

### Elimination

Managing clothes during toilet functions requires good dynamic standing balance. Otherwise this activity can be done in a sitting position by the patient, who leans from side to side in order to push undergarments off and pull them on.

### Bathing

Long-handled sponges with compartments for soap, washcloth mitts, hand-held shower hoses, and scrub brushes with suction cups are adaptive equipment items found to be most helpful for one-handed bathing. They can be purchased commercially. Toiletries in plastic containers and spray containers are easier and safer to use than those in glass containers with screw tops.

### Grooming

Evaluation of grooming skills involves asking the patient to use a toothbrush or hair brush, comb, and possibly a safety razor (without blade) and observing the patient's difficulties or any neglect of the affected side. Training in grooming usually includes such tasks as shaving, combing hair, and cutting nails. For shaving, electric shavers have been found to be satisfactory and safer for this activity than straight razors. If the patient needs to be sedentary he can be trained to use a mirror on a table at comfortable height. Stretching of the skin when the patient is unable to use the affected upper extremity may be done by blowing air into the cheeks.

For combing hair, the patient can sit the same way as for shaving if standing balance is impaired. Both activities may require repetition, especially if the patient is changing hand dominance. The patient should be made aware of grooming the involved side, and should be reminded to turn his head, particularly when there is hemianopsia present.

Cutting nails is a more difficult task to accomplish one-handed. (Foot-operated clippers can be purchased.) The patient can secure a nail file on a table with tape and use the file to shape and shorten the nails.

### Transfers

Points to consider in all transfers:
1. Allow the patient to do as much as possible for himself.
2. Before transfer, the patient should be correctly positioned with a wide base of support at the edge of the surface on which he is seated. He should move his center of gravity within the base of support.
3. The therapist should be positioned to give aid to the patient's affected side but should give only as much assistance as needed.
4. Transfer should always be accomplished toward the patient's *unaffected* side.

For positioning, the patient should be wearing his sling (if he has one) in order to keep his affected arm close to the midline and within his base of support. The patient's wheelchair (or chair) should be placed at a 90 degree angle, or the helper should slightly move acute angle to the patient's bed or other surface on the *unaffected* side.

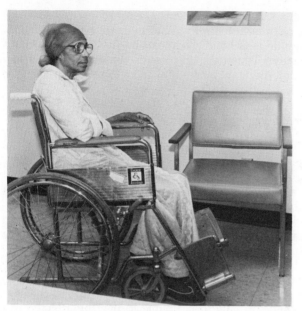

**Figure 1–39.** Patient transferring to armchair. Wheelchair and chair are placed at 90 degree angle with armchair on sound side. Note hemi-sling on affected side.

### Procedure

The patient is positioned at the edge of the bed or chair with feet apart. Demonstrate the procedure to the patient so that he *clearly understands* what he is expected to do. The patient should be flexed at the knees more than 90 degrees and flexed at the waist, bringing his head forward to shift his center of gravity within the base of support. The unaffected arm will aid in pushing up to standing.

Initiate transfer with a rocking motion to build up momentum on a count of 3. On 3, the patient pushes up with his unaffected arm and straightens his legs. You can assist with the affected leg by pushing on his kneecap with your knee.

Once standing, the patient should pivot on the ball of his unaffected foot and place his unaffected arm on the near armrest of the chair for support. While continuing the pivot he changes to the more distant armrest and *slowly* lowers himself into the chair.

Types of transfers are dependent, assisted, and independent with equipment.

The patient should be sitting on the edge of the bed or chair with his feet approximately shoulder width apart and knees bent, feet on the floor.

### Your Position

Stand directly in front of the patient. (Rubber-soled shoes with low heels are advisable to prevent you from sliding and minimizing strain to your back.) Keep your feet approximately shoulder width apart with one foot in front of the other for increased stability. The foot that is placed to the rear is pointed in the direction toward which you will transfer. This position allows you to shift your weight during the transfer while maintaining your center of gravity within your base of support.

Place one hand under the axilla of the affected side (or place both hands on either side of the patient if more assistance is required) to help lift the patient. *Do not pull.* With your hand(s) under the axilla, keep your elbows bent and arm(s) at your side(s).

Just before initiating the transfer, with your arms and feet correctly positioned, bend at the knees and the hips, keeping your back straight. Bending over causes unnecessary strain on your back and requires more energy.

Verbally cue the patient to stand and assist him only as much as needed. When standing you are positioned in front of him so that you may brace his knee on the affected side to prevent it from buckling. Also, your feet are positioned outside of his to widen your base of support and ensure safety. *Keep all distances as short as possible.*

### Dependent Transfer

In this transfer the patient is unable to assist to any degree. This is not the usual case involving stroke patients, but occurs on occasion because of other medical factors such as inability to bear any weight on either lower extremity, as in a patient who is highly confused.

Dependent transfers can be accomplished by the Hoyer lift or the two-man carry. A Hoyer Lift is a mechanical device that is operated by one person. In the two-man carry, the patient is placed in a sitting position with his arms crossed in front of him. One lifter is positioned behind the patient with his arms under the patient's axillae and grasping the forearms just below the elbows. The second lifter is positioned in front of the patient holding securely behind the patient's flexed knees. At a signal from the first lifter, both move the patient from one surface and transfer him to a second surface.

### Assisted Transfers

The three types are the sitting pivot, standing pivot 90 degrees, and standing pivot 180 degrees.

The *sitting pivot transfer* is the one used for the patient who is most dependent and has the least functional ability. Use of a wheelchair with removable armrests is advisable, positioned 90 degrees from the transfer surface. Position the patient for transfer (edge of seat, wide base of support, etc.) Properly position yourself.

Rocking to build momentum, give the patient the auditory cue "On three" to come to a semi-standing position. The patient pivots the ball of the unaffected foot toward the wheelchair. Place the patient's hand on the arm rest to make sure he is over the chair and he can assist in safely lowering himself onto the chair.

The *90 degree standing pivot* is used by a less dependent and much more functional patient. It is advisable that the patient have a more stable sitting balance than required in the sitting pivot transfer and also have the ability to bear weight fully on the unaffected leg. The amount of assistance provided to the patient ranges from the least, verbal cueing, to the most, maximum assistance.

*Verbal cueing* is reminding the patient of proper procedure and body alignment. *Contact guarding* is providing hands on the patient to prevent momentary loss of balance. *Minimum assistance* involves providing the patient with slight assistance in either the lift or the pivot. *Moderate assistance* is providing greater assistance in lift, pivot, or both. In *maximum assistance* you are providing more assistance than the patient can provide for himself throughout the transfer.

The procedure is performed as outlined under Procedure.

The *standing 180 degree pivot* is the most difficult of all the assisted pivot transfers, requiring more functional ability of the patient than any other type.

The patient may attempt this transfer when he can accomplish the 90 degree pivot with moderate to minimum assistance. Grading is the same as in the 90 degree pivot. The procedure is also the same, only in this transfer the two surfaces are 180 degrees apart and the patient pivots on the ball of his foot to that degree at the completion of his

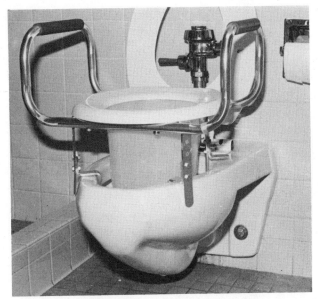

**Figure 1–41.** Raised toilet seat with arm rests.

transfer. The advantage of this transfer is that it is much more practical in tight spaces such as in a bathroom or small bedroom where there may not be sufficient room or where it may not be advantageous to place the wheelchair at 90 degrees.

### Independent Transfer with Equipment

This is for the patient who is able to perform pivot transfers from a wheelchair without the aid of contact guarding or verbal cues but requires additional equipment in the transfer. Some typical

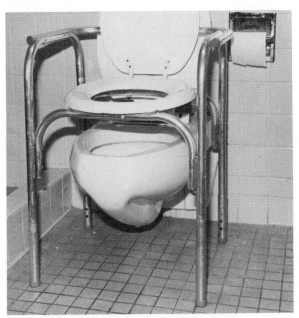

**Figure 1–40.** Bedside commode with pail removed may be used over toilet to provide arm rests and increase seat height.

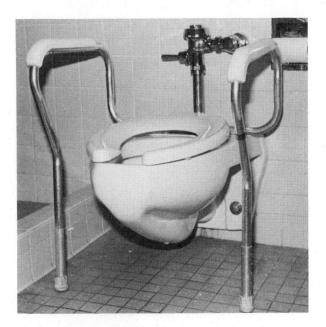

**Figure 1–42.** Toilet safety bilateral rails.

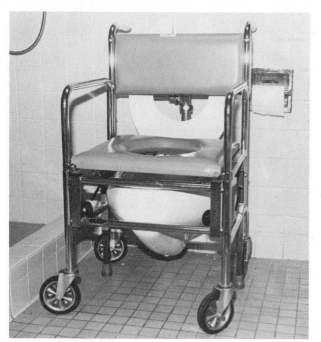

**Figure 1–43.** Bedside commode with casters may be used to transport patient to toilet or tub area if bathroom is not wheelchair accessible.

transfers; the equipment provides additional support.

Using the quad cane in transfers, the patient may use the pivot technique or for greater safety and control he should turn and back up to the transfer surface until he feels it at the back of his legs. Then he can reach back and slowly lower himself to the transfer surface.

### Wheelchair Mobility

The stroke patient will generally find it easiest to propel his chair using his sound hand and leg. The hand is used for propulsion and the foot is used for direction.

For the patient who is unable to use his foot for direction, a one-arm drive mechanism can be used. The patient should have good cognitive and perceptual function. (For a description of this mechanism see Chapter 25.) For the right hemiplegic patient, the rims would be attached to the left side of the chair. The inner rim would propel the chair to the right side, the outer rim to the left side. Both rims are pushed to go straight forward. The opposite is done for the left hemiplegic patient.

devices are: grab bars, toilet bilateral rails, raised toilet seat, tub seat, and quad cane.

In transfers requiring equipment, all of the same procedures are followed by the patient as in pivot

### Homemaking

As a part of discharge planning, the hemiplegic homemaker should be evaluated by the occupational therapist to determine if the patient can realistically return to the role of homemaker. An evaluation session in an apartment setting with a

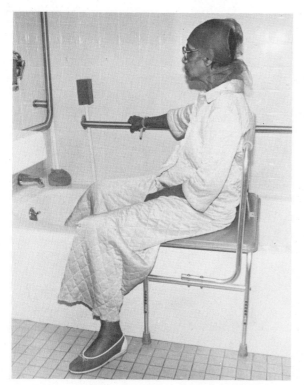

**Figure 1–44.** Bathtub transfer using transfer tub seat (and grab bars).

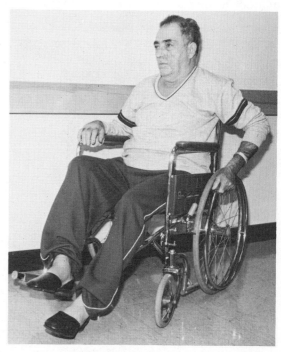

**Figure 1–45.** One-handed wheelchair mobility using sound hand and foot to propel wheelchair.

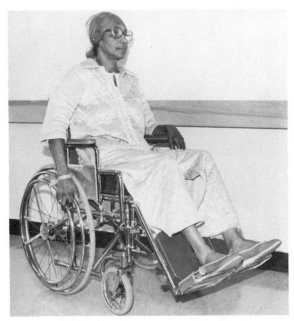

**Figure 1–46.** Patient using one-arm drive with sound upper extremity.

kitchen is the ideal; however, not every hospital provides this and the therapist may have to use ingenuity to perform an evaluation. Asking the patient to attempt a simple task such as preparing a cup of tea can provide valuable information. Through close observation, the therapist can evaluate the patient's judgment, motivation, endurance, problem-solving ability, and, in general, functional ability to perform homemaking tasks. The safety of the patient is a crucial factor.

The evaluation will determine whether the patient, with training, has the potential to perform independently or with supervision or with assistance by a family member. The occupational therapist may determine that all but the most simple tasks should be performed by someone else. If the hemiplegic patient is returning home alone or to an elderly spouse, hiring someone to help in the house may be recommended.

Once it is determined that the hemiplegic patient has the potential to perform homemaking in a safe fashion, training in a kitchen setting begins with the emphasis on work simplification and energy conservation. Family members should be included in training sessions so that they are aware of the patient's abilities as well as limitations.

Important questions to be answered in connection with training are: What were the homemaking responsibilities prior to the stroke? Who is available to provide assistance and to what extent? Is the patient totally wheelchair bound or can he or she stand briefly at the wheelchair to reach an object or perform an activity? What is the vertical reach in sitting and standing? How is the dynamic

balance in sitting and standing? For example, can she manage to open the refrigerator without losing her balance? Does she ambulate with an assistive device? If so, can she let go of the device long enough to perform an action safely? Can she manage if she stabilizes her body against a counter while working? For those who are not wheelchair bound, it is usually advisable to keep a chair in the working area. Sitting while working conserves energy and frequent rest stops are also recommended.

A home visit is recommended to see the layout of the kitchen and other work areas and the type of equipment the patient will be using. If this is not possible, the therapist may obtain a description of the home setting from the patient or family members. A diagram of the interior provided by the family can be used to aid the therapist in structuring training sessions to duplicate the home setting as much as possible.

The therapist should be prepared for frustration on the part of the patient during training and realize that much practice is necessary for competence, especially for the one-handed homemaker.

There are many commercially available adaptive devices, some of which can be constructed at home, which can bring optimal independence to the disabled homemaker. Many of these devices, along with work simplification and energy conservation hints, are discussed in the following paragraphs.

Kitchen storage should be organized so that everything is easily reached. Lazy susans are helpful. Vertically divided sections separating each pot and pan make it easier to reach these with one hand. Utensils can be hung on a pegboard within easy reach.

A 31-inch-high countertop is recommended as a comfortable working surface for a wheelchair patient. The counter should allow the knees to fit under the work area requiring, on the average, a 24-inch-high open space. If this is not possible through architectural adaptations, a modified work area can be set up on a table with an electrical outlet nearby. Portable kitchen equipment such as an electrical skillet, hot plate, and toaster oven can be used to prepare simple meals.

To conserve energy, it is usually advisable for the patient to sit while working at the kitchen sink. A higher than standard chair will provide a comfortable working distance to the sink. If the patient is wheelchair bound, the cabinet doors under the sink may be removed to allow the homemaker to sit at the sink. A shallow sink is easier to reach into if the patient is seated in a wheelchair or standard-height chair. A deep sink can be adapted by the addition of a rack onto which a dish pan can be placed. The hot water pipes should be insulated.

A rubber mat can be placed into the sink to prevent glasses from breaking. A bottle brush or small

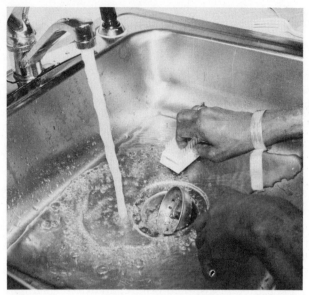

**Figure 1–47.** Nail brush with suction cups for one-handed washing.

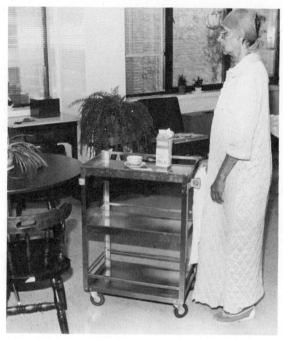

**Figure 1–48.** Cart with wheels for transporting items from one area to another.

nail brush with suction cups or both can be used for washing one-handed. Sponges can be squeezed with one hand to eliminate wringing washcloths, or a washcloth, if preferred, can be wrapped around the faucet to wring it out.

Reachers are useful for retrieving objects that fall unexpectedly on the floor or for reaching objects outside of arm's reach in cabinets or on counters. Pots and pans should be slid along countertops instead of being lifted. Light-weight stainless steel pots and pans with one handle are recommended.

A cart with wheels can be used to gather items and to transport them from one area to another if counterspace is not available to slide them along. It is also helpful to transport a finished meal to the eating area. A lapboard placed on a wheelchair can be used for this purpose as well. An apron with pockets can be used to carry small items. Velcro closures can be used for the apron to aid the one-handed homemaker.

Equipment can be stabilized by using a Dycem mat or sponge cloth or octopus suction cups. Jars, bowls, or packages can be wedged into a partially opened drawer for opening or for stirring one-handed.

Electric can openers that can be held with one hand; portable electric hand mixers are helpful. A Zim jar opener that attaches to the wall surface is recommended.

A cutting board with two stainless steel nails 1 inch apart can act as an extra hand to stabilize foods (fruit, meat, or vegetables) while slicing or chopping is done. Rubber suction cups underneath keep it from sliding. A Dycem mat or spongecloth could also be used. A right-angled attachment can be used at one corner to allow for stabilizing bread

while a spread is applied. If left open at the edge, the knife can go through to cut the bread.

Rocker knives as well as pizza wheel cutters are handy for one-handed cutting. A one-handed chopper with plunger action can be used to chop vegetables.

A peeler with a large looped handle is easier to hold than the standard one. Generally, larger handles are easier to hold; therefore, it may help to build up the handle of utensils such as a wire whisk or mixing spoon.

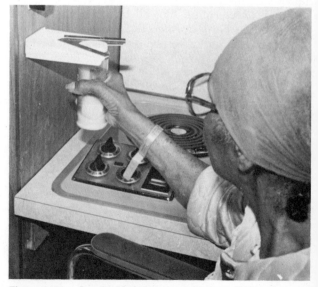

**Figure 1–49.** One-handed Zim jar opener.

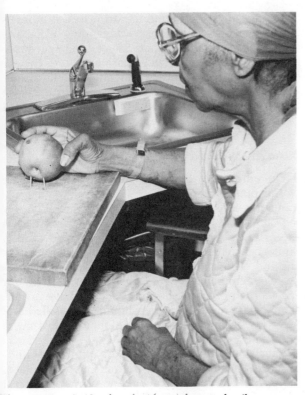

**Figure 1–50.** Cutting board with stainless steel nails.

Steps can be saved by using "mixed in one bowl" foods plus convenience foods where possible. Oven-to-table cooking dishes eliminate some extra work.

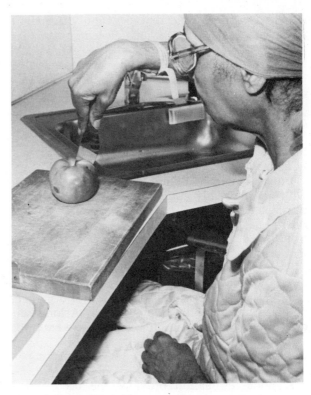

**Figure 1–52.** Rocker knife.

A pot handle can be stabilized in a device commercially available in chrome-plated steel with suction cups; this is an aid while stirring is done on the stove. It can also be constructed at home in

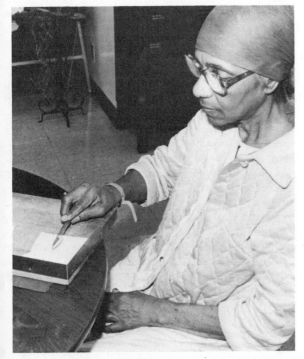

**Figure 1–51.** Right angle attachment on cutting board to stabilize bread while applying a spread.

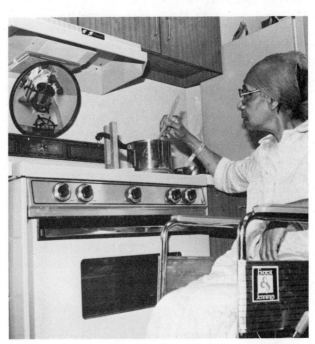

**Figure 1–53.** Pot stabilizer and mirror placed on slant over stove.

wood. A pot with a lid that locks into place eliminates the need for two hands when draining liquids.

A mirror placed on a slant over the stove will allow for a wheelchair bound person to check on the contents of pots on the burner.

Eggs can be broken one-handed using the "short-order cook" method.

A front-loading washer and dryer as opposed to top-loading is recommended for a wheelchair-bound homemaker.

Ironing should be done from a sitting position, with an adjustable ironing board used to obtain a comfortable working height. A portable ironing board used on top of a table is another idea. A travel iron may be easier to use because it is lightweight.

Soak dishes to avoid the need to scrub and let dishes air-dry instead of drying by hand. A self-cleaning oven, frost-free refrigerator, and garbage disposal make cleaning much easier. A long-handled sponge can be used for cleaning the bathtub.

### Home Evaluation

A home evaluation provides the occupational therapist with valuable information to use in structuring activities of daily living and homemaking training sessions in the hospital before discharge as well as allowing for effective discharge planning.

Two important considerations when performing a home evaluation are (1) the financial ability to make adaptations in the home (including resources such as insurance coverage) and (2) the psychological willingness to make changes on the part of either the patient or family members. Very often, denial of the disability exists; making changes in the home requires acceptance of the disability and the realization of its permanence. The therapist can only make recommendations and provide all the necessary information, such as the cost of equipment and sources for obtaining it.

Usually a home evaluation is necessary for a wheelchair patient returning home, but it is also helpful for a patient ambulating with equipment such as a walker or quad cane. A wheelchair, however, presents more of a problem in terms of accessibility. Ideally, the evaluation of the home and the evaluation for the wheelchair should be done at the same time, as one affects the other. If the patient already has a wheelchair, it is important to know the measurements before the home evaluation is performed.

### Wheelchair Facts

A wheelchair-bound person requires a minimum of 5 by 5 feet of clear floor space for mobility and transfer activities. The standard width of a wheelchair measured from one handrim to the other is 26 inches. The width varies depending upon the type of armrest and seat width. A chair with one-arm drive and a motorized chair are wider. The average overall length including footrests is 42 inches. The removal of footrests or legrests can decrease the length by 11 to 14 inches. Average seat height from the floor is 20 inches (see Chapter 25).

### Basic Areas for Concern

**The entrance.** How many steps to the entrance of the building and how high is each? What entrance is the most convenient? Is there a railing for the steps and if there is, is it on the right or left side? If the patient is wheelchair bound, can a ramp be installed? To negotiate a ramp safely and independently, a wheelchair-bound person requires a gradient of 12 inches of ramp length for each 1 inch of rise. The ramp should have a non-skid surface and hand rails should be installed at a height of 32 inches. The ramp should be a minimum of 36 inches in width.*

**The Type of Building.** Is it an apartment building with elevator, a walk-up apartment building, or a single-family home on one floor or several floors? Stair lifts are available to enable a wheelchair-bound patient to negotiate a flight of steps in the home; however, they are expensive to purchase and install. It is possible to rent them. The patient may consider the alternative of living on the main floor of the home. A dining room or part of the living room may be converted by the addition of bedroom furnishings. If a bathroom is not available on the main floor, the patient can use a bedside commode and can sponge-bathe in bed or by the kitchen sink.

If the wheelchair-bound patient needs to negotiate a flight of stairs to reach his apartment, he may have to accept the unfortunate reality that he will seldom be able to leave the apartment without the assistance of one to two people capable of carrying him up and down.

**Doorways.** Measure the width of all door entrances. The recommended door width for the wheelchair bound is 32 inches, though few homes provide this. If the patient's chair is just a few inches too wide, it may be possible to use a narrowmatic device on the wheelchair to allow for accessibility through the doorway. It may also help to remove the door from the hinges and replace it with a curtain to provide more room. The door sills should be noted and height measured. Ideally, they should be removed.

**Hallways and Floors.** Note the width of the

---

*Building Design Requirements For The Physically Handicapped. Eastern Paralyzed Veterans Association, Inc., 432 Park Avenue South, New York, NY 10016.

hallways. For easy turning into rooms, a wheel-chair-bound person needs a width of 48 inches. Floors should be level and in good condition. Scatter or throw rugs should be removed; thick or shag carpeting is not recommended for wheelchairs as it is very difficult and tiring to push over this type of surface.

**Location and Type of Furniture.** Five by five feet of clear floor space is required to turn a wheelchair 180 or 360 degrees. It may be recommended that items of furniture be rearranged or perhaps removed in order to allow wheelchair access to the bed, dining room table, desk, and so forth. The height of the bed should be equal to the seat height of the wheelchair to facilitate transfers. A firm mattress makes bed mobility and transfers easier. Generally, working surfaces (desks, tables, counters) should be about 29 to 31 inches high to be comfortable for the wheelchair-bound person; however, each person has to be considered individually. Wheelchairs with standard armrests require more clearance under the table than do those with deskarm style.

**Accessibility of the Bathroom.** Ideally, the bathroom door should open out to allow for more open space once the wheelchair is inside. The patient may consider replacing the door with a curtain, which is easier to handle and takes up less space. If the bathroom door is not accessible to a wheelchair even with the use of a narrowmatic device, the patient may have to use a bedside commode and sponge-bathe in bed or by the kitchen sink. Some hemiplegic patients may be able to leave the wheelchair outside the bathroom door and ambulate a few steps inside with the aid of an assistive device or with a family member's assistance. Once inside, the patient can transfer to a sturdy straight chair.

The bathroom sink should allow for a minimum of 27 inches clearance in height from the floor for the wheelchair-bound. The wall-hung type is better than the pedestal style. A sink with a vanity cabinet underneath will not enable the wheelchair-bound person to get close enough to use it.

Toilet transfers are easiest if the toilet seat height is similar to the wheelchair seat height. A remova-ble raised toilet seat is commercially available. Is there a wall adjacent that can support a grab bar? Certain bedside commodes, 20 to 22 inches wide, can be used over the toilet to provide bilateral grab bars. Safety frames that attach to the toilet are also available. They measure from 17 to 20 inches between armrests (adjustable in width). Towel racks should never be used as grab bars.

A shower stall is easier and usually safer for a wheelchair patient than a bathtub, which requires getting over the rim. Several different styles of bath benches and tub seats are available to eliminate the need to stand in the shower or get down into the bathtub. Consider where grab bars could be placed. Vertical, horizontal, and L-shaped bars are available. A soap dish should never be used as a substitute for a grab bar. Note where the faucets are in the bathtub. This will determine the direction the patient should transfer so that he is seated in front of the water controls.

In general, evaluate the amount of floor space available to maneuver the wheelchair and to perform transfers to the toilet, tub, or shower stall. If the ambulatory status permits, it may be preferable to leave the wheelchair outside the bathroom door and to assist the patient inside the door to a sturdy straight chair.

**Miscellaneous.** Where is the telephone(s) located? A phone next to the bed is recommended, especially for someone living alone. Can wall sockets and light switches be reached? It is advisable to lower the rod in closets so that the clothes are accessible for the wheelchair patient.

## SUGGESTED SOURCES

Marshall, E. (ed.): Occupational Therapy—Management of Physical Dysfunction. Syllabus materials compiled from data collected from occupational therapists and occupational therapy departments. Loma Linda University School of Allied Health Professions.

Trombly, C. A. and Scott, A. D.: Occupational Therapy for Physical Dysfunction. Baltimore, Williams & Wilkins, 1977. Chapter on arthritis.

Mealtime Manual for the Aged and Handicapped. Compiled by the Institute of Rehabilitation Medicine, New York University Medical Center. Foreword by Howard A. Rusk.

# Speech and Language Problems Associated With Cerebrovascular Accidents

*by Karen Joelson, M.A., C.C.C.*

Frequently, the most striking symptoms signaling the onset of a stroke are slurring of words, inability to speak, and difficulty in understanding. There may be physical distortions such as weakness or drooping on one side of the face. These may be transitory problems but, unfortunately, for many people some degree of speech or language deficit will remain. The speech pathologist is the professional on the rehabilitation team who is qualified to diagnose and treat these individuals.

In forming a diagnosis, the task of the speech pathologist is to determine the type and severity of the communication impairment. Some of the specific conditions related to patients who have suffered strokes are aphasia, dysarthria, apraxia, and agnosia. To ensure clarity throughout this discussion, each of these diagnostic categories is described briefly.

*Aphasia* is a disturbance in language functioning due to cerebral damage. Generally, lesions would be found in the left hemisphere, thus the association between aphasia and right hemiplegia or paresis. The possibility of aphasia following a right cerebrovascular accident (CVA) should not be excluded or overlooked, since this occurs in a minority of individuals. Expressive aphasia is a condition whereby the individual is unable to or has difficulty in using words to name objects, formulate sentences, and generate ideas verbally or by writing. Receptive aphasia is an impairment in the ability to recognize spoken or written words, to follow commands, to understand questions, and to interpret connected speech. These symptoms are not found in isolation; generally, patients will suffer some degree of both the receptive and expressive aspects. Arithmetic processes would also be impaired.

The speech-articulation problem found in stroke patients is called *dysarthria*. It is important to distinguish between the language and the speech problems because the needs of the patient and the treatment approach for each diagnosis are different. Language is a well-ordered system of rules by which thought, feelings, and ideas can be communicated. Speech is the medium or vehicle by which the speaker's language is passed from him to others. Most commonly, speech takes the form of sequences of vocal sounds known, of course, as words. Since a stroke can result in weakness in facial, oral, and laryngeal musculature, a person with dysarthria will have difficulty manipulating the tongue, lips, soft palate, jaws, and vocal cords. Articulated speech may sound slurred, labored, sluggish, weak and hypernasal. Neuromuscular control is impaired and, as a result, vegetative functions in chewing and swallowing may also be involved. Drooling is frequently associated with dysarthria.

*Apraxia* is the difficulty or inability voluntarily to use the organs of articulation to initiate sounds and place them in sequence to form words. In apraxia there is no muscular weakness or paralysis present to account for this. Characteristically, the person is able to perform an oral movement in a nonlinguistic situation but has great difficulty imitating or initiating similar movements in attempts to talk. For example, a woman may be able to blot her lipstick but be quite unable to produce the "m" sound on command or through imitation. What we have in this case is an individual whose language functioning may be more intact than would be suggested by her misguided fumbling and struggling attempt at speech.

Last, *agnosia* is an impairment in the patient's ability to recognize. It can exist in any of the sensory modalities but for communication, auditory and visual agnosias are most relevant. Although the patient may be able to hear, perhaps the sound of a dog barking would have no meaning or the patient might not recognize his own name. This is truly a profound perceptual disturbance.

## COGNITIVE AND BEHAVIORAL CHANGES OBSERVED IN APHASIC ADULTS

The person who has suffered a stroke has been traumatized in many ways. The reduction in the level of language usage available for communicating with others affects the facility with which the aphasic can communicate within himself. This implies a diminished awareness of self and of others. Patients are frequently poorly oriented to times, places, or persons and may have memory problems that impede carryover from day to day. Such an individual may have difficulty monitoring or controling his behavior and tolerating frustration. It may be observed that judgment is poor in various situations and that there may be a reduction in alertness and responsiveness to the environment. The patient may be confused.

Aphasic people, as well as others with brain damage, may appear interested in the present and in concrete, observable events only. Such patients may not be able to plan or concern themselves with a future occurrence and may even appear oblivious to all but their own immediate needs. There may be difficulty carrying out an intended activity or in attending to a task for a prolonged period of time. The individual who is aware that he has suffered damage may experience feelings of loss, mourning, and depression. He will have problems effectively adapting to the surroundings and the demands of a constantly changing environment.

## FAMILY INVOLVEMENT

The patient's family and close friends serve a vital and indispensable function. The familiarity, support, and comfort his own home provides contribute to the aphasic's personal resources, sense of self, and motivation. Family members face various problems also, such as feelings of deep concern, anxiety, confusion, and even anger at the situation they suddenly find themselves in. Uncertainty and fear about how to help that family member will undoubtedly arise. The following may be of assistance when communicating with an aphasic adult.

## APPROACHES TO COMMUNICATION

1. Encourage but accept any level of communication available to the patient.
2. Never isolate the patient except for rest and sleep. Maintain a sociable, stimulating, and verbal environment.
3. Maximize use of the patient's "good" periods, when he is most alert, rested, and comfortable, for therapy. The patient may be more responsive to particular friends or family members.
4. Learn to recognize stressful and frustrating situations by observing if he appears fatigued, anxious, or confused, and avoid these.
5. Speak in natural but clear and simple sentences.
6. Supplement your speech with gestures and demonstrations if necessary and encourage the same from the patient.
7. Ask questions that can be answered using "yes" or "no" or nods of the head.
8. Encourage and praise the patient in an adult and realistic manner.

9. Set goals for improvement with extreme patience.
10. Help ease stress on the patient by verbalizing what he may be feeling at a particular moment, but do not stifle his attempts to talk.
11. Treat the patient as the respected adult he is and avoid an oversolicitous approach. Involve him in as many daily decisions and events as is appropriate or possible.

### ACTIVITIES TO STIMULATE LANGUAGE COMPREHENSION AND EXPRESSION

**Verbal Comprehension.** Verbal comprehension refers to how well the aphasic individual understands what is said to or asked of him. This language skill depends upon the integrity of those centers of the brain developed to receive, interpret, and associate messages delivered through the ear. It is important first to assess how severe the involvement is by noting how well the patient can follow commands, understand questions, follow conversation, and so on. Generally, the speech pathologist is best able to form such a diagnosis; however, if none is available, the physician or family must make some judgment so that the treatment that follows is appropriate.

1. Place three or four common objects on a table and ask the patient to point to each after it has been named and its function described.
2. Ask the patient to show you a series of two or three items that are named in succession.
3. Ask him to point to the various parts of the body or to follow commands involving body movements. ("Close your eyes.")
4. Ask him to follow commands that require simple actions and manipulation of objects such as to put a spoon in a cup. Directions can be made more complex by lengthening the command or adding another object.
5. Read a simple paragraph and ask questions based on content. The same can be done using other media such as radio and television.
6. Make use of many daily situations to stimulate language and allow the patient to hear oral language. Involve him by posing questions and directions but also by commenting on his actions and your own as they occur. In this way, a steady flow of meaningful verbal stimulation is provided.

**Verbal Expression.** Attempting speech can be a laborious and frustrating experience for the stroke patient. A patient may have difficulty initiating speech, recalling what an object is called, and composing thoughts into sentences. Often a word associated with the one he is trying to say will be produced in its place. On the other hand, he may be able to utter only a seemingly irrelevant or repetitious word or phrase. At first, improved nonverbal communication, social appropriateness, alertness, and personal awareness may be the devices the patient uses to communicate his progress. These strides should be looked for and encouraged from the start.

1. Using familiar and meaningful objects or pictures, involve the patient in trying to name, repeat, or say the name in unison with you.

2. Pronounce the initial sound of a word to help the patient complete it ("Sss" _ _ _ _ [soap] ).

3. Use associations or common phrases to help trigger memory traces such as Bread and _____ . . . How are _____ ?

4. Make certain the patient can see your face and lips because these visual cues may aid him to form words himself.

5. Use visual and tactile stimulation to encourage the patient to generate words to describe the sensations he experiences.

6. At times aphasics have extreme difficulty forming verbal responses but may be able to point to printed words or pictures on a communication board (see p. 20) as a viable means of expression. Boards can be made to suit individual needs.

7. Sign language or a more informal system of gestures often can be devised and taught if the patient does not use meaningful hand signals spontaneously.

**Retraining Reading and Writing Skills.** Generally, language impairments affect all modalities so that reading and writing are disturbed to varying degrees. Complicating the problem may be paralysis of the dominant hand formerly used to write with, as well as apraxias, which hinder the use of writing tools. However, underlying the aphasic condition itself is a fundamental loss of spelling ability and difficulty generating words and ideas in writing. Reading disturbances may also be a function of various factors such as visual perceptual problems, agnosias, and the linguistic disturbance associating visual symbols with their conventional meanings.

1. Use activities involving matching identical printed words to each other, pointing to a printed word as it is named aloud, and pairing written words to a corresponding picture or object.

2. Tracing words, copying from a printed sample, and eventually writing them spontaneously to dictation should be encouraged. The patient may be forced to use his nondominant hand because of hemiplegia.

3. Always work toward a multimodality approach so that the aphasic patient has experience reading for comprehension and meaning. Frequently use of written material assists the patient in verbal expression.

4. The patient may be able to fill in completions to written phrases or select an appropriate word from a set of choices:

Grass is _____ heavy
green
book

5. More advanced activities may include writing sentences to describe something observable, writing a brief letter, and so on.

## REFERRAL SOURCES AND PERTINENT LITERATURE

There are many approaches available to vary, simplify, and individualize home therapy programs. With practice and some experimentation, family members will be able to manipulate activities to suit the patient's ability and frustration tolerance. Time for both the patient and family to adjust to their trauma is one of the most important considerations. Assistance from the physician, a psychologist, and a speech pathologist should be sought. The American Speech-Language-Hearing Association* can help locate licensed speech pathologists in any locality.

For families who have the major responsibility for language retraining, the following materials may also be quite helpful.

(1) *Adult Aphasia Program* by Kathleen Bullock and Judy McLoughlin.† This volume covers 14 language-deficiency areas with a short chapter followed by activity sheets for each area. There are also 117 program sheets with step-by-step lessons in each of the 14 areas such as auditory recognition, comprehension, naming, functional writing. It costs $13 plus $1.50 handling.

(2) *Workbook for Aphasia* costs $9.95 plus $1.00 handling.‡ This book contains exercises for the redevelopment of higher-level language functioning with areas in word usage, development of syntax, concrete and abstract reasoning, use of factual information, and so forth.

3. *Speech and Language Rehabilitation—Workbook for the Neurologically Impaired* by Robert Keith is available in two volumes at $5.95 each.§ These volumes are designed for the patient who is not able to receive continuous therapy by a speech pathologist and is meant to improve family and patient involvement.

4. *An Adult Has Aphasia,* also published by the Interstate Printers and Publishers Inc., 80¢ a copy. This booklet was written to help families better understand the nature of the aphasic's problems and make suggestions for assisting in his progress.

---

*10801 Rockville Pike, Rockville, Maryland 20852.

†Word Making Productions, 70 West Louise Ave., Salt Lake City, Utah 84115.

‡Wayne State University Press, 5959 Woodword Ave., Detroit, Michigan 48202.

§The Interstate Printers and Publishers Inc., Danville, Illinois 61832.

# Recreation Therapy

by Michael Chaiken, M.S., Roger Davis, B.S.,
Barbara Eisner, M.P.S., and Michael Levine, M.S.

When an individual suffers some form of incapacitation, his leisure time grows in scope, meaning, and importance to personal identity. With this understanding, the recreational therapist directs and emphasizes a positive attitude toward a most meaningful aspect of rehabilitation. Life becomes the focus of continued purpose and self-growth after a stroke. In this area, recreational therapy is the prime resource.

Within the recreational therapy field have been developed types of activities that can be classified as diversional, self-expression, creativity, educational, cultural, and spiritual. These activities will be discussed in more detail as to function. Each of these may or may not be utilized in the treatment of individuals, depending on the therapist's orientation and skills and the needs of the patient.

Most patients, and stroke victims in particular, who have been admitted to our rehabilitation institute, seem to share serious misgivings about the true value of therapeutic recreation. This prevalent attitude is highly regrettable, yet in a sense understandable, since the idea of "fun and games" may sometimes appear to be directly at odds with and in violation of our work ethic. It is not unusual to hear a patient say, "I came here to get better through therapy. I didn't come here for recreation!" In succeeding paragraphs are described some of the activities offered at our institute.

Scholars disagree on a singular descriptive term for recreation. For practical purposes, however, let us think in terms of recreation as both a process and a service offered, by which therapists attempt to help patients use their leisure time in a constructive manner, thus resulting in resocialization and a renewed self-image.

In focusing on recreation for the stroke victim, we must always bear in mind that it is not a prescribed therapy. Whereas some of our tools are interchangeable with occupational therapy or physical therapy, our goals and methods of utilizing them are influenced by our different backgrounds, philosophies, and professional training. Objectives of recreational therapists are many and varied, but basically they are reflected in short-term and long-term goals. An attempt is made in this section to put these in their proper perspective as some of the activities offered are discussed.

The typical stroke patient who requires hospitalization has a host of adjustments to make, the most obvious of which are physical. The exercise program offered at our facility is geared to minimize limitations and to maximize capabilities in a manner that is entertaining. We use simple exercises done to music. This not only promotes a positive, relaxing atmosphere but also enhances socialization and heightens the pleasure of the activity itself. Music is a universal language to which all can respond, and it is rewarding to observe how much fun the patients derive from exercising their upper and lower extremities to the accompaniment of popular tunes.

Stroke victims who have limited use of their upper extremities derive encouragement from seeing others with similar conditions who are involved in art therapy. This mode of treatment lends itself to free expression and originality, and there is also immense satisfaction to be obtained by the patient from something he has produced.

Two activities that require some degree of manual dexterity are ceramics and arts and crafts. Patients with varying levels of sophistication enjoy participating in these programs, which lend themselves to creativity and self-expression.

## THERAPEUTIC RECREATIONAL ACTIVITIES

One obstacle that faces the newly admitted stroke victim is a feeling of anonymity. It is difficult for him not to feel that he has become a cipher or "the patient in room 407B." One way of combatting this is through discussion groups, which furnish a learning experience, and the ideal forum for patients to air their social and political views. Ample opportunity is provided for personal expression, and, at the same time, sensitivity and a healthy respect for peer's opinions are encouraged.

The patient's newspaper at our institute also serves as a valuable outlet for self-expression and creativity. Because of physical limitations, the patient may be restricted in actually writing an article; this provides an opportunity for staff people or other patients to spend some time interviewing that individual and recording his thoughts for publication.

Religious and cultural activities are held in our institute under the auspices of the recreation division. We encourage patients to exercise their freedom of choice in following these pursuits.

Bedside therapy is a vital part of recreation.

Through this medium, we reach out to those patients whose conditions preclude their active participation in group programs. Some patients are so overwhelmed by their disability that they experience depression and self-pity and subsequently withdraw from others. The scope of bedside therapy may range from supportive counseling to providing the opportunity for the patient to engage in sensory stimulation. It may also encompass treatment to increase or stimulate cognitive functioning.

Although painting, ceramics, and music promote enrichment of living, recreational therapy utilizes all activities to enhance self-image and competency. For some stroke victims the investment in a leisure life style brings meaning and a purpose for their rehabilitation.

There are two organizations that represent the field of therapeutic recreation. The first, The National Therapeutic Recreation Society,* represents broad professional concerns and provides information. The American Association for Leisure and Recreation (AALR)† focuses primarily on sports and athletics.

## MUSIC THERAPY FOR THE STROKE PATIENT

Music therapy is usually a subdivision of creative arts therapy or recreation therapy. Its general goals, like those of recreation therapy, are to provide satisfying and enjoyable new leisure opportunities for the stroke patient. It offers to teach new tools for self-expression and socialization through music study, performance, and attendance at concerts. Music therapy for stroke patients provides stimulating physical and language development through the processes of learning to play an instrument or singing. The immense satisfaction and pleasure derived from music activities serve as sources of motivation and encouragement for the patient to continue efforts to improve his level of functioning and renew feelings of vitality and enjoyment of life. One of the major rewards of music therapy is that the patient can actually hear his strengths and skills increasing in the music he is able to master.

There are any number of instruments that are suitable for playing by the stroke patient, or can be adapted. The autoharp, for example, requires minimal use of the impaired hand to achieve adequate playing skills. The instrument can be used to accompany solo or group singing. With increased finger dexterity, the intricate and expressive qualities of the instrument may be enjoyed. The piano provides a wide range of opportunities for physical

growth, emotional satisfaction, and new social activities. A considerable repertoire of piano music for one hand presently exists. Additionally, many compositions are suitable for transcription to one hand, thereby allowing the hemiplegic to enjoy retained body functioning. The process of playing the piano helps the patient develop sitting balance, control of arm movement, and fine finger coordination. For patients having use of one hand only, a tape recorder can be used to record one hand's part of a composition. This can then be replayed while the patient plays the other hand's part "live," accompanied by the tape in the "music-minus-one" fashion. Family and friends may also join in the music making by playing the "other hand's" part, or with duets for four hands, when a patient has use of both hands.

For patients with minimal use of a hand, there are various small hand instruments that can be used to stimulate arm and hand motion and to provide meaningful music opportunities. There is a considerable amount of published music, arranged and/or written by music therapists, that utilizes tambourines, maracas, small hand drums, horns, and whistles. Many of the arrangements are of familiar ballads, folk songs, and spirituals. With instruments of this sort, it is important to stress that they should be of high quality so that they will have pleasing sounds and will not appear shoddy or infantilizing to the stroke patient. The patient whose physical control and concentration span are so limited is easily discouraged and insulted when asked to play instruments that are of poor quality or that look like children's toys. It would be a disservice and an insult to overlook the mental sophistication of patients and ask them to work with equipment that is childish and unpleasant-sounding.

Various wind instruments are suitable for the patient's leisure enjoyment and physical development. In most cases, for these instruments, however, it is necessary to have the use of both hands. Playing wind instruments causes strengthening of facial and tongue muscle control and helps the patient develop fine finger coordination. With some proficiency it is possible to join any number of amateur orchestras and chamber ensembles that are sponsored by music schools and community recreation organizations.

The therapeutic values of singing and voice training have been recognized for some time by speech therapists and otolaryngologists. Various techniques such as melodic intonation have been developed to stimulate language development in aphasics. Community recreational opportunities for amateur singers are plentiful, including local church choirs and choruses sponsored by recreation centers.

Musical study can be supplemented with attendance at concerts. For the person who is more of a

---

*1601 North Kent St., Arlington, Virginia 22209.
†1900 Association Dr., Reston, Virginia 22091.

listener, attending concerts can be a satisfying means of joining family and friends in social activities.

Music therapists who work with handicapped patients may be referred through music therapy associations and many colleges and universities. Further information about music therapy may also be obtained from these sources as well as from music therapy journals. Music therapy associations and university programs exist in several European countries as well as in North and South America. In the United States one may contact: (1) American Association for Music Therapy (AAMT), Education Building, New York University, New York City, N. Y. 10003; (2) National Association for Music Therapy (NAMT), University of Kansas, Lawrence, Kansas 66044; (3) *Journal of Music Therapy*, same address as NAMT.

## ROLE OF ART

Life for the stroke patient can be very frustrating. Art can relieve some of this frustration while providing much pleasure and satisfaction. The use of art as therapy for the stroke patient has many benefits, both physical and emotional. Through the manipulation of various tools such as brushes, pencils, pastels, and charcoal, the patient exercises his fine motor coordination. Activities such as drawing or painting can make exercise fun. Drawing or painting with acrylics or watercolors helps the patient develop the ability to grasp and control. Watercolor is a medium that demands patience and control. Typically, we see a patient with the use of only one hand who is frustrated by the lack of control of his other hand. This person learns that the hand he thought quite useless can be used most constructively. He can hold the paper down with this hand as he draws or paints with the other. The very basic techniques of drawing and painting provide exercise in fine motor coordination.

Art is a viable means of expression: it can deal with another aspect of a stroke, impairment in or loss of speech. For the person having difficulty with verbal communication, art provides an alternative—a nonverbal means of communication. Art provides an emotional outlet when words are unable to do this.

Participation in art therapy also encourages skill development. Finding new interests and learning new skills is extremely important to someone who has lost skills and as a result has lost interest in life. Art is an extremely broad subject, with many options open for someone who is reluctant to try something new. There is much satisfaction associated with learning how to draw, how to work with acrylics, how to control watercolors, or how the painting process works. In learning a new skill, one usually forgets other problems while concentrating on art form.

Art can provide the patient with a leisure activity. Art can be most relaxing, and for an hour or so a day can take the person away from his problems. Art can be play, breaking up the monotony of the day and providing the patient with sheer enjoyment.

Some people, no matter how much they try, cannot master the basic techniques of, for example, the use of brushes or the blending of colors. This can become just as frustrating as their physical disability, thus defeating the whole purpose of art therapy. For these people, there are art activities with built-in success. Some examples of these guaranteed success activities are blot painting, string painting, and sponge painting. Blot painting entails putting dots of paint or ink on a piece of paper, folding the paper in half, pressing down on the paper to spread the ink, and opening the paper to see a surprise design. String painting uses this same principle, but utilizes a string dipped in paint that is placed in between a folded piece of paper, then pulled out. In sponge painting small sponges are dipped in paint as opposed to brushes to produce designs in various colors. These are just a few examples of the use of art in building the patient's self-confidence.

Art activities can be used by stroke patients with all types of disability, from mild to severe. For those people with severe disabilities as a result of stroke, modifications can be made with the use of various adaptive devices. For example, a mouthpiece or a headpiece to which a pencil or a brush can be attached can be fitted to the individual.

Art is a perfect medium for instilling pleasure and a sense of pride, for there is no right or wrong in art—thus the options are limitless. Displaying a patient's work in some sort of exhibit is even further reinforcement of accomplishment. Family and friends can share in the art process by helping in the setting up and the cleaning up. Also, museum trips or visits to galleries helps to make art a shared experience. Family members taking an active interest in the patient's art efforts can give him the confidence and perseverance to continue.

For more information concerning art therapy and its applications the organization to contact is the American Art Therapy Association, Inc., 428 East Preston Street, Baltimore, Maryland 21202.

There is also a quarterly journal of articles, case studies, job and education information, and reviews of recent literature. The address is *American Journal of Art Therapy*, 6010 Broad Branch Road, N.W., Washington, D.C. 20015.

### CERAMICS

Ceramics can provide much satisfaction for the stroke patient. It is an enjoyable leisure activity that enables the patient to create something he can be proud of.

The first step in creating a ceramics piece is to pour the slip (liquid clay) into a mold. For the patient lacking strength, the slip can be poured a few ounces at a time, while a stronger patient may pour a few pounds at a time. After the slip sets for a while, the mold is emptied. The excess slip will pour out, while the slip that has hardened is left coating the inside of the mold. The mold is then opened, and the figure inside formed from the set clay is removed. This piece is called greenware. The greenware must then be cleaned. This process involves removing all of the seam lines and imperfections. The patient uses a variety of tools to do this, including a clean-up tool, a grit cloth, and a sponge. The piece can be placed on a foam rubber cushion to hold it steady or taped down to the table or to a paper plate. Cleaning the greenware helps the patient to develop fine motor control and concentration.

At this point, the project can be continued in one of two methods. In the first procedure, the patient can paint the finished piece a solid color. This is done with paint called glaze, a special substance that when fired in a kiln (baked in a special high-temperature oven) becomes glossy and hard. A brush is usually used to apply the glaze. Holding the brush and applying the glaze help to develop manual dexterity, eye-hand coordination, and concentration. After the piece has been finished and fired, it usually looks as good as or better than a ceramics piece bought in a store. The patient experiences considerable satisfaction upon seeing his completed piece.

The other way in which a piece can be finished is by using the greenware as a canvas on which the patient paints a picture. The glazes used for this method are different from those used in the first method. These glazes are used in a manner similar to water colors or acrylics rather than for solid color coverage. This technique requires a much greater degree of motor control than the first method. The patient can create an original picture or he can trace a design. As an alternative to using a brush, the glaze can be applied by dabbing with a sponge, spattering with a toothbrush, or rubbing on with a rag. The possibilities for other variations are many and depend upon the availability of materials and the imagination of the patient.

A small kiln can be bought for use in the home. However, if a patient does not wish to purchase a kiln, a neighborhood ceramics studio will usually fire pieces for about 4 or 5 cents per cubic inch. Similarly, if the patient does not wish to purchase molds, he can buy prepoured greenware from a ceramics studio. The patient can then do the cleaning and glazing and return the piece to the studio for firing.

An individual who wants to work at home without needing to fire his pieces can use air-hardening clay. This is available at most hobby stores. This clay can be formed through coiling, slab building, or sculpting. When the pieces are finished, they will harden when left exposed to the air for a few hours. They can then be painted with regular paints (not glazes). The finished pieces, however, are purely decorative and not for utilitarian purposes.

Organizations for stroke victims provide a valuable opportunity to develop positive feelings in an environment of peers. Many settlement houses or community centers offer therapeutic recreation programs that can provide meaningful activities for special populations. A final resource is the local parks and recreation department of municipalities. Since legislation has been passed regarding accessibility, many government recreation agencies provide opportunities for the disabled and often these programs are geared to stroke victims. Other resources for advice are local recreation professional societies and universities offering a recreation or adapted physical education curriculum.

# 2

# Upper Extremity in Hemiplegia

*by Rene Cailliet, M.D.*

The upper extremity, because of its intricacies and because distal dexterity must be restored in order for meaningful function to be regained, recovers poorly after a stroke. Ambulation in the lower extremity can be achieved with minimal hip extension with essentially simple forms of orthotic assistance. However, the upper extremity requires much more complicated shoulder function to place the hand into a position of function. The hand demands precise fine motion of the fingers with preservation of sensation if it is to perform as before.

Upper extremity functional return following a stroke depends on the degree of spasticity, the return of voluntary motor control, the extent of peripheral sensory loss, the presence of apraxia or perceptual loss, the extent of reversibility of reflex synergic patterns, if those patterns can be reversed, and the loss of intellectual impairment. Ultimately other factors influence functional return and these include pain, dystrophic changes, contractures of the fingers, elbow, and shoulder, and psychological impairment.

Spontaneous return of function—the natural history of the disease entity—has been documented in one study with the conclusion that "subjects who eventually recover full motor function regain their initial motion recovery during the first two weeks and always within the first month."[1] Of patients destined to recover, some regained active motion during the first four weeks and all by the third month. In patients destined to recover partially, improvement was noted during the first six to

seven months. Pertaining to the extent of recovery, these studies revealed that, in spite of *full voluntary* motion, some 40 per cent had residual impairment manifested by weakness, fatigue, sensory impairment, ataxia, and proprioceptive deficiency. The presence of spasticity usually indicates that recovery will be only partial.

Recovery of active motion is greatest in elbow flexion and extension, less in elbow supination and pronation, and usually significantly less in the shoulder.[2]

"Functional recovery" is variably defined. Carroll defined "recovery" as return of adequate sensation and coordination, not merely voluntary movement.[3] On the basis of these criteria, Carroll stated that a hemiplegic patient who did not recover within a week would not regain full use of the upper extremity. When recovery of the hand was achieved, this recovery was greatest on the radial side (thumb and index finger) than on the ulnar side. Practical functional recovery was noted in only two of a small group of 50 patients in this study.

Sensory impairment with some spontaneous recovery is a poor prognostic sign; recovery probably should not be expected within the first three months.[4] Sensory retraining has advocates, but the practical results remain unverified.

Twitchell,[6] in what is now considered to be a classic article, noted that, immediately after the onset of hemiplegia, total loss of voluntary function usually occurred, with loss or diminution of deep tendon reflexes. Seldom did a complete flaccidity exist, although there was decreased resistance to passive movement. Within 48 hours, the deep tendon reflexes returned and became increasingly more reactive. Clonus could be noted from the first to the thirty-eighth day.

Clonus is more noticeable in the lower extremities but could be noted in the finger flexors. Passive resistance is noted early in the adduction and internal rotation of the arm and the flexors of the forearm.

Twitchell also noted that return of voluntary function occurred between the sixth and thirty-third day, usually in the flexors of the shoulder. This flexion gradually evolved into a flexion synergy of the upper extremity. These synergies may become utilizable for gross movements but not for fine discriminatory movement. These synergies start proximally and spread distally. They are initiated or intensified by stimuli such as tapping, scratching, rubbing, pinching, stretching, and so forth. Progression may continue until only synergies are present or may plateau at any stage of development. Recovery to normal voluntary function may occur at any stage and return so that the only remaining neurological deficit is weakness, spasticity, or residual of a portion of the synergy.

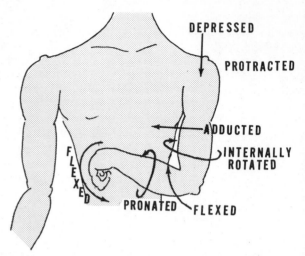

**Figure 2–2.** Flexor synergy of upper extremity. (From Cailliet, R.: The Shoulder in Hemiplegia. Philadelphia, F.A. Davis Co., 1980, p. 8.)

Brunnstrom designated the following six stages.[7]

State I–Flaccidity is present.

Stage II–Spasticity gradually develops, with beginning of synergies.

Stage III–Spasticity increases with some voluntary control of synergies as the patient improves.

Stage IV–(In improvement): spasticity declines with increasing control of components of synergy. Recovery may end at this phase.

Stage V–Synergies no longer control motor function (Fig. 2–2).

Stage VI–Individual joint movement develops.

The first three stages are progression of the illness process and the last three stages are degrees of recovery: all may stop at any stage. Because sensory impairment constitutes a major obstacle to recovery, complete and accurate testing must precede treatment prescription and formation of a prognosis.

## TESTING OF FUNCTION

Gross testing is performed for sharp and dull discrimination, position sense, two-point discrimination stereopnosis (identification of familiar objects, texture, contours, and so forth). Some assistance may be necessary to approximate the patient's fingertips to the object being tested when prehensile movements of the fingers cannot be performed.

Range of motion must be determined for the shoulder, elbow, wrist, and fingers. Meaningful functional ranges of motion must be ascertained, such as forward flexion of the shoulder, external rotation of the arm to sagittal position, elbow flexion, forearm pronation, finger extension to neutral, and thumb circumduction to position into opposi-

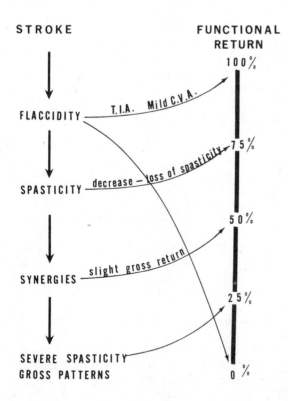

**Figure 2–1.** Estimate of spontaneous recovery from stroke. (From Cailliet, R.: The Shoulder in Hemiplegia. Philadelphia, F.A. Davis Co., 1980, p. 5.)

tion. If restriction by spasticity or by contracture is present, the range of motion is tested in regard to the restriction.

Voluntary control of motor function then is determined as to individual muscle function and coordinated grouping of motor function; another step involves elicitation of synergies that may be voluntarily initiated and may become at least partially useful. Motor function must be evaluated on a regular, sequential (preferably daily) basis because it may *change:* from a flaccid to a spastic state, and to synergies. Then it may reverse itself. Sensory function must also be determined frequently to ascertain any deterioration or improvement. Early in patient management determination of perceptual impairment is indicated, as its presence considerably influences potential ultimate functional recovery. If intellectual impairment is present, its extent must also be ascertained.

## TREATMENT

### PHYSICAL

The ultimate goal of treatment of the upper extremity is to promote return of function to improve activities of daily living (ADL), assist in transfer and ambulation, and when feasible bring about a return to gainful occupation. Some return of finger movement without return of shoulder or elbow movement to place the hand in a useful position is of no practical use. It may be appreciated also that some gross motor return with residual severe sensory deficit or severe perceptual impairment will be of limited value.

Exercises are often advocated using *simultaneous* voluntary movement of the *normal* areas to assist or retrain the hemiplegic side. Although this has been claimed to be a valuable adjunct to therapy, there is evidence that in most cases the contralateral "normal" extremity may also have some impairment: at least its simultaneous function may be impaired when attempted with voluntary movement of the paretic extremity.[8] The impairment of the normal side when action is performed with the paretic side[9] becomes more apparent when there is greater recovery and thus improved voluntary function of the paretic extremity.

Some techniques of "neuromuscular re-education" permit the gross use of reflex pattern: utilization of synergies or portions of synergies. These may be of value but fail to achieve fine intricate control of the hand and fingers. They may result in ability to perform such activities as dressing, transfer, ambulation, and independence in toilet function but deny the patient more precise and meaningful function.[10] The goal of treatment must be clearly established, the duration of treatment esti-

mated, and the efficacy of treatment techniques evaluated.

There are indications for treatment of the upper extremity that do not involve attempts at restoration of function but are directed to the control of pain. This is predominantly observed in the shoulder. As spontaneous improvement in function frequently continues, much of treatment is concerned with minimizing or preventing secondary disabling factors. These are contractures, subluxation, disease, and psychological despair and depression.

Numerous concepts and techniques of rehabilitation have been advocated and tested. The technique chosen is based on the stage at which the patient is first seen for rehabilitation, the degree and type of neurological deficit, the extent of sensory deficit, the degree of specificity, and the particular training, experience, and bias of the treating therapist.

In the early areflexive flaccid stage numerous sensory stimuli are centralized to initiate some movement, albeit reflex in nature and having no voluntary central control.[11] These modalities include stroking, brushing, stretching, and tapping. Stretching may initiate movement.

Use of electrical stimulation has had a resurgence in re-education as well as in spasticity prevention of joint contracture. (Biofeedback is discussed in another chapter.) Rancho Los Amigos in Downey, California has recently claimed great strides in muscle "re-education," a return of strength, prevention of joint contractures, and minimization of subluxation by frequent daily electrical stimulation of the motor points of afflicted muscles.[32]

As motion appears, much of it may be reflex; early synergy is essentially involuntary. Many of these reflex patterns are utilized in the treatment concepts of the following: Brunnstrom,[7] Bobath,[12] Progressive Neuromuscular Facilitation,[13] Rood,[11] and Fay.[14]

All techniques implement certain neurophysiological concepts:

1. Sensory input is necessary for initiation or inhibition of motor function.

2. Reflex activities may facilitate or inhibit voluntary motor activities.

3. Neurological sequential development from infancy to adult motor activity is the basis of motor development.

4. Repetition and frequency in each approach to treatment is mandatory.

5. Most important probably is the personal interaction of the patient and the therapist.

The Brunnstrom method takes advantage of the stages of recovery outlined by Twitchell, namely, the initiation by sensory stimulation of synergies.

These may develop and regress. Various tonic reflexes are utilized, with all movements made to act against resistance. As the synergies subside, if they do, the emerging voluntary isolated movements are emphasized. Good sensory function is mandatory.

Proprioceptive neuromuscular facilitation utilizes resistance of synergies initiated by sensory stimulation all done in *total diagonal patterns*. The stimulation of synergistic reflexes may be stretching, tapping, neck reflexes, and so forth, with strong emphasis on repetition, verbal commands, and bilateral co-contraction. Here, as in the Brunnstrom concept, the effort is to make motor control increasingly more voluntary by repeated involuntary reflex activity.

The Rood technique is essentially motor reaction to dermatomal stimulation of the same sensorimotor representation that is considered to be cortically represented. The sensory stimulation is by brushing, applying ice, or stroking. Rood's concept claims that reciprocal relaxation is attained from agonistic contraction.

The Bobath method utilizes proprioceptive and tactile stimuli by modifying postures, allegedly via central mechanisms.

Fay advocated re-educating the central nervous system by employing phylogenetic patterns of crawling and creeping.

The exact specifics of these techniques are beyond the scope of this presentation and require study of the original publications. As all these techniques involve sensory stimulation and the teaching of cortical control of subcortical reflexes, the advocacy of one or other of the methods is not intended. Peszczynski[15] tested the efficacy of these techniques and claimed equal success with simple active or passive exercises.

Relief of spasticity has been the focus of most treatment techniques; in these, exercise, drugs, modalities such as heat and cold, and surgical intervention have been used. Spasticity has been combated by utilization of neurophysiological mechanisms such as:

1. Antagonistic relaxation of the spastic muscles by attempting repeated and sustained contraction of the agonistic muscle groups. Because the agonists (prime movers) are often unable to be voluntarily contracted, pathological reflexes are utilized in most therapeutic techniques (Brunnstrom, Bobath, Rood, PNF, Fay, and so forth).

2. Slow, gradual, sustained stretching of spastic muscle groups has been shown to release the spasticity and thus permit greater agonistic activity. Spasticity release by these methods is short-lived and not of prolonged functional value.

## PHARMACEUTICAL

*Pharmaceutical* treatment of spasticity remains of limited value. However, drugs specifically for spasticity such as dantrolene sodium and baclofen have proved helpful in proper dosage. Drugs originally designated for their tranquilizing action (benediazine, diazepam) have also evoked antispastic action. The original enthusiastic support for curare and curare-like drugs has waned, but these have some limited value. Baclofen (lioresal) has a recommended dosage schedule of 5 mg three times a day for three days, 10 mg three times a day for three days, 15 mg three times a day for three days, then 20 mg three times a day. Dosage should not exceed 80 mg daily nor dosages rapidly changed. When relaxation is reached, the dose increase can be stopped; then the dosage can be gradually decreased to maintain maximum benefit with minimal dosage.

Dantrolene sodium (Dantrium) is usually begun with 25 mg, one daily, increasing to 25 mg twice a day, then up to 100 mg four times a day. Gradual increases not to exceed 400 mg daily are usually well tolerated. Again, as with baclofen, gradual tapering of dosages to maintain benefit is suggested. Valium (Diazepam) has, in my opinion, limited value in spasticity, as has Soma (carisoprodol). Amitryptyline (Elavil) in doses of 50 to 100 mg taken before bedtime appears to enhance the efficacy of baclofen.

## OTHER MODALITIES

*Other modalities* continue to be valuable adjuncts to physical therapeutic approaches. *Heat* possibly has its greatest value when pain or soft tissue contracture impedes rehabilitation efforts. Its value in overcoming or decreasing spasticity is limited. *Ultrasound* allegedly decreases nerve conduction time but has not been effective in decreasing spasticity.

*Cold* applied superficially directly to the spastic muscle group appears to be the most useful modality. Total immersing in an ice bath has been advocated and claimed to be helpful, but its beneficial effect has occurred before the deep tissue temperature has significantly decreased so that its effect is apparently upon the proprioceptors, the spindle cells, or the nerve fibers to the spastic muscles. Cold decreases the excitability of the muscle spindles and allows intrafusal elongation to proceed with greater facility. The type of spasticity determines whether ice will be of value through its spindle effect;[16] i.e., spasticity caused by hypersensitivity of the spindle cell will respond, whereas spasticity from alpha motor neuron activity will not. The beneficial effect of cold upon spasticity is brief; therefore, cold must be considered as an adjunct to other therapeutic approaches.

*Surgical intervention* has been advocated in overcoming disabling spasticity. Tenotomies of spastic muscle tendons with total or partial release are valuable.[17, 18] In the shoulder, where spastic internal rotation and adduction present a major problem, tenotomy of the subscapularis muscle is an accepted procedure.[19] For hands that have severe flexion spasticity of the fingers, partial release of the flexor tendons has been advocated.[18]

Surgical or chemical rhizotomies or neurectomies that interrupt the motor *or* sensory nerve supply to spastic muscles are very valuable. Chemical neurectomies have been successfully performed with dilute phenol injected near the peripheral nerve or into the myoneural junction. This form of injection creates a motor paresis (via alpha motor neurons) that may last for three to six months, then usually produces a complete regeneration.[20] During the paresis incurred from the phenol nerve blocks, the weaker agonist can be strengthened, contractures can be decreased, and functional training initiated. However, pain that can lead to a reflex sympathetic dystrophy may occur locally at the site of injection.

*Chemical nerve blocks* have not proved of great practical value in the upper extremity. Because the hand is so delicate in its mechanism, blocking of the hand flexors in the forearm releases the spastic flexors and permits greater extensor strength and range, but creates only a better "helping" hand at best.

## PREVENTION OF CONTRACTURE

Prevention of contracture in the hemiplegic is of primary importance. Return of muscular function of portions of the extremity that is contracted is not especially helpful. Much of nonsurgical treatment has prevention of contracture as its objective, with surgery being required when the program of treatment fails.

Connective tissue that forms the periarticular tissues is composed of cellular elements (fibroblasts and mast cells), fibrillar elements (collagen, reticulin and elastic) and ground substance. Connective tissue is composed of all these tissues in varying proportions, depending upon the required activity of that particular tissue site. Connective tissue undergoes constant change that depends on external forces.[22] For areas in which free motion is required, collagen and reticulin form a loose mesh that is sparcely attached; the greater the motion, the more distant are the sites of attachment. When motion is restricted, collagen becomes more dense and is arranged in sheets that attach at more frequent and shorter distances. The contracture represents reorganization, not the formation of more collagen. The collagen fibers do, however, become shorter and thicker.

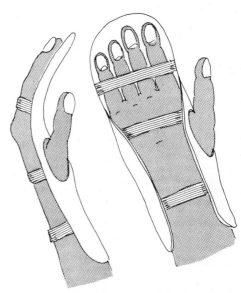

**Figure 2–3.** Static (rest) splint. This splint can be made of plaster, plastic, Polysar, orthoplast, or other materials and strapped with leather, Velcro, or webbing. It maintains the wrist and fingers in a physiological position. Among its uses are wrist drop from peripheral neuropathies and early flaccid stage of stroke. It prevents deformity, relieves pain, and avoids overstretching of flail musculature. (From Cailliet, R.: Hand Pain and Impairment. 3rd ed. Philadelphia, F.A. Davis Co., 1982, p. 218.)

Connective tissue *normally* tends to contract unless this process is thwarted by stretching forces. Without these stretching forces contracture can occur in one week. With the addition of trauma,

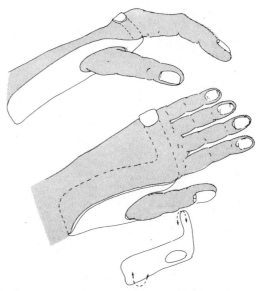

**Figure 2–4.** Rest wrist splint. This splint can be used as a rest or a semidynamic splint. Its purpose is to maintain the wrist in slight extension yet permit and assist finger and thumb movement. It can be made of any material. It has definite value in treating median nerve compression (carpal tunnel syndrome). (From Cailliet, R.: Hand Pain and Impairment. 3rd ed. Philadelphia, F.A. Davis Co., 1982, p. 219.)

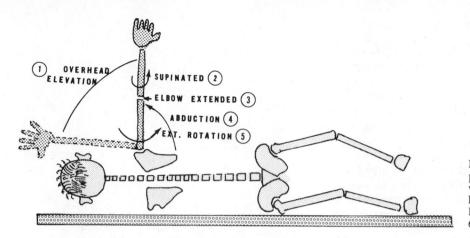

**Figure 2–5.** In passive exercise, the patient tries to hold the extremity in various positions (1–5). (From Cailliet, R.: The Shoulder in Hemiplegia. Philadelphia, F.A. Davis Co., 1980, p. 61.)

edema, and impaired circulation, it can occur in three days.

Collagen can elongate under moderate constant tension. This is the basis for treatment. An acute abrupt stretch is resisted by the tensile strength resistance of the tissue. If traction is prolonged and constant, it does elongate. The modality of heat applied during prolonged stretching of contracture enhances the facility of elongation. In the spastic hemiplegic, the local heat also relaxes spasticity. The type of heat applied varies with availability and applicability of heat appliances and with the treatment site. Hot moist packs (hydrocollator) or paraffin are accepted home modalities. In the clinic or hospital situation, ultrasound has the deepest penetration for the treatment of contracture.[22, 23] It has been demonstrated that continuing stretch is beneficial after the removal of the heat packs.[24]

Once extensibility of connective tissue has been regained, it must be maintained. In areas in which active muscular contraction is possible, this is relatively simply done by the institution of *active* range of motion exercises. When active contracture is not possible, frequent passive stretch is indicated, with splinting applied between the stretching sessions.

For the shoulder, the bed and chair positions must maintain abduction to approximately horizontal position (90 degrees) and keep the arm externally rotated.

The elbow must alternate between full extension and 90-degree flexion. As the tendency is for sustained (spastic) flexion, frequent extension must be passively or actively produced, then support splinted. Pronation of the forearm is predominant in the upper extremity synergies; this must be neutralized and supination produced.

The hand tends to flex at the wrist, with fingers and the thumb adducting into the palm.

Use of towels and splints, both dynamic and static, must be evaluated[16] and *specifically* prescribed and applied. Each patient differs as to the type, severity and duration of the problem, as to spasticity and its degree, and as to ability to expe-

rience sensation. Ease and availability of treatment methods also vary. Basic guidelines must be established. Whether the patient will receive physical or occupational therapy and by whom the treatment will be given must be determined.

The patient with a hemiplegic upper extremity may have the problem of *pain*. This pain predomi-

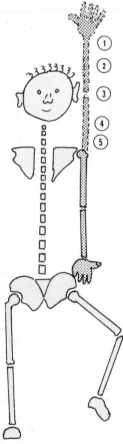

**Figure 2–6.** With patient supine, the extremity is gradually raised to the overhead position: 1 and 2, the forearm is supinated; 3, the elbow extended; 4, abducted; 5, the upper arm externally rotated. (From Cailliet, R.: The Shoulder in Hemiplegia. Philadelphia, F.A. Davis Co., 1980, p. 60.)

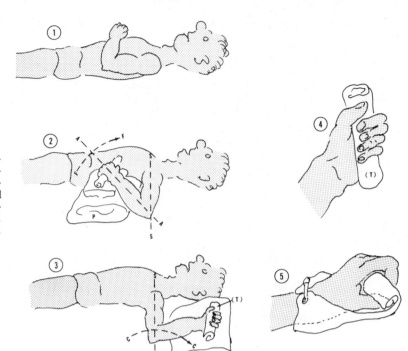

**Figure 2–7.** Shoulder exercises. With arm abducted to 90° and the hand held with wrist extended (4) and fingers cupped in some extension, the arm is rotated toward overhead position (3). This exercise regains and maintains shoulder range of motion. (From Cailliet, R.: The Shoulder in Hemiplegia. Philadelphia, F.A. Davis Co., 1980, p. 105.)

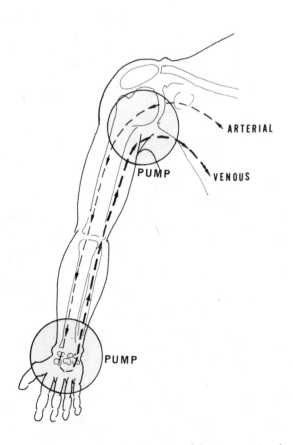

**Figure 2–8.** Venous lymphatic pumps of the upper extremity. (From Cailliet, R.: The Shoulder in Hemiplegia. Philadelphia, F.A. Davis Co., 1980, p. 108.)

nantly occurs in the shoulder and, to a slightly lesser degree, in the hand and wrist. In the shoulder, subluxation noted early in the flail stage is considered to be a common cause of pain. This is adequately discussed in the literature.[2] There are numerous causes postulated, from scapular downward rotation and functional scoliosis to cuff involvement at the glenohumeral joint.

In the early flail stage the use of a sling has general acceptance, but complete physiological or clinical benefit has not been established for this. Electrical stimulation of the supraspinatus, infraspinatus, and deltoid muscles has been claimed to be effective in prevention or correction of subluxation.[25]

As the shoulder becomes spastic and range of motion becomes impaired, the *hand-shoulder-finger syndrome* may develop. This is known by numerous terms such as minor dystrophy, causalgia, and reflex sympathetic dystrophy. The syndrome includes:

1. Limited shoulder range of motion (flail or spastic).

2. A swollen hand; the hand initially is edematous on the dorsum of the fingers, then the edema envelopes the entire hand.

3. Vasomotor changes of vasospastic or vasodilatation.

4. Possible ultimate involvement of the elbow.

5. A painless but "frozen" shoulder and a stiff atrophic hand.

6. Osteoporosis that develops with a flail shoulder.

A neurological vasomotor phenomenon probably initiates the syndrome. Some investigators believe the etiology and sequence of the syndrome is that of impaired arteriovenous lymphatic circulation of the upper extremity. When the shoulder becomes immobile and elevated above cardiac level, the "shoulder pump" fails to mobilize venous and lymphatic fluid from the arm.[2] As the hand fails to contract and relax, the "hand pump" fails to remove the venous and lymphatic fluid from the hand and swelling occurs. The edema appears initially on the dorsum of the fingers. (Venous lymphatic drainage is in the dorsum of the fingers; the arterial supply is in the palmar aspect). When swelling occurs, it impedes the elongation of the extensor tendon and ultimately of the collateral ligaments. The edematous fluid is fibrinoid and pro-

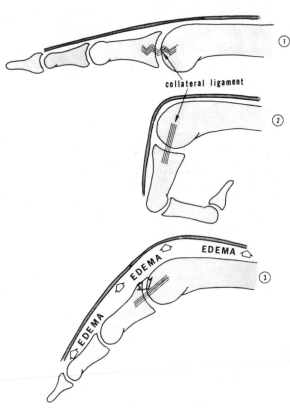

**Figure 2–10.** Finger changes in hand-shoulder syndrome. *1,* Normal extension of metacarpophalangeal joint with relaxed collateral ligament. *2,* Normal flexion of metacarpophalangeal joint with the collaterals becoming taut. *3,* Edema on dorsum of hand elevates the extensor tendons and prevents flexion. The collateral ligaments are never fully elongated and develop contracture. This further limits the "pump action" of the flexion of the hand. (From Cailliet, R.: The Shoulder in Hemiplegia. Philadelphia, F.A. Davis Co., 1980, p. 110.)

tein in nature and adds to contracture by causing further impairment of motion.

Osteoporosis rapidly occurs; its etiology is unclear. Undoubtedly disuse is a factor, as is a vasomotor element.

Pain may occur or be absent. The vasomotor component may be absent.[26] When present, the entity is termed *reflex sympathetic dystrophy syndrome* or *causalgia:* this produces the symptom of "burning pain" or hyperesthesia.

The time between stroke and the first symptoms of shoulder-hand-finger syndrome has been estimated and is given in Table 2–1.

Treatment is *preferably preventive.* Range of motion of the shoulder, wrist, and fingers must be regained and maintained. If there is indication of vasomotor changes noted objectively by cold, moist or warm redness, or a "burning-like" pain, stellate chemical ganglion block should be initiated early. Massage, hot packs, whirlpool treatments, and ice packs are usually poorly tolerated. Cool packs of 70° are soothing.

*Active* range of motion exercises for the shoulder,

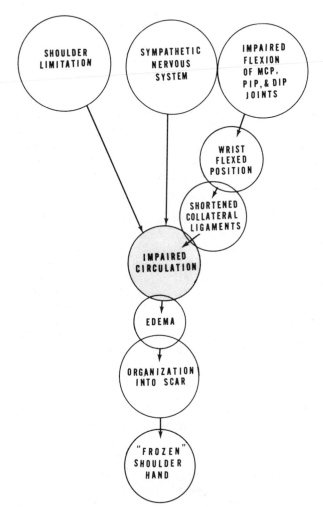

**Figure 2–9.** Sequences leading to frozen shoulder-hand-finger syndrome. (From Cailliet, R.: The Shoulder in Hemiplegia. Philadelphia, F.A. Davis Co., 1980, p. 112.)

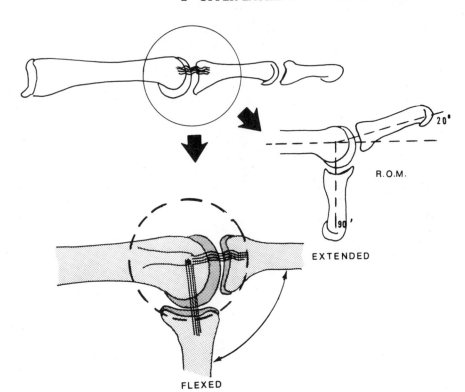

**Figure 2–11.** Normal flexion-extension of metacarpophalangeal joints. Due to the elliptical shape of the head of the metacarpals, the collateral ligaments are slack with finger extension and taut when the fingers are flexed. (From Cailliet, R.: The Shoulder in Hemiplegia. Philadelphia, F.A. Davis Co., 1980, p. 109.)

hand, and fingers should be started immediately. The part(s) that cannot be actively moved should be passively moved frequently or movement should be actively assisted. Intermittent vasopneumatic treatment as advocated by Jobst is used for the entire upper extremity. Compressive centripetal wrapping of the finger with ⅛ inch soft braided nylon can remove or reduce the edema.[27]

Oral steroids in large doses for brief course have been found effective, if these are not medically contraindicated.

Other painful conditions of the shoulder such as tendinitis and capsulitis can coexist with the hemiplegia.

When the patient arrives at the "frozen shoulder" stage, at which shoulder (glenohumeral) pain decreases or disappears and range of motion both actively and passively is not possible, surgical release of the subscapularis has been advocated.[28] A

frozen shoulder exists when range of motion is markedly curtailed and an arthrogram reveals a severely constricted capsule (allowing 3 to 5 cc of fluid or dye). "Brisement" therapy has been advo-

**TABLE 2–1.** TIME BETWEEN STROKE AND FIRST SYMPTOMS OF SHOULDER-HAND-FINGER SYNDROME

| Months | Percentage of Patients |
|--------|------------------------|
| 0–1 | 0 |
| 1–2 | 28 |
| 2–3 | 37 |
| 3–4 | 16 |
| 4–5 | 17 |
| 5–6 | 2 |

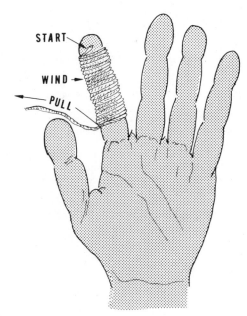

**Figure 2–12.** Removal of finger edema. Each finger is firmly wrapped with a heavy twine, beginning at the tip and moving towards the webbing. This procedure should be performed several times daily and can frequently be done by the patient using his uninvolved upper extremity. (From Cailliet, R.: The Shoulder in Hemiplegia. Philadelphia, F.A. Davis Co., 1980, p. 118.)

cated.[29] This involves injecting a large volume (40 cc) of dilute procaine HCl solution and triamcinolone under forceful manual pressure into the glenohumeral joint until the capsule tears and the arm can passively be abducted and externally rotated. This must be followed by active and passive range of motion exercises with splinting to maintain the shoulder at the newly acquired range of motion.

*Bracing* with specific rationale and indication has value in preventing contracture and deformity. There are very few functional splints currently of value in the upper extremity.

The patient who has impairment largely from sensory deficit, or who fails to benefit from therapy because of sensory loss, may benefit from sensory retraining.[30]

## REFERENCES

1. Bard, G. and Hirschberg, G. G.: Recovery of voluntary motion on upper extremity following hemiplegia. Arch. Phys. Med. Rehabil. 46:567–572, 1965.
2. Cailliet, R.: The Shoulder in Hemiplegia. Philadelphia, F. A. Davis Co., 1979.
3. Carroll, D.: Hand function in hemiplegia. J. Chronic Dis. 18:493–500, 1965.
4. Van Buskirk, C. and Webster, D.: Prognostic value of sensory deficit in rehabilitation of hemiplegia. Neurology 5:407–411, 1955.
5. Caldwell, C. B., Wilson, D. J., and Brown, R. M.: Evaluation and treatment of the upper extremity in the hemiplegic stroke patient. Clin. Orthop. 63:69–93, 1969.
6. Twitchell, T. E.: The restoration of motor function following hemiplegia in man. Brain 74:443–480, 1951.
7. Brunnstrom, S.: Movement Therapy in Hemiplegia: A Neurological Approach. New York, Harper and Row, 1970.
8. Cohn, R.: Interaction in bilaterally simultaneous motor functions. AMA Arch. Neurol. Psychiatr. 65:472–476, 1951.
9. Kausmanowa-Petrusewicz, I.: Interaction in simultaneous motor functions. AMA Arch. Neurol. Psychiatr. 81:173–181, 1959.
10. Stern, P., McDowell, F., Miller, J., and Robinson, M.: Effects of facilitation exercise techniques in stroke rehabilitation. Arch. Phys. Med. Rehabil. 51:526–531, 1970.
11. Stockmeyer, S. A.: An interpretation of the approach of Rood to the treatment of neuromuscular dysfunction. Am. J. Phys. Med. 46:900–956, 1967.
12. Bobath, B.: Abnormal posture reflex activity caused by brain lesion. London, William Keinemann Medical Books, Ltd., 1965.
13. Knott, M. and Voss, D. E.: Proprioceptive Neuromuscular Facilitation, 2nd Ed. New York, Harper and Row, 1968.
14. Flanagan, E. M.: Methods of facilitation and inhibition of motor activity. Am. J. Phys. Med. 46:1006–1011, 1967.
15. Peszczynski, M.: Rehabilitation of the Adult Hemiplegic Locomotor System. Fourth Annual Volume of Physiology and Experimental Medical Science, Calcutta, 1965.
16. Mossman, P. L.: A Problem Oriented Approach to Stroke Rehabilitation. Springfield, Charles C Thomas, 1976.
17. Mooney, V., Perry, J., and Nickel, V. L.: Surgical and non-surgical orthopedic care of stroke. J. Bone Joint Surg. 49-A: 989–1000, 1967.
18. Treanor, W. J. and Reifenstein, G. H.: Potential reversibility of the hemiplegic posture. Am. J. Cardiol. 7:370–378, 1961.
19. Mooney, V., Frykman, G., and McLamb, J.: Current status of intraneural phenol injections. Clin. Orthop. 63:122–131, 1969.
20. Halpern, D., and Meelhaysen, F. E.: Phenol motor point block in the management of muscular hypertonia. Arch. Phys. Med. Rehabil. 47:659–664, 1966.
21. Khalili, A. A. and Betts, H. B.: Management of Spasticity with Phenol Nerve Blocks. Final Report, R.D. 2529-M. Washington, D.C., Dept. HEW, Social and Rehabilitation Service, 1970.
22. Kottke, F. J., Pavley, R. L., and Ptak, R. A.: The rationale for prolonged stretching for correction of shortening of connective tissue. Arch. Phys. Med. Rehabil. 47:345–352, 1966.
23. Gersten, J. W.: Effects of ultrasound on tendon extensibility. Am. J. Phys. Med. 34:362–369, 1955.
24. Kottke, F. J., Stillwell, G. K., and Lehmann, J. F. (eds.): Krusen's Handbook of Physical Medicine and Rehabilitation. Philadelphia, W. B. Saunders Co. 1982.
25. Lehmann, J. F., Masock, A. J., Waven, C. G., and Koblanski, J. N.: Effect of therapeutic temperature on tendon extensibility. Arch. Phys. Med. Rehabil. 51:481–487, 1970.
26. Benton, L. A., Baker, L. L., Bowman, B. R., and Waters, R. L.: Functional Electrical Stimulation—A Practical Clinical Guide. Downey, Calif., Rancho Los Amigos Rehabilitation Engineering Center, 1980.
27. Moberg, E.: The shoulder-hand-finger syndrome as a whole. Surg. Clin. North Am. 40(2):367, 1960.
28. Cain, H. D., and Leibgold, H. B.: Compressive centripetal wrapping technique for reduction of edema. Arch. Phys. Med. Rehabil. 48:420–473, 1967.
29. Caldwell, C. B., Wilson, D. J., and Brown, R. M.: Evaluation and treatment of the upper extremity in the hemiplegic stroke patient. Clin. Orthop. 63:69–93, 1969.
30. Simon, W. H.: Soft tissue disorders of the shoulder. Orthop. Clin. North Am. 6(2):521, 1975.
31. Goldman, H.: Improvement of double simultaneous stimulation perception in hemiplegia patients. Arch. Phys. Med. Rehabil. 47:681–687, 1966.

# 3

# Nursing Rehabilitation of the Stroke Patient

*by Rosemary Murray, M.A., R.N.*

Patients who have experienced a stroke (also termed cerebral vascular accident, CVA, and stroke syndrome) comprise a major portion of the patient population requiring specific rehabilitation measures throughout the entirety of the treatment program.

Although a stroke may occur in childhood or early adulthood, the highest percentage of strokes occur in the middle to older age groups. This complicates the situation because of a number of conditions that can coexist in this older age group. First, one is likely to see the cumulative effects of one or more risk factors; smoking, obesity, hypertension and elevated serum cholesterol, lipoproteins, and triglycerides. Many patients are likely to have related or precursor diseases such as cardiovascular disease, diabetes mellitus, or polycythemia vera. In addition to age-related physiological and functional decrements, the stroke patient may also have impairments resulting from chronic disease such as arthritis and emphysema. Management of the stroke patient, therefore, must be comprehensive in scope and extended in duration.

Consideration must also be given to the patient's family, since its members will be significantly affected by the patient's response to the stroke and share in the achievements and failures of rehabilitation efforts. In addition, there is evidence of a familial factor in the incidence of cardiovascular disease (and the precursor diseases as well). Poor health habits that place all members at risk for cardiovascular disease may be present as the established family life style. Educating the patient and family concerning methods of coping with and adapting to the functional limitations imposed by the residual neurological deficit of a stroke is equaled by the need to educate the patient and family in adopting behaviors to promote and maintain health. To be successful, rehabilitation will require the compliance of the patient, the cooperation of the family, and the collective, collaborative efforts of many health care professionals. The patient, the family, and the health care professionals each are essential parts of the rehabilitation team. Rehabilitation goals, if they are to be achieved, must be established collectively, must reflect the priorities agreed to by each member, and must include the contribution of each member according to role and ability.

Although it would be unwise to venture specific predictions about return of function during the acute phase, the patient and family are offered an element of hope if they are made aware that complete recovery is rare but some degree of recovery is a very real possibility. From the beginning of the acute phase every effort should be made (1) to maintain muscle tone and strength and joint range of motion, (2) to preserve and promote function, and (3) to prevent complications so that restoration of normal function or adaptation to altered patterns of function will become a reality during the rehabilitation phase.

Once survival from the original neurological insult is assured, nursing concerns focus on assisting the patient to perform functions in the face of neurological deficits that will alter performance and to do for the patient those functions that he can no longer accomplish. All nursing interventions are designed to promote maximum recovery from the stroke. The nature and degree of the specific interventions will be determined by the individual patient and family. In this sense the nursing interventions will be unique to each patient. There are, however, some common problems and related nursing interventions that apply to many stroke patients. These problems concern adapting to motor and sensory dysfunction, learning self-care activities, promoting adequate nutrition and elimination, assisting with communication problems, dealing with emotional distress, and providing for patient safety.

## POSITION AND BODY ALIGNMENT

While in bed the patient's position should be changed every one to two hours around the clock in order to prevent pressure ulcers. After a stroke the patient is at risk for the development of a pressure ulcer because of decreased perception of pain indicating tissue ischemia caused by excessive and/or prolonged pressure, inability or limited ability to shift body weight, compromised skin integrity because of the presence of urine, feces, moisture, and bacteria, altered nutritional status, and decreased circulation.

Maintaining proper body alignment is necessary, regardless of the position selected, in order to prevent edema, joint pain, and deformity. Any bed activity for the stroke patient with hemiparesis or paresis will be facilitated if the mattress is firm or supported by a bedboard. A footboard should be attached to the foot of the bed as a support measure to prevent foot drop. Adjustable footboards are suggested, since they can be placed in any position along the length of the mattress and can provide adequate foot support for even the very short patient.

Side rails should be used when the stroke patient is in bed because they provide the patient with a sense of physical security and safety from falls. This is especially important if the patient's mental state is altered and in the presence of hemianopia, decreased proprioception, and poor balance. The patient can also use the side rails to assist in changing position and shifting body weight.

A trapeze can be used by the patient for turning and moving up in bed as well as an assistive device when lifting the buttocks to use the bedpan or to relieve pressure on the sacrum. Some find a pull rope helpful. The rope is attached to the foot of the bed and is of sufficient length that a patient can grasp it from a supine position and pull up until the sitting position is reached. Pull ropes can be made from any material, although muslin strips are readily available in most hospitals. Commercial devices are also available, as shown in Figure 3–1.

Turning a stroke patient with hemiparesis can be facilitated by the use of a turning sheet. It consists of a regular bed sheet folded widthwise in thirds. It should be placed under the patient from the shoulders to just below the buttocks. If the patient's trunk is long the sheet should be folded in half. Once the sheet is in place under the patient, equal portions of the sheet should be visible at each side. If the patient is to be turned from the supine position to his right side, the nurse rolls the sheet on his left side close to the trunk. The turn is accomplished by grasping the rolled edge of the sheet and turning the patient to the right. The procedure is reversed when the patient is turned to the left side. Using a turning sheet permits a smooth, easy change in patient position, especially if the patient cannot or should not assist in this change.

The stroke patient can be placed in the supine or prone positions or the left or right sidelying positions. There are, however, nursing considerations associated with the choice and use of each position as well as the fact that each of these positions can

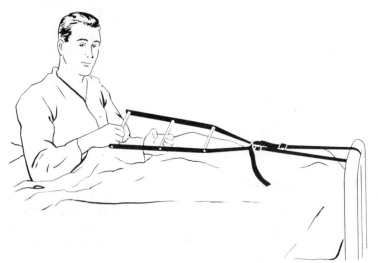

**Figure 3–1.** Pull-up device. (From Hirschberg, G. G. et al.: Rehabilitation: A Manual for the Care of the Elderly and Disabled. Philadelphia, J. B. Lippincott Co., 1976, p. 71.)

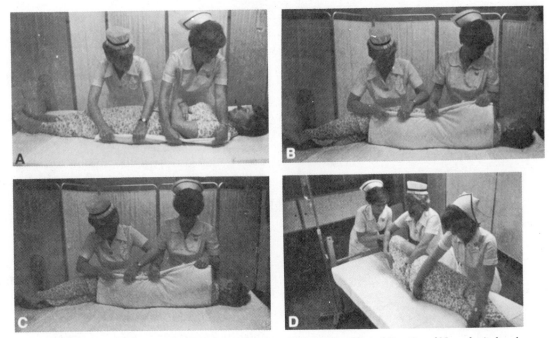

**Figure 3–2.** Using a turning sheet. (From Hickey, J. V. X.: The Clinical Practice of Neurological and Neurosurgical Nursing. Philadelphia, J. B. Lippincott Co., 1981, p. 304.)

be modified according to the requirements of the individual patient. The supine position may be contraindicated if the patient is unconscious or if gag or swallow reflexes are absent.

When the patient is in the supine position, the heels should be kept off the bed with a pillow and the patient's feet should be supported by a footboard. A pillow should be placed in the axillary region of the paretic arm to support the shoulder and one or more pillows should be placed under the length of the arm and hand to prevent edema.

Since the paretic leg tends to rotate externally, a trochanter roll should be placed from the ileac crest to the midthigh to prevent deformity. A simple trochanter roll can be fashioned by tightly rolling a towel or bathsheet. Sandbags can also prevent external rotation of the hip, but their use increases the amount of external pressure on soft tissue.

The prone position should not be used if the patient has severe musculoskeletal limitations because of injury, disease, or age or if the patient has a tracheostomy or gastrostomy tube in place. For those stroke patients with no contraindications, the prone position can be quite comfortable and will reduce the risk of hip flexion contractures. A pillow placed under the pelvis will increase the patient's comfort in this position. If the feet cannot hang freely over the end of the mattress, a pillow under the lower legs will prevent the toes from pressing against the mattress.

The sidelying or lateral position can be achieved

with relative ease. When the patient is placed on the paretic side, care should be taken to protect the affected arm. The shoulder should be moved forward so that the patient's weight is not directly on the shoulder. If necessary, the patient's hand can be elevated on a pillow. Enough pillows (usually two) should be placed between the legs to provide adequate support for the hip, knee, and ankle joints. Because the patient has altered pressure and pain sensation on the paretic side, he may not be aware of the early signals of tissue trauma from excessive or prolonged pressure or both. The nurse should evaluate the patient's skin response to pressure when he is placed on this side and determine when the position should be changed. It is not unusual, because of the stroke patient's compromised physical status, to limit the time spent positioned on the paretic side to no more than 30 minutes.

The purpose of maintaining good alignment is to prevent the development of deformities that will decrease the desired rehabilitation goals. Light splints are often prescribed to maintain normal joint position for the paretic wrist and hand, and the ankle and foot. These splints can be fashioned easily and inexpensively in the hospital occupational therapy department. Splints can also be made of "lite cast" material or from plaster of Paris. Inexpensive splints can be obtained commercially. When such devices are used, care should be taken to examine the skin frequently, and the devices should be padded to prevent excessive tissue pressure.

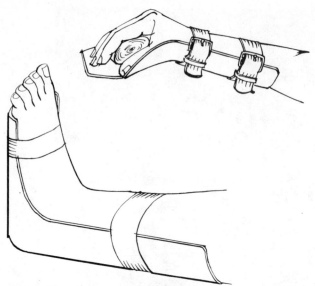

**Figure 3–3.** Wrist and foot splints. (From Luckman, J. and Sorenson, K.: Medical-Surgical Nursing: A Psychophysiologic Approach. Philadelphia, W. B. Saunders Co., 1980, p. 584.)

There are some additional measures that will improve the comfort of the stroke patient while in bed. Synthetic sheepskin is available for use as a bed pad. Heel and elbow protectors made with this material are also available. These products will protect the patient's skin from abrasion and will add to the patient's comfort. *However, under no circum-*

*stance will they relieve pressure or reduce the need for frequent position change or elevation of the patient's heels from the mattress.*

Pressure on the sacrum can be better distributed if the patient lies on an antidecubital gel pad, an alternating air mattress, or a water mattress. Again, it must be emphasized that pressure has not been eliminated but only more evenly distributed. Therefore, these products must be viewed only as adjuncts to the care of the patient, which still requires that pressure be minimized and *position changed frequently.* A more detailed approach to prevention of decubitus ulcers can be found in Chapter 6.

The stroke patient should be taught to change positions or encouraged to participate in changing position as soon as possible. Patients find it easy to turn onto the paretic side and this is one of their favored positions. They should be also encouraged to turn onto their unaffected side. This change in position will require supervision or assistance by the nurse, at least in the early attempts. To turn onto the unaffected side, the patient is instructed to bring the paretic arm across the chest using the unaffected hand. The unaffected foot is tucked under the paretic foot. The patient then grasps the side rail or edge of the bed with the unaffected hand and pulls the shoulders and upper trunk toward the unaffected side. Simultaneously, the patient turns both hips and legs toward the unaf-

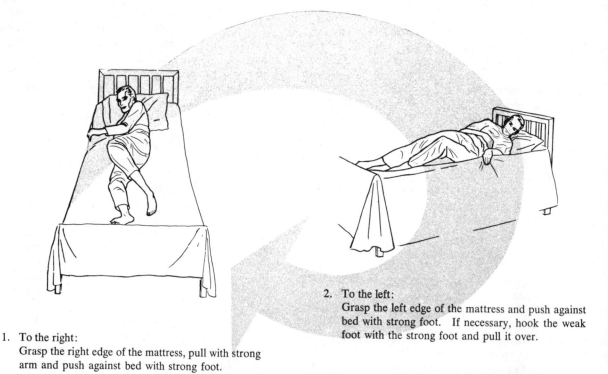

1. To the right:
   Grasp the right edge of the mattress, pull with strong arm and push against bed with strong foot.

2. To the left:
   Grasp the left edge of the mattress and push against bed with strong foot. If necessary, hook the weak foot with the strong foot and pull it over.

**Figure 3–4.** Patient turning in bed. (The terms in the illustration are appropriate for a lay audience and the illustration was taken from a teaching publication.) (From Up and Around, American Heart Association, p. 7.)

fected side. The paretic leg is moved passively by the action of the unaffected leg and foot.

The participation of patients in their care cannot be emphasized strongly enough. If they are able to contribute to the team effort of their care, they will begin to see the possibility for personal independence. Assisting in bed activities is an important step in this direction.

## EXERCISES

The stroke patient and the family should be made aware that the nursing actions are designed to provide for the patient's maximum recovery. Encouraging patient activity at the earliest possible time demonstrates this positive approach to the patient's situation. Unless contraindicated by the physician, passive joint range of motion for the paretic extremities and active joint range of motion for the unaffected extremities should be performed from the day the patient is admitted to the hospital. These exercises can be incorporated into many of the nursing tasks for the patient and performed, for example, when the extremities are moved during bathing and change of position. At this point, the physician, physical therapist, and the nurse should all be involved in the development, implementation, and evaluation of the patient's exercise program. Factors to be considered in any exercise program include pre-existing as well as current restrictions or limitations altering the usual range of motion, pain, spasticity, the patient's level of consciousness and comprehension, as well as endurance and fatigue levels.

As soon as possible, the patient is instructed in exercises for the paretic extremities. Initially, the nurse will provide the passive exercise for the paretic extremities. The patient is encouraged to actively exercise the unaffected extremities. Once the patient has become familiar with the normal joint range of motion, the nurse can begin instructing him on those passive joint range of motion exercises that he can perform. The nurse will reinforce the patient's role and responsibility in maintaining joint mobility through a daily program of self-exercises. These exercises should be performed at least three to four times a day. A gentle massage with a mild skin lotion can accompany the daily exercises. These activities provide an excellent opportunity to focus the patient's attention on the paretic side, which many stroke patients tend to ignore or deny.

Although full joint range of motion is the optimal goal for the exercises, care must be taken to avoid moving the joint beyond the limits of its usual range or in an abnormal pattern of motion. In addition to providing a demonstration of joint range of motion exercises that the patient can perform, the health professional should provide the patient with written instructions and, if possible, pictures of the desired exercises. A graph or exercise chart can be left at the patient's bedside and as each exercise is completed, this can be indicated on the chart. This provides a data flow sheet for quick reference; it also can be used to motivate the patient by marking progress and achievement.

## MOBILITY

Preparation for mobility begins with maintaining sitting balance. Some stroke patients will spontaneously regain trunk balance; however, the majority require some retraining in maintaining trunk balance. In a large number of patients this requires overcoming the listing phenomenon, which is seen as the trunk leans toward the paretic side when the patient is sitting upright without support or assistance. Normal symmetrical trunk posture in the sitting position can be facilitated by using several techniques.

Before any techniques are employed the patient should be assured that the nurse and or the physical therapist will protect him from falling. In fact, unless the listing is stopped, the patient will indeed fall to the paretic side.

Eliciting trunk balancing response is best achieved if the stroke patient is sitting on a straight-backed chair. The paretic arm is cradled by the unaffected arm as the patient grasps the elbow of the paretic arm with the unaffected hand and rests the paretic arm and hand on the unaffected arm. Optimally, the nurse and the therapist stand on each side of the patient. The patient is then gently pushed off balance laterally, first to one side and then to the other. The nurse and the therapist check the patient's fall but the patient is instructed and encouraged to attempt to regain trunk balance as soon as the push is felt. Particular attention should be paid to pushing the patient off balance toward the paretic side.

The balancing response can also be evoked in the backward and forward direction. The nurse and the therapist stand behind and in front of the patient. At first, the person behind the patient should lightly touch his shoulders to reassure him that he will not be permitted to fall completely backward. Gradually, the lateral and forward push can be more forceful and given without warning in order to improve the patient's balancing response.

Trunk stabilization and balance can be further improved by trunk bending and trunk rotating techniques. The stroke patient sits on a straight-backed chair and supports the paretic arm as in the trunk balancing technique. The nurse or physical

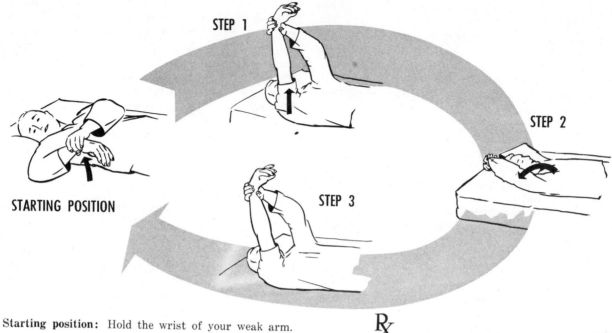

Starting position: Hold the wrist of your weak arm.

Step 1. Lift the hand up.

Step 2. Carry the hand back alongside your head.

Step 3. Lift the hand up and carry it forward to the starting position and repeat the exercise.

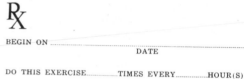

℞

BEGIN ON .............................................
DATE

DO THIS EXERCISE ............... TIMES EVERY ............... HOUR(S)

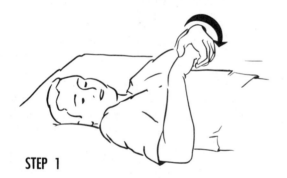

STEP 1

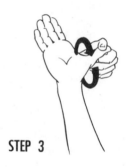

STEP 3

Step 1. Bend the fingers into the palm. Then bend the hand forward.

Step 2. Open the hand, straighten the fingers, pull the hand back keeping the fingers straight and repeat.

Step 3. Move the thumb in a circle.

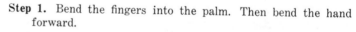

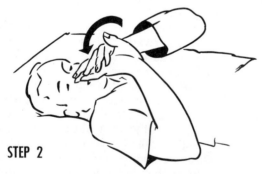

STEP 2

℞

BEGIN ON .............................................
DATE

DO THIS EXERCISE ............... TIMES EVERY ............... HOUR(S)

Figure 3–5. Joint range of motion exercises. (The terms in the illustration are appropriate for a lay audience and the illustration was taken from a teaching publication.) (From Strike Back at Stroke, American Heart Association. A, p. 23, B, p. 28, C, p. 29.)

Illustration continued on opposite page.

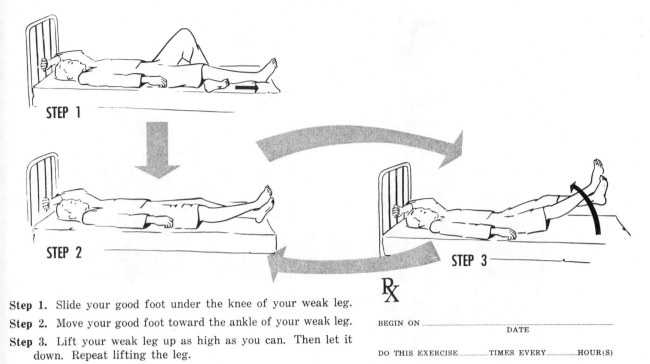

**Step 1.** Slide your good foot under the knee of your weak leg.

**Step 2.** Move your good foot toward the ankle of your weak leg.

**Step 3.** Lift your weak leg up as high as you can. Then let it down. Repeat lifting the leg.

**Figure 3–5** *Continued*

℞

BEGIN ON ................................................................
DATE

DO THIS EXERCISE..............TIMES EVERY..............HOUR(S)

therapist sits or stands facing the patient and guides the trunk forward by grasping the patient's elbows. The patient is continuously focused on controlling the trunk posture. Gradually, the patient may be able to perform the technique without assistance. The nurse should, however, always supervise the patient and maintain a safe environment. If the patient gains sufficient trunk control, he can be instructed to perform the trunk bending technique in the forward left oblique pattern and the forward right oblique pattern.

Trunk rotation is accomplished with the patient sitting and supporting the paretic arm as before. Since some swing motion is involved in this technique, the patient is instructed to maintain a firm grasp on the elbow of the paretic arm.

The nurse faces the patient and supports the trunk. The patient is told to rotate the trunk first to the left side and then to the right in a rhythmic fashion. The patient should return to the neutral position before rotating to the opposite side.

As greater balance is achieved the patient assumes more independence in performing the techniques. The nurse and the patient and the patient's family should mark each achievement and share in the pleasure of the patient's progress.

Getting out of bed is an important step in the rehabilitation process of the stroke patient. It provides relief from bedbound activities, reduces the risks associated with continuous, prolonged bed rest and improves the patient's morale by expanding the horizons of his environment.

Another important gain associated with getting out of bed is that it facilitates bladder and bowel functions. Because complete emptying of the bladder and ease of bowel evacuation are impeded by using a bedpan in bed, one of the first transfers to be attempted should be from the bed to the bedside commode. It is suggested that whenever possible (day and night) the patient be permitted to use the bedside commode or bathroom for bladder and bowel functions. Other transfers for the stroke patient include transfers to and from the wheelchair and the stationary chair, since the former provides a means of mobility and the latter will be used for trunk balancing exercises.

There are a number of physical and safety factors associated with transfer activities to be considered for every stroke patient with hemiparesis and possible visual and perceptual deficits. Before any transfer is attempted the patient's tolerance for sitting up and standing should be assessed. A baseline blood pressure reading should be taken and a pulse rate determination should be made. After the patient has sat at the edge of the bed for a few minutes the blood pressure and pulse should be taken. If the patient is markedly hypertensive or hypotensive or if the pulse rate and rhythm deviate significantly from the baseline, the physician needs to evaluate the patient's status before further activities are begun. If the patient tolerates this activity, progressively independent transfer activities can be instituted.

A sling is not recommended to support the pa-

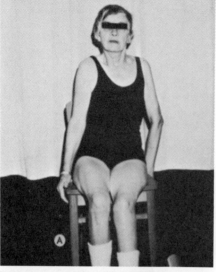
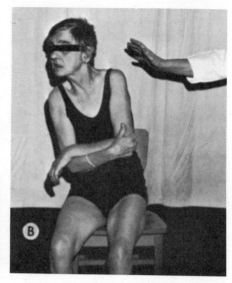
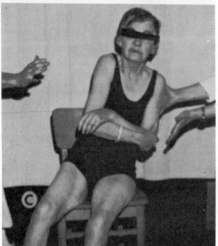

Figure 3–6. Sitting trunk balance. (From Brunnstrom, S.: Movement Therapy in Hemiplegia. Hagerstown, Harper and Row, 1970, p. 61.)

retic arm and hand unless there is a significant risk of subluxation of the shoulder caused by gravitational pull in the presence of flaccid paralysis. Once there is evidence of even a small degree of spasticity in the arm, use of the sling should be discontinued. If a sling is employed it should be worn only during transfer or ambulation activities. When the transfer or ambulation is completed, the sling should be removed. Whether the patient is resting in bed or sitting in a chair, the paretic hand, arm, and shoulder are supported best by the proper placement of an adequate number of pillows.

The knee and ankle joints of the paretic leg are usually unstable, particularly during the flaccid period, and the nurse should brace this knee and foot with her leg during any transfer.

Because of the neurological deficits from a stroke, the patient's paretic foot tends to slip forward during the transfer. Using rubber-soled slippers or shoes will help to reduce this sliding effect.

An important point to remember and to teach the patient, whether he is transferring to or from the bed, wheelchair, commode, or stationary chair, is that the unaffected side moves first in the transfer. Movement, therefore, is always in the direction of the unaffected side. It should be noted that during a transfer the stroke patient is basically pivoting on one foot, the unaffected foot, and that the general direction of movement is controlled by the unaffected limbs.

Although transfer activities for stroke patients may be the responsibility of the physical therapist, the nurse frequently assumes the responsibility of assisting the patient to transfer as well as teaching him safe methods of transferring. The stroke patient should not be permitted to transfer alone or unsupervised unless and until the nurse is certain that a correct and safe transfer has been learned. It is recommended that the patient demonstrate the learned transfer rather than verbally assuring the nurse because following a stroke the patient's ability to judge may be impaired. This is particularly

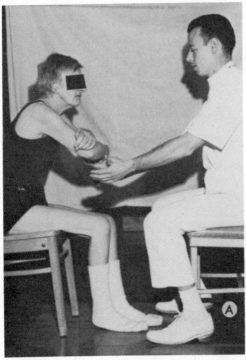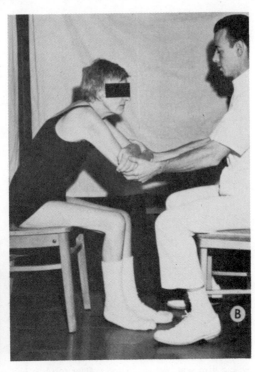

**Figure 3–7.** Trunk bending. (From Brunnstrom, S.: Movement Therapy in Hemiplegia. Hagerstown, Harper and Row, 1970, p. 62.)

true in patients following a right hemispheric infarction.

A brief review of the national statistics of accidents in health care institutions involving the elderly in general and stroke patients in particular confirms the need for vigilance for these patients' safety by all professionals caring for them. It is wise to alert family members to any alterations in the patient's cognitive and judgment abilities so that they too will be mindful of his safety needs. The nurse will identify the specific risk factors and the various methods that the family should employ to help prevent accidents and ensure a safe environment for the patient when he returns home.

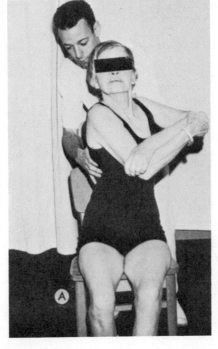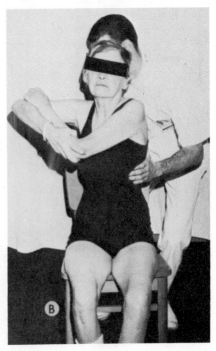

**Figure 3–8.** Trunk rotation. (From Brunnstrom, S.: Movement Therapy in Hemiplegia. Hagerstown, Harper and Row, 1970, p. 63.)

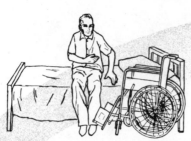

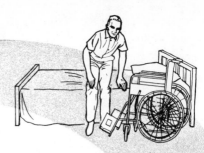

1. Place wheelchair at slight angle to bed, on patient's strong side, facing foot of bed. Keep the right front corner of the chair as close to the bed as possible as shown below.* Brakes locked. Footrests up.

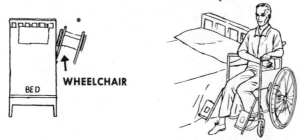

Note: An armchair can be used by the bed instead of a wheelchair. A chair that is heavy enough not to slide and with a firm seat that is not too soft or too low will be suitable.

2. Keep feet beneath body, lean forward placing strong hand near edge of bed and push to standing position keeping weight well over strong foot.

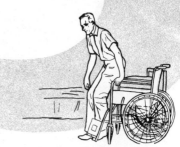

3. When standing position is steady enough for momentary release of support by strong hand, move strong hand to farther arm rest of wheelchair. Keeping body weight well forward, turn on strong foot and lower to sitting position.

1. Face wheelchair toward head of bed. Keep front corner of chair (on patient's strong side) as close to bed as possible as wheelchair is shown in No. 2. Position the wheelchair so the patient sits near the center of the bed, closer to the foot for a tall person. Lock brakes, lift foot rests.

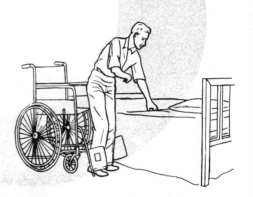

2. Assume standing position from wheelchair (as in Number 6).

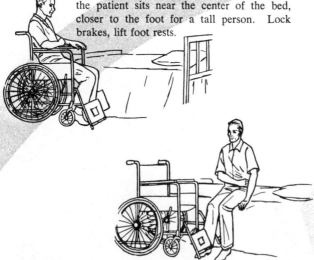

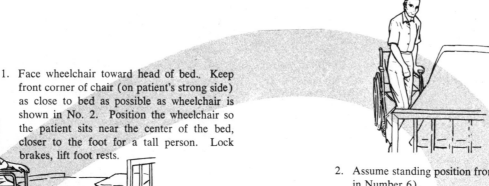

4. Lean forward, turn on strong foot and slowly lower to sitting position.

3. Move strong hand to edge of bed for support.

**Figure 3–9.** Transfer from a bed to a wheelchair. (The terms in the illustration are appropriate for a lay audience and the illustration is taken from a teaching publication.) (From Up and Around. American Heart Association, pp. 11 and 14.)

# AMBULATION

For some patients with limited recovery following a stroke mobility may be restricted to propelling the wheelchair using the unaffected arm and leg or using a one-arm drive wheelchair. Most patients, however, will be able to learn to walk following a stroke, and walking should be an appropriate goal for the rehabilitation of the stroke patient.

Preparation for walking begins with muscle-strengthening exercises, particularly of the quadriceps, and developing standing balance. Quadriceps exercises can be started while the patient is in bed and standing balance can be facilitated by using the tilt table. As soon as the patient can tolerate it, he can practice standing balance at the bedside by standing at the foot of the bed and holding onto the foot (or head) of the bed for support. Most stroke patients will develop an extensor reflex in the paretic leg that provides for sufficient knee extension to support their weight momentarily as the trunk weight is shifted from unaffected to paretic leg while walking.

To walk correctly, the patient must learn to bear full body weight on the paretic leg with the knee in a slightly fixed position. Frequently, the patient will hyperextend the knee as weight is shifted to the paretic leg, a stable but undesirable stance. The reverse can also be a problem. Until the patient learns to support full weight on the paretic leg, the knee may tend to buckle during weight bearing. The patient needs to practice shifting weight and relearn normal gait patterns. This is best taught using parallel bars; gradually the patient is able to shift greater amounts of body weight onto the paretic leg with the knee in slight flexion. The patient is instructed to keep the trunk forward over the feet.

If the paretic foot is too weak to prevent toe scraping, a dorsiflexion assist strap may be used to provide better positioning. In some cases the paresis may be severe enough to require short leg bracing to accomplish ambulation. In either case the patient should be able to learn to walk with minimal circumduction and appropriate heel-toe gait patterning. For those patients who have severe paresis or paralysis of the leg following a stroke, a long-leg brace will be necessary for ambulation.

Rhythmic gait training with reciprocal trunk and arm swing requires considerable re-education. This can be facilitated by the nurse or physical therapist walking in tandem with the patient, holding the patient's trunk. Another approach is for the nurse to walk next to the patient's unaffected side holding both of the patient's hands so that their arms cross over each other. The nurse and patient establish a similar cadence and the nurse is then able to support the patient and assist him in shifting his weight from one leg to the other.

Some, but not all, patients respond to rhythm in music. A melody played or hummed at an appropriate rate can frequently establish a gait rhythm for the patient in an effective and enjoyable manner. Some dance music is particularly helpful for the stroke patient in relearning normal rhythms. However, very fast rhythms and loud music are disturbing to the patient and may prove to be counterproductive by agitating him and increasing spasticity. The patient's response to music should be carefully evaluated and it should be used or not used according to each individual's response.

Safety remains a concern, especially during ambulation. The patient who has homonymous hemianopia must learn to scan the environment by turning his head completely to the left and right in order to see the total visual field. Also, if visual perceptual deficits exist, the visual field may appear to the patient to be tilted 15 degrees counter-clockwise. The patient needs to be taught to adjust to the alteration in perception. Depth perception may also be altered. The patient needs to learn other visual cues to compensate for these visual deficits. The family and patient can be taught to use contrasting colors and object size as cues to assist in compensation for visual deficits when the patient returns to the home. For example, painting door frames and door handles in contrasting colors will decrease miscalculation of distances. Using different color carpet sections on the alternating steps will aid in stair climbing. Increasing the lighting throughout the home will also improve the safety of the patient's environment.

Stair climbing depends a great deal on the degree of the neurological deficits of the patient and the condition of the stairs to be climbed. In this instance the patient's ability as well as cardiac status need to be carefully evaluated because of the physical strain of the activity.

Banisters on one or both sides of the stairs are extremely helpful. In the absence of banisters, the patient can use a cane or can climb or descend on his buttocks, one step at a time. The important point in stair climbing is that the patient's unaffected foot always leads when ascending the stairs and the paretic foot always leads when descending.

# NUTRITION

Providing adequate nutrition for the stroke patient is a complex situation because of the presence of a number of factors besides the patient's limited ability to manage the physical functions associated with eating. Consideration must be given to the patient's lifelong eating pattern and cultural food preferences, as well as to provision of sufficient nutrients to match the patient's energy requirements while the medically prescribed dietary restrictions and/or additions are adhered to.

Following a stroke some patients develop partial paralysis of the mouth, tongue, and throat, which causes some degree of difficulty in swallowing (dysphagia). This condition is frequently compounded because of altered or diminished sensations in the areas of partial paralysis. The patient's fear of choking or aspirating, therefore, is a significant factor to be considered in the effective management of dysphagia.

The patient should be assessed to determine the presence and degree of dysphagia. Classical signs are drooling, pocketing of food in the paralyzed side of the mouth, food getting stuck in the throat, choking and coughing while swallowing, and regurgitating if the patient lies down after eating. If the patient demonstrates poor protection of the airway while swallowing by coughing or aspirating and exhibits only marginal pharyngeal swallow function, successful treatment of the dysphagia is questionable and alternative methods of feeding, such as tube feeding or gastrostomy feeding, should be explored. Those stroke patients who are alert, with functional airway protection mechanisms and who can swallow voluntarily or in response to stimulation will generally respond quite well to techniques to manage dysphagia.

Whenever the patient is to be fed the nurse should provide a quiet, relaxed atmosphere and should approach the patient in a calm and unhurried manner. When possible the family should be instructed in the specific techniques that are successful with the patient; as the program progresses, they may be included in appropriate teaching sessions. For eating or drinking, the patient should always sit fully erect, whether in bed or in a chair, with his head slightly flexed; this facilitates swallowing. In order to reduce the possibility of regurgitation the patient should sit up for at least 30 minutes after eating.

The nurse and patient should focus on one of the three phases (biting, chewing, swallowing) of the eating process at a time. The swallow phase is usually dealt with first. Thus, food that requires little or no chewing is given so that the patient can concentrate on swallowing. A half-filled teaspoon of food (such as applesauce) should be placed on the midback portion of the patient's tongue. Once the food has been deposited on the patient's tongue the patient is instructed to move the food to the back of the tongue and swallow. As the patient swallows, his hand should gently rest against his throat to confirm that he is able to swallow.

Once the patient is able to swallow effectively, chewing activities can be started. Easily chewed foods such as cheese and sliced fruit should be introduced first. Foods should be chewed on the unaffected side of the mouth so that the patient can re-establish the normal rotary chewing pattern. Finally, the biting phase is focused on. Easily incised foods should be used in initiating this aspect of the eating process. Toast, fruit, and soft foods should precede the more difficult foods such as sliced meats.

Even though the patient may satisfactorily progress in eating, foods that are difficult to chew or swallow such as tough meats, stringy vegetables, and fruits with pits should be avoided. Milk and milk products tend to bond with the patient's saliva and increase its tenaciousness, which will make swallowing more difficult. It is best for the patient to avoid taking milk alone in the early training process. After eating, the patient's mouth should be examined for pocketed food, and the teeth (natural or dentures) should be cleaned.

As soon as the nurse is certain that the patient will not aspirate fluids, he should be encouraged to drink. The nurse should start by placing water on a spoon in the front of the patient's mouth behind the teeth. Once the patient learns to handle water without dribbling or aspirating, he can progress to drinking from a glass. For drinking as well as eating, the patient should be sitting fully erect with the head slightly flexed. The glass of liquid should never be more than half empty so that the patient can keep the head slightly flexed. A dysphagic patient tends to aspirate more readily if he tilts his head back to drink from a glass.

If the patient has difficulty sealing the rim of the glass with his lips, the liquid will run out the side of his mouth. In this situation the patient can learn to drink using a toddler drinking cup with a lid and drinking spout; this is helpful in eliminating dribbling of the liquid. Sucking through a straw requires considerable muscle function of the mouth; if straws are to be used they should be short, of large diameters, and bendable.

The use of a syringe for feeding the stroke patient is not recommended. If the patient's lack of awareness and functional disability are such that proper nutrition cannot be supplied with assistance, he is at risk for aspiration. The use of a feeding syringe only increases that risk, and other feeding methods should be used.

Finally, all nurses involved in feeding activities for the stroke patient with dysphagia should be familiar with the Heimlich maneuver in case the patient chokes on food. The nurse should also be familiar with the signs of aspiration and should teach the family the signs of choking and aspiration and appropriate methods of intervention. This should be taught in such a way as not to frighten the family. They should be assured that even in the event of choking they can handle the situation.

Self-feeding is an activity of daily living that can give the patient a sense of independence. Even if the dominant side is paretic, the patient can learn to feed himself using one hand with the assistance of devices and techniques.

A rocker knife can be used to cut meat with one hand. If a rocker knife is unavailable, the patient can be taught to cut meat by using the blade of a regular knife. Plate guards are inexpensive and can be attached to most plates. This allows the patient to push the food against the guard and onto the utensil. Double-headed suction cups keep plates and dishes stabilized and right-angled ledges hold bread, which can be buttered by one hand. There are numerous devices that are available to assist the patient in feeding as well as the other activities of daily living. The American Heart Association (local chapters), Institute of Rehabilitation Medicine (New York City), and the Sister Kenny Institute (Chicago) are known for their publications on devices and resources for the disabled.

The patient and the family must be prepared for the awkwardness and frustration of learning to eat with one hand, especially if it is the nondominant extremity. Spills and mishaps will characterize the early eating trials, and the patient and family will need to expect and accept these as usual events in the educative process.

Persistence, acceptance, calmness, and a sense of humor are necessary ingredients to the success of any aspect of the rehabilitation program. The patient, family, and rehabilitation professionals need to share these qualities as they strive for their common goal. Since eating has such a strong psychosocial aspect associated with it, it provides a unique opportunity for all the team members to share in the patient's accomplishments in an atmosphere in which the emphasis can be social and personal rather than institutional and medical.

## ELIMINATION

Following a stroke the most common bladder problems are frequency and urgency. If the patient is incontinent of urine it is usually because of decreased awareness, mild confusion, and an inability to reach appropriate toilet facilites in the face of urinary urgency. Urgency, frequency, and stress incontinence are bladder problems frequently encountered in the aged female, and perceptual and cognitive deficits from a stroke will only heighten these problems. Older men may be experiencing bladder problems from benign prostatic hypertrophy that may be further complicated by the neurological deficits resulting from the stroke.

Usually an indwelling catheter is inserted into the bladder during the acute phase of the stroke. Once the acute phase is over, the catheter should be removed and the patient is catheterized intermittently until the residual urine is less than 100 cc.

From the initial trial voiding the patient should use the commode or toilet in order to enhance emptying the bladder completely. Voiding attempts should be made every two hours. As continence improves the time between voiding can be increased to four hours. Restricting fluids at bedtime will reduce the risk of nocturnal incontinence, especially if the patient is confused or slightly disoriented at night.

The most common bowel problem of the stroke patient is constipation. Since many stroke patients are also hypertensive or have cardiovascular dis-

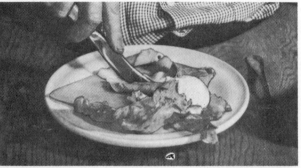
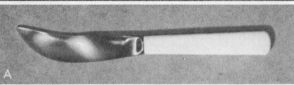
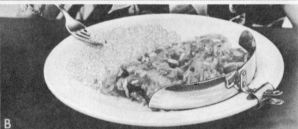
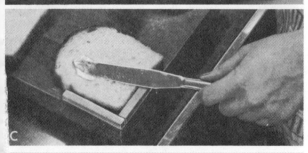
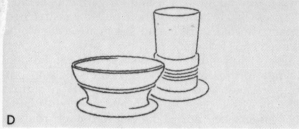

**Figure 3–10.** Eating assistance devices. A, Rocker knife; B, plate guard; C, Right-angled ledge; D, suction cups. (From Do It Yourself Again. American Heart Association, 1965, p. 9.)

ease, it is important that they avoid straining to have a bowel movement because the associated increase in blood pressure may precipitate another infarction.

A good bowel routine includes adequate fluid intake and a diet with sufficient residue to enhance bowel function (see Chapter 22). Stool softeners may be ordered to improve elimination. Elimination will be facilitated by inserting a glycerine suppository in the rectum about 30 minutes before the time desired for a bowel movement. If necessary, laxatives and enemas can be used, but caution should be exercised so that the patient does not rely on these methods as the only means to achieve regular bowel function.

The patient's bathroom at home may need some alterations to assist in use of the toilet. A hand rail may be installed next to the toilet (attached to the wall or floor) to assist the patient sitting down on and raising up from the toilet. Most toilet seats are too low to be managed easily by the stroke patient with hemiparesis. Raised toilet seats (available in various heights) may be easily added to the existing toilet. These simple bathroom adaptations will be very important to the patient's independence in elimination when he returns home.

## BATHING

Some patients need to learn how to bathe using only one hand. There are several ways this can be managed. Since the patient has only one hand to manage the soap and washcloth, the soap should be stationary. It can be attached to the wall with suction devices near the tub, shower, or sink; the patient soaps the washcloth by rubbing it against the stationary bar of soap. A number of pump soap dispensers are now commercially available. Soap pumps can be hand or foot operated. Using a terrycloth mitten is often easier than a washcloth. These mittens can be purchased or sewn easily. A sponge rubber bath brush with a soap pocket is also available. This brush is easy to use and, in effect, helps to extend the patient's reach for washing the back, legs, and feet. A terrycloth robe is an excellent help for drying after a bath or shower and reduces the risk of chilling, especially in cold weather.

For the stroke patient, safety in the bathroom should be a paramount consideration. Whenever possible the patient's bathroom should be evaluated for protective and assistive adaptations prior to discharge.

All faucets should be changed so that the mixture of hot and cold water emerges from one tap. If the patient has some sensory alteration he should be instructed to always test the water temperature with his unaffected hand.

Bathing activities for the patient with hemiparesis can best be performed in a stall shower with a shower stool or chair. A bar can be mounted on the wall of the shower to help the patient. Nonskid strips should be added to the floor of the shower to minimize slipping. Using a bathtub is more difficult and more dangerous for the stroke patient. It is advised that the patient have someone present to assist in moving in and out of the shower. It is mandatory for a person to assist the stroke patient moving in and out of the tub. Nonskid strips should be placed on the bottom as well as on the edge of the tub.

If the hemiparesis is significant, it is not recommended that the patient sit on the bottom of the tub because it is too difficult to lower and raise the body to this degree. Instead, a shower stool or chair should be placed in the tub for the patient to sit on. A portable shower or spray shower can be attached to any existing tub fixtures to be used for bathing.

As many handrails or assist bars as are necessary should be added to the tub and the walls next to the tub to assist the patient in getting in and out of it. If the patient can climb into the tub a detachable bar can be mounted on its edge. The important point to remember is that the assist bars should be mounted in a way that the patient can reach and use them from any position he may assume either sitting in the tub or moving into or out of it.

## DRESSING

Dressing can be accomplished by the stroke patient with hemiparesis as long as certain adaptations to singlehandedness and thoughtful clothing selections are made. (See the appendix to Chapter 13 on arthritis for adaptations that might be used for the stroke patient.)

The hemiparetic patient should wear garments with front closures. Zippers and Velcro closures are the most easily managed. Larger buttons are better than smaller ones. The patient may find that using clothing, especially shirts and blouses, a size or two larger than customary will be less cumbersome when dressing with the paretic arm. Material that gives should be selected for garments because it is less likely to tear when pulled or stretched. Elastic-waisted dresses and slacks are a wonderful convenience for women.

There are a number of devices that can be used as aids to dressing. Stocking holders help in putting on socks and nylon hose. Elastic on buttons eliminates the need to open and close shirt cuffs. Suspenders can replace the belt for men's trousers. Elastic shoe laces eliminate the need to tie and untie shoes. Shoes can also be laced with one hand if the patient receives proper instruction. Clothes

# SAFETY TIPS:

Getting into the tub
or shower

1. USE HELP!
2. TEST TEMPERATURE OF WATER WITH THE STRONG HAND!
3. WHEN IN TUB OR SHOWER, SIT ON A CHAIR WITH A BACK.
4. Rubber suction mat or safety tread tape can be used in the bottom of the tub to prevent slipping.
5. Grab bar on wall at side and head of tub.
6. Use a safety rail to fit on outside of tub.
7. Sit on side of tub while lifting legs into tub.
8. Use flexible shower hose.
9. Dry self and tub before getting out of tub.
10. Keep bathroom floor dry to prevent slipping.

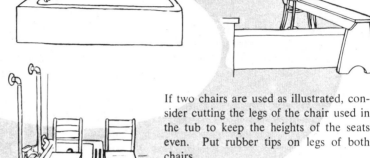

Detachable Bar

Various grab
bar suggestions

Hints for installing grab bars:
1. Place within reach of the patient for getting into as well as out of tub.
2. Fasten securely to the wall.
3. Place bar far enough out from wall for easy grasp.
4. Use bars made of rustproof metal.

If two chairs are used as illustrated, consider cutting the legs of the chair used in the tub to keep the heights of the seats even. Put rubber tips on legs of both chairs.
(This drawing was adapted from the booklet "Rehabilitation Nursing Techniques—1" published by the Kenny Rehabilitation Institute, Minneapolis, Minnesota.)

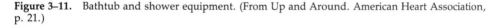

**Figure 3–11.** Bathtub and shower equipment. (From Up and Around. American Heart Association, p. 21.)

with big pockets are helpful for carrying small objects, money, and personal effects. Pocketbooks with shoulder straps should be used to keep the functional hand free. Adaptations for dressing are numerous and reflect the creative problem-solving approach of the occupational therapist and the stroke patient and family. Each patient will learn certain adaptations that meet specific needs and reflect personal taste and style preferences.

There are a number of companies that sell adaptive devices and clothing that would be particularly helpful to the stroke patient and family. A few such companies are listed at the end of the chapter.

It is important to teach the patient that the paretic extremities are always dressed or undressed first. The unaffected hand actually dresses the paretic extremities.

Slacks, trousers, and shirts should be put on while the patient is lying in bed. It is safer and easier to put these clothes over the legs and raise the buttocks lying in bed than sitting up. Shirts, blouses, and jackets should be spread on the patient's lap with the collar away from the body as the patient sits on the edge of the bed. The paretic hand is placed into the armhole and the sleeve is pulled up to the shoulder for the paretic arm using the unaffected arm. The rest of the garment is thrown behind the patient's back. The patient then reaches behind his back with the unaffected arm and puts his unaffected arm in the sleeve and then works the garment into proper position. The process is simply reversed to remove the garment (see Chapter 1).

Learning to dress using these techniques requires practice, energy, and patience. The patient and family should be instructed and should see a demonstration of the techniques. *Up and Around,* a teaching booklet on activities of daily living for the stroke patient, is available from the American Heart Association and is an excellent guide.

## COMMUNICATIONS

Stroke patients with an infarction in the dominant cerebral hemisphere, usually the left, will have dysphasia to some degree. Historically, dysphasia has been thought to be entirely receptive, a loss of ability to understand language, or expressive, a loss of the ability to speak. Clinically, the dysphasia following a stroke is a mixture of both decreased comprehension and speech reduction with a predominating receptive or expressive character to the communication disorder. There are some severely aphasic patients, with global aphasia, who have lost both receptive and expressive language abilities.

Language dysfunction needs to be carefully evaluated by a speech pathologist who is qualified to diagnose and treat the dysphasic condition. The nurse, physician, and speech pathologist or speech therapist need to work closely with the patient and family if an effective communication system is to be developed. It is important to focus on effective communication rather than on speech alone because if language dysfunction persists or improves only marginally, other communication methods may need to be used.

Everyone involved with the stroke patient must appreciate the devastating effect that dysphasia has on a person who is part of a society so heavily invested in speech for transmitting thoughts and feelings and as a means for self-identification. After a stroke the patient may not know what has happened and because of expressive dysphasia may not even be able to ask the one question that will supply the necessary information. Or, if the patient has receptive dysphasia, his fears and concern cannot be relieved because he cannot comprehend an explanation of the stroke. The stroke patient with dysphasia is usually anxious and fearful and frustrated as a result of the inability to communicate. When this is added to the physical insult of the stroke and the alteration in emotions and sensory input, irritability, frustration, and depression are understandable behaviors in the situation.

Although the speech pathologist and speech therapist will institute the specific therapeutics to rehabilitate the patient's communication function, the nurse can help the patient by continuing and reinforcing the techniques prescribed for him. There are some suggestions for the nurse and family to use for the stroke patient that will improve communications.

If the patient is predominately receptively dysphasic, one should speak more slowly than usual, use a lower tone of voice, and repeat the statement several times. Observe the patient's response carefully because his speech and behaviors are important clues to the content of the communication. Also speak directly to the patient and allow him to watch your lips while speaking. Use common, simple, and descriptive words that clearly relate to the idea or content of your communication. Use the patient's name and touch the patient frequently to maintain his attention.

If the patient is predominately expressively dysphasic, great attention must be paid to understanding what he is trying to communicate. If the person cannot name an object, for example, then show him various objects or identify them and ask him if that is what he wants to say. Try to identify the content area or class first (food, clothing, body, emotions) and then try to identify the specifics of that content area: "Are you hungry? Do you want to change your clothes? Does your shoulder hurt? Are you unhappy?" Attempt to simplify the amount of language needed by the patient to respond. Use whatever devices will help the patient express himself, such as pointing to pictures of items, using name cards, or, if the patient is able, writing his requests or responses.

The nurse's most valuable contributions to establishing effective communications in dysphasia are a positive approach to the patient, an open acceptance of him and his limitations, demonstrated attempts to communicate with the patient, a willingness to listen to him, calmness, and an unhurried manner. Any attempt to help the patient communicate is important because it indicates to him that the nurse wants to share thoughts and feelings. The nurse should encourage the family to follow her example and should emphasize that expressions of love and affection such as kissing and touching are important and necessary parts of communications between the patient and family.

## CONCLUSION

Most stroke patients and their families need the support as well as the therapeutic interventions of the rehabilitation team in order to achieve goals of re-entry into society functioning at the maximum capacity and participating in life as fully as possible. A number of personal accounts have been published of patients and families who have survived the physical, emotional, and financial impact of a stroke and emerged strengthened by the experience. *Pat and Roald*, published by Random House, is the true story of actress Patricia Neal's recovery from a series of strokes. It is a story of a stroke patient, the patient's family, and the rehabilitation team and triumph over the challenge of physical disability. This is important literature for rehabilitation professionals and their stroke patients because its message documents the reality of hope.

## COMPANIES SELLING SPECIAL DEVICES AND CLOTHING

There are a number of companies that sell adaptive devices and clothing that would be particularly helpful to the stroke patient and family. A few such companies are:

Be OK Self Help Aides, Fred Sammons Inc.
P. O. Box 32
Brookfield, Illinois 60513

Downs and Company
1014 Davis St., Dept. 469
Evanston, Illinois 60204

Everest and Jennings Co.
1803 Pontius Ave.
Los Angeles, California

Fashion-ABLE
Rocky Hill, New Jersey 08553

MED Inc.
19701 S. First Ave.
Maywood, Illinois 60153

Miles Kimball
Kimball Building
Oshkosh, Wisconsin 54901

Rehab Aids
P.O. Box 612
Miami, Florida 33144

Rehabilitation Products
Division of American Hospital Supply
40–05 168th St.
Flushing, New York 11300

Spencer Gifts
455 Spencer Building
Atlantic City, New Jersey 08404

Sunset House
151 Sunset Building
Beverly Hills, California 90213

# 4

# Biofeedback and Behavioral Medicine

*by John V. Basmajian, M.D., F.A.C.A., F.R.C.P.(C)*

Three main scientific sources flowed together to form the broad stream that is modern biofeedback. The first of these arose from my work in electromyography (EMG) with a long series of colleagues and students at Queen's University between the years 1957 and 1969. We found that when our subjects were provided with instant visual and acoustic feedback of the EMG signals arising from invisible and unfelt contractions of their muscles, they could learn to perform elaborate tricks with the tiniest units of muscle: the motor units.

Motor units are each supplied by a single nerve cell in the spinal cord. Hence it became apparent that we were training conscious control of individual motor cells in the spinal cord, a feat then considered by most neurologists to be impossible. Equally important, our subjects could put a single cell through elaborate tricks while completely inhibiting the activities of the surrounding cells; they consciously relaxed all the muscle fibers in a muscle (or even a whole limb) while activating the target motor unit "in isolation."

Not only can human subjects "fire" single motor nerve cells with an active suppression or inhibition of neighbors, but they can also produce deliberate changes in the rate of firing. Most persons can do this if they are provided with aural (and visual) cues from their muscles by means of electromyography.

The word *biofeedback* was coined only a decade ago, but it represents a widespread and exciting concept: Given instant and continuous electronic displays of their internal physiologic events (by means of meters, banks of lights, and various au-

diting devices), human beings can be taught to manipulate those otherwise unsensed events voluntarily. Biofeedback as it is now being practised is a scientific technique rather than a separate science, but the basic concept has stimulated the beginnings of a probable revolution in medicine—the discipline of behavioral medicine. Behavioral medicine emphasizes the use of behavioral techniques, especially self-regulation (including biofeedback), for the treatment of a host of behavioral disturbances, ranging from "simple" obesity through recurring tension headaches to severe cardiovascular problems. Since these three categories account for more than half of all symptom-complexes seen by physicians, it is easy to predict that in the next few decades behavioral medicine will come to occupy a central place in treating sick people. Meanwhile, the technique of biofeedback has already permitted useful and occasionally dramatic cures of serious medical problems.

While the word biofeedback is new and unifying, the origins are older and diverse. It first appeared in 1969 with the formation of a then small society at Santa Monica, California, the Biofeedback Research Society (now the 2000-member Biofeedback Society of America). A group of investigators (most of whom barely knew each other but who recognized a common theme in their studies) gathered to discuss biological feedback mechanisms, especially in psychotherapy. For convenience (and against my objections), "biological feedback" in the society's name became "biofeedback." Then the society gave its new name back to the subject that gave it birth.

## PSYCHONEUROLOGICAL MECHANISMS

Is biofeedback training based on volition or is it operant conditioning similar to that shown for experimental animals by B. F. Skinner? The evidence from various groups is contradictory and reflects their commitment to or rejection of the operant conditioning paradigm. Certainly biofeedback training is related to it. Conditioning can clearly be employed in modifying electromyographic responses.

As the general biofeedback stream widened and deepened, it became apparent that the EMG or muscle feedback portion developed at Queen's University was the most directly useful clinically. There were two broad areas to which it could be, and soon was, applied: medical rehabilitation and general relaxation therapy.

Ever since World War II, clinical electromyographers (including myself) occasionally used the diagnostic device to train handicapped patients more rapidly. Perhaps the fortunate disappearance of paralytic poliomyelitis more than any other factor slowed down the application of EMG feedback. Thus little work of any consequence was done to train handicapped people with feedback until the late 1960s. Then, along with other forms of feedback therapy, medical rehabilitation became a field of especially active usage.

Various forms of brain damage (strokes and cerebral palsy) result in both partial paralysis and spasticity. A number of medical research groups soon began reporting the efficacy of training the motor functions of a substantial proportion of previously "untreatable" patients. No miracles were wrought, but patients were able to discover and use within themselves motor pathways that apparently had survived the injury and had lain dormant. Other disorders of movement and posture are now also proving to be treatable.

## STROKE REHABILITATION

In rehabilitating stroke patients with biofeedback, three major symptom complexes have been our targets: footdrop (with or without spasticity), shoulder subluxation, and reduced hand function. Immediately following onset there is a total loss of voluntary movement in the involved extremities accompanied by a loss or diminution in the tendon reflexes. The resistance to passive movement is decreased because of the flaccidity of muscles. Usually within 48 hours the tendon reflexes become more active and a minimal degree of increased resistance to passive movement is manifested, signaling the onset of spasticity in the muscles. This increased resistance to passive movement continues for five to ten days and, concurrently, tendon reflexes become brisker and clonus may appear.

At this point, spasticity and other signs of exaggerated proprioceptive responses are at a peak in their capacity to influence motor action. Typical flexion and extension synergies in both extremities become evident. Volitional activity appears first in the proximal and later in the distal muscles of the involved extremities. Initially, between the command and execution of movement, a latent period of about two to five seconds occurs. Similarly, relaxation does not take place immediately, generally requiring one to three seconds. With recovery, improvement becomes obvious in the complexity of movements, the decreased latency period between alternating movements, and the increased resistance to fatigue.

### Rehabilitation Techniques

In his challenging Sixth Annual Walter J. Zeiter Lecture to the American Academy of Physical Medicine and Rehabilitation, Frederick Kottke pointed out the cost in dollars and cents of dependency and institutionalization following stroke. The maintenance cost in a nursing home for the patient with a nonfunctioning hand who must be fed is increased by $2300.00 per year (in 1974 dollars). Even limited improvement in self-care produces a significant economic advantage. The greatest costs involving stroke victims are produced by the necessity of maintenance of the patient who survives in the dependent state. Simple calculations indicate that savings through rehabilitation are tremendous.

While physical therapy in the treatment of hemiplegia is generally advocated, both physiatrists and physical therapists have been criticized for failing to demonstrate that simple, functionally oriented patient care is inferior to elaborate, expensive rehabilitation programs. Even with this expensive arsenal, we find little apparent effect on recovery of the hemiplegic arm. Apart from the goals of helping the patient either to attain a comfortable mobile upper limb or to optimize his spontaneous recovery, we conclude that active intervention ("aggressive physical therapy") has had limited value. Unless a new and unique approach that has demonstrated effectiveness can be provided, the fate of upper limb function in almost all surviving stroke patients is bleak. The introduction of electromyographic biofeedback has given workers in stroke rehabilitation a new hope of changing the outlook for their patients.

### FOOTDROP

The first significant demonstration of the usefulness of electromyographic biofeedback came with the treatment of footdrop of hemiparetic patients (Figs. 4–1 and 4–2). For example, in our first series

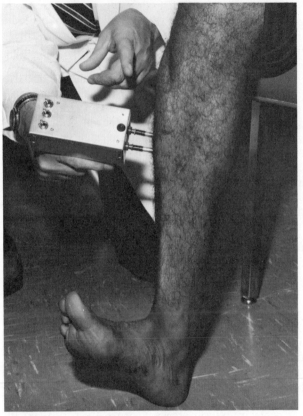

**Figure 4–1.** Portable EMG biofeedback device with probe electrodes for monitoring tibialis anterior activity and training dorsiflexion of the ankle.

of 25 patients 16 were able to discard their short leg brace entirely following 3 to 25 sessions (mean, 16.6 sessions). Each biofeedback rehabilitation training session lasted approximately one half hour. The remaining nine patients showed little or no improvement, sometimes for obvious reasons, such as poor motivation, severe spasticity, intercurrent illnesses, and early discontinuance of treatment. (Only three or four treatments were given in four of these nine patients.) Some of the patients

were even able to discard their canes for activities of daily living. Several now use their short leg braces intermittently when they are on their feet for long periods of time.

Fourteen patients with footdrop had reasonably good function at the ankle and had not been treated with braces. The aim of treatment was to produce sharp gains in function. After 3 to 17 sessions in biofeedback rehabilitation training, ankle function failed to improve in only two patients, while six had moderate to excellent improvement of strength and range of motion, which greatly improved their gait.

The patients' age apparently was not directly related to the effectiveness of biofeedback. Patients in both the 30- and the 60-year-old age groups were among those who discarded short leg braces. The proportion of men and women in whom treatment was successful was the same as in the general population studied. Neither failure nor success of treatment seemed related to the duration of footdrop. Failure occurred in patients with either recent or late stroke, while treatment was successful in patients who had had footdrop for periods ranging from three months to six and one half years.

Biofeedback for footdrop in the stroke patient is of undisputable value, especially if the patient is not confined to a chair and has mobility.

The neural pathways involved in this marked neuromotor improvement are unclear. There are two possibilities: either new pathways are developed (highly unlikely), or old persisting cerebral and spinal pathways are mobilized by introduction of the artificial feedback loop. The latter explanation is highly probable; the artificial internal awareness provided by acoustic and visual responses to a peripheral motor act appears to be a powerful reinforcer. Undoubtedly, new forms of cognition at the cortical level also are recruited. What is said about retraining paralyzed muscles is also apparently true of voluntary inhibition of spastic muscles.

In recent years, the process of motor learning and control has received increasing attention. Chil-

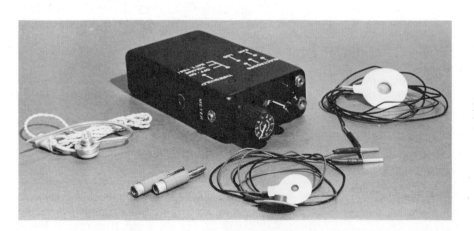

**Figure 4–2.** Miniature EMG device with electrodes and earphone for "private" acoustic signal if desired.

dren are born with a high level of anarchy in their motor control. As they mature, the overactivity disappears; it is absent in healthy adults. It appears in adults under psychological stress, but people can be trained to inhibit it to varying degrees. In patients with diseases and injuries of the central nervous system the normal inhibition pattern is lacking; then mass responses from local stimulation of the motor nerve cells in the spinal cord result in an exaggerated mass response described as *spasticity*.

## Inhibition of Spasticity

The inhibition patterning would seem to come in part from obscure processes in diffuse centers on the cerebral cortex. Since inhibition is a central feature, one must consider the possibility that brain stem centers (and perhaps the cerebellum) are critically important in the imprinting of the learning. It is simplistic to consider a schema in which an impulse is started in a tiny area of the cerebral cortex and is then passed directly along a facilitatory path to a desired set of spinal motor cells. The motor learning process probably employs a nerve network, with the "main" pathway for motor activation being almost a small part of the whole.

Stroke patients who succeed in inhibiting marked peripheral spasticity apparently use surviving pathways that increase the inhibition of overactive spinal centers. Using an "override mechanism," they must be succeeding in damping even the influence of the powerful reflexes otherwise unrestrained. In any case, our patients are able to voluntarily move one muscle while inhibiting the usual hyperactivity.

Relaxation therapy too has a major application, both targeted and generalized, in managing stroke patients who obviously are under great emotional stress. Functional improvement can be gained in stroke patients with general biofeedback and deep relaxation, just as psychosomatic ailments can be improved in the neurologically intact patient.

### SHOULDER SUBLUXATION

The treatment of shoulder subluxation by biofeedback seems related to that just discussed, and yet it also involves a mechanism that is quite different. In this case, patients are trained to mobilize an area by the usual biofeedback technique, which in turn results in the restoration of a passive (but effective) function of a joint. Much superior to the usual treatment of subluxation by the use of slings, this treatment technique relies on an understanding of normal anatomy. This permits the reversal of the sad effects of previous neglect of simple biomechanics.

The strategy in treating stroke patients who have a subluxed shoulder joint depends on remobilization of the scapula as well as the glenohumeral joint. Feedback from EMG electrodes on the upper trapezius (for elevation of the "lateral angle" of the scapula), and middle and anterior fibers of deltoid is emphasized. These muscles are easily monitored and relate to movements the patient understands.

After applying the electrodes, the therapist starts by asking the patient to attempt a shrugging of both shoulders with or without resistance. The acoustic response of the biofeedback equipment is obvious to the patient even if movement is minimal (or perhaps absent). Then work is concentrated on abduction of the shoulder (middle deltoid) because this automatically recruits scapular rotation upward caused by many other muscles. Subluxation is the result of the drooping lateral angle, that is, the glenoid cavity. By repeated sessions of exercise with biofeedback reinforcement, the therapist helps the patient to restore the normal scapular orientation with a resultant elimination of subluxation in more than half of all patients treated.

### HAND FUNCTION

Much of the problem in hand function is not simply the obvious paralysis; muscle spasticity is equally disabling. Combining inhibition training with neuromotor retraining of the weak hand and forearm muscles seems a logical approach—at present the only approach. It is being thoroughly investigated in many clinics.

As pointed out by Baker in *Biofeedback, Principles and Practice for Clinicians*, a most consistent problem in the hemiplegic hand is flexor spasticity; this interferes with extension. Therapists find that monitoring the finger flexors with electrodes widely spaced is a good beginning. With improvement, electrodes may be placed much closer to monitor individual muscles. After mastering flexor spasticity, the patient starts to learn active extension.

Various physical therapy modalities (e.g., vibration) are used as reinforcers. Electrodes for pickup from the extensors are used as monitors for the voluntary contraction while electrodes over the flexors are used to monitor relaxation. Baker discusses the various strategies therapists employ in obtaining improvement in hand function. In our experience, hand function can be substantially improved, but no patient has had a cure of the hemiparetic hand. The reason for this seems to be that the primary Betz cells in area 4 that control fine finger movement are incapable of regeneration.

## Course After Surgical Restoration

Electrokinesiologic devices coupled with EMG biofeedback promise to greatly enhance the recov-

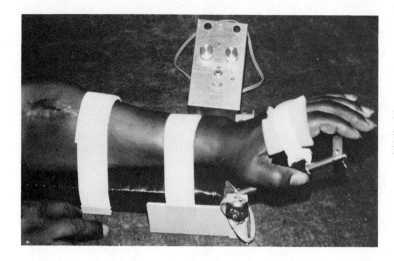

**Figure 4–3.** One form of biofeedback wrist electrogoniometer. (From Basmajian, J. V.: Biofeedback, Principles and Practice for Clinicians. Baltimore, Williams & Wilkins Co., 1979.)

ery of hands that have had trauma or surgery involving the tendons or nerves. Electrogoniometers, pressure transducers, and microswitches give patients instant and accurate feedback of their attempted responses. Still in the infancy stages of development, this approach to hand rehabilitation is gaining widespread use among occupational therapists who work in hand clinics (Figs. 4–3 to 4–7).

## MUSCLE RELAXATION THERAPY

The other main use of EMG biofeedback has been relaxation therapy. As unexciting as this training might appear, it has stimulated thousands of clinicians in several continents—mostly psychologists and psychiatrists—to apply biofeedback for the relief of various symptoms of stress. Tension headache, chronic back problems, and anxiety are prime targets, and the literature on their management with biofeedback relaxation is expanding rapidly, as evidenced by the many articles in the new journal *Biofeedback and Self-Regulation*. The main problem in this area is confusion about "placebo effects," always a bugbear in psychosomatic medicine. Nevertheless, many patients have received substantial benefit when all earlier treatments have proved ineffective. In volumes 1 and 2 of the aforementioned journal long-term success rates have been reported that are more than double the short-term placebo rates of 32 per cent cynically cited by critics for all novel treatments.

Relaxation training for the treatment of psychosomatic ailments actually predates biofeedback, going back a half-century to the work of Edmund Jacobson, who developed the technique known as *Progressive Relaxation*. In the 1920s and 1930s, Jacobson became the enthusiastic proponent of a

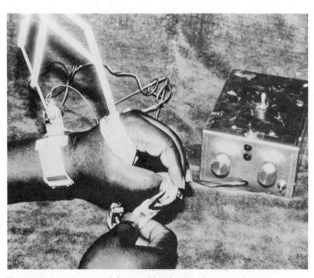

**Figure 4–4.** A second form of biofeedback wrist electrogoniometer. (From Basmajian, J. V.: Biofeedback, Principles and Practice for Clinicians. Baltimore, Williams & Wilkins Co., 1979.)

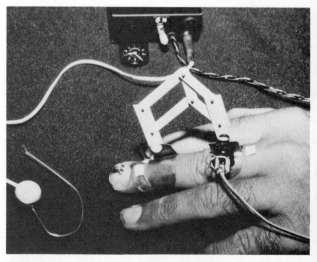

**Figure 4–5.** Finger electrogoniometer that feeds a biofeedback device. (From Basmajian, J. V.: Biofeedback, Principles and Practice for Clinicians. Baltimore, Williams & Wilkins Co., 1979.)

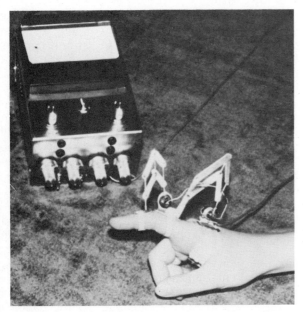

**Figure 4–6.** Double finger goniometer. (From Basmajian, J. V.: Biofeedback, Principles and Practice for Clinicians. Baltimore, Williams & Wilkins Co., 1979.)

clinical form of EMG biofeedback that has finally found new acceptance. Limited by the apparatus available at the time, Jacobson developed methods of electrical measurement of the muscular state of tension and employed these measurements to facilitate progressive somatic relaxation for a variety of psychoneurotic syndromes. Fortunately, in this decade he has seen the exuberant revival of his life's work along modern lines.

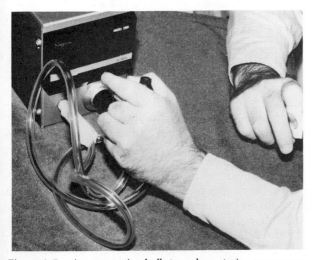

**Figure 4–7.** A compression-bulb transducer to improve grasp. Connected to the child's radio, it must be squeezed to keep the radio operating; hence it is a motivating device as well as a biofeedback device. (From Basmajian, J. V.: Biofeedback, Principles and Practice for Clinicians. Baltimore, Williams & Wilkins Co., 1979.)

Meanwhile in Germany, J. H. Schultz developed a technique, Autogenic Training, which is both similar and different. This method has been widely popularized by the Montreal physician Wolfgang Luthe. Biofeedback has simply provided an instrumental method to constantly monitor the level of relaxation achieved by the patient. To it must be added an improved style of daily living, which is practiced at home and at work. Other related self-regulation techniques such as Transcendental Meditation and the Relaxation Response (invented and publicized by Herbert Benson of Harvard) appear to have substantial benefits for many people.

Studies in many centers have shown that the EMG (among other parameters) is altered during relaxation. Relaxation is in some way associated with a controlled decrease in "arousal level," with retention of consciousness. A comparison of hypnotic suggestion and brief relaxation training showed the superiority of the latter in reducing subjective tension and distress.

## NONSPECIFIC EFFECTS

Only a naive person believes that nonspecific effects do not play an important part in the treatment of disabilities that are seen in a rehabilitation clinic. However, even an experienced physician may be surprised at the extent to which nonspecific effects become apparent in the treatment of patients with severe physical handicaps. The placebo response is not confined to patients with the usual types of psychosomatic ailments. It is found throughout all of physical medicine and it often is the most significant element in the treatment of patients with severe musculoskeletal problems.

Even before the appearance of biofeedback and similar therapeutic modes in the treatment of neurological disabilities, specialists in rehabilitation have known that many ailments are alleviated by the nonspecific effect. Especially in the hands of skilled therapists, the element of improvement through suggestion or other nonspecific effects has been an important part of physical therapy, occupational therapy, and related methods. Of course, rehabilitation does not stand alone in the use of, and even dependence on, the ancient art of suggestion for the improvement of illness.

The "magic" element in touching and manipulating the patient is a particularly powerful one in the rehabilitation clinic and may indeed surpass the effects of pills and injection. However, physicians have ignored rehabilitation techniques and have spent time in elaborating the concepts of pharmacology and related therapeutic methods. Organized medicine is gradually awakening to the need to evaluate the specific and nonspecific effects of occupational therapy and physical therapy.

This comes at a time when personnel in therapy groups themselves are anxiously seeking scientific answers. The problem is accentuated by the fact that practicing therapists generally have had little or no training in research or even intensive education in understanding the effects produced by what they do.

Many of the therapeutic methods used in rehabilitation have been developed and introduced by some authoritative or authoritarian clinical specialist and handed down to (or seized by) the therapists. The latter sometimes have accepted some of these procedures enthusiastically, especially if they have had a patina of scientific jargon attached to them. Thus over the past three or four decades, therapists have hopped from massage to manipulation to electrical and other physical treatments on the basis of the limited success of these various treatments. Each method in its time has been a great wonderment to many therapists and their patients. However, little advance research has been done before treatment systems are introduced; these systems have sometimes dominated activities in rehabilitation centers for many years before being abandoned. Today, therefore, many rehabilitation therapists have become skeptical about some methods while holding onto clinical approaches that succeed in their own hands.

## The Machine as Placebo

The nonspecific effects that we attach to placebo pills can also be produced by the milieu of the rehabilitation center and the various machines employed in it. In a rehabilitation setting the surroundings, the equipment, and the assured way in which therapists handle the equipment must have a strong and similar influence upon a patient. The effect may be achieved through a placebo effect or through improved compliance by the patient that enhances the therapeutic efficacy of the physical treatment.

In addition to the equipment, the attitude and the apparent skill of the therapist are essential in this placebo response. If the therapist appears to be knowledgeable of the procedures employed, confident, and (above all) comes in close contact with the patient, some success must occur in over 30 per cent of all patients with almost any treatment. If the therapist touches and manipulates the patient, this greatly enhances the effectiveness—regardless of whether the current fad treatment is carried out correctly or incorrectly. Hence many patients will recover from disabilities of the musculoskeletal system by having what is actually an "improper" manipulation or traction rather than the "proper" manipulation that happens to be advocated by some presently popular charismatic healer.

In this decade, transcutaneous electrical nerve stimulation and acupuncture are enjoying a special place as techniques of physical therapy. It appears that some successes are due to a specific effect; but for many cases it is quite obvious that the response is of a nonspecific nature because the techniques used by some therapists are quite eclectic and "unscientific." Further, the effects wear off at about the same rate as placebo response to placebo pill treatments wears off. After a week or two, the transcutaneous electrical stimulation loses its potency in most cases.

What about the serious ailments caused by clinically apparent lesions of the central nervous system and musculoskeletal system? It is beyond question that therapists in their clinical practice perform many training procedures that are highly effective—for example, gait training of amputees, stroke patients, and cerebral palsy patients. However, this is not really "therapy"; it is *re-education* of the innate capabilities retained by the patients who are actually doing the "therapy" (learning) themselves with the assistance of a trained teacher. That is education or re-education and I do not consider it to be therapy in the classical medical model. When physical therapists and occupational therapists are engaged in that kind of work, there still may be some overlay of placebo response because even education is subject to nonspecific effects. However, the main effect is one of learning rather than of therapy.

Complex modalities in which the therapist applies something to the patient such as heat and cold, water treatments, noninvasive internal deep therapies such as ultrasound and radiant energy in general, vibration, manipulation, and so on, probably have the highest placebo responses. They are treatments as opposed to training. Most of them have evolved gradually rather than arising from clear-cut research showing their value as specific therapy. They are highly successful in some clinics because of the relationship between therapist and patient, in which the positive effects of the personality of the therapist flow to the patient and enhance any specific effect that may be present.

The nonspecific effects of the various modalities used in rehabilitation settings now require enormous amounts of research that most therapists are not in a position to do. Few physical and occupational therapists have any training in research, and those who have are overwhelmed by practical considerations involved in specific problems. Rehabilitation physicians with scientific training are relatively few. Their constant echoing of skepticism about what their therapist colleagues do simply alienates them from the therapists who are seeking increasing professional recognition. Thus the professional rehabilitation specialists who have some training in research, that is, the physicians in rehabilitation, must either stand by helplessly or continue to carp at the lack of scientific rigor employed by the therapists in their everyday practice.

For physical and occupational therapists to point out correctly that probably just as high a percentage of what physicians do is nonspecific does not alter the facts. In the case of all the rehabilitation specialties, whether they are medically oriented or not, the greatest specific effects are in the retraining of function rather than in the significant modification of tissue responses by the physical agencies employed.

Is biofeedback a special placebo in such cases? This would hardly seem to be the case. If it is not a nonspecific effect, what are the pathways for its specific effect? Little work has been done to establish the pathways that must be employed. Intuitively, I believe that improved retraining depends upon recruitment of existing pathways with which the patient's cognitive functions could not link when only standard therapies were employed prior to biofeedback. Apparently the feedback instruments provide a *cognitive loop* that permits the patient to respond more directly and strongly to the request of the therapist to activate specific muscles or to inhibit spasticity in the spastic muscle. Centers in the corpus striatum and in the thalamus well may be involved, but the main center for improved function seems to be within the cortex itself. Thus the patient is provided with an improved input to cortical areas that can be reflected as improved control of motor ability in the periphery. This implies that there is a redundancy in the corticospinal pathways that previous techniques of retraining had not been able to exploit. If there is a nonspecific effect in biofeedback for the training of the neurologically handicapped, its nonspecificity is our lack of understanding of the specific pathways that must be employed. Further, it might be argued that multiple pathways are used to circumvent the lesion that has obstructed the normally direct corticospinal tract.

Little doubt should persist that nonspecific effects blend with specific effects in physical restoration of handicapped people in a rehabilitation setting. Even in the retraining of patients with neurological losses there is at least some element of placebo effect. The greatest nonspecific effects appear to work in disturbances of the musculoskeletal system, in which a substantial psychosomatic factor is clearly suspected by all physicians. The significant superiority of biofeedback relaxation methods in relieving discomfort of such disturbances must still be explained.

## REFERENCES

Baker,: Basmajian, J. V. (ed.) Biofeedback: Principles and Practice for Clinicians, Baltimore, Williams and Wilkins Co., 1979.

Biofeedback and Self Regulation (Journal), Vols. 1–5. New York, Plenum Press, 1976–80 et seq.

Ray, W. J., Raczynski, J. M., Rogers, T. and Kimball, W. H.: Evaluation of Clinical Biofeedback. New York, Plenum Press, 1979.

# 5

# Geriatric Rehabilitation

*by J. B. Redford, M.D.*

The popular view of old age is not pleasant. Often, it is viewed as a gradual loss of physical and mental abilities with an increasing fight to maintain mobility and independence. Old age may be even equated with chronic disease and disability. The famous passage from Shakespeare's *As You Like It* that begins "All the world is a stage" ends with this bitter description of old age:

> Last scene of all
> That ends the strange eventful history,
> Is second childishness and mere oblivion;
> Sans teeth, sans eyes, sans taste, sans everything.

Ferguson Anderson, the distinguished Scottish geriatrician, has deplored this picture of old age. He argues that Shakespeare's and others' literary descriptions are pictures of sick old age—not old age per se. Many elderly persons enjoy a vigorous, active life until death comes. Nevertheless, there is little doubt that chronic disability is much greater in the elderly than in the young, and United States studies have shown that about 40 per cent of persons over 65 experience some limitation of activity related to chronic disability. With modern methods of rehabilitation, this may well be improved in the future even though the general age of the population continues to rise. Chronic illness can probably be postponed by changes in lifestyle, and it has been shown that some of the "markers" of aging may be altered.[1] According to a recent report by Fries, the challenge of chronic disease in elderly people is not simply to rage against it but to accept impairments as a partly unavoidable fact of life and apply every measure of modern medical technology to alleviate disability.

If one examines the physiologic and pathologic reasons for limitation of activity in the elderly, it could be summarized as primarily deficiencies in the body systems concerned with motion—namely, the nervous, the musculoskeletal, the cardiovascular, and the pulmonary systems. All of these systems decline in function with age and a disorder in one usually ultimately affects the others. Multiple-system impairments in disabled elderly persons is the rule rather than the exception. Furthermore, environmental factors in today's fast-paced world tend to aggravate or accelerate these impairments.

Physical medicine and rehabilitation is a medical specialty primarily concerned with disorders of human motion. Thus, specialists in this field seek to improve motor performance and curb physical disability in the elderly. The major goal of geriatric rehabilitation is to keep loss of mobility from becoming a cause of social withdrawal and decline. Therefore, functional activity is stressed by physiatrists and others concerned with care of the aged. As chronic diseases of old age are generally degenerative and incurable, techniques used in rehabilitation are not to cure but to prevent secondary complications and relieve symptoms. This is what many elderly patients expect: help with performing their activities of daily living, not a complete cure or merely a "diagnostic label."

A successful rehabilitation program for a geriatric patient depends on a precise description of the disability. This requires not only an evaluation of the cause of the disability but also an assessment of how physical impairment affects the person's ability to move about, communicate, live at home, and engage in social and recreational activities. It is the physician's responsibility to assess the problem and judge what is needed to set a realistic goal in each case, and physiatrists have particular expertise in this area.

## THE VICIOUS CIRCLE OF AGING AND DISEASE

Much has been written about the multiple problems of the elderly. Fear of becoming dependent on others because of chronic disease is perhaps the greatest cause of anxiety in older people. Clearly, the longer a person lives, the greater the possibility of developing a chronic illness or disability. This in turn may lead to a vicious circle that, if not interrupted, increases dependency and ends in confinement to a nursing home—a prospect that most people dread. It is impossible to discuss in detail all factors in this vicious circle, but they can be summarized in a diagram (Fig. 5–1).[2]

Several factors in this vicious circle of aging stand out.

*Infections and other acute illnesses* in older people often do *not* present with typical signs and symptoms. For example, many older persons may experience no pain with an acute myocardial infarction; no fever may be present with pneumonia; nonrecognition of dehydration may occur with mild illness or hot climatic conditions because older persons notice thirst much less than the young and so may fail to drink enough liquids. Physical disease in an older person may present as an acute confusional reaction, that is, sudden disorientation and disturbed ability to communicate may be the first sign of pneumonia, cardiac failure, coronary occlusion, electrolyte imbalance, or anemia. The musculoskeletal pain signaling serious illness such as cancer for which a younger person seeks medical opinion, an older person may pass off as "arthritis" or just one of the penalties of growing old. It has been the experience of many geriatricians that most elderly patients underplay their symptoms rather than exaggerate them. Obviously, unless such conditions are recognized promptly, the older patient may develop serious secondary complications or irreversible pathological conditions.

*Multiple disorders* are well-known characteristics of disabled elderly persons. Many systems can go wrong at one time in the elderly, chronically ill patient. What physicians and others may not appreciate is how minor disorders that are inconsequential in youth prolong recovery or prevent it in major illnesses in the aged. Foot disorders, for example, may make ambulation painful or impossible if left uncorrected. Mild osteoarthritis of the spine or hip may be aggravated by bed rest for pneumonia or after a myocardial infarction and create serious barriers to resuming normal self-care activities. The lowly decubitus ulcer, which starts perhaps from a minimal pressure or skin trauma after a stroke, if unattended, may cost thousands of dollars in nursing care. These minor problems may be overlooked by the organ system specialist whose only focus is on the acute illness. A competent practitioner in geriatric care and those assisting him must foresee, forestall, discover, and treat all the physical disorders encountered in the elderly, no matter how minor they may seem. This is the essence of geriatrics: the discovery and management of problems simultaneously. To treat these problems systematically, an important tool is the problem-oriented medical record. Such a record treats each problem in turn as it is uncovered—not only diagnostic problems but problems in functional recovery. An excellent review of its use in geriatrics is found in Chapter 3 of *The Geriatric Patient* by Reichel.[3]

*The decreased financial resources* and resulting economic insecurity of an older person may underlie the reason for his failure to seek medical help for illness. Even if an excellent program to preserve health and counteract disability has been developed, the patient may not be able to afford the expensive medication, special diet, or custom-made self-care equipment so vital to preserving his independence. Obviously, medical social workers and home health personnel working in close cooperation with the physician play a key role in finding financial assistance and other help when this is needed. One would hope that future economic planning in the health care field will shift dollars from expensive and often unnecessary multiple diagnostic procedures in hospitals to programs that provide the financial help needed to maintain people independently in their homes. Concerned phy-

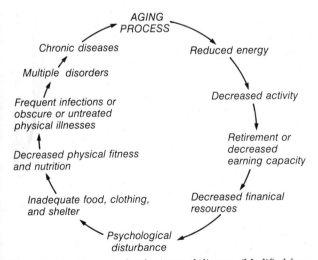

**Figure 5–1.** Vicious circle of aging and disease. (Modified from Rao, B.: The team approach to integrated care of the elderly. Geriatrics 32:88–89, 95–96, 1977.)

sicians should play a vital role in supporting political decisions advocating more sound economic policies in the distribution of health care dollars for the elderly, namely, more funding to maintain patients in their homes instead of keeping them in the hospital.

*Physical and social isolation* and the resulting psychological disturbances are unfortunately all too common especially among the indigent aged. Decreased physical activity, architectural barriers, loss of family and friends through separation, migration or death, and alienation from many of today's concerns all contribute to the older person's physical and social isolation. Difficulty in using public transportation and fear of criminal attack associated with living in urban areas are particularly poignant causes of social withdrawal in the disabled elderly. Of course, a physician working in isolation cannot solve many of these problems. However, he should be sensitive to their existence and when they are uncovered during an initial medical interview, he should refer the patient to concerned persons or agencies. He should not be content simply to treat the disease or disability in isolation. In other words, a physician practicing geriatric rehabilitation is inevitably and inexorably connected with many other health care specialists. Close cooperation and working relationships with various paramedical professions are of paramount importance in any geriatric practice. This field more than any other in medicine involves a team effort. For example, in addition to one or more medical specialists, the elderly patient may require help from nurses, psychologists, nutritionists, speech therapists, audiologists, physical therapists, and occupational therapists; other services may be needed as well as prosthetics, orthotics, housekeeping, transportation, home food service, and recreation.

## ROLE OF REHABILITATION MEDICINE IN CARE OF THE ELDERLY

Many authors have commented on the general lack of interest among physicians in looking after elderly patients, particularly if a practice involves almost exclusively geriatric care. Some of the reasons suggested are a lack of glamor and financial reward in caring for the elderly. Another reason for lack of appeal is that diseases are rarely "cured" in older people. Unless a physician is prepared to accept something less than complete restoration or cure in dealing with illness, he should refer his chronically ill geriatric patients to someone else.

Specialists in rehabilitation are usually very capable of providing such care. Their primary goal is to return older disabled persons to their homes and communities; studies of persons in nursing homes have shown time and again that if rehabilitative services had been provided early in the course of their illnesses, confinement to custodial institutions could have been avoided. Unfortunately, all too frequently the primary attending physician is not only unaware of the value of physical and occupational therapy in the elderly but also of the value of orthotic and prosthetic devices and special equipment available to help patients become partially independent or even possibly restored to full independence in a wheelchair.

The premise of this book is that primary physicians need a guide to current methods used in rehabilitation medicine. This chapter stresses how these services can be applied to aging—particularly, failure of systems concerned with motion. Elsewhere in the book are given detailed discussions of specific techniques as applied to disorders such as stroke, musculoskeletal disease, peripheral vascular disease, and amputations. Therefore, in this chapter, only the more general aspects of geriatric rehabilitation will be dealt with.

The physiological systems under discussion are the nervous system, the musculoskeletal system, the cardiovascular system, and the pulmonary system. Obviously, classifying disorders of the elderly in such a way is artificial, even simplistic. In a given patient, all systems interact—disorders of one system affect all others and alter the overall functional abilities of the individual. In fact, in the elderly disabled, it is much more important to have a functional classification rather than a diagnostic one. In other words, "What can this patient do for himself?" is much more significant than "What chronic diseases does this patient have?" Nevertheless, aging in each bodily system presents certain unique challenges in applying restorative or preventive techniques and so these will be discussed in turn rather than collectively.

## DISORDERS OF PHYSIOLOGICAL SYSTEMS

### NERVOUS SYSTEM

It has been said that a man is as old as his arteries, but perhaps the real key to the aging process lies in the nervous system. The nervous system is composed of nonmitotic cells, which means that they are irreplaceable. Thus, during life, there is a steady decrease in the number of nerve cells and during aging, the central nervous system actively shrinks in size. Bullough[4] suggests that the reason for this loss is to set a limit on life span. All living creatures have a predetermined length of life that seems necessary if evolutionary processes are to continue. In animals, as the many controlling and regulating functions of the brain decline, other systems slowly deteriorate.

Other histologic characteristics of aging are an increase in number of senile plaques and neurofibrillary tangles and an increasing quantity of pigment granules in the neurons and glial cells. Alterations in brain chemistry such as a decrease in water and lipids also occur. All of these changes lead to a progressive reduction in the individual's capability to recognize and process a wide variety of external stimuli. Slowing of nerve conduction and decrease in processing internal stimuli are also characteristic of the aging nervous system. Associated with these age changes are slower learning capacity, easier fatigue, decreased motor skills, and altered sensory perception. Particularly significant to the individual are losses in vision and hearing. Therefore, any rehabilitation program prescribed for an elderly person must take all of these changes into account.

As more restorative techniques involve primarily learning new skills to replace lost abilities, more detailed instruction and more time for repetition must be allowed in elderly persons. When problems arise in rehabilitation treatment, psychological testing with assessment of learning capabilities and emotional responses are most important in planning treatment goals. As most learning involves the special senses—vision and hearing—these abilities must be carefully assessed in all older patients. Corrections may have to be made for any deficiencies even before rehabilitation can be started. Tight schedules that force all patients to be rationed the same amount of therapy time should be altered to give extra time to the elderly. Rehabilitation personnel should learn special attitudes and communication skills needed in working with old people. The alert therapist will seek clues suggesting organic mental changes such as sudden behavior alteration that may herald the onset of an acute illness.

Unfortunately, irreversible chronic organic brain change with memory loss and behavior disorders is one of the contraindications to extensive application of rehabilitation techniques such as activities of daily living skills as taught in occupational therapy. Unless the behavior or abnormalities are very severe or the patient has an irreversible degenerative central nervous system disorder, if at all possible all elderly disabled should have a trial of rehabilitation for at least a week or two before intensive therapy is withdrawn.

Of all the changes in the aging nervous system that may affect mobility, perhaps the most significant one is loss of balance control. This may ultimately lead to a fall and major injuries that, in the elderly, may result in prolonged periods of immobility followed by a long, difficult rehabilitation. Cape in his excellent book on aging has noted, "Falling precipitates loss of mobility and to the old person, mobility is as precious as life."[5] In fact, for many in the ninth and tenth decades of life, the secondary complications of a fall ultimately lead to death. It is most important to investigate the cause of a fall in an older person, whether it is nervous system disorders, cardiovascular changes, other intrinsic diseases, or external environmental factors. This is as essential, in fact, as investigating the cause of a seizure in a young person.

With this problem of falling, prevention is all important; it depends partly on removal of environmental factors and partly on correction or adjustment of the patient's activities to allow for the physical impairment.

Services in rehabilitation departments play a vital role in such prevention by providing canes or other walking aids or developing exercise programs to improve righting reflexes or muscle strength and coordination.

## MUSCULOSKELETAL SYSTEM

Musculoskeletal complaints are extremely common in the aged. It is estimated that by age 70, 80 per cent of the population has some rheumatic complaints. In fact, musculoskeletal complaints are so prevalent in the elderly that they seem almost characteristic of aging. Thus, it is of great importance for the primary physician to distinguish rheumatic complaints requiring a thorough investigation from those that can respond symptomatically to simple methods of rest, physical modalities, exercise, and mild analgesics. Muscle weakness without pain is not so common but it too must be investigated as to whether its origin is in the nervous or muscular system.

Damaged muscle cells, like nerve cells, do not replace themselves, but unlike in nerve cells there is little evidence that individual muscle cells are lost throughout life. Therefore, those individuals who are robust physically and who keep in training throughout life maintain their bulk and strength well into the sixth and seventh decades. Then, perhaps only because other aging processes in connective tissue and endocrine function and in the cardiovascular and nervous systems start to affect muscle function, does muscle strength diminish.

These considerations are important because it has been thought by some gerontologists that strength in aged muscles cannot be increased. However, studies have shown that muscles in healthy persons in the seventh and eighth decades respond to graduated resistive exercise programs in the same way as in younger adults. In one study, repetition of resistive exercises three times a week increased strength in selected muscle groups until a plateau of strength was noted, usually at the end of six weeks.[6]

The aging process in the connective tissues, bones, and cartilage differs from that in muscle because there is a gradual change in these tissues throughout life. Much of the change appears to be caused by loss of body water: we literally dry out as we grow older. With this change, there is a gradual loss of connective tissue flexibility; joints become stiffer, skin becomes thin and develops wrinkles, posture becomes more rigid, and full ventilation of the lungs is impeded.

Osteoporosis, a condition in which bone resorption exceeds bone replacement, is a well-recognized accompaniment of aging, particularly in postmenopausal women. The loss of calcium from the bone, oddly enough, is accompanied by calcification of cartilages and ligaments, leading to more restriction of mobility, particularly in the spine.

Although these connective tissue changes are universal, the rate of change varies from person to person: heredity, work, environment, dietary habits, and degree of physical activity all have definite effect on accelerating or decelerating these changes.

### Exercise Programs

One fact stands out: muscles and joints, whether diseased or healthy, become less flexible if unused for extended periods. Consequently, joint range of motion diminishes and muscle weakness increases. We suspect that many of the changes in joint mobility that in the past have been attributed to aging are in reality caused by misuse or underuse of the organs of voluntary motion.

These observations have profound implications, particularly for residents of custodial institutions. Preventive range of motion and resistance exercises on a regular basis for such patients would appear to be a sound method of retaining functional ability and reducing nursing care needs. Fortunately, this is now being recognized and many nursing homes are providing such preventive exercise programs. A good example of a simple series of exercises has been proposed by Liss.[7]

Liss has described a simple exercise program for elderly persons that has the advantage of requiring only minimal equipment, namely, a standard chair and a six-inch step. Participants are monitored using the technique recommended for screening for physical fitness programs. The radial pulse is determined at rest, immediately after exercise, and in the two-minute phase after exercise recovery. Supervisors of the program, who may be nonprofessionals, are trained to take pulses. Potential participants whose resting pulse rates exceed 100 beats per minute or are less than 60 beats per minute should not be included without the approval of their personal physician.

In a group exercise setting, the exercises are divided into three phases:

1. The group performs a series of breathing exercises, stretching exercises, and range of motion exercises such as those employed by physical educators in "warming up." Usually this is done with groups sitting in chairs or benches. It includes mobilizing the neck and active motion of the various joints with the arms and legs as well as the trunk.

2. The stand-up, step-up program consists of a series of exercises performed standing up from a chair and stepping up and back on one step. There are several graduated levels of exercises beginning with five stand-ups from an average chair and five step-ups to a six-inch high step. Then participants progress at their own rate and rise only to their own maintenance level. Resting and postexercise pulse rates are carefully monitored. (See Reference 7 for details.)

3. After the participants have completed the stand-up step-up program and have acceptable pulse rates, they are then asked to walk at a comfortable pace around a room or a gymnasium in a group. Participants start this by walking only a few laps, but as they improve, they pick up the pace of walking and increase the number of laps.

In this group exercise program, the participants are asked to attend classes three days a week but perform their stand-up step-up program at home daily until they have reached the level of exercise consistent with current physical condition. Once this level has been reached, a class three times a week is considered sufficient to maintain the level of conditioning required. If at the beginning the participant cannot get up from a chair without using his hands, one or more telephone books may be placed in the chair or a slightly elevated stool or chair can be used as a start. The number of books can be gradually reduced during the exercise program as the strength of the lower limbs improves until the participant can rise unassisted. The stand-up step-up program is gradually increased from 5 to 15 repetitions or within various levels until a person reaches an acceptable pulse response without symptoms of discomfort. Guidelines and acceptable pulse rates are recommended by the American Heart Association. These are related primarily to age, except in patients with known cardiac disease. These should only undertake exercise programs recommended by their personal physician.

This series of exercises have proved very popular in several nursing homes, park and recreation centers, and retirement centers. Initially it was thought that special entertainment, awards, guest speakers, and other special activities would be needed to keep the exercise program from becoming monotonous, but participants have been enthusiastic and regularly introduce newcomers into the program without any additional stimulus. As in many exercise programs, music as an adjunct to keep up the interest of the participants certainly could be used. This has been done for many years in the various exercise programs sponsored by volunteer agencies such as the YWCA and YMCA.

In developing treatment programs for musculoskeletal deficiencies in elderly patients, several points need emphasis. It is important to evaluate strength and joint range of motion, paying particular attention to certain joints. For example, (1) Limitation of neck range of motion is very common and often a major bodily impairment. (2) Loss of flexion and abduction of the shoulder caused by a worn-out rotator cuff affects all functions of the upper extremity and may impede many activities of daily living. (3) The elderly person immobilized in bed for a long time develops a very straight, stiff lumbar spine that greatly affects bed mobility and sitting. (4) Hip flexion tightness is easily overlooked, but it is a cause of the decreased stride length and poor posture in the elderly. It is aggravated by prolonged sitting and often accompanied by knee flexion contracture. (5) Foot pain and deformities must be evaluated and relieved before any extensive walking can begin. Physicians need to appreciate that improper footwear and poor foot hygiene may be a significant cause of misery in many older people.

Exercise programs impose considerable physical demands and may overtire an aged patient unaccustomed to physical effort. As well as a general assessment, the status of a patient's cardiac and pulmonary systems must be carefully evaluated before specific exercise programs are attempted, particularly if isometric resistive type exercises are to be employed. Active assistive range of motion exercises are always better than passive stretching techniques. However, if stretching is used, forced sudden stretches should be avoided. Ligaments, tendons, and muscles are less elastic and and more subject to injury; osteoporosis increases the risk of fracture. Use of low-resistance stretching with weighted pulleys or sand bags applied over a long period and accompanied by heat to the affected tissues is the best approach in any program designed to increase range of motion.

The best exercise programs for the elderly are those designed with a functional goal in mind. Passive range of motion or electrically stimulated muscle contractions may have a place, but if precious therapist time is spent in using these techniques in place of functional exercise training under supervision, the disabled person is being cheated in time and money. For example, if treatment time is limited, it is much more important for a hemiplegic patient to learn wheeling and transferring from the wheelchair than to spend time on such activities as passive shoulder and arm manipulation, progressive resistive exercises to the quadriceps, and heel-cord stretching.

In any treatment program for an elderly patient with rheumatic complaints, emphasis should be placed on balancing rest against activity. Any functional activity or exercise program that causes pain persisting for 12 hours or into the next day is too vigorous. Often, arthritic patients need as much instruction on which activities to avoid as they do in learning exercise programs.

In this regard, occupational therapists are specifically trained to instruct patients in general principles of joint protection, e.g., use of assistive equipment to save time and energy or use of dynamic orthoses for pain relief or use of environmental adaptations that reduce stress on muscles and joints.

### Physical Modalities

Physical modalities such as heat, cold, electricity, massage, and water in treatment of degenerative musculoskeletal problems have wide appeal to the public. Rehabilitation departments are notable for an impressive array of physical agents. Unfortunately, graded physical activities and the judicious use of orthotic and self-help devices may be much more important than any of these modalities for the elderly arthritic. Use of physical agents in an indiscriminate manner over a long period of time without good clinical indication is all too frequent and certainly no substitute for a well-rounded rehabilitation program supervised by a physiatrist.

Particular care should be taken with deep heating modalities in older patients. The possibility of impaired circulation or a decrease in sensation in the part being treated should not be overlooked. As there is no way of measuring how much energy is delivered to the tissues by shortwave or microwave diathermy, the sensibility of the patient is critical. Extensive deep or superficial heating may also have considerable autonomic nervous system effects on elderly persons with cardiovascular or pulmonary disorders.

As a general rule, it is better to use cold or local superficial heat applications for specifically limited periods of time in relieving rheumatic pain in older people than the expensive heating devices found in physical therapy departments.

During the past few years, the use of safe and convenient transcutaneous electric nerve stimulators has made a significant difference in relieving musculoskeletal pain in older people. This modality seems most effective for acute pain, particularly of rheumatic origin. It can even be used to reduce joint pain during exercise routines. For example, the current can be passed across the skin of a painful shoulder joint during an active assistive exercise. A trial lasting one or two days should always be made before the units are prescribed for more prolonged use. The patient should be carefully instructed in placement and maintenance of the electrodes and the electric stimulator. Contraindications to use of the transcutaneous nerve stimulators are only two: Avoid use in patients with skin disorders that may be aggravated by the electrode placement and in patients with cardiac pacemakers or other internally placed electronic devices that may be affected by the electrical pulses.

## CARDIOVASCULAR SYSTEM

Cardiovascular disease is responsible for almost one third of the deaths in older people, and poor circulation from hardening of the arteries is regarded as the main factor causing most chronic disability in the aged. Nevertheless, in elderly persons who have escaped the ravages of arteriosclerosis, the heart shows few differences from that of young adults. In aging, the heart muscle volume relative to fatty tissue decreases and many muscle cells show lipid pigment accumulation. This is accompanied by slower myocardial contractility and a reduction in cardiac output. In the very old, defects of the conducting system may occur independently of ischemic heart disease so the incidence of cardiac arrhythmias also increases with aging. Arterial walls generally become more rigid after age 50, causing an increase in circulation time and a steady increase in peripheral resistance with rising blood pressure.

Because of these changes, persons with aged but not diseased hearts can tolerate most therapeutic exercise programs very well. Vigorous or rapid forceful exercises should be avoided, as should activities involving isometric work. Isometric tasks increase cardiac afterload, may be associated with ectopic cardiac activity, and do not produce a cardiovascular training effect. Generally, the slower the active muscle contraction, the greater the amount of activity that can be tolerated by the elderly individual. If an elderly person with a mild degree of heart disease, for example, inquires about physical exercise, little reason can be given to stop usual activities, but they should be carried out more slowly for shorter periods. In fact, physicians should be encouraging recreational activities in which a person can pace his effort and not have to perform in vigorous spurts. For example, gardening, fishing, bicycle riding, golf, bowling, and recreational swimming all can be well tolerated by elderly persons.

Maximum heart rate and maximum oxygen consumption decrease steadily with advancing years. Those persons who have exercised regularly show less rapid decline in these physiologic parameters of fitness than those who have not. In the unfit person, the cardiovascular and respiratory systems adapt to effort more slowly, and more time is required for the heart rate to return to resting level after exercise stops. Consequently, fatigue sets in earlier for a given amount of work.

These well-known physiological facts have produced a remarkable recent surge of interest in fitness exercise programs, particularly among middle-aged adults. Training for fitness depends on the use of large muscle masses with repeated contractions at submaximal loads. Therefore, most programs to improve fitness emphasize jogging, swimming, or other moderately vigorous activities involving the lower extremities, performed for 20 to 30 minutes at least three times per week. Such programs should be medically supervised for anyone over 60 and certainly for persons who have a history suggestive of a cardiovascular disorder. Injuries resulting from stress on the musculoskeletal system have been common in those who have embarked on jogging programs without medical advice.

Details of cardiac rehabilitation programs are described in another chapter and so will be omitted from this section. However, a few comments concerning fitness programs for the elderly patient with or without known heart disease should be made.

Heart rate and blood pressure changes are usually a reliable guide in estimating work capacity of healthy adults. The maximum heart rate depends on age and does not increase with training. Nevertheless, a fitness exercise program carried out for one to two months will lower heart rate for a specific submaximal workload. A study by DeVries has shown that physiological improvements from exercise regimens can be measured even in elderly persons who have not been trained vigorously in youth.[8] The greatest improvements were in oxygen utilization, but physical work capacity and resting blood pressure also improved after a program lasting from six to ten months. Therefore, persons even of advanced age can benefit from cardiovascular fitness programs.

Training prevents fatigue and enables patients to adjust better to additional exercise loads often needed during rehabilitation such as the use of braces, crutches, or artificial limbs. Therefore, elderly patients in rehabilitation programs should carry out some activities designed primarily to improve physical fitness with the precaution that their response to these exercises is carefully monitored.

Older persons often ask if fitness exercises will prevent or improve heart disease. It has not been scientifically proved that heart disease can be prevented by physical fitness programs, but there is much suggestive evidence. Furthermore, longitudinal studies imply that chances for recurrence or death from myocardial infarctions are reduced in patients who exercise regularly. Most of these studies have been retrospective, but a recent Canadian multicenter prospective study definitely suggests that fitness exercises have a beneficial effect on long-term survival from heart disease.[9] Another recent study has concluded that physical conditioning augments the fibrinolytic activity occurring in response to venous occlusion. This could be an important mechanism in the beneficial effect of habitual physical activity on the risk of cardiovascular disease.[10]

For patients known to have heart disease who participate in rehabilitation programs, certain precautions are critical. Therapists and others exercising patients must know the symptoms and signs of overtaxed heart such as anginal pain, shortness of breath, cyanosis, and complaints of dizziness or faintness.

In moderately rigorous exercises, the heart rate should be monitored (this is now made easy by electronic gadgetry) and any change in rhythm, excessive rise during activity, or failure to return to normal levels after exercise must be brought to the attention of the attending physician. Physiatrists and others in charge of rehabilitation programs must be familiar with cardiopulmonary resuscitation procedures. Although cardiac arrests in rehabilitation departments have been rare in my experience, they seem to occur mainly in patients walking in the parallel bars or exercising in the gymnasium; therefore, these areas should be carefully supervised. Anyone involved in cardiac rehabilitation should also be aware of the pharmacology of cardiovascular drugs such as digitalis, diuretics, antihypertensives, and antiarrhythmic agents. Many older people are either overmedicated on drugs that can cause side effects by adverse interactions or underdosed because they forget to take their medication. Recent developments in pharmacology that permit measurement of serum drug levels have made drug prescribing much more efficient in older people.

The diet of the cardiac patient may also need supervision by the physiatrist and staff. Many elderly patients and their families have great difficulty following a low-salt regimen and need encouragement by persons other than just the attending physician. In fact, efforts to involve the cardiac patient in his medical order care and instruct him not only in exercises but in all aspects of managing heart disease should be made by all rehabilitation team members. As a vascular or cardiac problem is frequently complicated by coexisting diabetes, even more special dietary and drug instruction may be necessary.

## PULMONARY SYSTEM

Age changes and disease in the respiratory system are intimately linked with those in the cardio-vascular system. However, unlike the heart, which may show little change in healthy aging, the pulmonary system declines in an almost linear fashion with advancing age. A combination of intrinsic lung changes and alterations in the configuration of the thorax is responsible for these changes. Ventilation and maximum breathing capacity are reduced so that by age 80, the latter is only 40 per cent of the person's capability at age 20. Emphysema, which is most simply defined as loss of alveolar walls, increases in incidence with age. Autopsy studies show that by age 90, nearly all persons have some degree of emphysema pathology, although most have few obvious symptoms.

Normal activities in an older individual may not be restricted by these changes, but they do limit vigorous exercise. As in other bodily functions, the older person who has followed a regular exercise program and who has not smoked finds fewer restrictions in breathing capacity in old age than does his unfit contemporary.

A significant number of elderly persons have clinical manifestations of pulmonary emphysema and chronic bronchitis—usually conveniently lumped together as chronic obstructive lung disease. Distinguishing these two conditions clinically is difficult, as they usually coexist. In any person complaining of cough and chronic dyspnea, there is an airway constituent—bronchitis, bronchiolitis, edema, and secretions, and a mechanical constituent—the collapsing airway and increased work of breathing. Details of management of these conditions are beyond the scope of this chapter and are given in many standard texts.[11] Other chronic lung diseases may be present but they are far less common in older people.

As in many chronic diseases, the emphasis in chronic obstructive lung disease is on patients with education. Patients need a review of the physiology of breathing, factors that aggravate their symptoms, and therapeutic regimens. They also need an understanding of their psychological responses to dyspnea.

From the standpoint of rehabilitation, the elderly person with lung disease needs retraining in his patterns of breathing. Many chronic obstructive lung disease patients have very inefficient rapid, discoordinated breathing with overuse of the accessory muscles of respiration. They can learn to control this with slow deep breathing ("pursed-lipped" breathing) combined with relaxation of the overtaxed accessory muscles and contraction of the abdominal muscles for more effective expiration. However, this takes individual instruction and practice supervised by trained physical therapists or respiratory therapists.

In addition to specific exercises, physical reconditioning with some simple graded exercises stressing normal walking has definitely produced improved mobility in many patients with chronic obstructive lung disease. In some cases, low-flow oxygen in portable tanks may be needed to start on reconditioning programs. Such rehabilitation programs must establish definite goals for mobility to be increased each day or each week. An organized program supervised by concerned therapists and physicians is necessary for success in any pulmonary rehabilitation program involving the aforementioned exercises. Such programs also incorporate instruction in how to conserve energy in daily activities using special equipment. Instruction in postural drainage, details of diet, medication, and avoidance of adverse environmental factors is also stressed.

Although pulmonary emphysema unfortunately is an irreversible disease process, many patients can avoid admission to hospitals and live happier, more productive lives if given two to three weeks of instruction in a rehabilitation department. They also need outpatient follow-up of their rehabilitation program and periodic reassessment of their respiratory functions.

## HOME CARE

Rehabilitation of the aged disabled patient with several coexisting diseases presents particular difficulties. As noted earlier, usually many problems must be managed simultaneously. We have said nothing about bowel and bladder difficulties, but these often cause almost insurmountable problems. In any geriatric rehabilitation setting, a close working relationship with urologists is an absolute necessity.

For many reasons, the goals that are set for the elderly disabled patient must be circumscribed. Restoration of function so that the patient can return to his home and family is the most common objective.

Steinberg has given a useful guide to conditions permitting a patient to be managed at home.[12]

1. He must be able to walk or at least transfer from bed to chair without having to be lifted.

2. He must have normal or nearly normal excretory function.

3. He should be able to take care of all or at least an essential part of his personal needs such as eating, dressing, and bathing.

4. His mental condition should be adequately clear.

In spite of these considerations, perhaps much of the rehabilitation process may be better carried out at home. It is widely recognized that disabled older people do not respond well to treatment in an institutional setting. For a particular case, some performance goals that the rehabilitation staff predict are possible must be reached in a home setting because the elderly person may not connect the goal with his hospital routine. Even if ambulation and self-care skills are adequately learned and performed under supervision in a hospital, they can be lost if no home follow-up program is initiated. Focus in geriatric rehabilitation, therefore, seems more and more on home treatment settings. Such settings may have such disadvantages as lack of special equipment and limited time availability for service, but this may be outweighed by the social and psychological advantages. Furthermore, home is where environmental adaptations are best observed and carried out. Often this is a task for the visiting nurse or occupational therapist because it cannot be easily performed by those working in hospitals.

Most major metropolitan areas now have provisions for home rehabilitation services. Underutilization may be more of a problem than lack of availability. Frequently this problem arises from poor discharge planning practices and lack of coordination with community health agencies by practicing physicians. Many hospitals have nurse practitioners whose responsibility is to ensure that no chronically ill patient leaves an acute care center without a home follow-up treatment plan. In time, it is hoped that all hospitals will have such a service. Home care has been shown to lower medical costs and reduce hospital admissions. Such conclusions were drawn, for example, from a study of stroke patients seen for home care programs in New York City in 1972.[13]

In conclusion, I must emphasize the need for early restorative measures in those advanced in years who are stricken. Early treatment is imperative for the vulnerable sick older person. If the practicing physician takes too long going down the many byways leading to obscure diagnoses without ordering concurrent exercises or other rehabilitation measures, much of the value of the rehabilitative techniques may be lost or wasted. The hip or knee contracture after amputation, the painful, stiff hemiplegic shoulder, and the rigid arthritic spine can all be avoided or ameliorated by rehabilitation measures. Time in hospital for the elderly patient should be kept to a minimum. The strategy of more home care for the elderly and less hospitalization is an idea whose time has come. It not only saves more money but promotes improvement in human welfare and happiness.

## REFERENCES

1. Fries, J. F.: Aging, natural death and the compression of morbidity. N. Engl. J. Med. 303:130–135, 1950.
2. Rao, B.: The team approach to integrated care of the elderly. Geriatrics 32:88–89, 95–96, 1977.

3. Reichel, W.: Multiple Problems in the Elderly. *In* Reichel, W. (ed.): The Geriatric Patient. New York, HP Publishing Co., Inc., 1978, pp. 17–22.
4. Bullough, W. S.: Aging of mammals. Nature 229:608–610, 1971.
5. Cape, R. L.: Aging: Its Complex Management. Hagerstown, Harper and Row, Inc., 1978, p. 114.
6. Perkins, L. C. and Kaiser, H. L.: Results of short term isotonic and isometric exercise program in persons over sixty. Phys. Ther. Rev. 41:633, 1961.
7. Liss, S.: A graded and monitored exercise program for senior adults. Texas Med., 72:(6), 58–63, 1976.
8. DeVries, H.: Physiological effects of an exercise training regime upon aged men. J. Gerontol. 25:325, 1970.

9. Rechnitzer, P. A.: The Role of Exercise in the Prevention of Complications Following Myocardial Infarction. Ann. R. Coll. Surg. Can. 13:219, 221, 1980.
10. Williams, R. S. et al.: Physical conditioning augments the fibrinolytic response to venous occlusion in healthy adults. N. Engl. J. Med. 302:987–991, 1980.
11. Rodman, J. and Sterling, F. H.: Pulmonary Emphysema and Related Disease, Part II. St. Louis, C. V. Mosby Co., 1969.
12. Steinberg, F. U.: Rehabilitation Medicine. *In* Steinberg, F. U. (ed.): Cowdry's The Care of the Geriatric Patient. St. Louis, C. V. Mosby Co., 1976.
13. Bryant, N. H., Candland, R. and Loewenstein, R.: Comparison of care and cost outcomes for stroke patients with and without home care. Stroke 5:54, 1974.

# *Section II*

# PAIN

# 6

# Treatment of Myofascial Pain

*by Hans Kraus, M.D.*

Of the many orthopedic complaints, pain in the skeletal muscle is the most common. In fact, over 83 per cent of back pain is of muscular origin, as was seen at a multidisciplinary back clinic at Columbia-Presbyterian Hospital in which over 3000 patients were examined.[2, 9] Treatment of muscle problems resulted in complete relief of pain in 82 per cent of 233 patients, followed 2 to 8 years.[9]

Muscle pain is present in almost every sprain, strain, and fracture; in each case it should be treated appropriately. Therefore, treatment of muscular pain must be preceded by an appraisal of its type. Muscular pain may be caused by (1) muscle spasm, (2) muscle tension, (3) muscle deficiency—weakness or stiffness, and (4) triggerpoints (discussed on p. 135.) (See also Chapter 8.)

Since muscle pain is part of every orthopedic condition, proper evaluation of muscle status must be part of every orthopedic examination. This is especially important in examination of patients with back and neck pain.

## MUSCLE SPASM

Muscle spasm is characterized by severely painful contraction of a muscle. Movement increases the pain; pain, in turn, increases the contraction; the cycle becomes one of pain, spasm, and increasing inability to move.

Painful muscle spasm can be caused by lesions of the central nervous system or by injury to the muscle proper—or to joints, bones, or, in fact, to most tissues of the body. In this chapter we are dealing with muscle spasm caused by strains, sprains, fractures, direct muscle trauma, or overtaxing of muscles. Painful muscle spasm can also be a symptom of pathology such as disc disease; in this case treatment is only palliative if it is successful at all.

Muscle spasm responds best to local treatment and is rather refractory to analgesics or muscle relaxants. Hot packs are helpful, but we find the use of surface anesthetics,[13–16, 29, 30] especially ethyl chloride spray, preceded by electrotherapy and followed by gentle limbering movements, to be the most effective approach.[10, 17] Analgesics are of limited help; however, tranquilizers and muscle relaxants are valuable when tension is a precipitating factor.

Cocainization of sphenopalatine ganglion (Ruskin) is described in Chapter 7 and merits special attention.

Local injection of procaine HCl may relieve pain, but it has several drawbacks. It may mask pathology and therefore permit aggravation of an injury. Frequently the relief of muscle pain by injection of anesthetics is followed by an even more painful rebound. I recommend the following procedure:

Place the patient in a comfortable position.[10, 17] Use tetanizing current for ten minutes followed by sinusoidal current for ten minutes, with the electrodes placed at the painful area. After electrotherapy, which relieves some of the spasm, spray ethyl chloride over the painful muscle and begin gentle limbering exercises. Continue spraying to different areas as the pain shifts while gradually increasing movements as long as they can be controlled with the spray. Do not continue to spray in an area after white frost has formed. I have found that ethyl chloride spray is much more effective than any other cooling sprays such as Fluorethane (or ice). However, we sometimes recommend that the patient use ice massage at home. Several sessions of treatment on successive days are usually needed to accomplish complete relief. Mild cases may respond in one or two sessions.

We recommend frequent repetition of exercise sessions at home, with the patient making each movement learned at the treatment session only one or two times, but at intervals of one or two hours, to keep muscles from tightening up again.

Back pain[17] patients are rarely ordered to bed. We reserve bed rest for only the most severe cases—and then, if possible, bed rest is combined with gentle exercises.

Patients with injuries to the lower extremities[8, 12] should not walk until they can do so without limping. If needed, partial weight-bearing with crutches is prescribed, along with rest and elevation. Prolonged standing, walking, and sitting must be avoided until the spasm has been completely relieved.

Surface anesthetics are self-limiting, but they do not mask major pathology. Although some of the pain recurs after treatment, it is not as severe as previously and gradually disappears on successive treatments.

## MUSCLE TENSION

Most of us are tense. Our sedentary, overmechanized lives rarely give us a chance to complete the fight-or-flight response, constantly triggered by our surroundings. Tensing in constantly repeated positions will shorten muscles and finally cause tension pain.[21] Squeezing the telephone between shoulder and ear, constantly leaning to one side while writing, and sitting stoop-shouldered at a desk will eventually cause muscles to tense and stiffen. On a particularly aggravating day, a sudden motion may overstrain a muscle and tension pain will cause a relapse into muscle spasm.[7]

I appraise tension by placing the patient in a comfortable position and observing the patient's responses to simple orders. The examiner lifts the patient's arm and asks that the patient let go and do nothing. Very tense patients will lift an arm before the examiner even starts to grasp it. Others will keep the arm elevated until the examiner lets it drop. A relaxed person lets gravity take over and drops the arm as the examiner stops holding it.

Tightening of the shoulders and adduction of the shoulder blades, along with tense movement patterns, may often be evidence of tension, making further examination for tension unnecessary.

Tension pain, be it manifested as tension headache, neckache, or backache, or caused by tension in any other muscle, frequently yields to muscle relaxants, analgesics, and tranquilizers. Muscle spasm does not.

Treatment of muscle tension[10, 17] must include recognizing and controlling its causes. Changing working habits or working posture may be indicated; eliminating or diminishing stress in family or work situations should be encouraged. Some patients may be advised to seek psychiatric help.

Relaxing exercises should be part of every exercise program. They are of the utmost importance in combatting repeated tension pain. A simple exercise consists of having the patient lie supine in a comfortable position with a pillow under the knees and eyes closed. The patient is asked to inhale through the nose and breathe out slowly through the lips. The patient continues to breathe in and out while concentrating on the act of breathing and listening for the humming sound that should be produced by exhaling. Then the patient is asked to shrug the shoulders and let go; drop the head left, then right, then let go; then breathe again and let go. The patient is asked to tighten a fist and to be aware of the tension and then to release it. The procedure should be repeated with the other arm, with a leg, with the neck—always noting the letting go and relaxing of the muscle. The patient may be asked to let the whole body or an arm or a leg go loose; this procedure is continued until a general state of relaxation is achieved. Teaching patients how to achieve muscle relaxation is often difficult because ingrained habits have to be reversed, and relaxation is a skill that is hard to learn.

Other ways of relaxation training include biofeedback (see Chapter 4), self-hypnosis for relaxation,[27] Schultze's autogenic training, Jacobson[4] relaxation, and Transcendental Meditation (TM). When possible, I try to confine treatment to simple relaxation exercises, leaving other methods for resistant cases.

## MUSCLE DEFICIENCY

Muscle deficiency, weakness, and stiffness may be caused by underexercise inherent in our mechanized way of life. Prolonged disuse of muscles induced by bed rest or immobilization may produce the same result. In this chapter the discussion of weakness is confined to the aforementioned causes and to weakness resulting from nerve root compression or peripheral nerve lesions.

Muscle strength and flexibility are appraised by manual muscle testing. Muscles of the extremities are rated for their ability to overcome gravity, to offer resistance, or merely to contract without producing movement. For appraisal of neck and back pain I use the Kraus-Weber tests.[9, 17]

Trunk muscle strength is best gauged by appraising the performance of key posture muscles. The Kraus-Weber tests, which I use, are as follows:

1. Position: Supine, hands behind neck, feet held down.
   Directions: "Keep your hands behind your neck and roll up to a sitting position."

2. Position: Supine, hands behind neck and knees bent. The examiner holds the patient's feet down on the table.
   Directions: "Keep your hands behind your neck and roll up to a sitting position."

3. Position: Supine, with hands behind neck and legs extended, feet held down.
   Directions: "Keep your knees straight and lift your feet ten inches off the table. Hold that position for ten seconds."

4. Position: Lying prone, with pillow under abdomen, hands behind neck. The examiner holds the patient's feet and hips down on the table.
   Directions: "Raise your trunk and hold that position for ten seconds."

5. Position: Prone over pillow. The examiner holds the patient's back and hips down on the table.
   Directions: "Lift your legs, hold that position for 10 seconds."

6. Position: Standing erect in stockings or bare feet, hands at sides.
   Directions: "Put your feet together, keeping the knees straight. Slowly reach down as far as you can."

Exercises to restore strength should be prescribed *individually* as the *individual* patient requires. Exercises should start with easy movements through full range in the warm-up period, then gradually increase to movement against gravity, and later, when extremities are involved, against resistance. Only when full range has been reached may weight exercises be added. Exercises should be performed slowly, with few repetitions—three or four repetitions of one movement only. After several different movements are performed, the first one may be resumed. This sequence should be repeated up to but not beyond the point of fatigue. Gentle easy motions are finally used as a cool-off.

Fatiguing a muscle will cause discomfort and decrease strength for three to four days[20] if the fatigue exercises are continued. Then a quick in-

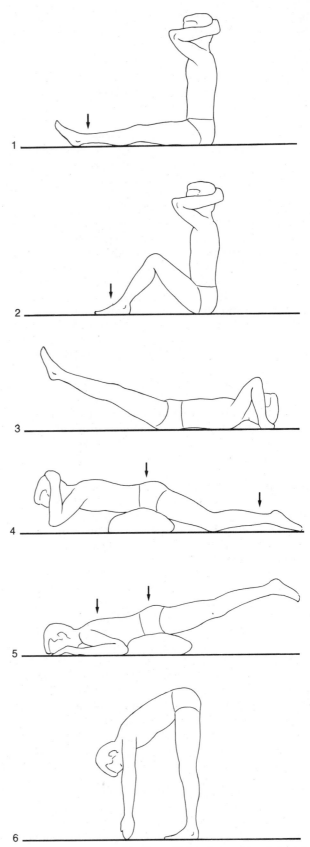

**Figure 6–1.** Positions for Kraus-Weber tests of trunk muscle strength.

crease of muscle strength will occur. In a muscle below normal potential, the improvement pace will not be reached. The patient will be unable to exercise, will require rest, and will then have to start at the initial level. Persistent repetition of the same procedure will result in no progress, muscle stiffness, pain, and discouragement.

Exercises to restore flexibility must be preceded by relaxation and limbering exercises.[10, 17] Relaxation exercises may consist of having the patient lie supine, with eyes closed, knees supported by a pillow. The patient should then breathe slowly and concentrate on breathing and relaxing with every breath. In other exercise the patient may tighten the muscles of one arm, then let loose, and repeat with the other arm; tighten one leg, then the other, and repeat the procedure with the neck, the back, and the whole body. In another the patient may feel that the limbs are getting heavy or loose or floating—whichever feels inevitable and right. Then gentle movements of one extremity after the other within easy range will limber the muscles. Finally, active stretching, while still supine and prone, should be followed by standing, stretching movements.

Relaxing and stretching exercises are essential to attain and maintain full flexibility of a muscle. Relaxed and stretched muscles will not easily be strained or torn. Many back strains or strains of extremity muscles can be avoided by properly warming up and stretching before activity.

Constant strain of a muscle by overwork will cause pain, such as strain of back muscles in pregnant women when abdominal muscles are inadequate. The same pattern occurs in persons out of condition who suddenly overexercise when other key posture muscles may be weakened or are relatively weak and inadequate to meet the imposed demands. Pain caused by excessive demand is especially evident after injury and the necessary immobilization of the lower extremity. When the injury to the bone has healed and the bone is ready for weight-bearing, the muscles may not yet be ready; if the muscles are returned too soon to full weight-bearing—that is, without prior reconditioning—they will be strained. This strain will cause pain and stiffness, and if continued weight-bearing and walking are permitted, the result will be stiffness, limitation of motion, triggerpoints, and inability to return to full normal function without adequate treatment.

Summarizing the basic rules of an exercise program:[10, 17]

1. Exercises should be prescribed for the needs of the individual.

2. An exercise routine must be preceded by relaxation exercises, because tension is almost always present in these patients.

3. Gentle limbering exercises should then be fol-

lowed by gentle strengthening exercises, warming up the muscles. Then gentle stretching exercises are followed by more demanding strengthening and stretching exercises. This sequence should be reversed as a cool-off.

Exercises should be repeated only two or three times during a session. This is especially true in cases of neck and back pain, for multirepetition of exercises will produce stiffness and pain.

In patients who have already made some progress, especially in patients with extremity problems, repetitions can be more frequent but should still be limited to no more than 10 or 20; then the patient returns to another movement and still another movement until finally the first movement is repeated again.

Exercises should be performed through the full range. When stretching is needed, active stretching should first be performed by the patient by using the antagonists, then only gentle added passive stretching should be done by the therapist. Any violent stretching is to be avoided. The movements should be performed slowly and each should be followed by a brief intermission and relaxation period before the next movement is started.

Isometric exercises are sometimes helpful, such as those to strengthen the quadriceps. More often they add to stiffness, especially if used by themselves without relaxation and isotonic exercises.

## TRIGGERPOINTS

Triggerpoints were first extensively described by Max Lange, a Munich orthopedic surgeon, in 1921.[18] He refers to authors who mention "rheumatic nodules" as far back as 1880. Lange not only mentioned most of the frequently found locations of triggerpoints but measured their resistance to pressure above that of normal muscles. He produced triggerpoints experimentally in animals and described their histology. As treatment, he advocated "crushing" massage with knuckles or wooden rods, a practice still used by some lay healers. He further used injection of glucose.

Biopsies were later performed by two other investigators, Glogowski and Wallraff,[3] who found triggerpoints to be small nodules of degenerated muscle tissue.

Miehlke[19] and co-workers biopsied the upper trapezius to study stages of gradual change. They found normal tissue in "psychogenic rheumatism"—our tension pain—and also found gradually increasing histological and biochemical changes in "hardened" muscle, and finally degeneration into what is known as triggerpoints.

More recently, several American authors have reported on triggerpoints: Steindler,[28] an orthopedic surgeon who coined the word, Travell,[29, 30] and Bonica[1] are among the most noted.[10, 17, 24, 25]

I first learned of the clinical disorder of trigger-points through Lange's work and have written extensively about the topic. Clinically, triggerpoints are tender spots that develop in skeletal muscle, more often close to the insertion of origin. Pressure will cause sharp pain, often simulating the pain complained of by the patient. Triggerpoints can be identified by the history given by the patient, who can very often localize the pain in one particular spot and describe the typical radiation of the trig-gerpoint. The patient will report that certain movements, often an unexpected movement, will result in pain and often in an episode of spasm. In a patient who seeks relief when in acute spasm, the spasm must be treated before the triggerpoints can be effectively identified and treated. Palpation of a thin individual with soft muscles sometimes permits the examiner to actually feel those nodules, or triggerpoints. On palpation, the patient expresses pain when a triggerpoint is touched and pressed and often makes an evasive twitching motion to avoid the pressure (Gillette). A pressure gauge devised by A. Fisher makes it possible to state if the pressure tolerance is normal in the triggerpoint areas, these areas usually being one third or less tolerant than normal muscles (see Chapter 8).

*Typical locations of triggerpoints* are posterior neck muscles and suboccipital muscles, with pain often leading to occipital headaches. Triggerpoints in the sternomastoid as well as in the neck sometimes cause dizziness on change of position. A bite problem[23] often causes triggerpoints in the masticatory muscles, and from there triggerpoints spread in the neck and upper back area. Triggerpoints in sca-

lenus or spasm in these muscles may be caused by peripheral nerve entrapment[5] with numbness, paresthesia of fingers, and numbness of arm and forearm. Triggerpoints in the trapezius and the infraspinatus as well as in the supraspinatus are frequent. Triggerpoints in the infraspinatus radiating to the lateral aspect of the arm are frequently a factor in athletic injuries, and are quite often associated with triggerpoints in extensor and supinator muscles of the forearm and at the lateral epicondyle of the forearm.

Triggerpoints in the intrascapular muscles are often produced by tension. Those in sacrospinal, gluteal, and tensor muscles and in the gluteus medius often cause radiation along the lateral aspect of the thigh and leg down to the ankle. Sometimes they cause peripheral nerve entrapment of the cutaneous femoris lateralis. Especially important is a triggerpoint in the piriformis, which quite frequently occurs and produces peripheral nerve entrapment of the sciatic nerve. This is accompanied by true neurological loss, loss or diminution of achilles tendon reflex, and weakness of the anterior tibial group, the peroneus, and the calf muscle. Triggerpoints in the lower extremities are not necessarily caused by disc disease but are frequently the result of problems with the feet—flat feet or even minimal foot inadequacies, now seen with increasing frequency in runners and joggers. In the acute phase, before the triggerpoint is formed as a result of long-standing muscle spasm and tightness, the same symptoms may appear and then may yield to local spasm-relieving therapy.

In a chronic back pain patient presenting in the acute phase, we first treat muscle spasm. Only after the spasm has been completely relieved is the patient examined for triggerpoints, muscle weakness and stiffness, and tension; and then a program is drawn up accordingly. The patient receives an injection and is treated three times in succession using electrotherapy, sinusoidal current, and ethyl chloride spray as a preliminary to help relaxation and to make exercises more comfortable. Only mild limbering exercises are used in these three follow-up treatments on successive days after injection of triggerpoints.

## TREATMENT OF TRIGGERPOINTS

The old method of crushing triggerpoints by hard massage has been replaced by injection[10, 17] and needling. The aim is to physically destroy the little nodules of degenerated muscle tissue. The fluid used for injection is lidocaine or saline. I have found it unnecessary to use steroids because the results of injection do not depend on the biochemical effect of the injected solution but on the actual hitting of the targeted triggerpoint. I prefer lidocaine to saline only for its anesthetic effect, which

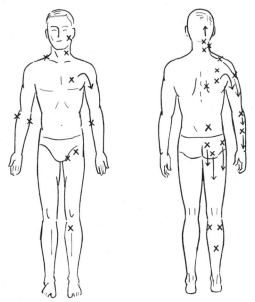

**Figure 6–2.** Typical locations of trigger points.

gives the patient an hour or two of relief. After identification of the triggerpoint by palpation, corroborated by the patient's expression of discomfort, the spot is marked with a scratch of the needle, then the area is cleaned three to four times with alcohol. After scrubbing, I insert the needle, fanning out in circular fashion and injecting whenever the patient feels pain. Ethyl chloride spray is used to make the insertion of the needle painless. The needle does not cause discomfort in normal muscle but does cause sharp, stabbing pain when hitting the triggerpoint.

The patient is warned to avoid prolonged sitting, standing, and walking, to avoid exertion in general, and to avoid exertion of the treated extremity for the next three to four days. The extremity should be moved gently at frequent intervals to avoid stiffening of the muscle. Injection is followed on three successive days by use of sinusoidal muscle stimulation; pads are applied to the injected area and gentle limbering movement is performed. Ethyl chloride spray is used to relieve discomfort (see under discussion for muscle spasm). Only one triggerpoint is injected at a time. An exception to this is made if triggerpoints are in the same anatomical vicinity such as the occiput, posterior neck muscles, or lateral epicondyle and forearm extensors; then more than one point can be injected simultaneously.

An exercise program is started only after all triggerpoints have been injected. Continued treatment of injected areas is often necessary. Since triggerpoints present with only the most advanced form of a muscle lesion, usually the rest of the muscle is also affected. Besides electrotherapy, exercise, and ethyl chloride spray, kneading and gentle point massage are needed to gradually restore the muscle to normal pain-free function.

Triggerpoint injections rarely afford immediate relief. More often the treated muscle is more painful than before. The patient must be apprised of this fact beforehand.

Contraindications for injection of triggerpoints are excessively low pain threshold of the patient, emotional instability of the patient, inability of the patient to comply with follow-up treatment, and acute muscle spasm. Patients who are on anticoagulants should not receive injections; a large ecchymosis and hematoma may follow.

It is understood that local treatment of any muscular problem will be only part of the attempt to help the patient. The history taken before treatment must be complete. An exploration should be included of all possible sources of tension from commuting and business problems to family and emotional difficulties. The history must explore the patient's working and movement habits, physical activities and participation in sports or lack of it, and attitudes and frame of mind. It is important to ask these questions, in addition to the usual questions asked on a history as to previous disease and special inquiries into a possible endocrine disturbance.

Endocrine imbalance frequently results in muscle pain[22, 26, 31] and ultimately in muscle spasm and triggerpoints. Patients who are not restored to normal endocrine function will continue to have recurrences of their muscular problems. The most frequent endocrine imbalances we find are estrogen deficiencies in women, which normally occur after a certain age with menopause but sometimes are present at an earlier age, and hypothyroidism in both sexes. Hyperthyroidism is much more rare in the course of muscle deficiency.

Two examples of treatment are presented:

**Example 1: Sprain of a Knee Joint.**[8] The patient is placed in a comfortable position with a pillow under the knee; sinusoidal current is applied to the vastus medialis and to the popliteus area and used for 15 minutes to tolerance until good, quick contraction of muscle is achieved. Then gentle motion, flexion, and extension of the knee are started with the use of ethyl chloride spray to relieve pain. Motion is kept within pain limits, but the range is gradually increased as the pain subsides with the use of the spray. After treatment, if the patient is able to walk without pain, permission is given to do so. However, if the patient limps or walking is too painful, walking is restricted. Then the patient is requested to return the following day, after doing the exercises several times for the remainder of the first day and avoiding standing and walking. However, in less severe cases the patient may stand and walk with crutches, simulating normal steps with the injured extremity. In more severe cases the patient must be on crutches; in still more severe cases, he must be recumbent for a few days. The treatment is continued daily for a week or 10 days, and by the end of that time the patient should be comfortable. Now rehabilitation of the weak muscles, mainly quadriceps and especially vastus medialis, is started, with gradually increasing resistance exercises and later with weight exercises. Return to full normal strength is necessary for permanent good results. This return occurs much faster after immediate mobilization than it does after prolonged immobilization. Return to full normal function is particularly important in injured athletes and injured workers who perform physical labor.

**Example 2: Treatment of a Painful Back.**[11, 17] When the patient has pain in the low back and some radiation down one leg, he is placed in the prone position with a pillow under the hips and legs. Electrodes are usually applied to sacrospinal muscles and gluteal muscles of the affected side. Ten minutes of tetanizing current and ten minutes of sinusoidal current to tolerance are used. Then the patient is started on gentle exercises while ethyl chloride spray is used to relieve discomfort. In the prone position, gluteal tightening and relaxing is started, then the patient is rolled over to one side and both knees are flexed. One knee is gently slid up to the chest, straightened out, and brought back to the semiflexed position. Ethyl chloride spray is used until pain is controlled, then the other side is treated the same way. Other exercises are added as tolerated. In more severe cases the patient may have to rest part of the day. Total bed rest should be avoided whenever possible. Prolonged bed rest is extremely disabling and rarely necessary.

When the acute phase has passed, the patient is re-examined. While the ailment is in the acute stage, the examination, if possible, is restricted to a neurological review. Afterward, x-rays are taken and Kraus-Weber tests performed. Tension is assessed and triggerpoints searched for. Assuming that triggerpoints are found in gluteal, gluteus medius, or tensor and piriformis areas as well as in sacrospinal muscles, we would first inject and treat the triggerpoints and then start a program of exercises. Assuming the Kraus-Weber tests show weakness of abdominals, stiffness of back and hamstrings, and a certain degree of tension, the program illustrated on the following pages is prescribed. Instructions to the patient accompany the illustrations.

## Exercise 1

Position yourself comfortably on the floor with both knees bent. Close your eyes. Take a deep breath and exhale slowly. Slide one leg out and slide it back. Slide the other leg out and slide it back. Take another deep breath. Tighten both fists, then let go. Repeat once more. When you do this exercise at the end of your exercise session, make sure that you include the alternating movement.

Take a deep breath—exhale slowly. Now shrug and breathe up. Exhale as you let go of the shrug.

Turn your head all the way to the left, then return it to the normal front and center position, and let go. Turn your head all the way to the right as far as you can, return to normal position, and let go. If you have a stiff neck, also do this exercise in a sitting position. Repeat three times.

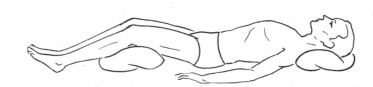

## Exercise 2

Flex your knees and slowly draw your right knee up as close to your chest as you can comfortably. Return your foot to the floor, slide the leg out, and slide back. Now bring the other leg up to the chest. Return the foot to the floor, slide the leg out, and slide it back.

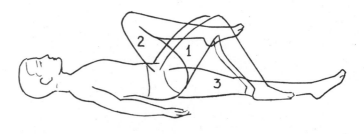

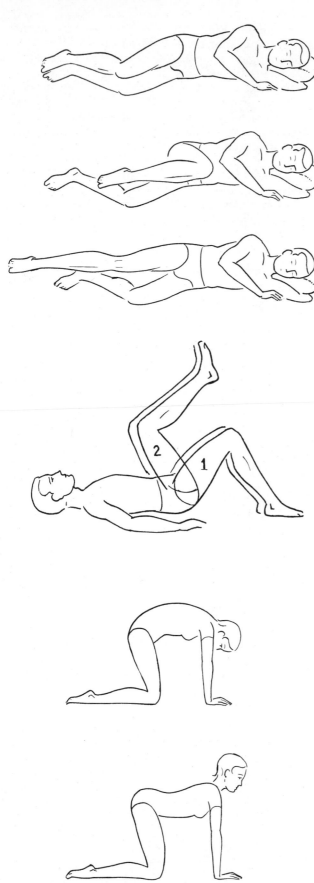

### Exercise 3

Lie on your left side with your head resting comfortably on arm. Keep both knees flexed and hips slightly flexed. Slide your right knee as close to your head as is comfortably possible, then slowly extend the leg until it is completely straight. The leg is dead weight. Do the exercise three times, then turn to your right side and do the exercises with your left leg. Remember the top leg is dead weight.

### Exercise 4. Double Knee Flex

Lie on your back with both knees flexed. Pull both knees up to your chest. Then lower your legs gradually to the floor in the flexed position. Do not raise hips off the floor.

### Exercise 5. Cat Back

Assume a kneeling position, resting on your hands and knees. Arch your back like a cat and drop your head at the same time. Then reverse the arch by bringing up your head and forming a U with your spine.

## Exercise 6. Head Up, Supine

Lie on the floor, with knees flexed, hands loose by your sides. Raise your head and shoulders off the floor, bring them down slowly, and let go. Remember that fingertips should touch the top of the knee.

## Exercise 7. Bend Sitting

Sit on a chair, feet apart on the floor. Let your neck droop, then drop your shoulders and arms and bend down between your knees as far as you can. Return to an upright position, straighten up, and let go. Do not force your downward bend.

## Exercise 8. Sit-up, Knees Flexed

Lie on your back with your hands clasped behind your head, knees flexed. Tuck your feet under a heavy object that will not topple over (a chest of drawers, bed, or heavy chair). Sit up, then lower yourself slowly to a lying position. You should sit up gradually, starting by raising your head, then your shoulders, and then your chest and lower end of the spine. Do not sit up by holding your trunk stiff and jerking your weight up. If you cannot do this exercise with your hands behind your neck, try to do it with your hands at your sides. Later, cross them over your stomach, and still later, when you are stronger, bring your crossed arms up to your chest and, finally, behind your neck and head. If you are unable to do this exercise at all, continue with the earlier exercises until you have gained enough strength to manage this one. Before the exercise, take a deep breath and exhale as you curl to a sitting position.

## Exercise 9. Bend-Sitting Rotation

Sit on a chair; bend forward as far as possible, dropping your head and shoulders. Bend down to the left, then gradually straighten up and rest. Do the exercise again, bending to the right.

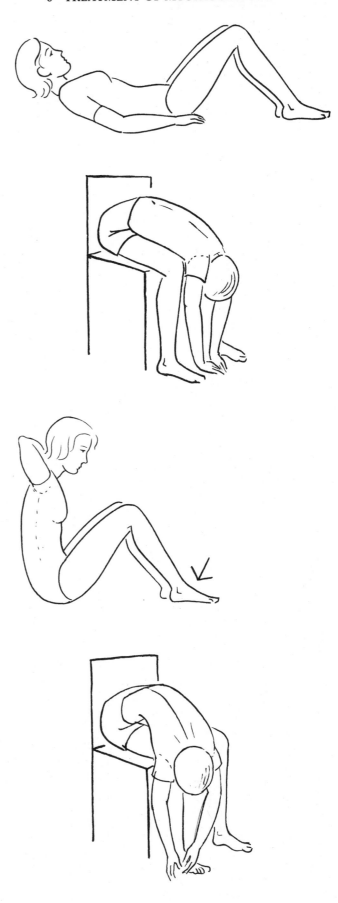

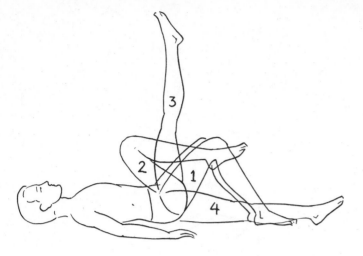

### Exercise 10. Hamstring Stretch

Lie on your back, both knees flexed, arms at sides. Bring one knee up as close as possible to your face and extend the leg, pointing the toes toward the ceiling. Keep the knee locked. Lower the straight leg to the floor. Slide the leg back to a bent position. Do the same for the other leg. Bring the other leg to the shoulder. As you extend the leg, cup the heel. Lock the knee, lower the straight leg to floor, and slide the leg back to a bent position. Do the same for the other leg.

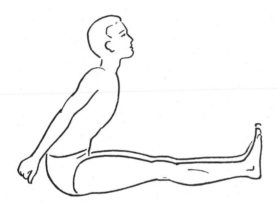

### Exercise 11. Hamstring Stretch

Stand up, and with feet together, clasp your hands behind your back, keeping your back and neck straight. Bend forward from the hips. Gradually lower your trunk and go down as far as you can, raising your head until you feel stretching in the back of your legs.

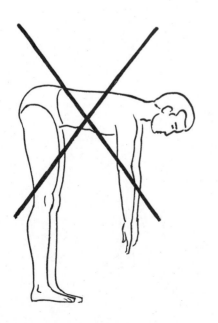
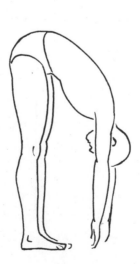

### Exercise 12. Floor Touch

This is the peak exercise given in all programs. Stand and keep the feet together. First relax by inhaling and exhaling deeply. Drop your neck gradually and let the trunk "hang" loosely from the hips. Drop the shoulders and then the back gradually. Let gravity help you. Do this two or three times. When you are completely relaxed, "hanging from the hips," try to reach down as far as is easily possible. Relax again, straighten up, then repeat. Now reverse the order of exercises, going from 12 to 1.

The patient visits the office for treatment two to three times a week and receives sinusoidal current to still-uncomfortable areas; the exercise program is given gradually. In the first session the patient is able to do three or four of the first exercises, which include relaxation. Then one exercise, rarely two, is given on successive days, provided that the patient can perform the exercises properly and with ease. Gradually the whole program of exercise is given. The patient is requested from the beginning to do the exercises at home every day at least once; in the beginning, when the program is very short, the exercise should be done twice a day.

A comprehensive preventive program is used by more than 1000 YMCAs. The program is known as "The Y's Way to a Healthy Back."

Over 83 per cent of patients with back pain examined in the Columbia-Presbyterian Back Clinic[2] had not disease but had strictly muscle problems; even patients with true disc or spinal abnormality always had associated muscle problems. Therefore, examination of a patient with back or neck pain without thorough assessment of the muscle status is incomplete.

The same principles apply to rehabilitation of patients after fracture,[12] whether it be fracture of extremity or back. The muscle status of these patients must be thoroughly evaluated. Reconditioning in fractures without major displacement that does not require immobilization must be based on the results of this evaluation. The evaluation must include assessment of tension and muscle function after relief of muscle spasm, and investigation for triggerpoints.

Patients with injuries to the lower extremities must not be permitted to walk unaided until they can walk painlessly without limping. Countless permanent disabilities have been unnecessarily incurred when patients were encouraged to walk in order to attain function when they were still in pain and incapable of walking properly. Damage to the upper extremities should be avoided by prohibiting movements that exceed the patient's muscular potential. There are especially dramatic consequences of too-early return to work by injured persons who have not been reconditioned to full strength and flexibility. These patients are subject to repeated recurrence of injury—and often to permanent disability.

## REFERENCES

1. Bonica, J. J.: Management of myofascial pain syndromes in general practice. JAMA 164:732, 1957.
2. Gaston, S. R.: Preliminary Report of a Group Study of the Painful Back. Low Back Clinic, Columbia Presbyterian Medical Center, New York. Personal communication, undated.
3. Glogowski, G., and Wallraff, J.: Ein Beitrag zur Klinik und Histologie der Muskelharten (Myogelosen). Z. Orthop. Grenzgeb. 80:238–268, 1951.
4. Jacobsen, E.: Tension Control for Businessmen. New York, McGraw-Hill, 1963.
5. Kopell, H. P. and Thompson, W. A. L.: Peripheral Entrapment Neuropathics. Baltimore, Williams & Wilkins, 1963.
6. Kraus, H. et al.: Back pain correction and prevention. N.Y. J. Med. 77:No. 7, 1977.
7. Kraus, H.: The need for relaxation in athletics, J. Sports Med. 3:No. 1, 1975.
8. Kraus, H., Mahoney, J. W. and Weber, S.: Immediate mobilization of certain ligamentous injuries of the knee. General Practice Vol. XXIV, No. 4, October, 1961.
9. Kraus, H.: Diagnosis and Treatment of Low Back Pain. General Practice Vol. 5, no. 4, April, 1952.
10. Kraus, H. Therapeutic Exercise. Springfield, Ill., Charles C Thomas, 1963.
11. Kraus, H.: Backache, Stress and Tension. New York, Simon & Schuster, Inc., 1965.
12. Kraus, H. and Mahoney, J. W.: Fracture Rehabilitation. In Donald A. Covalt (ed.): Rehabilitation in Industry. New York, Grune & Stratton, 1958.
13. Kraus, H.: Neue Distorsions Behandlung. Wien. Klin. Wschr. 48:1014, 1935.
14. Kraus, H.: The use of surface anesthesia in the treatment of painful motion. JAMA 116:2582, 1941.
15. Kraus, H.: Behandlung akuter Muskelharten. Wien. Klin. Wschr. 50:1356, 1937.
16. Kraus, H.: New treatment for injured joints. Abstract, JAMA 104:1261, 1935.
17. Kraus, H.: Clinical Treatment of Back and Neck Pain. New York, McGraw-Hill, 1970.
18. Lange, M.: Die Muskelharten (Myogelosen). Muchen, J. F. Lehman Verlag, 1931.
19. Miehlke, K., Schulze, and Eger, W.: Klinische und experimentelle Untersuchungen zum Fibrositis Syndrom. Zeitschrift fur Rheimaforschung Vol. 19, August 1960.
20. Peder, H.: Neue Versuche uber die Bedeutung der Ubung fur die Leistungsfahigkeit der Muskel. Scand. Arch. Physiol. 27:315, 1912.
21. Sainsbury, P. and Gibson, T. G.: Symptoms in anxiety and tension and the accompanying physiological changes in the muscular system. J. Neurol. Neurosurg. Psychiat. 17, no. 3, August, 1954.
22. Schwarz, G. A. and Rose, E.: Neuromyopathies and thyroid dysfunction. Arch. Intern. Med. 112:555–568, 1963.
23. Schwarz, L., Laszio, and Daniel P. Tausig, D. P.: Temporomandibular joint pain. NY State Dent. J. 20:219–223, 1954.
24. Simons, D. G.: Muscle pain syndromes—Part I. Am. J. Phys. Med. 54:289–311, 1975.
25. Simons, D. G.: Muscle pain syndromes—Part II. Am. J. Phys. Med. 55:15–42, no. 1, 1976.
26. Sonkin, L. and Cohen, E.: Treatment of the menopause. Mod. Treatment 5:545–563, 1968.
27. Spiegel, H. and Spiegel, D.: Trance and Treatment. Basic Books, INc. 1978.
28. Steindler, A.: Lectures on the Interpretation of Pain in Orthopedic Practice. Springfield, Charles C Thomas, 1959.
29. Travell, J.: Basis for multiple uses of local block of somatic trigger areas (procaine infiltration and ethyl chloride spray). Miss. Valley Med. J. 71:13–21, 1949.
30. Travell, J. and Rinzler, S. H.: Pain syndromes of the chest muscles: Resemblance to effort angina and myocardial infarction, and relief by local block. Can. Med. Assn. J. 59:333–338, 1948.
31. Wilson, J. and Walton, N.: Some muscular manifestations of hypothyroidism. J. Neurol. Neurosurg. Psychiat. 22:320, 1959.

# 7

# Treatment of Pain, Spasm, and Psychosomatic Symptoms Mediated Through the Sympathetic System, Including Sphenopalatine (Nasal) Ganglion Blockade

*by Asa Ruskin, M.D.*

It is common knowledge that muscle spasm and associated pain are strongly affected by psychosomatic factors and that tension spasm alone is probably one of the most common of all physical complaints, closely followed by a wide variety of common disorders whose psychosomatic etiology is widely recognized.

It is my belief that the underlying physiological mechanism of all these disorders is mediated through the sympathetic nervous system and its control of vasomotor responses in the effector organs. Symptoms such as muscle pain and spasm are provoked or prolonged by localized micro-

ischemia and relieved by relaxation of this focal vasoconstriction, allowing a return of homeostatic metabolic conditions in the muscle necessary for relaxation of the fibers. An understanding of this mechanism and its far-reaching implications may be gained from the abundant medical literature that has evolved from empirical observations on the easily accessible sphenopalatine ganglion.

A review of the literature dating back to the beginning of the century shows that the nasal ganglion (Meckel's ganglion or sphenopalatine ganglion) has been implicated in the therapy of such disparate syndromes as pain of the head and neck, facial pain, abdominal pain, diarrhea, asthma, angina pectoris, intractable hiccup, low back pain, sciatica, menstrual pain, hyperthyroidism, blindness, glaucoma, metallic taste in the mouth, as well as muscle pains of the shoulder, upper extremity, neck, and low back. There is also a group of publications on its use in ophthalmological conditions including ophthalmic migraine, blindness associated with arterial spasm, glaucoma, and ophthalmic herpes.[2, 5, 8, 12, 16, 17, 28–30] One connecting thread of all these conditions is the fact that on occasion they may be psychosomatically induced.

## ANATOMY

The sphenopalatine ganglion (SPG) is the largest collection of neurons in the head outside of the brain itself. It is located in the pterygopalatine fossa. One is immediately struck by the extensive territory to which this ganglion distributes branches and by its major connections with the trigeminal nerve (via the sphenopalatine nerves), the facial nerve (via the greater superior petrosal nerve), and the internal carotid artery plexus, providing also direct communication with the superior cervical sympathetic ganglion.

From a physiological standpoint, the SPG can be treated in conformity with the other sympathetic ganglia of the head in describing three types of roots: motor (visceral motor), sensory, and sympathetic. This is a convention, because the roots usually are of a mixed character. However, one or the other type of fibers usually predominates.[2–5, 9]

Figure 7–1 shows fibers of a sensory afferent type passing through the SPG to the maxillary branch of the trigeminal nerve. There is also evidence that some axons of postganglionic neurons (motor sympathetic) with cell bodies located within the SPG pass by way of the sensory route to be distributed with the somatic sensory fibers of the maxillary nerve (No. 10, Fig. 7–1).

The visceral motor or parasympathetic fibers arising in the medulla oblongata pass through the geniculate ganglion, joining the SPG via the superficial petrosal nerve. It has also been established that a number of somatic sensory neurons with cell bodies located in the geniculate ganglion are also part of the so-called motor root of the SPG, passing through the greater superficial petrosal nerve. These sensory nerves serve areas of the soft palate and adjacent parts of the pharynx, where they are concerned with gustatory function and some general sensation. There is also evidence of sympathetic afferent neurons with cell bodies located in the geniculate ganglion, the peripheral processes of which follow the same course as the somatic sensory neurons but have a much wider distribution, including other parts of the nasal cavity.

The sympathetic root of the SPG is the great deep petrosal nerve, which is, in a sense, a direct extension of the carotid plexus. The great deep pe-

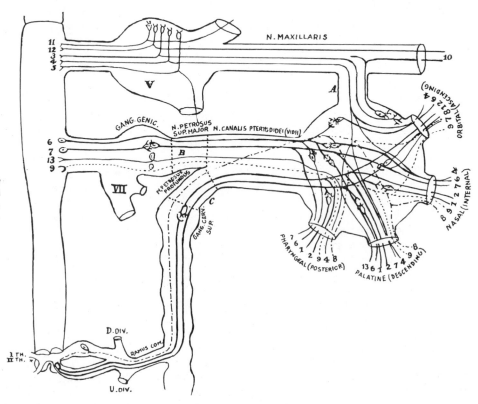

**Figure 7–1.** Connections of the sphenopalatine ganglion. (From Sluder, G.: Nasal Neurology. Headaches and Eye Disorders. St. Louis, C. V. Mosby, 1927.)

trosal nerve may be considered the connecting fasciculus between the superior cervical sympathetic ganglion and the SPG. Most of the fibers are postganglionic, arising from cell bodies located in the superior cervical sympathetic ganglion. Some of the fibers are peripheral processes of preganglionic nerve neurons from cell bodies located in the ventral horns of the upper thoracic spinal cord segments.[2, 3, 5]

Branches to the orbit and lacrimal gland, as well as branches to the other sympathetic ganglia, have been described. There is also evidence that some sympathetic fibers accompany the sensory fibers of the facial nerve in its distribution to the posterior scalp, neck, and external ear.[6] Zacharias[7, 8] described direct branches from the SPG to the anterior lobe of the pituitary, visible microscopically, their function described in his paper on pseudopregnancy following extirpation of the sphenopalatine ganglion in the rat.

We can see that at least in lower animals the SPG, situated as it is, constitutes an autonomic system crossroads, linking four major systems, three neural and one humeral: the trigeminal, facial, autonomic, and pituitary. Before considering the pathological and therapeutic implications of this superficially located major autonomic ganglion, let us try to understand why it exists where it does.

Developmentally, the nose in lower animals is probably the greatest factor in the preservation of the species. It has a wide variety of physiological functions, ranging from regulation of temperature to recognition of the presence of enemies. The success of its adaptation is dependent on reflex mechanisms as well as the direct effects of nasal stimuli. However, it is probable that an equally important role is played by stimulation of the trigeminal, facial, and autonomic nerves and perhaps the endocrine system by direct action on the nasal ganglia. The chemical presence of an enemy not only immediately arouses the sympathetic system but reflexively induces change in facial expression, used by some animals to strike fear into their enemies, as well as an increase in sensitivity of the face and increase in acuteness of hearing and sight. All of these phenomena can be mediated via the SPG and have been shown in certain pathological states in humans, including the provocation of hyperacusis and an effect on the accessory muscles of accommodation of the eye.[5]

## PATHOLOGICAL CONSIDERATIONS

For a long time, various pathological conditions throughout the body were ascribed to phenomena in the nasal pharynx. Nineteenth century and early twentieth century physicians spoke of rheumatism and other disorders ascribed to foci of infection in the nose or buccal cavity and ascribed manifestations at a distance to the effects of mysterious toxins.

The father of nasal neurology, if such a title were to be given, would be Greenfield Sluder, who was clinical professor and director of the Department of Otolaryngology at Washington University School of Medicine in St. Louis. Sluder's textbook *Nasal Neurology, Headaches and Eye Disorders*, which appeared in 1927, carried an extensive modern description of the various neurological aspects and complications of rhinology, with a lengthy discussion of "The Syndrome of Nasal (Sphenopalatine-Meckel's) Ganglion Neurosis." The term neurosis was equivalent to the currently used term neuralgia. He also referred to this syndrome as "lower half headache." While most modern texts dealing with headache make brief mention of this syndrome, it behooves us to review it in more detail.[2]

Sluder indicated that a past history of coryza occurs but the condition is often so slight that the patient may have forgotten it. The pain begins at the root of the nose and is felt about the eye, upper jaw, and teeth and sometimes the lower jaw, teeth, and ear. It frequently radiates backward to the occiput and the neck and may extend to the shoulder blade and shoulder. In severe attacks, it can radiate to the arm, forearm, hand, and even the fingertips. Rarely it is accompanied by a stiff or aching sensation in the throat and a feeling that the "teeth are too long." A metallic taste is occasionally noted and mild cases exist that are described as a sense of tension in the face and stiffness or "rheumatism" in the shoulder and neck. Sluder also reported that the syndrome just described is sometimes supplemented by a sympathetic syndrome "very wide in its distribution and wonderously complex," a prominent part being vasomotor and secretory phenomena.

The sympathetic syndrome occurs less often than the painful syndrome, but a sharp division is impossible because they are often mixed together and may alternate in the same patient with the same etiology. The onset may be explosive, with the patient seized by severe and protracted sneezing, accompanied by marked nasal congestion and very abundant thin secretions. There is marked redness and swelling of the external nose. In addition to these symptoms there is abundant tearing, redness, and congestion of the eyes, and occasionally dilatation of the pupil. Photophobia, asthma, vasomotor rhinitis, hay fever, and paroxysmal sneezing may all be seen. A given patient may have all these symptoms or just one, in greater or lesser severity. Sluder emphasizes that all of these symptoms are stopped by blocking the SPG with cocaine or other topical anesthetic. In severe cases he used 2 per cent silver nitrate solution or 2 per cent mercurochrome. He found that isolated symptoms of the sympathetic syndrome, including glossodynia, otalgia, nausea, parageusia, vertigo, scotoma, photophobia, rhinorrhea, and asthma, were all controllable by similar blocking of the SPG.

Simon Ruskin in 1929, in an article titled "The Neurologic Aspects of Nasal Sinus Infections,"[5] pointed out that the symptoms described by Sluder, as well as other symptoms at a distance, seemed to be related to irritation of the nasal sympathetic system by chronic postinflammatory hypertrophy of the nasal mucosa. He believed that the face and head pains secondary to SPG irritation and amenable to SPG blocking could be divided into two categories, an anterior group of trigeminal type with a neuralgic quality and caused by direct sensory involvement and a posterior type with a more myalgic quality that seemed to follow the distribution of the facial nerve. He thought that this latter category was caused by vasomotor spasm resulting from irritation of cranial autonomic fibers that accompanied branches of the facial nerve. He suggested that the vasomotor spasm, by interfering with the microcirculation of the muscle, allowed accumulation of metabolic wastes that evoked a low-grade spasm and at the same time created a vicious cycle so that the spasm itself induced further vasomotor disturbance. This, he noted, would also explain the relief accorded by vigorous massage, diathermy, and various forms of heat. He postulated that a more diffuse effect on the involuntary nervous system was responsible for the relaxation of muscle spasm that could be noted in other muscles of the trunk and extremities.

Ruskin was not alone in utilizing this technique for treatment of muscle spasms at a distance. Byrd in 1930[10] reported using it in treating low back pain, sciatica, asthma, angina, and Buerger's disease. Heitger reported its use in brachial neuritis in 1925; Byrd and Byrd[11] reported in the Archives of Internal Medicine in 1930 a lengthy list of conditions with over 10,000 treatments having been given in 2000 patients. It is interesting that they indicated that lumbago was relieved in three fourths of the cases and sciatica in one fourth to one fifth. Dock[12] reviewed the literature in the Journal of the American Medical Association in 1929 and gave an essentially similar list of cases to those already mentioned.

In 1938, Larsell, Bonds, and Fenton[13], in the Archives of Otolaryngology, also reported that Sluder's syndrome was due to vasomotor changes in areas of pain caused by reflexes secondary to irritation of the nerves in the region of the SPG producing local ischemia in the painful muscles. They indicated that pain in Sluder's syndrome can be relieved by procaine injection in the skin loco dolenti and substantiated their findings by experimental studies in rabbits. Faradic stimulation of the SPG produced vasoconstriction of the ear. This vasoconstriction would occur even after section of the maxillary branch of the trigeminal nerve. However, it was abolished by section of the cervical sympathetic chain or of the cervical cord. Fenton wrote on the pathways of referred pain from the nose in 1938[6] and emphasized also referral of pain to the neck, ear, and occipital area corresponding to sensory fibers in the facial nerve as postulated by Ramsey and Hunt following their description of herpes oticus.

An interesting aside that I noted in reviewing the literature was an article by Stewart and Lambert in 1930,[14] in which they disagreed with Ruskin on the anatomy, stating that if remote effects occur, it must be by a central mechanism, with the general tone of their article being highly skeptical. Stewart and Lambert[15] published an article in 1934 entitled "Further Observations on the SPG" in which they reported having done a controlled series using cocaine with epinephrine to limit the area of application. They reported the successful treatment of lower half headache, facial pain, asthma, and ear, neck, and shoulder pains, as well as a case of sneezing attacks.

The role of the SPG in causing systemic diseases, including pain in the hip, colitis, asthma, and multiple autonomic complaints including visceral pain, depression, and nervousness, was outlined by Van Osdol in 1931[16] who reported on the systemic effect of nasal hyperplasia as it affects the nasal ganglia.

There is a separate literature concerning the sphenopalatine ganglion in ophthalmology. Dubois-Poulsen[17] described a nasal facial reflex very similar to the description of Sluder's, with tearing and erythema of the eye and face, dilatation of the pupils, and paresthesias in the upper extremities spreading to the neck and occipital area. He also reported a nasocardiac reflex producing syncope and noted that while he did not find alterations in intraoccular pressure, there were marked changes in retinal artery pressure. He described irritative effects on the eye as secretory, vasomotor, and sensatory, and responding to anesthesia of the SPG. He also reported a case of optic atrophy that improved subsequent to SPG block. This was attributed to improved circulation.

I submit as a medical curiosity the 1935 report of Sparer,[18] whose paper described the cessation of convulsive seizures following injection of alcohol into the SPG in three cases. In each case there was significant nasal pathology with impacted turbinates. Sparer postulated that the seizures were due to vasomotor spasm by irritation of cranial autonomics.

## PAIN AND SYMPATHETIC INNERVATION

At the International Symposium on Pain in 1974, several papers were presented concerning pain and the autonomic nervous system. Gross noted that it is "lack of neurotomal distribution that has delayed recognition of this group of disorders as clinical entities" (Bonica[25]). He also quoted Leriche, who observed that certain types of pain disappeared after localized resection of the sympathetic chain and that stimulation of the cervical sympathetic trunk during surgery produced "very strong painful anxiety and produced strong pains in the lower jaw teeth and behind the ear on the same side."[1] These radiations did not correspond to the known topography of spinal nerves. Citing these and many other studies, Gross concluded that the sympathetic pain syndromes corresponded to vascular zone topography. Studies dating back as far as 1935 showed that excision of pelvic autonomic nerves gave pain relief in advanced pelvic carcinoma.[26]

Procacci[27] reported a study of cutaneous pain threshold changes after sympathetic block in reflex dystrophies. He indicated that, in the opinion of some current investigators, an abnormal sympathetic reflex activity is present in many diseases differently classified. This activity induces and maintains trophic disturbances, pain, and other sensory alterations. This mechanism is operant, for instance, in some limb vascular diseases and in some rheumatic diseases, as in muscular rheumatism with myalgic spots. He indicated that in his own research dealing with 30 patients suffering sympathetic reflex dystrophies of the upper or lower limb, all patients had myalgic spots, often having the well-known characteristics of triggerpoints. He carried out pharmacological block of the sympathetic chain, ipsilateral to the affected limb, and found that not only was the causalgic pain relieved but the "triggerpoints" became less painful to pressure or completely disappeared, even in the limb contralateral to the sympathetic block.

He pointed out that concepts regarding sympathetic control are:

1. Efferent sympathetic discharge is under the control of ipsilateral and contralateral neuronal systems located at different levels in the CNS. Every change of the afferent cutaneous muscular and visceral input to the CNS sets up variations of the sympathetic discharge through spinal, bulbar, and suprabulbar somatosympathetic and viscerosympathetic reflexes.

2. The efferent sympathetic fibers to somatic and visceral structures and most of the visceral afferents pass through the sympathetic ganglia, as well as some afferent somatic fibers. He concluded that pharmacological block of the sympathetic ganglia produces an interruption of the efferent sympathetic and afferent visceral fibers of the blocked side. His research also showed that the sympathetic system controls the cutaneous pain threshold and sympathetic block induced changes, not only in the skin but also in ipsilateral and contralateral deep tissues "as shown by the disappearance or attenuation of the muscular triggerpoints."

## AUTONOMIC SYSTEM AND PSYCHOSOMATIC DISORDERS

The list of disorders that have been shown to be amenable to sympathetic block, principally at the sphenopalatine ganglion, includes in addition to those already mentioned various dermatological conditions including psoriasis and essentially every condition for which a psychosomatic etiology can at times be implicated. This does not mean to imply that these conditions are always or even in most instances psychosomatic, but simply that they can be, and that in those instances in which they are of psychosomatic etiology, the sympathetic innervation appears to be implicated. In 1978 I postulated that one of the roles of the sphenopalatine ganglion in lower animals, located as it is in the nose with nerve connections far exceeding those necessary for simple control of local secretory processes, might be as a trigger declenching the rage reaction.[31, 32] I stated at that time that psychosomatic disorders could be looked on as highly attenuated segments of a rage reaction and amenable to physiological dampening by topical anesthesia of the sympathetic mechanism underlying the physical manifestations of the complaint.

While the role of sympathetically mediated vasoconstriction may be most dramatic in the provocation or maintenance of muscle spasm, it is easy to conceive of this mechanism also being applicable to a variety of effector organs bringing about all the pathological conditions noted previously. We may also speculate that microspasm of the vasonervorum could underlie other forms of pain and paresthesias arising from either organic or psychosomatic causes. In 1964 we demonstrated that the small nerve fibers were differentially more susceptible to ischemia than the larger myelinated fibers[33] and also the effect of topical anesthesia on sensory nerve conduction.[34]

The role of vasoconstriction in muscle spasm is further borne out by recent thermographic studies showing that muscle in chronic spasm is cooler than surrounding normal muscle (see Chapter 8, section on thermography), and what appears to be an underlying unity in the mechanism of action of the common treatment modalities.

## UNITY OF MECHANISM UNDERLYING COMMON MODALITIES OF TREATMENT FOR MUSCLE SPASM

The oldest and most common first aid treatment for muscle spasm is heat with attendant vasodilatation, supplied externally or by deeper penetration achieved with diathermy or ultrasound. The use of a rubifacient in the form of a poultice, a mustard plaster, or a more modern topical ointment is also an old standby. Massage produces vasodilatation, either by direct physical mechanical effect or by reflex mechanism, depending on the technique used.

The use of superficial cold by ethyl chloride spray may seem at first contradictory, but it is well established that this technique, while causing a superficial vasoconstriction of the skin, evokes a reflex vasodilatation of the deeper muscle tissue for its beneficial effect.

The injection of procaine, a potent vasodilator, is often used to relieve myofacial triggerpoints and muscle spasm with effects far outlasting its transitory anesthetic action.

One of the effects of acupuncture has been shown to be the production of a brief local vasoconstriction followed by a reflex vasodilatation (see Chapter 9), although this might not be the only mechanism of action of this technique.

High-voltage electrical stimulation is another electrotherapeutic method of provoking vasodilatation (see Chapter 10).

Several reports strongly suggest that chiropractic manipulations may owe whatever efficacy is attributed to them to the provoking of local segmental

sympathetic reflexes having mechanisms probably not unlike all the other treatment modalities.[35]

Figure 7–2 summarizes the conception of psychosomatic mechanisms and the loci of therapeutic intervention. It is important to further emphasize, however, that these treatment techniques may be effective even though the symptoms arise from a purely organic cause or, as in many instances of chronic pain, are due to a combination of factors. As shown in Figure 7–2, going counterclockwise, there is a continual reciprocal cybernetic relationship between the brain and the neuroendocrine or the autonomic nervous systems, or both, and it is at this level that psychotrophic drugs can exert their effect.

In order for the mental processes to be manifest, be it as muscle spasm, asthma, urticaria, and so forth, I have postulated that transmission needs be made via the autonomic nervous system and principally the sympathetic chain, and it is at this level that the various treatment modalities discussed exert their primary influence. The sphenopalatine or other types of sympathetic block work at a greater distance and, in the case of muscle spasm, the physical therapy modalities and heat work directly at the level of the sympathetically innervated microcirculation.

The various effector organs subject to psychosomatic disorder can respond to the usual chemical symptomatic treatments common in general medical practice.

Psychoanalytic concepts consider that the symptoms produced in a given individual by psychosomatic mechanisms have symbolic significance for that individual. I would postulate a reciprocal relationship between the individual and the symbolic representation of the symptoms as being the site amenable to therapeutic intervention by psychotherapeutic and cultural approaches.

The syndrome of sympathetic reflex dystrophy with causalgia can almost be looked upon as a naturally occurring experimental demonstration of these mechanisms. In that little-understood syndrome, the existence of a strong psychogenic factor has long been commonly accepted. The sympathetic reflex dystrophy syndrome is usually initiated by a relatively minor but painful injury to an extremity such as a pinch or crush injury to a finger or toe, followed by development of sympathetic reflex changes over succeeding weeks that involve the entire limb with vasomotor changes characterized by vasoconstriction of the smaller vessels causing a decrease in surface temperature, progressive swelling of the limb, atrophic changes of the skin (which becomes shiny), and a paralysis frequently with contracture of the fingers into a fist. This syndrome can often be relieved by sympathetic block, the usual technique being injection of the cervical chain at the stellate ganglion. It also

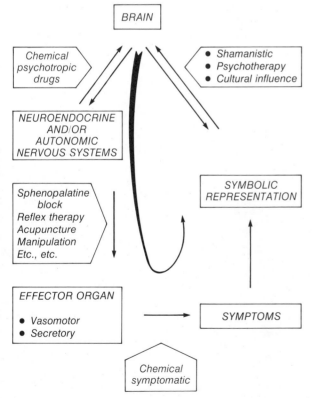

**Figure 7–2.** Psychosomatic mechanisms and locations of interventions.

may respond favorably to a series of sphenopalatine blocks. I have observed that following sphenopalatine block, the skin temperature of the affected hand will increase by 3 or 4 degrees and the patient will report a reduction in pain. The optimal treatment is to combine sympathetic block with a physical therapy regimen designed to reduce edema, improve circulation, and increase range of motion.

## TECHNIQUE FOR PERFORMING SPHENOPALATINE BLOCK

Early technique involved direct injection of the SPG, often utilizing alcohol or application of silver nitrate. Various techniques for direct needle application existed and are described by Sluder.[2] Simon Ruskin,[5, 9, 23, 24] who also used SPG anesthesia to perform tonsillectomy, developed a technique of direct injection through the posterior palatine canal utilizing a specially designed needle. While this technique worked well in his hands, it does leave the less experienced operator subject to the very undesirable possibility of intraorbital injection by error.

The most satisfactory technique currently utilized is to affix a small pledget of cotton to a wire metal applicator and apply a topical anesthetic directly to the SPG area and the adjacent descending nerves (Figs. 7–3 and 7–4). This can best be accomplished by using two applicators, one directed upward behind the middle turbinate and the second under the inferior turbinate, as noted in Figure 7–4. Any topical anesthetic is effective. Tetracaine (Pontocaine) in 4 per cent solution is satisfactory but takes longer to act than cocaine 25 per cent,

which is the most rapid. The patient is always questioned regarding sensitivity, and the initial application, if cocaine is used, may be a lower percentage, such as 10 per cent. Only one or two drops of anesthetic are necessary on a pledget directly applied. This amount does not produce systemic effect.

It is important that the cotton pledget be affixed to a metal applicator, the last centimeter of which has been twisted in spiral so that the cotton may be firmly affixed with a clockwise rotation of the applicator and removed by counterclockwise rotation. This essentially eliminates the risk of loss in the posterior nasopharynx. Under no circumstances should a wooden applicator be utilized, as a broken applicator could be extremely difficult to remove from the nose. In the very unlikely event that the cotton on a metal applicator becomes dislodged, the nasopharynx should be irrigated abundantly with normal saline or plain water, allowing the cotton pledget to be swallowed, because trying to remove it directly with forceps could provoke serious damage. We have also found it useful to have the patient suck on a piece of hard candy during the treatment. This stimulates a constant flow of saliva that will wash the anesthetic from the posterior pharynx if it should drip down, and avoid the occasional suppression of the gag reflex that may cause the patient momentary anxiety.

In my experience of 25 years, and the experience of Simon Ruskin extending for 40 years prior to that time, there have been no serious incidents of idiosyncratic reaction to the use of cocaine or other topical anesthetic. Mild to moderate anxiety reactions may occur during the first or second treatment in the same manner that such reactions

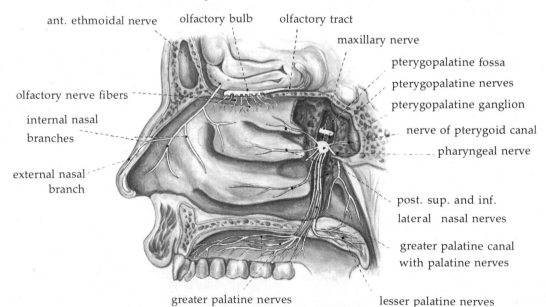

**Figure 7–3.** Nerves of the lateral nasal wall. (From Langman, J. and Woerdeman, M.W.: Atlas of Medical Anatomy. Philadelphia, W. B. Saunders Co., 1978.)

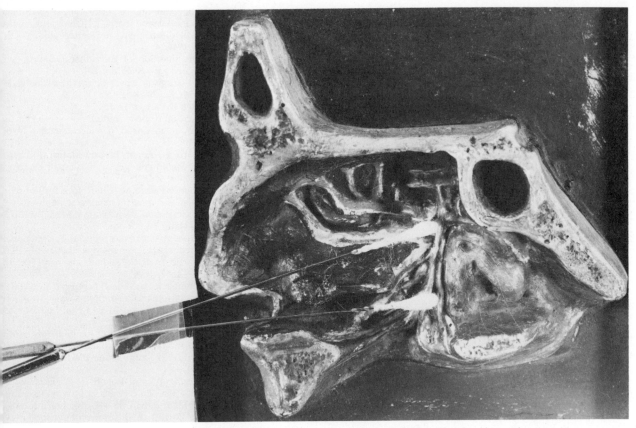

**Figure 7–4.** Model of lateral nasal wall showing cotton-tipped applicators in place for performing sphenopalatine block.

sometimes occur in some individuals who undergo any injection or medical procedure. For this reason it is extremely important to explain the procedure carefully to the patient before the initial treatment and emphasize that no needles will be used and no injection will be given. The patient should be advised that the procedure will cause a peculiar sensation or tickling of the nasal passage but is not painful. The patient should be warned in advance that he might experience an unpleasant taste or a momentary inability to swallow and for these reasons the candy has been given.

Sphenopalatine block has been shown to reduce blood pressure in hypertensive individuals, and reports of its use in the treatment of hypertension were published in the 1930s prior to the development of the modern pharmacological antihypertensive agents. Some patients will manifest a symptomatic drop in blood pressure with typical perspiration forming on the forehead, mild tachycardia, and a "light-headed" sensation. In all instances it has been sufficient to remove the applicators and have the patient lie down for 15 to 20 minutes. Patients who experience a light-headed feeling are advised to have a cup of coffee and relax before going home.

Before the applicators are placed, the nasal pas-

sages should be examined utilizing a lighted nasal speculum or a head mirror. One must observe for a deviated septum, nasal polyp, or any other condition that could impede entrance or withdrawal of the applicator or otherwise complicate the procedure.

This technique has been readily learned by the residents in our department and is within the capability of any physician who wishes to learn it.

## REFERENCES

1. Leriche, R.: La Chirurgie de la Douleur. Quoted by Gross, D.: Advances in Neurology, 4:93, Raven Press, New York, 1974.
2. Sluder, G.: Nasal Neurology. Headaches and Eye Disorders. St. Louis, C. V. Mosby, 1927.
3. Schaffer, J. P.: The Nose. Paranasal Sinuses, Nasolacrimal Passageways, and Olfactory Organ in Man. Philadelphia, Blakiston, 1920.
4. Paparella, M. M. and Shumrick, D. A.: Otolaryngology, Vol. 1. Philadelphia, W. B. Saunders Company, 1973.
5. Ruskin, S. L.: The neurologic aspects of nasal sinus infections. Arch. Otolaryngol. 10:337–383, 1929.
6. Fenton, R. A.: Pathways of referred pain from the nose. Am. J. Surg. 42:194–198, 1938.
7. Rosner, S., Shelesnyak, M. C. and Zacharias, L. R.: Nasogenital relationship II. Pseudopregnancy following extir-

pation of the sphenopalatine ganglion in the rat. Endocrinology 27:463–468, 1940.

8. Zacharias, L. R.: Further studies in nasogenital relationship. J. Comp. Neurol. 74:421–445, 1941.

9. Ruskin, S. L.: Contributions to the study of the sphenopalatine ganglion. Laryngoscope, Feb. 1925, pp. 3–24.

10. Byrd, H.: Sphenopalatine test. J. Mich. Med. Soc. 29:294–298, 1930.

11. Byrd, H. and Byrd, W.: Sphenopalatine phenomena; present status of knowledge. Arch. Int. Med. 46:1026–1038, 1930.

12. Dock, G.: Sluder's nasal ganglion syndrome and its relation to internal medicine. J.A.M.A. Sept. 7, 1929, pp. 750–753.

13. Larsell, O., Barnes, J. F. and Fenton, R. A.: Relation of irritation in region of paranasal sinuses to certain vasomotor changes. Arch. Otolaryngol. 27:266–274, 1938.

14. Stewart, D. and Lambert, V.: Sphenopalatine ganglion. J. Laryngol. Otol. 45:753–771, 1930.

15. Stewart, D. and Lambert, V.: Further observations on sphenopalatine ganglion. J. Laryngol. Otol. 49:319–322, 1934.

16. Van Osdol, H. A.: Systemic effect of nasal hyperplasia as it affects nasal ganglion. J. Indiana Med. Assoc. 24:3–8, 1931.

17. Dubois-Poulsen: Le ganglion sphenopalatin et l'oeil. Annales d'Occulistique 174:217–248, 1937.

18. Sparer, W.: Cessation of convulsive seizures following infection of alcohol into the sphenopalatine ganglion in three cases. Laryngoscope 45:886–890, 1935.

19. Ruskin, S. L.: The role of the coenzymes of the B complex vitamins and amino acids in muscle metabolism and balanced nutrition. Am. J. Dig. Dis. 13:110–116, 1946.

20. Ruskin, S. L.: The control of muscle spasm and arthritic pain through sympathetic block at the nasal ganglion and the use of the adenylic nucleotide.

21. Ruskin, S. L.: The dynamics of muscle tones and its relationship to circulatory failure. Am. J. Dig. Dis. 15:261–271, 1948.

22. Ruskin, S. L.: A newer concept of arthritis and the treatment of arthritic pain and deformity by sympathetic block at the sphenopalatine (nasal) ganglion and the use of the iron salt of the adenylic nucleotide. Am. J. Dig. Dis. 16:386–401, 1949.

23. Ruskin, S. L.: The injection of the sphenopalatine ganglion. Laryngoscope July 1935, pp. 1–7.

24. Ruskin, S. L.: The surgical aspect of the nasal ganglion. N.Y. State J. Med. 25:929–940, 1925.

25. Bonica, J. J.: Quoted by Gross, D. (1).

26. Behney, C. A.: Excision of pelvic autonomic nerves for the relief of pain from advanced pelvic carcinoma. Ann Surg. 101 (1); 1935.

27. Procacci, P., Francini, F., Zoppi, M. and Maresca, M.: Cutaneous pain threshold changes after sympathetic block in reflex dystrophies. Pain 1:167–175, 1975.

28. Amster, J. L.: Sphenopalatine ganglion block for the relief of painful vascular and muscular spasm with special reference to lumbosacral pain. N. Y. State J. Med. Pp. 2475–2480, Nov. 15, 1948.

29. Ruskin, S. L.: Herpes zoster oticus relieved by sphenopalatine ganglion treatment. Laryngoscope 35:301–302, 1925.

30. Ruskin, S. L.: Toxic hyperthyroidism of nasal origin J.A.M.A. 83:1586–1587, 1924.

31. Ruskin, A. P.: Sphenopalatine (nasal) ganglion, a review of its role in "psychosomatic" symptoms, rage reaction pain and spasm. Arch. Phys. Med. Rehab. 60:353–359 1979.

32. Ruskin, A. P.: Sphenopalatine (nasal) ganglion, its role in pain, spasm and the rage reaction and possible relationship to acupuncture. J. Acupuncture Electrotherapeutics Res. 4:91–103, 1979.

33. Ruskin, A. P., Jocson, A. and Rogoff, J. B.: Effect of ischemia on conduction of nerve fibers of varying diameter. Arch. Phys. Med. Rehab. 48:304–310, 1967.

34. Ruskin, A. P. and Rogoff, J. B.: Study of sensory nerve conduction and the effects of topical anesthetic. Arch Phys. Med. Rehab. 45, December 1964.

35. Korr, I. M.: The Neurobiologic Mechanisms in Manipulative Therapy. New York, Plenum Press, 1978.

# Diagnosis and Management of Chronic Pain in Physical Medicine and Rehabilitation

*by Andrew A. Fischer, M.D., Ph.D.*

This chapter summarizes a personal experience of almost 10 years in differential diagnosis and management of painful conditions in various clinical settings, including in my private office and in a pain clinic. The types of patients include private patients, those involved in workers' compensation cases, patients treated under the New York State no-fault automobile insurance program, and veterans with full benefit for free treatment. Both inpatients and outpatients, those with ambulatory acute conditions and patients suffering from chronic pain syndromes with typical and atypical psychological changes were treated and followed.

Since the documentation and differential diagnosis of pain seems to be the first logical step in the management of these patients, we must first consider methods for quantitative and objective documentation of physical findings. Thermography, heat imaging of the body, seems to be the most important method in documentation of pain and its differential diagnosis. My colleagues and and I found that thermography can be used for diagnosis of several painful conditions, including myofascial pain syndromes and triggerpoints. Another method useful for documentation of pain is pressure threshold, which measures the minimum force or pressure inducing local discomfort or pain

and represents a quantitative measure of local tenderness. Pressure tolerance is a clinical method useful for assessment of patients' sensitivity, tolerance to pain and is measured by the maximum force (pressure) that a patient can tolerate over the tibia or deltoid muscle. Muscle spasm is a frequent phenomenon accompanying and signaling pain. A new method has been developed, the tissue compliance measurement, that expresses the consistency of soft tissue. Tissue compliance can be used for objective and quantitative documentation of muscle spasm, spasticity, swelling, tumors, and other soft tissue pathology. Finally, ambulatory monitoring for a 24-hour period, including the sleep hours, proved to be useful for detection of muscle spasm and activity during the day and night.

After a description of these methods and of our approach to the evaluation of the pain patient are given, the physical diagnosis and treatment of pain syndromes will be described. The most important conclusions from our experience with various patients can be summarized as follows: Pain originating from muscles, ligaments, tendons, bursae, and periarticular structures, in a vast majority of cases, is concentrated in small circumscribed areas that are very tender on palpation and are extremely sensitive to pressure. These exceedingly tender spots are called *triggerpoints* (see pp. 106 and 135); if their irritation induces pain in a remote area, they are called the *referred pain zone*.[1, 19, 32, 33, 36] If there is no obvious referred pain from a sensitive point, the "tender spot" is a more appropriate name. The diagnosis and treatment of tender spots and triggerpoints play a major role in the management of chronic pain, since it can usually be alleviated utilizing a special technique of injection to the most painful triggerpoint causing the patient's present complaint. The triggerpoint injection consists of careful needling of the tender spot combined with infiltration by local anesthetic. This technique is described in detail later in the chapter.

The second major conclusion of our experience based on treatment of a large number of chronic pain patients is that the vast majority, in our estimate at least 80 per cent of patients with chronic pain, suffer from undiagnosed or improperly treated myofascial pain syndromes with triggerpoints or tender spots. We discovered the reason for this fact from our experience in training resident physicians. A considerable amount of time is required in order to train a person to detect triggerpoints even under the direct personal supervision of a clinician experienced in the field. Training in technique of triggerpoint injections and their combination with proper physical therapy is even more time-demanding and usually takes six months.

## HISTORY

This chapter deals primarily with treatment. However, at least some highlights of history and physical examination of the patient with chronic pain should be mentioned, because they are the two most important methods for diagnosis and differential diagnosis of chronic pain conditions. Very often they are the only way to identify the cause and pathophysiological mechanism of pain.

It is obvious and quite recognized in all other disciplines of medicine that a condition cannot be treated successfully and properly without identification of its etiology. Nobody would seriously consider treating patients with a diagnosis of chest pain without identifying whether it is of coronary origin or whether it arises from pleurisy, pneumonia, embolism, bone metastasis, or is pain originating in muscles of the chest wall. In comparison, consider the number of patients we see with the diagnosis of "chronic low back derangement," "low back pain," or "neck sprain," without identification of the exact source of discomfort. Often the origin of the pain, which is so crucial for treatment, is not identified, as to which ligament, muscle, joint, root, or nerve, or specific area is involved. Interestingly, the tremendous progress in

diagnostic methodology, particularly noninvasive techniques including computerized tomography, thermography, and electromyography, has not reduced the importance of the history and physical examination. On the contrary, the contributions of these new technologies to the analysis of painful conditions only reaffirmed the unique value of the history and physical examination. One of the reasons for this conclusion is the fact that techniques that document anatomical pathological changes, including myelography and computerized tomography, frequently show positive findings even in areas without clinical symptoms. Therefore, the results of all diagnostic procedures should be carefully correlated with physical findings and history in order to assess the clinical significance of anatomical changes.

A complete history provides information not obtainable by any other means. I find the use of a "Pain Questionnaire" extremely helpful. This contains a body picture on which the patient marks the sites of pain, its extension and intensity, as well as the areas of numbness, parasthesia, or loss of sensation. The intensity of pain is carefully noted. A simple way to define it is to ask the patient, "If the worse pain you can imagine is worth $100, how much pain are you having now?" The scale essentially reflects the severity of pain on a 10-step scale: 9 or 10 or 90 to 100 would be extremely severe pain, 7 or 8 very severe, 5 or 6 severe, 3 or 4 moderate, 1 or 2 minimal to mild pain. I find the 10-step scale more valuable because on a 5-step scale patients were unable to express less dramatic changes such as can take place after physical therapy.

Important information may be obtained when inquiring regarding the character of the pain: Is it throbbing, boring, burning, dull, sharp? The duration of pain is also important for the evaluation of the patient's progress. Often the patient may continue to complain, but on careful evaluation we find that the intensity and frequency have decreased and the duration of the pain has shortened. The time of the day that pain occurs and its development is a useful cue. If pain, accompanied by stiffness, occurs in the morning hours after the patient gets up, activity and a hot shower or local heat applied usually bring relief. In the subacute stage, pain occurs following a certain amount of physical activity. As the patient improves further, pain no longer occurs on mild activity, and bed rest gives complete relief. At this stage, pain usually occurs in the afternoon only after prolonged activity, indicating that the main problem is weakness and lack of muscle endurance. The muscles are able to hold the spine in proper position for a limited time only. Eliciting this information during history-taking and understanding its meaning will provide guidelines for the goal and method of treatment in each particular stage of recovery. As improvement occurs its meaning is explained carefully to patients so they understand that progress to a new, advanced stage in pain control has been achieved. Accordingly, an adjustment in physical activity and therapy is then necessary to utilize the increased functional capacity and upgrade the intensity of treatment.

Similarly the question, "What brings on the pain?" is essential for selecting treatment. Radicular pain and symptoms such as tingling or pins-and-needles feeling are frequently related to a certain position of the back or neck and can be alleviated with proper mechanical support. This support may gradually become less effective during the day and the pain may become worse with activity such as walking, sitting, and standing. Morning pain and stiffness, which are alleviated by mild activity but recur in the afternoon with fatigue, are typical of myofascial pain syndromes. Mild activity usually relaxes and relieves tension in the muscle by stretching, while more intensive or sustained activity induces pain.

Stretching of a painful area by bending or other movements is extremely useful in differential diagnosis of the origin of pain. Most of the painful conditions originating in muscles are relieved by stretching. The muscle spasm that usually accompanies the pain is also alleviated. Exceptions to this rule are very severe muscle spasm, tenderness, and acute muscle sprain or acute inflammatory reaction. These conditions are usually obvious and do not represent a diagnostic dilemma. The time the patient spends in bed, sitting, standing, walking, or working is carefully recorded. A useful question to ask is, "What can't you do that you would like to do?" Limitation of activity by pain has a completely different nature and significance for a housewife who can pace activities than for a working person who is forced to perform continuously. Limitation also differs in an executive who can take breaks during the day when the pain occurs. A person may put in a full-time work day without great difficulty but, if his main hobby is tennis, which he cannot play because of pain, he may still feel disabled. If sports are an important part of the patient's life, necessary for enjoyment and relaxation, the expectation to return to the favorite recreation activity becomes an essential goal. Otherwise, functional limitation by pain is very individual and depends on patient's life style, expectation, interests, and personality.

## PHYSICAL EXAMINATION

The purpose of physical examination of the patient with chronic pain, similar to the purpose with acute pain, is to establish the cause. Unless the cause of pain is established, effective treatment cannot be prescribed and the examination is of little value for the patient. On physical examination, we are looking for limitation of motion, weakness, and functional limitations. Gait analysis of pain is helpful. Observation of the patient's movements and their limitation often presents clues to the problems. A complete neurological evaluation is done with particular attention to the sensory changes, with determination of whether changes consist of decrease or increase in sensitivity to pinprick, touch, etc. If changes in sensation are established, their relation to dermatomes and to innervation areas of peripheral nerves is evaluated. Loss of sensation usually indicates chronic nerve compression, rarely neuropraxia. Hyperalgesia indicates acute irritation of the nerve structures and represents an important warning against the use of strong stimulation. The therapist should proceed with caution from a very mild degree of physical therapy and increase it gradually.

Complete functional muscle testing is done as soon as the pain allows. This is essential for documentation of the patient's condition as well as for diagnosis of segmental or peripheral nerve involvement. Testing of strength in painful muscles often leads to the false impression of partial tear.

One of the most important parts of the assessment is to determine whether the pain originates in active tissue, such as muscle, or passive tissues supporting the joints, such as ligaments, bursae, and tendon sheaths. Pathologically sensitive passive (noncontractible) tissues produce pain on elongation by passive stretching, but no pain is caused by active muscle contraction against resistance. Exceptions are conditions in which passive tissue is pulled by the muscle, as in the attachment of a tendon to the bone, or the tendons themselves, or when the passive tissue is squeezed by muscle contraction, as in suprapatellar bursae and some other bursae.

Pain produced in damaged muscle is aggravated on active movements only. Exceptions include very tender acute partial muscle damage. In this condition stretching may induce pain because of reflex contraction, hyperirritability, and inability of the muscle to relax and to follow the stretching force by passive elongation. This situation of tender and severely damaged muscle or severely spasmodic muscle induced by acute pain is usually easy to differentiate from a chronic pain condition in which the rule applies that pain induced by active contraction originates in muscle, while pain on passive stretching is usually caused by damage to passive tissues, usually ligaments. The sensitivity of damaged ligaments on passive stretching can be demonstrated easily in ankle sprain, in which the lateral ligaments are usually sprained without muscle involvement and pain typically occurs on passive inversion with supination. Similarly, a sprain of the supraspinous and interspinous ligaments is typically aggravated by flexion of the trunk, which induces stretching of the above structures. The significance of this differentiation for therapy cannot be overemphasized. Stretching of painful muscle, particularly when the pain is the result of triggerpoints, tension, or fatigue, often brings relief. The effect of stretching is enhanced when it is combined with cold or heat, and the combination yields good therapeutic results. Conversely, the stretching of an already damaged ligament always induces further aggravation of the sprain and pain and is contraindicated.

Series of tests are done routinely for neck pain and upper extremity pain. The head compression test, in which the head is pressed caudad, tests the root irritation secondary to a narrowed disc space in advanced discopathy. Lateral bending of the head with a slight rotation to the opposite side and pressure applied to the head caudad encroaches on the cervical foramina if they are narrowed. These tests are considered positive only if the solicited pain has radicular character.

In low back pain and lower extremity pain, I use a combination of tests that can be performed efficiently without causing the patient discomfort. The straight-leg raising test is done, followed by extending slightly the hip with a still-straight knee. The forced ankle dorsiflexion maneuver after release of the stretch of straight leg raising, sometimes is called Braggard's or Lasègue's sign, and is essential for differential diagnosis of the origin of pain. On straight-leg raising, pain may originate from stretching of the sciatic nerve, from tight hamstrings, or from the sacroiliac joint. In the latter instances Braggard's sign is negative. The FABERE (flexion, abduction, external rotation, extension), or Patrick's sign, is then tested for. I combine this test with pressure over the opposite anterior superior iliac crest, thereby stressing the sacroiliac joints. Hyperflexion of the hip and full knee flexion is then done, with rocking of the back to test each sacroiliac joint. The opposite leg is held extended on the examination table so that the sacroiliac joint on the side of hip flexion is put under stress. If this test is positive, further testing of the sacroiliac joint can be done. The examiner presses his elbow on the iliac crest with the patient lying on the side. Pressure on the sacrum of a prone patient also places stress on sacroiliac joints.

The lumbosacral junction is then tested by hyperflexion of both hips and knees simultaneously and by rocking of the pelvis. In the same position with hyperflexed knees and hips, after the degree of flexion is reduced somewhat, both legs are held firmly together and twisted laterally right and then left. This maneuver places stress on the lumbar facet joints. In the aforementioned sequences the straight leg raising is combined with stressing of hips and lumbosacral, sacroiliac, and facet joints.

The last step in noninstrumental physical examination is usually the most productive in diagnosis of the origin of pain; it consists of careful palpation for tender areas and for muscle spasm. The technique of palpation is really an art that can be learned only with extensive experience and most efficiently under direct supervision of an experienced teacher who shows the student where to palpate, what to feel for, and what to concentrate on. Without this direct instruction it is extremely difficult to learn to diagnose muscle spasm or some sensitive points, particularly in the deep tissues such as buttocks or lumbar or cervical paraspinals.

It is likewise important to learn how to differentiate a bunch of contracted and tender muscle fibers from other structures. Palpation is the most sensitive method for pain diagnosis and for the identification of its source. Since in the majority of patients with chronic pain the immediate cause lies in tender spots or triggerpoints, palpation is the only productive diagnostic method. The patient is asked to point with one finger where the pain is located and where the pain comes from. The area is then palpated carefully with the fingertips, and if tenderness cannot be found, greater pressure is applied, either by the thumb or by two superimposed digits. Special positions are necessary for palpation of certain muscles such as deep paraspinals and of ligaments.

# Documentation of Pain and Tenderness: Thermography, Pressure Threshold, and Tolerance Measurement

Important progress recently has been achieved in the documentation of pain and local tenderness. The pressure threshold is the minimum pressure or force that induces local discomfort or pain. I introduced this testing method to evaluate tender spots and triggerpoints.[5, 6] The method has been used for assessment of arthritic joints. Pressure threshold measurement (PTM) is a clinical method valuable in many aspects for documentation of tender spots. This quantitative documentation is useful in the diagnosis of myofascial pain syndromes and also to prove to patients the differences between the normal and the involved areas, which sometimes is necessary to convince them that tenderness is present. PTM is also helpful in the documentation of a patient's progress when different methods of treatment are evaluated. Finally, the method is essential for medicolegal documentation of triggerpoints and related pain.

The technique of PTM is easy to master. The patient lies or sits relaxed. We ask where the pain is, and palpate carefully for the most sensitive spot. Usually it corresponds to known sites for triggerpoints.[19, 36] Then the rubber disc attached to the pressure gauge is applied to the area (Figs. 8–1 and 2). The patient is told, "I'm going to increase the pressure gradually; please say yes when you start to feel discomfort or pain. I will stop pressing immediately so it won't hurt you." The pressure is increased gradually by 10 Newtons per sec, which is approximately 1000 gm per sec, until the patient indicates discomfort or pain. Usually the maximum hold position is used, but an automatic zeroing of the dial is available for rapid scanning (Fig. 8–1). Normal values have been established for nine areas where triggerpoints occur often and in the middle deltoid muscle, which is used as normal reference area because it seldom becomes tender. The normal values for males and females were established over the following areas: supraspinatus, infraspinatus, teres major, pectoralis, lumbar paraspinals 2 and 4 cm from the midline at L4 level, and gluteus medius.[7] Clinical experience confirmed by many physicians has proved PTM to be a useful clinical method.[20]

Pressure threshold measurement is useful for documentation of triggerpoints or tenderness in any kind of tissue, particularly in superficial tissues. When the tenderness is located deeply, relatively more pressure is needed in order to induce pain; therefore less impressive differences between both sides do not necessarily represent normal values. Considerable side-to-side differences (over 30 Newtons (N) per sq cm) are therefore more significant than lesser differences. Although the side-to-side differences are more reliable, deviations from normal values can be diagnosed using our standards. A side-to-side difference of 20 N per sq cm is considered pathological and a difference exceeding 30 N is definitely pathological, in our experience.

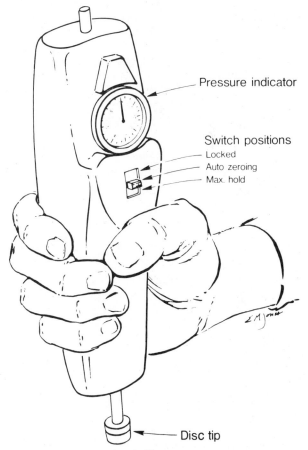

Pressure indicator

Switch positions
- Locked
- Auto zeroing
- Max. hold

Disc tip

**Figure 8–1** Pressure threshold meter.

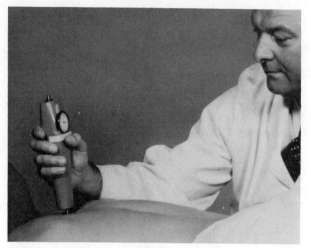

**Figure 8–2.** Use of pressure threshold measurement in thoracic paraspinal area.

Figure 8–3 represents the effect in a patient with psoriatric arthritis of triggerpoint injections on pressure threshold, which is displayed on Y axis as opposed to the day of follow-up (X axis). The right teres minor showed a pressure threshold of 50 N on the first day; this increased immediately after the injection to 70 Ns. The follow-up shows that after the first few days when local tenderness secondary to the injection decreased the pressure threshold, the reading increased, and again at 140 days after the injection it stayed at over 70 N (full line). The dotted line and open circles show the pressure threshold at T1 level over paraspinals, which equaled 40 N on the initial examination. Immediately after the injection to the same areas, marked X, the pressure threshold increased to al-

most 100 N. This indicates that the entire trigger-point has been anesthetized. In the follow-up the pressure threshold has leveled at 60 N, which is normal. In the lower part of the graph the triangles connected by the interrupted line show a pressure threshold of 20 N at the tip of the xyphoid process. This increased immediately after injection to 56 N but then decreased again; therefore, on the 140th and 150th day it was the same as at the time of the injection. This demonstrates the failure of the trig-gerpoint injection to improve the condition. At this time the patient complained of pain only at the tip of the xyphoid process. There was no pain in the right teres minor and T1 paraspinal level; this improvement was demonstrated by increase in pressure threshold.

Figure 8–4 demonstrates the use of pressure threshold measurement for evaluation of physical therapy. The patient was a 54-year-old women with low back pain secondary to a fall; the pain was worse on the left side. Subjectively, the patient felt improvement of 1 on a 5-step scale of pain after the therapy.

The site of measurement is indicated on the figure. Pressure threshold in Newtons per sq cm is indicated on each side before and after the administration of physical therapy consisting of hot packs, stimulation with sinusoid current, massage, and exercises.

Figure 8–5 shows changes of pressure threshold after physical therapy and their relationship to pain rating. The pressure threshold before (filled circles) and after treatment (open circles) is presented for a period of 24 days. The triangles represent the patients' *pain rating* on a scale of 0 to

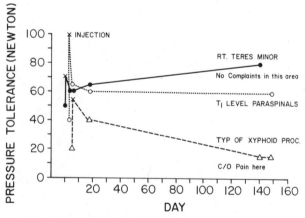

**Figure 8–3.** Effect of trigger point injections on pressure threshold.

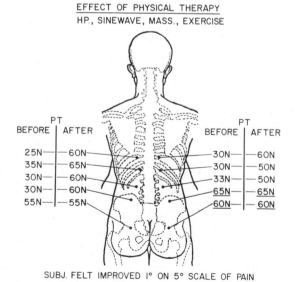

**Figure 8–4.** Effect of physical therapy on pressure threshold.

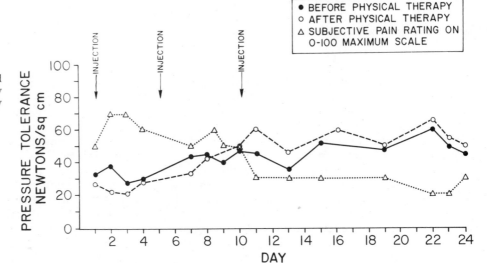

**Figure 8–5.** Pressure threshold before and after physical therapy session and pain rating by patient.

100. Note that the pressure threshold decreased regularly after physical therapy (i.e., the pain became worse) during the first week of treatment. This indicated that the treatment was too strenuous for the patient's acute condition. After the eighth day, when the pain rating decreased from 60 to 30, the reaction of pressure threshold to physical therapy demonstrated a reversal: with decrease of pain and of sensitivity, the same type and amount of physical therapy had a positive effect and the pressure threshold increased with each treatment. The pressure threshold measurement indicated that the therapy was inappropriate in the first week and that the treatment became effective when the patient's condition improved and his sensitivity decreased.

**Pressure tolerance** is the maximum pressure tolerated by the patient in clinical conditions. The technique is similar to that of pressure threshold, but the patient is asked to indicate when the operator is to stop increasing the pressure. A gauge with a higher force range is used. Pressure tolerance measurements provide information on the patient's pain tolerance (sensitivity to pain) that cannot be found by any other clinical method. The

measurement can be performed easily as part of the physical examination. For clinical purposes measurement over the mid-deltoid area, representing soft tissues (muscle), and over the anteromedial aspect of the shin bone, expressing sensitivity over bones, is suitable.[13] Normal values for males and females were established.[13] Pressure tolerance is higher in males than in females and higher over muscles as compared to bones. The range of force gauge required for these measurements is 0 to about 17 kg per sq cm. Decreased pressure tolerance over bones and muscles indicates low pain tolerance in general and is found in some patients with chronic pain syndrome. Decreased pressure tolerance over muscles usually indicates endocrine disorders, such as hypothyroidism or ovarian insufficiency.

In patients in whom pressure threshold–documented triggerpoints correspond to the patient's complaints and in whom there is a normal pressure tolerance, one may conclude that the tenderness developed in an area that prior to injury had been normal. The conclusion can be drawn that the triggerpoints are the results of injury to a previously normal area.[13]

# Tissue Compliance Recording in Documentation of Soft Tissue Pathology

Tissue compliance is a new method that was developed in the Veterans Administration Medical Center, Bronx, N.Y. The compliance is the quality of a material that allows it to yield to pressure. Compliance can be expressed by its reciprocal value, which is elastic resistance to deformation. Tissue compliance measures quantitatively the softness or firmness of the tissue, which usually is appreciated only by the subjective method of palpation. Amazingly, when palpation fails to reveal differences in consistency, tissue compliance demonstrates identical measurements on opposite sides of different comparable areas. When palpation reveals a difference in tissue consistency, the tissue compliance recording demonstrates the findings quantitatively and objectively.

The tissue compliance meter consists of a rubber disc with a surface area of 1 cm similar to the pressure threshold meter. However, the force applied is recorded through an electronic transducer on the abscissa of an XY plotter. The depth of penetration of the rubber disc is recorded also on the Y axis from a larger plastic disc that slides on the axis of the pressure transducer. When the force disc penetrates into the soft tissue, without damaging the skin, of course, the plastic disc stays on the surface of the body and the transducer records the depth of penetration of the force-measuring disc.[9]

Tissue compliance measurement is useful for the objective and quantitative documentation and diagnosis of changes in soft tissue consistency resulting from muscle spasm, swelling, tumors, lumps, hematomas, and so forth. The earliest signs of healing and resolution of soft tissue pathology, including injuries, are manifested in changes of consistency prior to any quantifiable alteration in the size of the structure.[15] Tissue compliance measurement is the most sensitive and the earliest objective indication of either healing and resolution or occurrence of complications in soft tissue pathology.[15]

Figure 8–6 shows a tissue compliance record from a lumbar paraspinal area in which spasm was palpable on the left side. The X axis represents the force used for pressing the rubber tip of the tissue compliance meter into the tissue and is calibrated in Newtons. The Y axis displays the depth of penetration of the same rubber disc. The lower record demonstrates the tissue compliance of the spastic left paraspinal muscles. Note that the penetration with the same force is much less on the left side than on the right, which is represented by the upper tracing.

An interesting approach still in the research stage is the 24-hour monitoring of muscle activity by recordings of electromyography. Using this method, spasm of lumbar paraspinal muscles was documented even during sleep in patients with low back pain.[10]

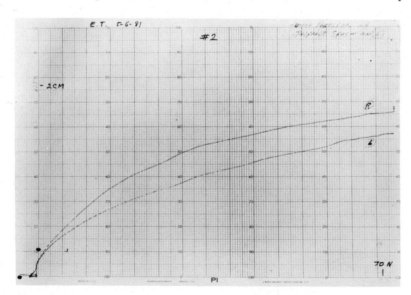

**Figure 8–6.** Tissue compliance record from lumbar paraspinal muscles. The lower record represents the spasmodic side.

# Thermography in Differential Diagnosis and Documentation of Painful Conditions

Thermography is a method of recording the distribution of surface temperature. Two systems of medical thermography are in current usage. Electronic (tele or noncontact) thermography is done with the use of scanning mirrors that reflect the infrared (IR, heat) radiation on an IR-electronic transducer. The IR pattern is then displayed on a black and white and/or color cathode ray tube from which it can be photographed. Contact thermography uses liquid crystals coated on a flexible sheet (Flexitherm system). Each of a possible seven colors represents a different temperature on an absolute but nonlinear scale. The sensitivity of clinical thermography is 0.1° C but 1° C sensitivity/color is usually employed, since a difference of at least 1° C is commonly considered clinically significant. Skin temperature depends mainly on local blood flow; it depends less on heat generated by deeper tissues. Anatomical configuration of surface (skin folds, gluteal cleft), and other factors also affect the picture.

## TECHNIQUE OF THERMOGRAPHY

Thermograms are taken in a draft-free room maintained at 65° F (21° C). Standardized views include about 35 pictures covering the entire body. The procedure is repeated in 15 to 20 minutes for proof that findings are not transient. Thermography is a noninvasive procedure. Since only the heat generated by the body is picked up and there is no exposure to radiation, repeated investigation can be undertaken without adverse effects. Comparison of repeat pictures increases essentially the reliability of thermography by helping to rule out false and questionable findings or confirming pathology.

Thermogram is considered abnormal if a side-to-side asymmetry occurs exceeding 1° C and affecting more than 25 per cent of the area. Changes in known physiological heat distribution patterns, such as the diamond shape in the lower back and the tadpole in the upper back, are also diagnostic.

Clinical use of thermography was introduced for study of breast carcinoma but is spreading steadily and has been established in a variety of diagnostic applications.[25, 29, 35, 37] In arthritis the extent and intensity of inflammation can be documented and the effect of therapy can be assessed quantitatively.

Thermography is used for diagnosis of peripheral arterial disease as well as evaluation of cerebral vascular dysfunction.[41] It is of utmost value in discovering, locating, and evaluating the course of thrombophlebitis.[41] Decubitus ulcers can be evaluated. Their early detection is possible, as is delineation of necrotic tissue and monitoring of risk areas.

Thermography may contribute to selection of a site of amputation and management of infected or sensitive stumps, the fitting of prostheses, and foot care in neuropathies.[8]

Thermography can document soft tissue injury,[12, 21, 31] infection, and inflammation. It is useful in preemployment screening for back disorders and in identifying persons at high risk for back problems.[18] Metastases, even into the spine, and osteosarcoma can be detected by thermography. Thermography in diagnosis of disc disease and radiculopathy is more sensitive than electromyography[14, 39, 40] or myelography.[27]

Triggerpoints (tender spots) are seen on thermography as discs with increased IR radiation (hot areas) of 5 to 10 cm in diameter (Fig. 8–7). Thus triggerpoints, the hallmarks of myofascial pain syndromes, can be studied objectively. Our results based on thermography and pressure threshold measurement indicate that the vast majority of back, neck, shoulder, and other soft tissue pain is related to triggerpoints.[8, 11]

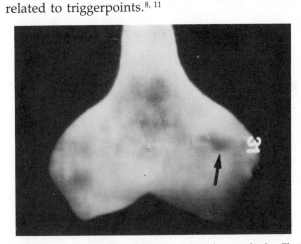

**Figure 8–7.** Liquid crystal thermogram taken with the Flexitherm system, showing the back of a 45-year-old woman with pain in the right shoulder blade area. The hot spot at right corresponds to a triggerpoint, which was tender on palpation.

Painful areas occur as hot zones on thermography in the acute stage but convert to cold zones in chronic pain. The shape of asymmetric (cold or hot) areas is of great diagnostic value. Stripes corresponding to dermatomes or portions thereof are diagnostic of segmental involvement. Irregular areas are often seen over injured tissue. Heat from active muscles is conveyed to overlying skin by vertically directed veins and can be recognized on thermography to be grouped in myotomes. Pathology in areas supplied by a peripheral nerve (carpal tunnel syndrome and other conditions) can be identified on thermography as such. Pain related to local infection or inflammation can be differentiated from ischemic pain in stumps and other areas. The presentation of pain in thermography thus has multiple facets, and interpretation always requires close clinical correlation.

Thermograms do not show a "picture of pain," since pain includes a subjective psychological experience. However, physiological correlates of pain induced by changes in vasomotor activity can be documented objectively and quantitatively. Thermography adds a new important aspect to documentation and differential diagnosis of pain originating in soft tissue not achievable by any other method.

Interpretation of thermal pathology related to pain requires a considerable experience in reading thermograms and knowledge of pain syndromes so both can be correlated with clinical findings.[8]

Figures 8–8 through 8–11 illustrate the use of thermography in selected cases. Figure 8–8 shows a thermogram of a tennis elbow. Findings include a hot area over the posterior aspect of the right elbow, with a localized hot spot on the area of the lateral epicondyle. The findings are compatible with local inflammation. The patient was a 47-year-old man, a regular tennis player, who had recurrent pain over the right elbow, especially in the lat-

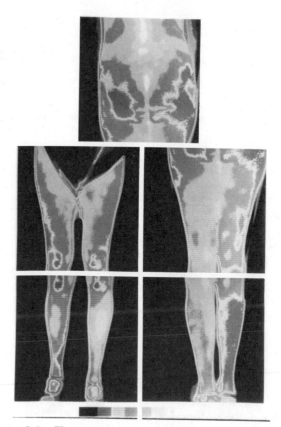

**Figure 8–9.** Thermogram showing L4,L5, S1,S2 radiculopathy.

eral epicondylar area. Clinical diagnosis was tennis elbow with triggerpoints in extensor muscles of the forearm. Findings were confirmed by pressure threshold measurements, by pain on triggerpoint injections, and by the course of recovery.

Figure 8–9 shows a thermogram of a patient with low back pain. Findings include bulging of heat emission at the level of L4–5 area bilaterally; this is suggestive of discopathy. Also seen were a colder lateral aspect of the right thigh (L5 dermatome), a colder anterior right leg (L4,5 dermatome), and a colder right calf (S1,2 dermatome). These findings are compatible with L4,5, S1,2 radiculopathy. The patient was a 57-year-old woman with chronic low back pain radiating to posterior aspect of the right lower extremity. Neurological evaluation revealed hypoactive ankle jerks. Electromyogram showed L5, S1 radiculopathy.

Figure 8–10 is a liquid crystal thermogram of lower extremities. The patient was suffering from chronic low back pain and underwent lumbar laminectomy. Note the difference over the anterior aspect of legs, one side being darker (warmer) than the other. The dorsum of the right foot is darker (warmer) than the left. The second to fifth digits on the left side are cold. The Flexitherm thermograph was used. Findings are compatible with L5 radiculopathy. The conclusions of thermography were confirmed by segmental block of the left L5 root, which alleviated the pain.

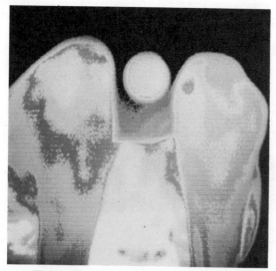

**Figure 8–8.** Thermogram of a tennis elbow.

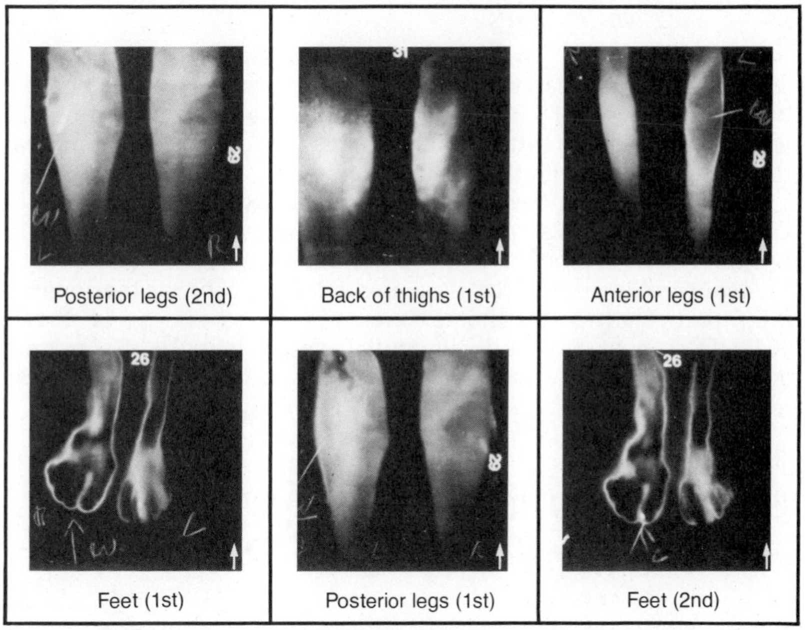

| | | |
|---|---|---|
| Posterior legs (2nd) | Back of thighs (1st) | Anterior legs (1st) |
| Feet (1st) | Posterior legs (1st) | Feet (2nd) |

**Figure 8–10.** Liquid crystal thermogram showing L5 root lesion.

Figure 8–11 shows photographs and thermograms of a stump ulcer. Findings include colder spots inside the ulcer suggestive of poor circulation. Transmetatarsal amputation failed to heal for three months. Thermogram suggested ischemia preventing healing.

## SUMMARY

Thermography in management of the pain patient can be used as follows:

1. Thermography can be used to document the presence of the pain. This applies for clinical documentation as well as for medicolegal uses, which are becoming more and more important. It is often useful to show the patient that pain is real and also the type of pain being treated. Frequently this is

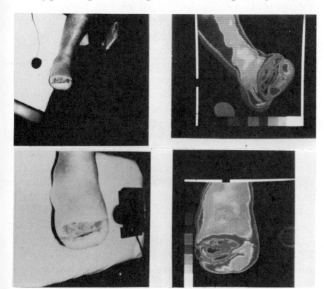

**Figure 8–11.** Photographs and thermograms of a stump ulcer.

necessary because chronic pain patients usually come to us after seeing many specialists, most of whom express different opinions. Patients are confused, and an objective method for diagnosis is needed. Very important is that we never suggest a diagnosis to the patient. We ask him, "Does this picture mean anything to you?" There is no suggestion in this question.

2. Thermography is important in ruling out or documenting segmental spinal cord involvement, and/or radiculopathy, disc disease, and pathology involving the spinal cord on a segmental level.

3. It has a unique role in documentation of soft tissue injuries such as whiplash injuries and sprains and low back sprains, which do not show up with any other method.

4. It is the only completely objective method to document triggerpoints and tender spots and so-called myofascial pain syndromes, which are a frequent cause of chronic pain.

5. Thermography is the method of choice for follow-up of patients with pain under any therapeutic regimen.

6. It is the method of choice for documentation of ischemia as a cause of pain. This is particularly useful in evaluation of stumps, ulcers, and non-healing and painful wounds.

7. Thermography is also the method of choice for documentation of any inflammation such as arthritis, bursitis, tendinitis, epicondylitis, and tennis elbow.

8. Thermography is the only method available for documentation of sensory nerve involvement that cannot be assessed by other methods when small branches are affected.

9. The diagnosis of thrombophlebitis is probably done easiest by thermography; the method provides high sensitivity and reliability.

10. Peripheral arterial vascular disease can be diagnosed and its extent assessed by thermography.

Similarly, cerebral vascular disease can be detected by thermography. Thermography is useful for selection of level of amputation in ischemic limbs and for evaluation of stump problems.

11. Visceral pain has been documented by us. Differentiation of this type of pain is extremely important when segmental root or peripheral nerve involvement is considered as a possible cause of pain, particularly in the thoracic area.

12. Documentation and differential diagnosis of so-called referred pain are important parts of man-agement of pain. The clinical hallmark of referred pain is that the painful areas show no local pathology on palpation and on testing of function. We were able to document referred pain on thermography.

13. Temporomandibular joint dysfunction can be documented objectively and its extent assessed by thermography, according to my experience.

14. Breast cancer risk evaluation is being done by thermography; however, the method is not considered of primary use in diagnosis of breast cancer.

# General Principles for Treatment of Patient with Chronic Pain

Chronic pain develops when treatment in the acute stage was incomplete or not effective. Since the primary goal of treatment is not only to alleviate the pain but to remove and possibly cure its cause, the therapy should be aimed specifically at the etiology.

Equally important, the goal of treatment is restoration of function, which includes prevention of functional deterioration, restoration of flexibility and range of motion, and maintenance of muscle power and endurance. The minimal grade of muscle performance necessary for a patient's usual recreational and vocational activities should be achieved. It is obvious that functional rehabilitation cannot be accomplished by use of painkillers and anti-inflammatory drugs and that the recovery of performance is hindered or prevented by long periods of bed rest. Therefore, bed rest is used only in the acute stage of pain, particularly in lower back problems, when root compression symptoms or signs are present requiring protection of the root from damage. As soon as the condition improves and allows, the patient is mobilized, first intermittently, sitting, standing, or walking to the point of discomfort but never to pain level. If this occurs, a pain-spasm-pain cycle may begin. The patient then gradually resumes activity, using a low back support. Exercises for relaxation, reduction of tension and anxiety, maintenance of flexibility, prevention of stiffening, and stretching to relieve spasm are encouraged even for the bedridden patient. Any movement that hurts is avoided.

In management of any pain condition, local treatment is most effective and takes priority over use of oral or parenteral medication that affects the entire body. Of course, a combination of local and general therapy is often necessary, and each poten-tiates the effect of the other. However, any treatment that does not utilize local modalities completely should be considered inadequate. Effective local treatments include heat or cold, cooling spray, ultrasound, massage, exercises, stretching, local injections, including triggerpoint injections, and local and regional nerve blocks.

The principle of specific treatment for various conditions is frequently ignored; this leads to failures. Kraus[19] described at least four conditions in patients with lower back pain, each requiring special prescription: Four are muscle weakness, muscle spasm, tension pain, and triggerpoints.

**Weakness.** This can be detected easily by the Kraus-Weber Test (see Chapter 6); it requires prescription for strengthening exercises. We usually start with development of endurance by repetitive movements with intervals of rest in between. Exercises done at home three or four times daily are part of the program. The strengthening and endurance exercises are concentrated on the muscle groups that showed weakness on the Kraus-Weber Test. Use of general exercises without a focus on the problem is evidently less effective and often the target muscles are missed entirely. This is particularly true in sports injuries and in patients active in recreational or competitive sports.

**Muscle Spasm.** This is frequently a cause of pain or a correlate of pain. Muscle spasm can be defined as sustained involuntary muscle contraction; it cannot be relaxed completely by voluntary control. The condition is frequently induced by pain,[10] and when sustained for a long period of time spasm itself induces pain by constant irritation of proprioceptors and by strangulation of the blood circulation. If severe spasm develops or even less severe spasm lasts for a long time, local ischemic changes may occur and triggerpoints may develop secondary to local tissue damage. Therefore, it is important to break up the spasm as soon as possible and with maximum efficiency. Relaxation of the muscles that are in spasm will prevent the vicious circle of pain-spasm-pain and the anatomical damage that may occur secondary to ischemia.

Effective means to relax muscle spasm is by local cold application, particularly with ethyl chloride spray. I have found fluoromethane spray less effective than ethyl chloride. Local moist heat is usually prescribed, along with electric stimulation using tetanizing current for 10 minutes. Sinusoid surging current or reciprocal stimulation is used for another 10 minutes. High-voltage stimulation sometimes is also effective in relieving muscle spasm (see Chapter 10). If noninvasive techniques fail (this may occur in very severe muscle spasm), local nerve block, particularly paraspinal block, will relieve the contraction promptly and usually will alleviate the pain completely. Two or rarely three segments are blocked to achieve the result. Paraspinal blocks are effective and the procedure is simple, particularly in the lower back area. It can

be performed with a 21-gauge 2-inch needle or with a 21 gauge 3-inch needle.

Muscle spasm and its relief can be documented promptly by recording of tissue compliance.

**Tension Pain.** Sustained stimulation with no relaxation of muscles from psychological stress causes this pain. Relaxation exercises, biofeedback, and stress management with counseling are adjuvants to physical modalities in treating tension pain.

Meditation and hypnosis are sometimes effective in chronic pain.

Sphenopalatine blocks often relieve pain, particularly in the acute stage[30] (see Chapter 7).

**Triggerpoints.** Treatment of triggerpoints is one of the most important types of therapy; it is usually rewarding. Triggerpoint injections combine injection and infiltration by a local anesthetic. The treatment of triggerpoints will be discussed in further detail, since the technique is crucial for success. Triggerpoints is the most frequently treatable condition causing pain. The failure to diagnose and treat the condition properly usually leads to development of chronic pain.

# Myofascial Pain Syndromes and Triggerpoints, the Most Frequent Causes of Musculoskeletal Pain

Myofascial pain syndromes constitute a group of disorders characterized by very sensitive small areas called *triggerpoints,* which are located in a muscle or connective tissue. Further characteristics include muscle spasm, tenderness on pressure, stiffness, limitation of motion, and weakness.[19, 32, 33, 36]

## What Are Triggerpoints?

Triggerpoints are small circumscribed hypersensitive areas in muscles or in connective tissues (ligaments, joint capsules, tendons, and so on) that have a specific and typical area of referred pain. The triggerpoint is so called because its stimulation, like the pulling of the trigger of a gun, "shoots" the pain into a distant zone called the reference (or target) area.

Pain usually is originated from triggerpoints in conditions diagnosed as myalgia (muscle pain), muscular or nonarticular rheumatism, myositis (myofascitis, muscle inflammation), fibrositis (in-

flammation of fibrous tissues), and fibromyositis. Similarly, in bursitis, capsulitis, tendinitis, and particularly in sprains, the pain is concentrated in the triggerpoints. Triggerpoint injection with a local anesthetic in these conditions usually results in prompt and long-lasting relief; this proves that the pain originated in the triggerpoint.

## What Induces Triggerpoints?

Any kind of local injury to myofascial structures (muscles, ligaments, and related tissues) can induce triggerpoints. Even slight injuries, blows, or sprains will induce triggerpoints if not treated promptly and properly. Traumatic triggerpoints are usually the cause of pain in ankle, back, or neck sprains.

Besides acute injury, chronic repetitive minor stresses are frequent causes of triggerpoints. Postural abnormalities, the stresses of daily activities that involve using the same muscles constantly, abnormal stress distribution in lower limbs (flat feet, knock knees, and so forth) are examples of these chronic irritants.

Another cause of triggerpoints is inflammation as in arthritis, myositis, rheumatism, and other connective tissue disease, and chronic infection. Nerve injuries and disorders, including nerve compression as in slipped intervertebral disc, induce triggerpoints, which may persist long after the compression has ceased. Endocrine dysfunction, particularly low ovarian and thyroid activity, and metabolic disorders, psychogenic stress, and exhaustion, are predisposing factors.

Muscle spasm (long-lasting contraction of muscle) can be caused by pain of any origin[10] and in turn induces pain that maintains the spasm. A cycle of pain-spasm-pain develops, which can be broken up promptly by infiltration with local anesthetic. However, if the cycle is allowed to continue, spotty ischemic muscle damage can occur. Metabolites that induce pain are trapped in the tender spots and become a source of constant irritation to the brain, thus forming the triggerpoint. Spasm persisting long after the original cause of pain has subsided can induce permanent damage to muscle tissue in the form of triggerpoints.

Psychological tension (inability to relax the muscle) may induce the pain-spasm-pain cycle.

### What Is the Best Treatment for Triggerpoints?

In suitable cases these should be treated by injection because no other method of therapy can reverse the pathological process so promptly, completely, and permanently. Other treatments of triggerpoints include ultrasound (a deep heating device) and deep kneading massage. Both methods are very painful and less effective than injections.

Once a chronic triggerpoint develops with fibrotic scar formation in the muscle, the most effective and best treatment is a triggerpoint injection. This consists of needling of the entire triggerpoint combined with infiltration with local anesthetic (lidocaine). Properly performed, a triggerpoint injection relieves the pain instantly and completely by breaking up the scar tissue so that the blood circulation removes the entrapped irritating metabolites. The difference between acupuncture and triggerpoint injection lies mainly in their effects. While acupuncture may induce relief of pain in some cases, once pathological changes have developed in the tissue, they cannot be rectified by this method. However, triggerpoint injections induce permanent relief by making possible the healing of the local pathology.

### Treatment After Triggerpoint Injection

After triggerpoint injection the muscle still tends to develop spasm and therefore spasm-relieving physical therapy (usually three sessions per week after each injection) is important. Heating, electric stimulation to relax the muscle, manual massage by a therapist, and relaxation and stretching exercises are irreplaceable after treatment of triggerpoints by injections. Gradually, as the pain improves, the intensity of exercises is upgraded to develop more flexibility, progressing to development of endurance and muscle strength.

The injection is followed by electric stimulation to decrease edema, improve circulation, reduce sensitivity to pain, and promote conditions for healing after the needling. We use the Medcollator or similar devices to apply sinusoid surging current or reciprocal stimulation to the injected area. Sometimes automatic stimulation, which includes a series of tetanizing currents combined with pulsating and sinusoid current, is preferred. The electric stimulation is combined with heating using hydrocollator packs, which cover the electrodes. An electric moist heating pad may be employed for easier handling.

The stimulation is set for about 15 minutes. The heating continues for 20 minutes and is followed by relaxation and stretching exercises. The session is then concluded by deep massage, ending with smoothing massage. After the triggerpoint injection the patient is requested to rest, and local heat or cold can be applied, whichever the patient prefers. Heat or cold decreases the pain and prevents the sore muscle from going into spasm. If the legs or buttocks are injected, the patient should limit walking for one day. Every one or two hours the patient should get up and walk for about five minutes to prevent stiffness. The patient is instructed in stretching exercises that are specific for the injected muscle, such as after injection to the gluteus medius the knee is pulled to the opposite shoulder and to the opposite flank, in lying, sitting, or standing position. (See Chapter 6 for stretching exercises.) The stretching exercises are specifically aimed at the injected muscle to induce relaxation and prevent development of spasm. Stretching is carried out for 6 to 10 seconds and is repeated on each side 10 times during a session. Stretching sessions are recommended every two hours after injection. This stretching regimen is very effective; patients feel the relaxation immediately. The regimen of limited use of the injected muscle is continued as long as local soreness after the injection persists, usually two to three days. However, the stretching exercises are beneficial and can be continued as long as the patient has any problem. Stretching is effective also for reduction of tension, stiffness, and prevention of spasm.

### Stages of Recovery
### After Triggerpoint Injection

1. Local anesthesia, one hour after the injection.
2. After the anesthetic wears off, numbness is re-

placed by local soreness that usually lasts two to three days or rarely longer. There is relief of "toothache-like" pain in the injected triggerpoint and often there is partial or considerable relief of pain in others.

3. After two to three days, in the case of generalized pain relief, patients begin to detect the presence of other triggerpoints. The impression is that of a "migrating pain."

4. The last stage is healing of the triggerpoint, allowing functional use of the injected muscle, which had been limited by the pain, stiffness, and other symptoms. For optimal functional recovery physiotherapy is essential.

The usual course of recovery after injection consists of four stages as just summarized. Immediately after the injection the local anesthesia is complete and there is no pain. Frequently pain from other triggerpoints also ceases temporarily, probably by lowering the total amount of irritation to the brain below the pain threshold. The patient feels relieved usually for two to three days.

About an hour after the injection the anesthetic wears off and local soreness from the mechanical effects of needling occurs. The soreness is perceived as a bruise in contrast with the original triggerpoint pain, which is similar to a deep toothache. The soreness can be controlled by mild pain killers. After two to three days the soreness usually subsides.

After triggerpoint injection there may still be pain present. Even properly executed injection affects only the injected triggerpoint permanently. In the area close to the injection many other triggerpoints may still be active. Only thorough examination of local tenderness can establish the site of origin of the pain. The triggerpoints close to the injected one usually are the source of persisting pain.

Frequently patients become concerned with pain occurring in an area that had not been painful prior to the injection. While a very painful triggerpoint exists in one area (for example, over the shoulder blade), it overshadows a less intense pain (in the neck) and the patient perceives only the most intense pain. When the more intense pain (in shoulder in this case) is eliminated by injection, the less severe pain in the neck becomes the one perceived. The patient is under the impression that the pain is migrating. It is important to realize that the triggerpoints that begin to be perceived are less painful and the shifting of pain is definite evidence of improvement.

### Outcome of Untreated Triggerpoints

If the triggerpoints are left untreated, or if conventional nonspecific therapy is used, the pain can be relieved, but the triggerpoint persists. Its sensitivity may be decreased gradually but it usually remains a constant source of irritation—the patient favors the area and pain occurs on minor stresses or exertion. Favoring the back or a sprained ankle with persisting triggerpoints induces increased stress to the other side or to the compensating structures.

Triggerpoints also disturb sleep, making the patient irritable and depressed, expanding and aggravating the adverse effects. Therefore, it is important to cure the triggerpoint by injection and not to allow further worsening of a condition that cannot rectify itself but deteriorates steadily.

### TRIGGERPOINT INJECTION

Hans Kraus, on my first visit to his office, taught me that meticulous adherence to minute details in injection technique makes the difference between complete failure and complete success. Many years of experience and thousands of injections given by me and many other physicians under my supervision have confirmed Kraus' conclusion.

The technique of triggerpoint injections will be described as I modified it during seven years of experience with intensive use of this fascinating modality. First, the exact location of the triggerpoint is identified by asking the patient to point to the spot where his pain is or where it comes from. The area is then palpated carefully. If light pressure fails to induce local pain, which is the case in triggerpoints located in deep muscles, particularly lumbar paraspinals and buttocks, pressure with the thumb or two superimposed fingers is necessary. Then pressure threshold measurement is performed, when indicated. Pressure threshold measurement is useful not only for finding the most sensitive spot exactly but also for documentation of the immediate effect of the injection. It is particularly useful for follow-up and documentation of the long-term effect.[3–5] Often this measurement is necessary to convince the patient that the injections have been effective, even if there is no immediate dramatic change in pain perception because the other non-injected triggerpoints are still painful. Decrease of pressure threshold reading in the injected area on follow-up visits proves that the injection was effective but more shots are required to bring complete relief of symptoms.

### SELECTION OF THE SITE OF INJECTION IN CASES OF MULTIPLE TRIGGERPOINTS

The most sensitive triggerpoint from the area is usually selected for injection; however, exceptions to this rule exist. In cases of multiple chronic triggerpoints when the difference in sensitivity is not remarkable and the subjective complaint is not prevailing in any part, the patient does not express preference for alleviation of pain in a certain area. The best results are achieved by treating the triggerpoints in the areas that are most important functionally. One of these is the gluteus medius, a muscle active during ambulation and often affected by triggerpoints. Other triggerpoint areas that take precedence in treatment when prevailing pain does not occur in one single area are the levator scapulae in the shoulder blade area and the midlevel cervical paraspinals for neck pain.

In acute sciatica secondary to disc disease, triggerpoint injections are amazingly effective when given together with paraspinal nerve block at the L5 to S1 level. Usually several painful triggerpoints are found and since the patient is supposed to be confined in bed to alleviate pressure on the nerve and to decrease or prevent pain, several triggerpoints can be injected in the first session according to the patient's tolerance. The next day and then in two-day intervals the remaining triggerpoints can be injected gradually; this often brings dramatic improvement in pain and in function. The following case serves as illustration.

### CASE REPORT

A 33-year-old man had acute excruciating low back pain that failed to react to chiropractic treatment and physiotherapy using ultrasound and electric stimulation. On initial examination patient was lying on the examination table moaning and complaining of excruciating pain in the lower back and over the posterior aspect of the left leg. The patient had a long history of recurrent back pain. Neurological examination, myelogram, and thermogram documented disc disease with radiculopathy. After lumbar paraspinal block and three injections to the most sensitive triggerpoints the patient was able to walk with minimal pain. Further injections to the remaining triggerpoints and physical therapy alleviated the pain gradually. The patient became ambulatory with only discomfort after ten days but was instructed to continue intermittent bed rest.

## TECHNIQUE OF TRIGGERPOINT INJECTION

After selection of the site of injection the exact location is marked, either by a needle scratch or by pushing the thumbnail into the skin. The injection is performed under sterile conditions, after careful washing of hands.

### EQUIPMENT USED FOR INJECTION

Betadine spray or sterile gauze soaked in Betadine.
Sterile 4 × 4 4-layer gauze pads for cleansing the injection area.
Sterile Band-Aids.
Sterile disposable needles—I prefer to use disposable needles.

16 G 1.5″—For withdrawal of lidocaine from the vial.
25 G 1.5″—For very sensitive areas, sometimes in temporandibular joint muscles, otherwise these needles are too thin for breaking up pathological changes.
22 G 1.5″—Used often for cervical paraspinals and suboccipital, scalp, arm, shoulder, elbow, forearms, leg, temporandibular joint muscles (pteryogoids and so on). Ideal for needling and injecting acute injuries such as muscle sprains and tears. Excellent for ligament sprain injection anywhere, particularly supraspinous and interspinous ligament sprain, extremity ligaments or small tendons or bursae.
21 G 2″—Excellent for paraspinal blocks at lumbar level or injections to superficial areas of the back, buttocks, and thigh and for large legs, muscular arms, shoulders, and shoulder blade muscles.
Sterile reusable needles—Some sizes are not available in disposable form with sufficient quality, therefore reusable needles are selected.
22 G 3″—Most frequently used for buttocks, lumbar paraspinals, sacroiliac joint, sacrotuberous and sacrospinous ligaments, thighs; also used in deep paraspinal blocks. This type of needle can be obtained as a disposable spinal needle or a 20 G 3″ size can be used. Best results are obtained with reusable needles; they are sterilized and stored in sterile envelopes.
25 G 2″—This is a long thin needle used in deep, painful, or delicate areas such as the gastrocnemius, which is very sensitive to injection, and in obese or muscular individuals sometimes for the back, shoulder blade muscles, or forearm muscles.
1 per cent Xylocaine, vials.
2 per cent Carbocaine vials (for cardiac patients) since Carbocaine has no effect upon the heart muscle.
A plastic box containing 2 or 3 needles of each size and a 10 or 12 cc syringe filled usually with 8 cc of 1 per cent Xylocaine.

Betadine-soaked gauze pads (4 × 4 multiple ply) and a bottle of ethyl chloride spray are taken into the patient area. The site of injection is marked on a body picture chart with the date of injections. The area is cleansed carefully, with the gauze pad exchanged at least twice.

The entire procedure is explained to the patient: "After cleansing the skin I will spray it with the coolant; this will decrease the pain. When the needle moves in normal tissue you won't feel any pain. When it hits the damaged tissue in the triggerpoint you will feel a short pain, then the anesthetic will take effect and the pain will be gone."

The proper needle is then attached to the syringe, which is held in left hand. The patient is alerted "This is cold" and the area is sprayed with ethyl chloride from a distance of 18 inches until white frost appears on the skin. During spraying, patients are instructed to breathe in and out as deeply as possible and to concentrate on the breathing so they will not feel pain. The instruction is repeated several times to reinforce it and to distract the patient from the procedure.

The skin is then pulled apart from the injected point to diminish the number of sensory endings and the needle is inserted by a fast movement to pierce the skin in the middle of the frosted spot.

The needling is then commenced. Patient is asked to say "yes" if pain occurs, indicating that the needle has penetrated the damaged tissue. The technique of needling is the critical part of the triggerpoint injection and will determine success or failure. The most frequent mistake is to inject the anesthetic the moment that the painful area has been penetrated. This usually gives only temporary relief while the entire damaged tissue or part of it is left in place. The basis of chronic irritation remains intact and the patient will continue to have recurrent pain, limited movement, stiffness, weakness—all symptoms of persistent triggerpoints.

Complete and long-lasting results can be achieved only by breaking up the damaged tissue. This is done by careful systematic inserting and withdrawing of the needle, almost millimeter by millimeter. It is useful to extend the needling to the border of the triggerpoint into normal nonpainful tissue on both sides of the damaged tissue. This method ensures that the entire triggerpoint area is needled until the surrounding normal tissue is reached. Also important is to withhold the injection of anesthetic until the triggerpoint area has been reached by the needle, otherwise the surrounding region becomes anesthetized and the patient is unable to feel the penetration of painful damaged tissue. Amazingly, penetration of normal deep tissue does not induce pain. Patients' cooperation by indicating pain on movement of the needle is often critical for location of the triggerpoint, particularly for less experienced physicians.

With experience, the operator develops a feeling for when the needle penetrates the triggerpoint. The syringe is held gently like a pen and resistance can be noticed by the fingertips. The character of resistance is "fibrotic" in chronic muscle triggerpoints and "induration-like" in pain with local tissue swelling. In ligament damage, on the other hand, the resistance to needling is abnormally slight, like soft butter. The feeling of resistance is a good guide as to where to needle and inject. About 10 to 15 progressions of the needle is usual, depending on the tenderness and size of the triggerpoint, the patient's pain tolerance, and the possibility of treatment after injection. A small deposit of Xylocaine is injected whenever the tender spot is penetrated.

## COMPLICATIONS OF TRIGGERPOINT INJECTION

There are very few complications of triggerpoint injections and usually these are not significant. A significant iatrogenic injury is piercing of the lung when the procedure is improperly done over the chest. A patient who was injected by me repeatedly took an injection by another physician, a specialist in another field who allegedly was experienced with triggerpoint injections. The right lung was pierced by an injection given to the supraspinatous area.

Chest pain radiating forward and aggravated by breathing occurs occasionally after injections into the chest wall. Females with very thin thoracic walls may develop this reaction. After an injection a patient reported pain going forward in belt shape to the sternum. Next day the pain had become severe and was aggravated by breathing. An analgesic with codeine improved the symptoms promptly and the pain subsided in few days. In one case after injection to the scapular area, excruciating pain was reported in the sternum. Palpation revealed an exquisitely tender triggerpoint in the sternocostal junction; this was injected, bringing instant relief of pain. The existence of this acute triggerpoint can be explained by severe muscle spasm induced by segmental pain. The injection interrupted the pain-spasm cycle, inducing prompt relief.

Another complication of triggerpoint injections is bleeding from the skin wound, which can be stopped by compression with gauze. Deep bleeding with formation of hematoma is rare; it occurs in patients with a tendency for bleeding. Riboflavin, 100 mg BID, a vitamin that decreases capillary permeability, usually prevents bruising. The patient should take riboflavin as long as injections are necessary.

Bluish discoloration occurs sometimes at the injected site. If the discoloration is large, tender, and cosmetically or functionally important, it is treated as an injury and needled. I recommend needling only half of the area in cases of first occurrence. (This is to prove to the physician and to the patient the amazing effect of needling.) Often the discoloration disappears even in deep hematomas within a few days in the needled area, while in the remaining untreated part the discoloration may persist for weeks. In a second session a few days or a week later the remaining discolored areas can be needled. The effect of needling that improves hematomas comes about through opening of the area to the circulation and piercing of the local edema so that the hematoma can be resolved and absorbed.

Extensive injection of triggerpoints in arms, thighs, or legs sometimes induces migrating discoloration, extending distally along fasciae or intermuscular septa. The area sometimes becomes sore, but the condition is harmless and resolves usually within a week.

An alternative treatment for hematomas is local ultrasound (1.5 W per sq cm for 5 minutes). This can be used also as treatment after needling of a hematoma.

## MECHANISM OF ACTION OF TRIGGERPOINT INJECTIONS

A considerable amount of discussion has been published on the hypothesis of how triggerpoint injections work. Melzack assumes that the effect of triggerpoint injections consists of a short-duration painful stimulus to induce relief of pain for several days.[22] The mechanism involved is probably the release of endorphin-like substances or neurological inhibition or both. I believe that this might be one component of the effects of triggerpoint injections. However, clinical experience has showed that when a triggerpoint is present and the needle misses it even by a few millimeters, long-term pain relief does not occur.

Local pathology in triggerpoints is often detectable in the form of a palpable "rope sign," which indicates constantly contracted, very tender bunches of muscle fibers. Fibrotic nodules or localized circumscribed exquisitely tender areas, often combined with puffiness as a sign of autonomic nervous system involvement, may be present in triggerpoints. These signs of local pathology do not disappear if the injection has missed the triggerpoint. The long-term effect of pain relief that lasts months cannot be induced only by intensive pain stimulus. The mechanism described by Melzack of relieving pain after brief intensive painful stimulus might be activated by some triggerpoint injections because often the patient reports complete or almost complete relief of pain from all triggerpoints for a limited period of three or four days after the injection. However, after the three-day period of generalized pain relief the patient usually complains of other triggerpoints that have not yet been injected. I believe that this generalized pain suppression for a few days following the injection might be the result of the intensive painful stimulus connected with the triggerpoint injections. However, the long-term effect that is the primary goal of the triggerpoint injection can be achieved only by careful needling, which breaks up the pathology, or by other mechanical means, as for example sudden injection of a sufficiently large amount of fluid, which have a similar mechanical effect.

It can be concluded that triggerpoint injection achieves the effect mainly mechanically: The needling breaks up the local pathology and opens the area for circulation to improve the inflammatory reaction. This explanation of a mechanism relieving the pain and abolishing local inflammatory reaction including edema is supported by the fact that the injection of a sufficiently large amount of saline without using any anesthetic and even without needling often has similar effects. Needling without use of anesthetic also has almost the same long-term effect as a combination of needling with infiltration by local anesthetic.

Besides the long-term effect in chronic triggerpoints, needling is also extremely effective in inducing immediate relief of pain in acute injuries, particularly muscle and ligament sprains or tears. Needling limited to part of the sprained area, with selection of the most painful and most affected zone of sprain, is useful. Such limited treatment also provides a model for understanding the effect of the procedure. There is usually immediate relief of pain and regaining of use of the injected part. Patients are warned that in spite of the ability to use the sprained muscle, it should not be used because the injury has to be protected for at least two weeks in order to achieve proper healing. When the injected area is compared with the noninjected part on follow-up, it will be obvious that the nontreated sprained areas become more swollen, painful, and distended. The pain is constant, often disturbing the patient's sleep at night. The sprained part that has not been injected is usually very tender, spastic, and tense from swelling, while the properly needled and injected part of the sprain is soft, without pain or tenderness, inflammatory reaction, or swelling. The muscle is relaxed and there is no spasm. The difference between the injected and the noninjected part of the sprain becomes evident immediately after the injection but is more prominent after two or three days and one or two weeks following the injections. In my opinion, the described differences in development and recovery indicate that needling of a sprained area combined with infiltration by local anesthetic prevents the development of inflammatory reaction by allowing the circulation to remove the irritative substances produced by the tissue damage. The healing after injection is less painful and is achieved in shorter time. The functional recovery is enhanced; functional losses in terms of limitation of motion and decrease in muscle power are also reduced.

## MEDICATION IN MANAGEMENT OF PATIENTS WITH CHRONIC PAIN

The basic rule is to use as little medication as possible. However, patients should be made comfortable and functioning if there is no risk involved for damage to nerve roots or to sprained structures. The danger of addiction is well known; I have seen many patients with chronic pain who became addicted to pain killers and tranquilizers. However, when the pain had been alleviated by triggerpoint injections, many reduced medications gradually without problems.

This experience emphasizes again the importance of causal treatment in chronic pain whenever it is possible. However, patients with untreatable pain, such as that secondary to arachnoiditis or similar conditions, are unable to give up pain medication that offers them at least some temporary relief. In the usual patient only seldom is use of strong pain killers necessary, and only in the acute stage or acute exacerbation when the patient is in excruciating pain even at rest. Much more effective in alleviation of pain and also more helpful functionally are nerve blocks, particularly paraspinal somatic blocks, including the sensorimotor roots related to the painful area. If paraspinal blocks are not feasible because of lack of equipment or inexperience of the physician, coating of the painful area with local anesthetic, particularly the side facing the nervous system, often is effective. Infiltration by local anesthetic of the painful area can be combined with nerve blocks or used independently. The nerve blocks and local alleviation of pain is superior to any other medication because pathological reflexes and vasospastic reaction will be abolished, and often pathology will improve when the circulation removes the irritative substances. A very strong pain medication is not supposed to be used for an ambulatory or working patient; suppression of the biologically important pain signal can lead to damage. We prescribe bed rest with a strong pain killer (Demerol) for the minimum period possible. Even in bed patients are encouraged to perform relaxation exercises to maintain mobility using movements that do not involve painful structures.

The next step is the use of pain killers of lesser strength. I have found Darvon to be useful; the patient may add Bufferin or a similar buffered or coated aspirin. Darvocet 100 mg is also useful starting with half a tablet TID or QID allowing to increase occasional doses to one entire tablet TID.

Often a combination of anti-inflammatory and analgesic effect is useful, particularly in diffuse pain. Motrin 400 mg TID or QID often helps. Other similar medications can be used. As soon as the acute stage is over we try to take patients off medication or reduce it. Buffered aspirin is useful following triggerpoint injections to reduce the inflammatory reaction, promote healing, and control discomfort.

Patients with depression and generalized high sensitivity to pain react well to antidepressants such as Elavil. The medication also improves sleep in the pain patient. Sinequan or other antidepressants are similarly effective.

Pain medication is prescribed to be taken PRN with a maximum limit not to be exceeded. I do not believe in giving patients pain killers regularly in a higher than needed amount, just to prevent addiction. I feel it is more effective to advise the patient of the maximum amount of medication he needs and is allowed, giving him the option to reduce the frequency of the drug when the pain is not severe.

The cocktail with gradually decreasing doses of pain medication as described by Fordyce[16] has proved helpful in detoxification of addicts with chronic pain. The method was successful mainly in patients in whom triggerpoint injections and physical therapy had relieved the pain.

# Physical Modalities in Management of Chronic Pain

Physical therapy modalities include electric stimulation using the Medcolator with different types of settings, such as automatic switching of different types of currents and sinusoid current stimulation. High-voltage stimulation is also useful, particularly in acute cases; it has the advantage that the current is not perceived by the patient. High-voltage stimulators, some combined with ultrasound, are manufactured by several companies. Another interesting modality is interference stimulation. The idea of the system is to use a medium frequency about 4000 Hz current, which readily penetrates into the deep soft tissues without any sensation to the patient. This current is applied through four electrodes attached to opposite aspects of the body. One pair of opposite electrodes carries a current adjustable from 4000 to 4100 Hz.

By mixing—interference—of the two medium-frequency currents, biologically active low-frequency pulses are generated within the tissues. The low-frequency current can be so generated deep inside the body. Cooling by ethyl chloride while moving the painful part is one of the most effective therapeutic uses of cold. Icing is also effective.

We use transcutaneous electrical nerve stimulation (TENS) with machines of different manufacturers. Sometimes switching to a different type of current is effective. The "pain suppressor" is also useful for office therapy. We consider a trial for a minimum of 2 weeks necessary before giving up TENS. Moving the electrodes and trying different types of stimulation and combination with heat or cold are sometimes effective.[23, 24]

Adverse consequences of immobilization include

both psychological and physical effects; anxiety, depression, loss of flexibility, loss of muscle power, deterioration of cardiopulmonary fitness, loss of postural cardiovascular reflexes, and so on. Therefore, we return the patient to activity as soon as possible, if only for short periods of time intermittently. We recommend that the patient lie down or sit down as soon as discomfort develops before pain or sensory symptoms in the form of tingling, paresthesia, or numbness develop, so the compressed roots are protected against damage in instances of possible radiculopathy. Muscle spasm, if present, should be relieved immediately by spray, therapy, or nerve blocks.

Low back supports are useful for allowing patients to return to activity and to work. The elastic low back support with individually thermo-molded solid insert is preferred. This type of support can be used as an elastic binder only or with the insert as solid support. We try to taper the back support as soon as endurance and strength of low back and abdominal muscles become adequate. Initially, the use of support is reduced by one or two hours in the afternoon; later it is gradually limited to half a day until the patient can be completely free of any support except for long car trips or strenuous activities.

Another important part of low back pain management is the "back school," in which body mechanics are taught to prevent or reduce the load upon the lower back. Regular lectures on body mechanics have helped to decrease the incidence of low back disability significantly in a significantly affected group of workers, the nurse aides in our hospital. The speakers concentrated on instructions for proper turning and moving of patients; this work causes most of the low back disabilities.

# Psychological Interventions With Patients Having Chronic Pain

Recently, clinicians from a wide variety of disciplines have been examining the influence of psychological and social factors on health and health care.[2, 16] Proponents of this new field of behavioral medicine are thus bringing a new perspective to diverse disorders, including chronic pain. The behavioral medicine orientation regards physiological and psychological components of disease as equally important, and emphasizes issues of patients' self-involvement in disease course and treatment.[16] It is within this context that psychological intervention is germane to chronic pain patients. The following section examines psychological intervention in more detail, including psychological evaluation, assessment of pain-coping strategies, stress management, and biofeedback as it is practiced in my pain center by a psychologist.

## PSYCHOLOGICAL EVALUATION AND ASSESSMENT OF PAIN-COPING STRATEGIES

Every physical pain induces psychological reactions, including tension, anxiety, depression, and suffering. These stress reactions, in addition to interfering with the well-being of the patient and family, can exacerbate pain. It is thus important to assess the psychological distress of the patient, the aspects of life that the patient finds stressful (including but not limited to pain), and coping strategies the patient may have developed to try to relieve pain and stress.

The initial interview, in addition to focusing on the patient's history, is designed to determine salient stressful situations that are occurring or have occurred in the patient's life. Special consideration is given to those situations that the patient feels he can do nothing about, since a feeling of having no impact on the environment is a major source of stress that can lead to increases in tension, anxiety, depression, and pain. Although most patients cite pain as the primary (or only) source of stress, we are interested also in the aspects of a patient's life style that are distressing, formerly enjoyable activities that are no longer pursued, and things that a patient feels can be done to improve his life situation.

During the intake interview, patients fill out a short paper-and-pencil inventory of psychological distress, the Brief Symptom Index (BSI).[4] The BSI is a 53-item measure that gives quantitative information on nine clinical scales: somatization, obsessive-compulsiveness, interpersonal sensitivity, depression, anxiety, hostility, phobic anxiety, paranoid ideation, and psychoticism. It is used in the psychological evaluation to pinpoint problems that may be a focus of treatment and to provide information concerning changes in psychological functioning over the course of treatment.

Examination and evaluation of coping strategies is consistent with the notion that how one responds to a stressor such as pain is an important part of the impact of that stressor on one's life. Coping strategies have been investigated and certain ones found to be influential in reducing the stresses of everyday life[26] and in recovery from surgery.[3] In acute situations, similar results have been obtained.[34] However, investigation of coping strategies characteristically used by chronic pain patients has largely been ignored. In pain syndromes, consideration must also be given to the patient's coping patterns and life style. To fill this void, and to assess the effect of coping strategies of chronic pain patients on the course of their disorders, Wagner devised the Chronic Pain Coping Strategies (CPCS) questionnaire.[38] This evaluation technique assesses response styles characteristically employed by chronic pain patients in coping with their pain. Factor analysis of this questionnaire has indicated that the multitude of strategies employed by pain patients (e.g., take medications, use a heat pack, lie down, change positions) can be reduced statistically to five major coping styles: (1) distraction techniques, (2) reliance on traditional medical remedies, (3) relaxation techniques, (4) stoicism, and (5) resignation and/or isolation.

Since distraction and relaxation strategies are developed during stress management and biofeedback training, this is a useful assessment device for measuring the degree to which patients spontaneously engage in these techniques, as it provides an indication of motivation for biofeedback training and compatibility with the orientation of the training regimen—that of self-management of the condition. In addition, preliminary analysis of outcome results indicates that those patients who rely primarily on stoicism and traditional medical remedies as pain-coping strategies tend to have more prolonged duration of pain, take more medication, and stay out of work longer than patients who use these techniques less. Thus it becomes important to gain a comprehensive picture of patients' coping styles, so as to discourage use of ineffective or deleterious strategies and to help each patient develop better means of dealing with pain. These evaluation techniques also help to enlist potentially successful candidates for biofeedback and stress management training.

## PSYCHOLOGICAL INTERVENTIONS: STRESS MANAGEMENT AND BIOFEEDBACK

Pain, according to a multidisciplinary group of scientists, is defined as "an unpleasant sensory and emotional experience associated with actual or potential tissue damage . . . (it) is always a psychological state even though we may well appreciate that pain most often has a proximate physical cause." Pain is also part of a vicious circle. A person who continually experiences pain is also bound to feel tension, stress, anxiety, and, as a result, more pain. As an adjunct to physical treatments for pain, stress management focuses on ways to break this vicious circle. While biofeedback is a component of stress management, we believe that the use of biofeedback for teaching voluntary control of physiological functioning may not be sufficient, since patients not only must control their physiology but they must be capable of dealing effectively with their environment.

Dealing effectively with the environment means recognizing that, in addition to pain, there are numerous sources of stress—economic, occupational, and interpersonal—that affect various aspects of our functioning. The effects of stress on a chronic pain patient are magnified considerably, especially if the patient feels relatively helpless in dealing with life's demands. In stress management, information gained in the psychological evaluation and the self-management orientation of the training program coincide. Stress is conceptualized as an interaction between the demands of a situation and a person's resources to handle it. For example, a skillful driver may know how to control a skidding car, whereas an inexperienced driver may panic under the same circumstances. By addressing the "demands of a situation," that is, those situations that the patient finds stressful, and the person's resources—coping strategies, psychological strengths, and motivation—stress management attempts to reduce the gap between demands and resources. Specific stress management intervention strategies include cognitive restructuring, coping skills training, assertiveness training, and biofeedback.

Cognitive restructuring is based on the fact that there are thoughts, feelings, and ways of looking at situations that may result in increased stress, tension, and perhaps pain. By "restructuring," that is, by discussing and learning different ways of interpreting stress and stressful situations, a patient can reduce the effects of stress. For example, being given an overload of work can be viewed as a stressful situation that may lead to feelings of anger and resentment, increased tension, and the thought that "I'll never be able to get all this done." However, this situation may also be viewed as a vote of confidence in one's ability, and this view may alleviate some of the pressure to perform in a "superhuman" way. In the same manner, patients learn to view pain less as an unwelcome houseguest and more as a *cue* that they should either slow down or employ some newly learned coping skill.

Skills training includes teaching distraction strategies such as use of imagery, use of relaxation techniques such as progressive relaxation, ordering of priorities and time management, and pacing of activity as a countermeasure to many people's tendency to "push on" and overdo—which often results in increased stress and pain. As an example of a specific intervention strategy, a secretary who had a tendency to type for hours at a time without taking a break (lack of pacing) was, during a session, instructed to type. By prearrangement, the telephone would ring at random intervals, a situation that she said occurred frequently at her job. She was taught that at the end of every phone call she could engage in brief relaxation exercises that slowed her work pace without a decrement in performance and made her more aware of her body. In addition, she gained a sense of control over her environment—the ultimate objective.

Assertion training is also an intervention strategy designed to increase the sense of control over one's environment. Here, patients are made aware of the importance of expressing feelings and desires directly in attempts to change situations that are less than acceptable. Included is the importance of the ability to say "no." Role playing in the office is used to improve patients' ability in these techniques and reduce the anxiety that usually accompanies interpersonal conflicts and the fear that may prevent one from asserting oneself.

The biofeedback component of stress management is conceptualized both as a specific relaxation coping skill that can be used in moments of anxiety and in stressful situations and as a "prototype" of the sense of control that can be achieved in both the physiological and environmental domains. Biofeedback is a technique through which patients learn to become aware of and reduce the level of muscular tension that usually occurs with and contributes to chronic pain. In this office, electromyographic (muscle tension or EMG) feedback is used. Tiny electric signals emanating from muscle groups in which pain and significant muscle tension occur are picked up by surface electrodes (so there is no discomfort to the patient). These are amplified and converted into acoustic and visual signals. This information is then "fed back" to the patient. By becoming aware of muscle tension that cannot be sensed without this equipment, patients can develop specific relaxation strategies and be immediately informed as to their success. Home relaxation practice exercises are delineated and emphasized as essential to gain the maximum effectiveness of biofeedback training. Weekly "homework" assignments (e.g., charting the frequency of home practice and its effects) are discussed and modified as necessary. Patients are told that relaxation is a skill, and like any other skill, it becomes easier and more effective with practice.

All components of stress management and biofeedback are integrated and individualized within the therapeutic sessions. The purpose, in general, is to foster a sense of mastery and self-control, and to assist people in acquiring new skills and resources to cope with and change life's stresses, including, but not limited to, pain.

## CASE REPORT

A 37-year-old man experienced lower back pain since 1973 and underwent an L4, L5 laminectomy and discectomy. He had been out of work since 1980 and began stress management training in June, 1981. Psychological testing on the Brief Symptom Index indicated significant elevation of the depression and phobic anxiety scales. He confirmed that he had a variety of "phobias," primarily relating to his back problem, that focused on the anticipatory fear that "something would happen" to his back while driving, taking a shower, or when away from home. Thus he tended to avoid many activities that gave him pleasure and remained relatively isolated—a situation that contributed to his depression. Similarly, on the chronic pain coping strategies questionnaire, he scored high on the resignation-isolation and medical remedies scales, indicating that much of his life centered on physicians' offices. When not directly pursuing medical treatment, he tended to respond to pain by increasing his isolation. Responses on this questionnaire were consistent with those on the BSI.

Stress management training focused primarily on two areas. First, electromyographic biofeedback training was initiated for general relaxation and presented as a coping strategy that could be employed during times of increased anticipatory anxiety concerning his back. Biofeedback training was important not only as a specific muscular relaxation technique but to foster an internal sense of control that was antithetical to the helplessness he felt when anxious and "panicky" about his back. For example, he was afraid to drive when his back was tense or painful since he was fearful of spasm and subsequent inability to get home or get off the highway. This anxiety surrounding the situation tended to make him more tense, contributing to the outcome he wanted to avoid. With increasing skill at relaxation and with use of his skills during this and other situations, he was able to reduce tension and anxiety concerning driving, and felt increased comfort. In addition, with increased sense of control of his own mobility, he tended to get out of the house more, visit friends, and enjoy more activities. Thus his depression was ameliorated. Coping skills training was consistent with biofeedback and was designed to decrease his isolation, inculcate an internal sense of control over events, and increase the use of distraction and relaxation as specific coping strategies. He was encouraged to socialize more rather than less when he had pain, and he found that the distracting element of being around other people helped his pain. This encouraged him to socialize more and keep in touch with his friendship network. In addition, he was taught to employ pleasant imagery as a coping strategy he could use when alone or to engage in some enjoyable activity. Through the course of training, he began using his relaxation skills before going to bed and reported sleeping much better, without use of medication. He increased his socialization, helped by his ability to drive without anxiety. On post-training testing, his depression and phobic anxiety scores were within normal limits. On the coping strategies questionnaire, his score on the resignation-isolation scale was below the mean for chronic pain patients, although his medical remedies score was still slightly elevated. He is currently making plans to return to work.

# REFERENCES

1. Bonica, J. J.: The Management of Pain. Philadelphia, Lea & Febiger, 1953.
2. Bonica, J. J.: Basic principles in managing chronic pain. Arch. Surg. 112:783–788, 1977.
3. Cohen, F. and Lazarus, R. S.: Active coping processes, coping dispositions, and recovery from surgery. Psychosom. Med. 35:375–389, 1973.
4. Derogatis, L. R.: The brief symptoms index. Baltimore, Johns Hopkins University Press, 1978.
5. Fischer, A.: Pressure tolerance measurement in assessment of musculofascial pain and its treatment. Exhibit at American Congress of Rehabilitation Medicine, New Orleans, 1978.
6. Fischer, A.: Pressure tolerance measurement—a quantitative method for diagnosis and evaluation of treatment in muscular fascial pain syndromes. Third Congress of the International Rehabilitation Medicine Association, Basel, 1978.
7. Fischer, A.: Pressure threshold over muscles of person without pain. The American Pain Society Second General Meeting, New York, 1980.
8. Fischer, A.: Thermography and pain. Introductory lecture on invitation. American Academy of Physical Medicine and Rehabilitation. Arch. Phys. Med. Rehabil. 62:542, 1981.
9. Fischer, A.: Tissue compliance recording—a method for objective documentation of soft tissue pathology. Arch. Phys. Med. Rehabil. 62:542, 1981.
10. Fischer, A. and Chang, C.: EMG evidence of paraspinal muscle spasm during sleep in patients with low back pain. Third World Congress on Pain of the International Association for the Study of Pain, Edinburgh, 1981.
11. Fischer, A. and Chang, C.: Deep tissue temperature and thermography in trigger points and painful areas. Third International Congress of Thermology of the European Association of Thermology. Bath, England, 1982.
12. Fischer, A.: Thermography in differential diagnosis and documentation of neuromuscular and skeletal disorders. 4th World Congress of the International Rehabilitation Medicine Association. San Juan, 1982.
13. Fischer, A., Criscuolo, R. and Sosa, D.: Pressure tolerance over muscle and bones in normal subjects. 4th World Congress of the International Rehabilitation Medicine Association. San Juan, 1982.
14. Fischer, A., Chang, C. and Kuo, J.: Correlation between thermogram, physical findings and EMG in low back and neck pain. American Thermography Society. Washington, D.C., 1982.
15. Fischer, A.: Objective evaluation of soft tissue injuries: tissue compliance, thermography, pressure threshold. World Congress on Sports Medicine. Vienna, 1982.
16. Fordyce, W. E.: Behavioral Methods for Chronic Pain and Illness. St. Louis, C. V. Mosby Co., 1976.
17. Gottlieb, H., Strite, L. C., Koller, R., Madorsky, A., Hockersmith, V., Kleeman, M. and Wagner, J.: Comprehensive rehabilitation of patients having chronic low back pain. Arch. Phys. Med. Rehabil. 58:101–108, 1977.
18. Karpman, H., Knebel, A., Semel, C. J., et al.: Clinical studies in thermography. II. Application of thermography in evaluating musculoligamentous injuries of the spine—a preliminary report. Arch. Environ. Health 20:412–217, 1970.
19. Kraus, H.: Clinical Treatment of Back and Neck Pain. McGraw-Hill, 1970.
20. Kraus, H.: Musculofascial pain. In: Pain Control: Practical Aspects of Patient Care. Masson Publishing, 1981.
21. Lelik, F. and Kezy, G.: Contact thermography in sports medicine. Acta Thermograph. 4:24–29, 1979.
22. Melzack, R.: Prolonged relief of pain by brief, intense transcutaneous somatic stimulation. Pain 1:357–373, 1975.
23. Melzack, R., Guite, S., and Gonshor, A.: Relief of dental pain by ice massage of the hand. CMA J 122:189–191, 1980.
24. Melzack, R., Jeans, M. E., Stratford, J. G., and Monks, R. C.: Ice massage and transcutaneous electrical stimulation: comparison of treatment for low-back pain. Pain 9:209–217, 1980.
25. Mintz, J.: Thermography in medicine today. Appl. Radiology 8:2–7, 1979.
26. Pearlin, L. I. and Schooler, C.: The structure of coping. J. Health Soc. Behav. 19:2–21, 1978.
27. Pochaczevsky, R., Wexler, C. E., Meyers, P. H., Epstein, J. A., Marc, J. A.: Liquid crystal thermography of the spine and extremities. J. Neurosurg 56:386–395, 1982.
28. Rask, M. R.: Thermography of the human spine. Orthop. Rev. 8:73–82, 1979.
29. Raskin, M. M. and Viamonte, M., Jr. (eds.): Clinical Thermography. American College of Radiology, Chicago, IL, 1977.
30. Ruskin, A. P.: Sphenopalatine (nasal) ganglion: remote effects including "psychosomatic" symptoms, rage reaction, pain and spasm. Arch. Phys. Med. Rehabil. 60:353–359, 1979.
31. Schmitt, M. and Guillot, Y.: Thermography and muscular injuries in sports medicine. Third International Congress of Thermology. March 29–April 2, 1981. Bath, England.
32. Simons, D. G.: Muscle pain syndromes-part I. Muscle pain syndromes-part II. Am. J. Phys. Med. 54:289–311, 1975; 55:15–42, 1976.
33. Simons, D. G.: Myofascial trigger points: a need for understanding. Arch. Phys. Med. Rehabil. 62:97–99, March 1981.
34. Spanos, N. P., Horton, C. and Chaves, J. F.: The effects of two cognitive strategies on pain. J. Abnormal Psychol. 84:677–681, 1975.
35. Tichauer, E. R.: The objective corroboration of back pain through thermography. J. Occup. Med. 19:727–731, 1977.
36. Travell, J. and Rinzler, S. H.: The myofascial genesis of pain. Postgrad. Med. 11:425–434, May 1952.
37. Uematsu, S. and Long, D. M.: Thermography in chronic pain. In Uematsu, S.: Medical Thermography, Theory and Clinical Applications. Los Angeles, CA, Brentwood Publishing Co., 1976.
38. Wagner, J.: Coping strategies in response to chronic pain: effects on illness course Unpublished doctoral dissertation, Graduate Faculty, New School for Social Research, 1982.
39. Wexler, C. E.: Lumbar, thoracic and cervical thermography. J. Neurol. Orthop. Surg. 1:37–41, 1979.
40. Wexler, C. E.: Thermography. Tarzana, CA, Thermographic Services, Inc., 1981.
41. Winsor, T. and Winsor, D.: Thermography in cardiovascular disease. Applied Radiology, Nov–Dec 1975.

# A Dynamic Approach to Pain Management

*by Asa Ruskin, M.D.*

Much has been written in the modern "pain" literature about development of the "chronic pain syndrome." The general tendency has been to consider that if a patient has not responded to treatment for pain and develops a "chronic pain syndrome," its cause must lie deep in the patient's psyche and relate to that individual's adaptive behavioral pattern, method of coping, or perhaps the influence of factors of secondary gain, either monetary or psychological. This general point of view has a number of important advantages, not the least of which is that it places the blame for the chronic pain syndrome directly on the patient. My late father, after more than 40 years of medical practice, used to tell me that if patients got better, he took the credit, but if they got worse it was undoubtedly their fault.

While I am certain that the psychobehavioral mechanisms apply to a certain number of cases, I strongly suspect that a very large number of chronic pain syndromes develop because the initial medical treatment is either inadequate, incorrect, or excessive and frequently a combination of all three. Furthermore, I believe that this occurs in part because too many physicians do not understand the underlying mechanisms of trauma and do not properly conceptualize the dynamics of its physical consequences.

Some months ago I attended a symposium on pain at which a football team physician described the horrendous carnage of a typical Sunday afternoon with the multitude of bruises, contusions, strains, and sprains that you can easily imagine. He recounted that by Wednesday, these injuries were well on the mend and by the following Sunday, the vast majority of players were back on the field with only a few held over for a second week. At the time I thought that this was a magnificent testament to human willpower and motivation with perhaps an element of psychic healing. But let us look a little more closely at what happens to these gridiron gladiators when they come off the field. The sprained neck, shoulder, etc., is immediately packed in ice, and appropriate precautions and techniques are utilized to prevent or reduce the development of edema. Within a day or two after injury an exercise and mobilization program is initiated that further aids in preventing edema and maintaining normal local flow of tissue fluid. Early sedative massage further helps maintain mo-

bility, and aggressive use of anti-inflammatory medications including steroids consolidates the miracle. It is a rare athlete who develops chronic pain syndrome, and then it is only after a lifetime of repeated trauma or a truly catastrophic event.

Let us contrast this level of care with the average civilian injury. A typical patient following a minor automobile collision is brought to a hospital emergency department with perhaps some complaints relative to the neck or low back. Frequently symptoms do not develop until several hours or a few days later, and only rarely is the probability of the victim's developing these anticipated and planned for. Our typical patient will, after waiting several hours for treatment, have a set of negative x-rays taken and then be given some Tylenol with an appointment to return to the orthopedic clinic two weeks hence. This inadequate approach is frequently compounded by incorrect advice such as to apply a hot compress or hot water to the acutely injured neck or back, the effect of which will be to increase the local swelling and edema, perhaps causing a nerve root compression and almost certainly resulting in a greater degree of back pain and immobilization. The cervical injured "whiplash" victim is all too frequently advised simply to "buy a collar," the application of which is left to the surgical supply store salesman or the patient's Uncle Harry. Almost invariably it is applied incorrectly, with the smallest part of the collar in back and the patient's chin raised in a position of hyperextension. This has two common results. First, it reduces the size of the cervical foramina, constricting the nerve roots and causing or aggravating any tendency to cervical radiculopathy. It further prevents the mobilization and muscle contraction that might help relieve the edema and facilitates the development of fibrosis and ligamentus contracture, setting the stage for a truly chronic neck condition.

When an analogous chain of events has occurred in the low back region, it is not infrequently topped off by two or three myelograms and a few surgical procedures, the efficacy of which in manufacturing chronic pain syndromes is all too well known.

Another very excellent way to manufacture a chronic back pain is to recommend two or three weeks of bed rest. If you think for a moment how many of us have a bit of backache after a single night of "bed rest," two or three weeks of strictly observed bed rest will do a wonderful job in shortening the tendons, creating fibrosis, and helping to set the stage for a "chronic back," not to mention the devastating effect that this has on the body generally, with a 50 per cent decrease in general strength, a decrease in cardiovascular tone and endurance, as well as widespread metabolic changes. Not the least of these is hypercalcemia produced as calcium leaves the bones, which are no longer subject to the normal stress of weight bearing, and contributes instead to the development of urinary calculi.

In order to approach the treatment of pain in a rational manner, we must visualize the pain syndrome as a complex multifactorial dynamic event that is continuously changing, both as to mechanism and manifestation. The basic medical school training, reflecting as it does the mechanistic philosophies of the 19th and early 20th centuries, develops a way of thinking that emphasizes a linear relationship of cause and effect. One pinches a nerve and gets radicular pain. A joint is sprained and a local pain occurs, and so on. Of course we know intellectually about the inflammatory process and edema, but we rarely think much beyond that, and often the intellectual knowledge is not translated into a conceptualization that alters the plan of treatment.

Let me describe an illustrative case. A prominent individual suffered a typical lumbar disc herniation. The diagnosis was correctly made and confirmed by myelogram, and the patient underwent surgery. Following the operation, which immediately relieved the sciatic syndrome, the patient spent two weeks in bed and another week or two convalescing. When the patient began to resume his normal activities, which were those of a typical executive and primarily sedentary, he complained of renewed radiating pain down the right lower extremity, the pain being most intense from the buttock to the knee. The patient was soon reduced to essentially hobbling about with a cane and was seen by a succession of eminent physicians with great reputations in the care of low back conditions. He was given all manner of expert physical therapy to the low back and was on the verge of a second surgical intervention when I first saw him. Physiatric examination revealed good mobilization of the back but markedly restricted range of motion of the right hip on attempted external rotation and moderate limitation in range of motion of the left hip. A course of treatment designed to produce relaxation of muscle spasm as well as increase the range of motion of the hips resulted in complete relief of symptoms, the patient being able to discard his cane and walk normally after about 8 to 10 weeks of treatment. The problem that had existed in this patient's management resulted from the various physicians' tendency to fixate on the initial cause-and-effect phenomenon, disc herniation producing sciatic pain, and not to recognize that the period of immobilization had caused contracture of soft tissues and ligaments about the hip so that they did not recognize that the patient's postoperative complaints came from a totally different mechanism from that which was applicable initially.

Let us look further at some of the mechanisms that can contribute to the pain syndrome. It is my opinion that ischemia is probably the most important and least appreciated of these.

The vast majority of pain syndromes include a component of muscle spasm. For a contracted muscle to relax, active metabolic energy must be expanded. However, the prolonged contraction or spasm itself is accompanied by spasm of the microcirculation, producing a relative state of ischemia, inhibiting the relaxation and setting up a vicious cycle in which the spasm feeds upon itself, creating a chronic state of contraction. The clinical importance of this was emphasized by Simon Ruskin in a series of articles on the dynamics of muscletonus in the 1940's. This underlying mechanism is supported by the most advanced findings of thermography, which have shown chronic painful spastic areas to be cooler than normal adjacent muscles.

Essentially all of the treatments that are used to reduce muscle spasm work by promoting vasodilatation. Everyone recognizes that this is the case when the therapeutic modality is heat in its various forms, either superficial by heat pack or deep by diathermy or ultrasound. It is also widely recognized that massage, vigorous rubbing, or the use of superficial irritants by topical application do likewise. It is less often recognized that use of superficial cooling, such as ethyl chloride spray, produces a reactive deep vasodilatation or that acupuncture and acupressure cause brief local vasoconstriction followed by more extensive, deeper vasodilatation. Electrical stimulation has the same effect, and it has also been shown that manipulation techniques have produced local sympathetic reflex inhibition that would promote relaxation of constricted muscles. Interestingly, direct injection with Procaine acts from the combination of the chemical vasodilator and the reflex response to the needle itself. Rapid and often dramatic relaxation of muscle spasm often follows direct blocking or ablation of the sympathetic chain regionally, or the much more easily performed office procedure of topical anesthetization of the sphenopalatine ganglion in the nose (see Chapter 7). Blocking of sympathetic outflow, while not producing vasodilatation in normally relaxed blood vessels, will inhibit active constriction of the blood vessels, producing a return to normal flow in areas of vasoconstriction.

On diagnosis, all too many physicians seem to fall into a rut and tend to diagnose any localized pain in or near a joint as arthritis except, of course, for the shoulder, which is invariably labeled bursitis. Radiating pains are all ascribed to "pinched nerves" in the neck or back, and when they exist in the lower extremities, they can only be caused by a "disc." There is a disconcerting lack of imagination and originality evidenced by the repetitiveness with which we see these catch-all diagnoses. Certainly they are occasionally correct, but all too often the actual cause of the pain is muscular, vascular, or other, and the erroneous diagnosis of "arthritis" is thought to be confirmed when some arthritic changes compatible with the patient's age are observed on x-rays.

The diagnosis of musculoskeletal pain must be approached in a holistic fashion, taking into account the patient's entire medical history and being on the lookout for contributory factors such as mild hypothryoidism, menopausal endocrine insufficiencies, diabetes, and other metabolic conditions that could predispose to the development of myofascial triggerpoints and musculoneuritic symptoms. The patient's occupation as well as diversional activities must be looked to as possible causal or aggravating factors, and these must be integrated with the patient's psychosocial situation. For example, a cashier or bookkeeper may be sitting on an inappropriate chair with a bad posture. While this alone might explain backache in many instances, another similar patient might have been using the same chair and posture for several years without incident, only to develop back pain when a new supervisor or other stressful occurrence is superimposed.

Many of these radiating pains so often labeled "disc" are in reality radiation of pain from myofascial triggerpoints, tendinitis, or an unexpected trochanteric bursitis. Nerves can also be pinched at many sites other than the vertebral foramina, with nerve entrapments such as the pronator teres syndrome not being uncommon at numerous points or at the supracondular process in the upper extremities, or at many sites in the lower extremities, including the popliteal fossa.

The role of ischemia as a causative agent for pain is not limited to muscle spasm. Most of us have experienced the painful dysesthesias caused by application of a tourniquet or blood pressure cuff. It seems to me quite likely that some of the more subtle neuritic pains and paresthesias might well be secondary to spasm or obstruction of the vasa nervorum and I have occasionally had gratifying therapeutic results when these were treated. Again, in these instances, there are multiple factors and it is impossible to separate out what portion, if any, of a given complaint might relate to a reversible ischemia as opposed to metabolic damage and actual axon degeneration.

We also should not forget that while full-blown intermittent claudication is an easy diagnosis to make, many cases begin with just an occasional pain in the calf that radiates upward, as might incidentally a myofascial triggerpoint in the gastrocnemius. Also, early signs of a Leriche syndrome caused by stenosis of the lower aorta and iliac arteries can be manifested as unusual neuritic radiating pain in the upper half of the lower extremities.

No discussion of pain syndrome can be complete without some consideration of the psychogenic factors.

It is common knowledge that psychological factors contribute to the development and maintenance of muscle spasm. We all accept the psychosomatic etiology of the common tension headache, neck and low back spasms, but rarely do we consider the physical mechanics that must underlie manifestation of these spasms. It is my belief that psychogenic muscle spasm as well as numerous other psychosomatic symptoms are mediated through the autonomic nervous system and can frequently be relieved by sympathetic block. Again, this is most easily performed at the sphenopalatine level but in some instances is equally amenable to regional blocking or use of sympatholytic drugs.

Figure 7–2 (p. 119) summarizes our conceptions of psychosomatic mechanisms and the loci of therapeutic intervention. It is important to further emphasize, however, that these same treatment techniques may be effective even though the symptoms arise from a purely organic cause, or as in many instances of chronic pain, are caused by a combination of factors.

As shown in the illustration, going counterclockwise, there is a continual reciprocal cybernetic relationship between the brain and the neuroendocrine and/or autonomic nervous system, and it is at this level that psychotrophic drugs can exert their major effect.

In order for the mental processes to be manifested, be it as muscle spasm, asthma, urticaria, and so on, I have postulated that transmission needs to be made via the autonomic nervous system and principally the sympathetic chain. It is at this level that the various treatment modalities discussed exert their primary influence.

The various effector organs subject to psychosomatic disorder, be it vasomotor or secretory, can respond to the usual chemical symptomatic treatments common in general medical practice.

The syndrome of sympathetic reflex dystrophy with causalgia can almost be looked upon as a naturally occurring experimental demonstration of these mechanisms. In that little-understood syndrome, the existence of a strong psychogenic factor has long been commonly accepted. The sympathetic reflex dystrophy syndrome is usually initiated by a relatively minor but painful injury to an extremity such as a pinch or crush injury to a finger or toe, followed by development of sympathetic reflex changes over succeeding weeks that involve the entire limb with vasomotor changes characterized by vasoconstriction of the smaller vessels causing a decrease in surface temperature, progressive swelling of the limb, atrophic changes of the skin, which becomes shiny, and a paralysis frequently with contracture of the fingers in a fist. This syndrome can often be relieved by sympathetic block, the usual technique being by injection of the cervical chain at the stellate ganglion. It also may respond favorably to a series of sphenopalatine blocks. I have observed that following sphenopalatine block, the skin temperature of the affected hand will increase by 3 or 4 degrees and the patient will report a subjective reduction in pain. The optimal treatment is to combine sympathetic block with a physical therapy regimen designed to reduce edema, improve circulation, and increase range of motion.

Psychoanalytic concepts consider that the various symptoms produced in a given individual by psychosomatic mechanisms have symbolic significance for that particular individual. I would postulate a reciprocal relationship between the individual and the symbolic representation of the symptoms as being the site amenable to therapeutic intervention by psychotherapeutic and cultural approaches.

## REFERENCES

Ruskin, S. L.: Role of coenzymes of B complex vitamins and amino acids in muscle metabolism and balanced nutrition. Am. J. Dig. Dis. 13:110–122, 1946.

Ruskin, S. L.: Control of muscle spasm and arthritic pain through sympathetic block as nasal ganglion and use of Adenylic Nucleotide: contributions to physiology of muscle metabolism. Part II. Am. J. Dig. Dis. 13:311–320, 1946.

Ruskin, S. L.: Dynamics of muscle tonus and its relationship to circulatory failure: Part II. New approach to treatment of hypertension and circulatory failure by use of iron salt of adenylic nucleotide. Am. J. Dig. Dis. 15:261–271, 1948.

Ruskin, S. L.: Newer concept of arthritis and treatment of arthritic pain and deformity by sympathetic block at sphenopalatine (nasal) ganglion and use of iron salt of adenylic nucleotide: dynamics of muscle tonus. Part IV. Am. J. Dig. Dis. 16:386–401, 1949.

Korr, M.: The Neurobiologic Mechanisms in Manipulative Therapy, New York, Plenum Press, 1978.

Ruskin, Asa P.: Sphenopalatine (nasal) ganglion: Remote Effects including "Psychosomatic" Symptoms, Rage Reaction, Pain and Spasm. Arch. Phys. Med. Rehab. 60, Aug. 1979.

# 9

# Management of Pain

by Masayoshi Itoh, M.D., M.P.H., Mathew Lee, M.D., M.P.H., F.A.C.P.,
Alice L. Eason, M.P.A., R.P.T., Gail M. Herring, M.S.W., A.C.S.W.,
and Etta Rybstein-Blinchik, Ph.D.

Pain is perception of noxious sensation. There are many hypotheses on pain stimuli, transmission of stimuli, perception, and localization. In addition, pain is an extremely subjective matter. A reliable method of measuring pain quantitatively and qualitatively has not been found. Pain is the most common, usually unpleasant and disabling condition about which so little is understood. Management of pain, particularly chronic pain, is a challenging subject in clinical medicine.

## EPIDEMIOLOGY OF PAIN

While many studies in neurology, neurophysiology, and neurochemistry are focusing on the question of pain mechanisms, some guide to a practical management plan may be obtained through an understanding of the epidemiology or natural history of pain. Pain is caused by simultaneous interaction of three causative factors: host, agent, and environment (Fig. 9–1). The host is man, who has various characteristics (Table 9–1). While many physical characteristics may be related to causation of "acute pain," psychosocial characteristics seem to be more closely related to development of "chronic pain."

The agent of pain can be extremely complicated. A primary agent is responsible for causation of acute pain. The external forces listed in Table 9–2 are primary agents. The direct cause in production of painful stimuli is instantaneous and of brief duration. The response of the host to the primary agent is perception of pain as well as of tissue reaction. The tissue reaction is one of the secondary agent. The secondary agent is responsible for pain during the recovery state of acute pain and perhaps causation of chronic pain. Obviously, the activity of the agent and its frequency and duration interacting with the host are important considerations in the causation of pain.

The physical environment (Table 9–3) is more directly related to the primary agent interaction, or acute pain, than to the secondary agent. However, climate or humidity or both are known to be related to chronic pain. The patient's psychosocial,

TABLE 9–1 HOST FACTORS OF PAIN

| PHYSICAL | PSYCHOSOCIAL |
|---|---|
| Visual acuity | Memory |
| Coordination | Judgment |
| Pain tolerance | Experience |
| Body constitution–genetic | Education–cultural |
| Age | Dependency |
| Sex | Anxiety |
| | Expectation |
| | Ego strength–coping ability |

TABLE 9–2 AGENT FACTORS OF PAIN

| EXTERNAL FORCES | INTERNAL FORCES |
|---|---|
| Mechanical | Patho-physiological |
| Chemical | Psychogenic |
| Electrical | |
| Thermal | QUANTITY/DOSE |
| Radiation | |
| Infectious | DURATION |
| Oncogenic | |
| | FREQUENCY |

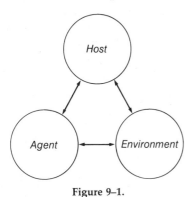

Figure 9–1.

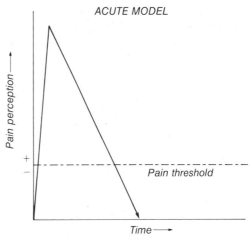

Figure 9–2.

economic, and occupational environment often influence causation of chronic pain.

## ACUTE PAIN

Acute pain is the direct result of the primary agent interaction. Pain stimuli are formed and the host perceives sharp pain. This initial interaction of the host and the agent produces the secondary agent. The secondary agent remains for a considerable time at the site of the body that was affected by the primary agent. During this period, the host perceives less pain than at the onset, and pain decreases progressively. The most outstanding characteristic of acute pain is that the duration of the syndrome usually is empirically predictable (Fig. 9–2).

## CHRONIC PAIN SYNDROME

In general, chronic pain may be observed in two forms, an acute to chronic model (Fig. 9–3) and a recurrent chronic model (Fig. 9–4). The former model is applied to the case of a patient who had acute pain but did not recover within an expected period. The recurrent chronic pain model is the case in which at one time a patient might have ex-

perienced acute pain and recovered completely, but after an unspecified period the patient re-experiences pain in the same anatomical location in which the acute pain existed. Pain in this model may recur repeatedly. The duration of chronic pain is unpredictable, and the severity of pain is usually less than acute pain, or it may fluctuate. Chronic pain may subside with or without treatment, and there is a tendency toward recurrence without identifiable agent interaction.

Some investigators claim that there are three types of pain: acute, chronic, and malignant. Malignant pain is pain of a malignant tumor, particularly in its terminal stages. It is chronic pain and often very severe. Intensity of pain may change from time to time.

It is important to note that the agent of chronic pain is very often the secondary agent. Identification of psychogenic force as the agent must be made with utmost care. Table 9–4 shows a comparison of acute and chronic pain.

**TABLE 9–3** ENVIRONMENTAL FACTORS OF PAIN

**PHYSICAL**
 Meteorological–climate, temperature, humidity, etc.
 Visibility–darkness, lighting, etc.
 Condition of ground or floor
 Noise level

**PSYCHOSOCIAL**
 Relation with family and/or friends
 Social norm
 Politico-Judicial
 Mechanization

**ECONOMIC AND OCCUPATIONAL**
 Disability compensation
 Job market
 Enforcement of occupational safety

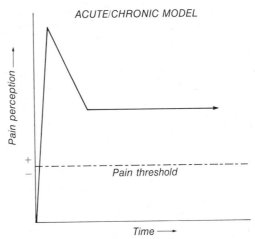

Figure 9–3.

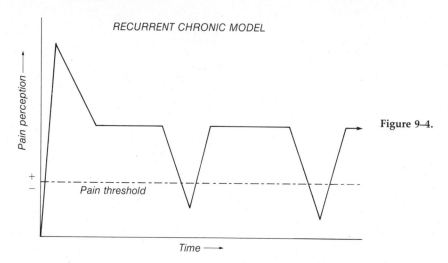

Figure 9–4.

## ASSESSMENT OF PAIN SYNDROME

The first step in the management of pain, acute or chronic, is to identify the pathology that may be responsbile. This task is relatively easy in acute pain. The history of pain, its location, various symptoms associated with it, and diagnostic tests are main components of diagnosis of acute pain.

Diagnosis of the causative pathology of chronic pain is often a very complex task. For example, physical abnormality found through diagnostic procedures may or may not have a cause-and-effect relationship with the pain the patient is complaining of. In some instances, in spite of a complaint of pain, no physical abnormality may be found. In such a case, thorough evaluation of diagnostic procedures performed is warranted in order to identify the true nature of the agent causing pain. It is wrong to generalize that pain without identifiable pathology is caused by the secondary agent, particularly psychogenic force.

The approach to assessment of chronic pain must be multidisciplinary, including but not limited to physician, physical therapist, social worker, psychologist, and vocational counselor. A patient with chronic pain syndrome tends to seek medical advice or information from more than one medical source. This should not be interpreted as the patient's distrust of the medical profession but as his anxiety and self-interest.

A physician seeing a patient with chronic pain must obtain detailed information from the patient as well as the physicians who treated him previously. This information should include the history of pain, medical findings, and treatment regimen administered by previous physicians. Such information is vitally important to establish a plan of clinical investigation of the patient's complaint. An objective assessment of previous medical findings and procedures for this patient will be the basis for planning the renewed diagnostic approach. Such information-gathering must be started from the pa-

**TABLE 9–4** COMPARISON OF ACUTE AND CHRONIC PAIN

| VARIABLES | ACUTE PAIN | CHRONIC PAIN |
| --- | --- | --- |
| Agent | Usually identifiable | Not always identifiable |
| Onset | Sudden or increased intensity, rapidity | Slow or incidious increase |
| Intensity | Extreme at onset and gradually decreasing | Usually moderate, may fluctuate; some may report as excruciating |
| Duration | Empirically predictable | Unpredictable |
| Physical disability | Always present | Always present |
| Anatomical and pathophysiological changes | Identifiable | Not always identifiable |
| Macroenvironmental factors | No influence | May influence |
| Social factors | No influence | May influence |
| Economic factors | No influence | May influence |
| Psychological factors | No influence | May influence |
| Cultural factors | May influence | May influence |
| Prognosis | Good if managed properly | Guarded |
| Recurrence | No | Often recurs |
| Response to treatment | Generally good | Uncertain |

tient. However, sometimes the patient may become suspicious of the motive of the current physician when being asked the name of physician(s) who treated him previously. Thus, the physician must first establish a good rapport with the patient and clearly explain why such information is necessary.

Unless there are overwhelming reasons, the diagnostic procedures that have been previously carried out should not be repeated. If repetition is absolutely necessary, again the physician must explain the reason to the patient very clearly. Even if a new procedure is indicated, the patient must be informed of the reason and what can be expected as an outcome.

## PHYSICAL INFORMATION

The information concerning the patient's physical condition is usually obtained by a physician and a physical therapist and is fundamental to assessment of chronic pain. this information includes:

1. History of present illness, including previous medical findings and treatment.
2. History of previous illness and traumatic conditions
3. Occupational history
4. Physical examination
5. Neurological examination
6. Radiological examination
7. Clinical laboratory tests
8. Electrocardiogram
9. Electromyogram
10. Conduction velocity study
11. Electroencephalogram
12. Measurement of active and passive range of motion
13. Muscle strength testing
14. Splinting by a patient as protective mechanism during a specific activity
15. Muscle atrophy
16. Muscle spasm
17. Spasticity
18. Rigidity
19. Gross functional deficiency
20. Sensitivity to light touch or pressure by palpitation
21. Deficiency in activities of daily living
22. Coordination or incoordination

Although both physician and therapist are seeking information concerning physical disabilities caused by the chronic pain syndrome, they can also observe the patient's behavior pattern under different circumstances and in different environments.

## PSYCHOSOCIAL INFORMATION

The chronic pain syndrome is often related to psychosocial factors with which clinicians are less familiar. The relevance and significance of the social history does not lie strictly in the factual data but must be viewed in the larger context of ethnicity, culture, environment, and social status.

**Ethnicity.** It has been said that individuals of a certain ethnic and/or cultural group—of Northern and Western European extraction—exhibit less emotion and complain less of pain than do those of Southern European or Latin groups. However, such generalizations are dangerous and misguiding. Instead of labeling pain and patient solely on the basis of the ethnic and cultural background, the investigator should rely on history and clinical data.

**Role of Learning.** The beginning of behavior associated with pain has roots in childhood. The young child learns to avoid pain and then gradually exhibits behavior that reflects familiar and wider cultural influences. The child may learn that pain can bring him affection or can be used to manipulate others. While these are normal behavior patterns in themselves, if they are seen in the history as patterns progressing into adulthood, then one might suspect some serious psychological problems.

Learning has relationship to the meaning of pain, and the history taker must look for learned pain behaviors and their meaning to the patient in his familial, ethnic, and social context.

**Ego Functioning and Emotion.** The "feeling" tone with which the history content is related must be evaluated and can be used as predicator of ego functioning. The history taker is concerned here with some assessment of the patient's judgment, level of anxiety, and, in particular, coping ability. Coping patterns are significant to ego functioning and to personality structure in general. Another element of emotion or feeling is that of the history taker. He must assess his own attitudes, biases, and feeling toward the patient.

**Personality.** Personality structure and functioning is highly relevant to the diagnosis and treatment of the patient's psychological problems. One of the most frequently used methods of personality evaluation of the patient with chronic pain is the Minnesota Multiple Personality Inventory (MMPI). MMPI may be administered by any paramedical professional, but its interpretation, practical application for diagnosis and treatment is in the domain of a psychologist.

**Pain Measurement.** The measurement of pain is essential for evaluation of pain control methods. However, it is quite difficult to measure pain directly qualitatively and quantitatively. Because of the lack of a universally acceptable definition of pain, it is necessary to establish pain parameters. The McGill Pain Questionnaire is used to specify the patient's subjective pain experience. The method of computation on this questionnaire is:

1. A pain-related index based on a patient's total rank values, derived from the sum total of the

rank values of all the words chosen in a given category; in this scoring system, the word in each subclass implying the least pain is given a value of 1, the next word a value of 2, and so on.

2. The number of words chosen is obtained.

3. The present pain intensity is derived from the number-word combination chosen as the indicator of overall pain intensity at the time the questionnaire is administered. We have found that the McGill Pain Questionnaire is a rather reliable and sensitive measuring method.

## TREATMENT

### ACUTE PAIN

The fundamental principle of management of acute pain is elimination of the basic causative pathology. However, this does not preclude application of various methods to lessen pain for comfort. Depending upon the basic pathology responsible for acute pain, a surgical or a conservative treatment plan must be established. Surgical approach may be utilized when resection, drainage, repair, or fixation is indicated. On the other hand, conservative treatment may be necessary for cases in which pharmacological treatment with anti-inflammatory agents, anti-microbials, anti-spasmodics, or other medications is chosen.

### Analgesics

1. Analgesics should not be used in acute pain prior to identification of the basic pathology responsible.

2. Once the diagnosis of the pathology is established, definitive surgical intervention, if indicated, may be performed under local or general anesthesia.

3. During the postoperative period, an appropriate analgesic may be administered for comfort for a limited period, say three to five days. Prolonged use of habit-forming analgesics during this period may result in drug dependency.

4. When pharmacological treatment is applied for elimination of the pathology, the choice of analgesics must be made carefully because some medications being used may have an analgesic effect. In addition, consideration must be given to the possibility of drug interaction.

5. When the use of analgesics is indicated, narcotic or non-narcotic analgesics can be used liberally. If the psychological component such as anxiety or tension is the predominant symptom, benzodiazepine may be prescribed for a limited duration.

6. Some acute pain may fit the acute/chronic pain model. An acute phase of rheumatoid arthritis or gout is such an example. In these cases, the use of narcotic analgesics should be restrained. Instead, a specific treatment regimen such as salicylates or corticosteroids or both for the former and colchicine for the latter is the choice for control of acute pain.

### Immobilization

1. Immobilization is an effective treatment to reduce acute pain.

2. When pain exists, the affected part of the body tends to decrease its mobility by increasing muscle tone. This is natural immobilization.

3. Bed rest is a common method of immobilization of the body in general. Prolonged bed rest may result in joint contractures; therefore, the patient should be encouraged to change body position as often as possible. However, if the purpose of bed rest is to conserve energy expenditure, passive range of motion exercises may have to be administered by a nurse or a physical therapist for prevention of joint contracture.

4. A part of the body may be immobilized by means of an Ace bandage, splint, or plaster of Paris cast. When this immobilization technique is used, the position of the body part, particularly joints that must be immobilized, has to be carefully determined.

5. Unless it is absolutely necessary, no joint should be immobilized at its maximum range of motion, i.e., in fully extended or flexed position.

6. Commonly used immobilization angles of the joints, such as 5 to 10 degrees of flexion at the knee and 90 degree at the ankle, are found in orthopedic textbooks.

7. The reason for using such angles is not for pain control but to facilitate easier and faster restoration of joint mobility after immobilization is no longer required.

8. The duration of immobilization should be limited and as short as clinically necessary because prolonged immobilization causes muscle atrophy, joint contracture, and osteoporosis, and a longer period will be needed to restore function.

### Cryotherapy

Cryotherapy is often an effective means of reducing acute pain such as low back pain or pain of acute bursitis. However, indiscriminate use of this therapeutic modality is dangerous. For example, an intra-abdominal inflammatory process such as acute appendicitis or pelvic inflammatory disease may be aggravated by the application of cryotherapy because of its analgesic effect. Therefore, the pathology must be properly identified prior to the application of this therapy.

Cryotherapy is applied in the form of an ice pack usually during the first few days after onset of pain. The treatment may last from 15 to 20 minutes at each session and may be applied two or three times a day.

## Heat Therapy

Heat therapy is another common form of treatment for reducing pain. After the pathology has been diagnosed and four to five days have elapsed since the date of the onset of pain, moist heat may be applied to the local area from 15 to 20 minutes two or three times a day.

## Transcutaneous Electric Nerve Stimulation (TENS)

TENS may be applied in traumatic cases such as whiplash injury or acute low back pain, even on the day of onset. TENS may be applied for an hour, and relief of pain may be observed up to two to three hours afterward. It may be repeated twice or three times (See Chapter 10).

## Mild Massage

A patient may experience pain and discomfort in the traumatized area. Some of the pain may be caused by increased muscle tension. In such cases, gentle massage may be helpful to reduce discomfort. However, massage should be given approximately one week after such trauma.

## Hydrotherapy

During the recovery stage of traumatic conditions, restorative treatment must be started. There may be pain on movement of body parts during the postimmobilization stage. In such cases, hydrotherapy has often been found to be useful to reduce discomfort. If an extremity is involved, perhaps whirlpool treatments may be sufficient. If total body immersion is necessary, the Hubbard tank may be used. The temperature of the water as well as its buoyancy may reduce discomfort.

One of the most important aspects of the management of acute pain is the proper selection of a treatment regimen or a combination of regimens, and the timely application of these.

## Psychosocial Therapy

Unlike in the chronic pain syndrome, psychosocial aspects play a minimal role in the management of acute pain. However, those who are in acute pain often experience anxiety and sometimes depression. These emotional conditions may aggravate pain perception. The physician in charge must explain to the patient his findings, the diagnosis, the treatment regimen, the prognosis, and the approximate time for recovery as clearly and as soon as possible. Much of the emotional turmoil that occurs during acute pain is because of fear of the unknown and uncertainty about the future. Clear and precise explanations by the physician, perhaps reinforced by a nurse, would often eliminate such anxiety and depression. Obviously the patient's family should also receive the same information from the physician.

## CHRONIC PAIN

As mentioned previously, the pathology responsible for the chronic pain syndrome may or may not be identifiable. To further complicate matters, abnormality found during examinations may or may not be directly related to the cause of pain. Consequently, although it is ideal to eliminate the pathology, it often is not possible. Therefore, an approach to the management of chronic pain is to reduce the amount of pain that a patient perceives, to decrease disability due to pain, and to teach the patient how to live with minimum discomfort.

On the basis of these concepts, the management plan for chronic pain must be thoroughly assessed. Surgical correction of any existing abnormality is most often unsuccessful. A conservative treatment plan utilizing multidisciplinary approach must be considered.

## Pharmacological Treatment

1. At the onset of pain from terminal malignant tumor, acetylsalicylic acid or acetaminophen in a large dose may be of value. However, non-narcotic analgesics soon become ineffective for control of pain of invasive expansion of primary or metastatic lesions or new metastatic lesions.

2. In such a state, the liberal use of narcotic analgesics must be considered without regard to development of addiction. Codeine, morphine, and sometimes heroin are often used. These medications should be made readily available at the patient's demand for relief of pain or to make pain tolerable. Use of narcotics on demand basis is not contraindicated for terminal patients who may have a relatively long duration of survival.

3. It is often observed that a patient develops drug tolerance when a single narcotic analgesic is used. In such cases, an increase in dosage is necessary, or sometimes alternate administration of analgesics such as morphine and methadone is useful. Brompton mixture (morphine, codeine, alcohol, a syrup, and chloroform water) or a simple aqueous solution of morphine is well tolerated for a long period by the patient without increased dosage.

4. Nausea, vomiting, constipation, and drowsiness are common side effects of these narcotic analgesics. If such side effects are observed, appropriate symptomatic treatment is necessary and a change of medication should be considered. Methadone seems to be relatively free from these side effects.

5. The value of neuroleptics and tricyclic antidepressants for control of pain in terminal cancer patients is inconclusive.

6. According to the definition of chronic pain (not including malignant pain), the duration of pain is unknown. Thus, any analgesics with habit-forming tendency should not be prescribed. If pain is very severe but intermittent, less addictive analgesics such as pentazocaine, propoxyphene, or a combination of propoxyphene with acetylsalicylic acid may be effective. The patient should be well advised of the nature of the analgesic in use, and should be advised not to take it regularly but only when pain is very severe.

7. Effects of and tolerance for analgesics may differ greatly from one individual to another. A particular analgesic that is markedly effective for one patient may not necessarily be as effective or tolerable or both for other patients. Various analgesics may have to be tried on a given patient until suitable ones are found. When there is a specific drug therapy for a painful illness, such as carbamazepine in trigeminal neuralgia or salicylates in rheumatoid arthritis, this drug is the one of choice.

8. Analgesics are not a single entity of chemical substances. While narcotics are used almost exclusively to control pain, other drugs that belong to the group of analgesics have various pharmacological effects other than analgesics, e.g. anti-inflammation, vasodilation, vasoconstriction, muscle relaxation, diuresis, and so on. Thus selection of appropriate analgesics should be guided by pathophysiology of the painful illness and the pharmacological effects of a particular analgesic.

9. Depending upon the nature, frequency, and severity of pain, medication sometimes may be prescribed on an as-needed basis. It is often useful to combine analgesics with one another or with other drugs, but prescribing too many drugs to a patient should be avoided.

10. A patient with chronic pain may have other unrelated illnesses for which certain medications or diets have been prescribed. Thus, before analgesics are prescribed, the possibility of drug interaction or detrimental effects to therapeutic diet must be considered. For example, a combination of acetylsalicylic acid with anticoagulants may result in hemorrhage. Sodium salicylate is detrimental to the patient on a sodium-restricted diet.

11. The use of analgesics for chronic pain is expected to be for a prolonged period. Even if an effective analgesic is found for a patient, as time passes its effectiveness may decrease. In addition, a precautionary approach must be taken for prolonged use of such drugs because cumulative effects as well as side effects may develop.

## Heat Therapy

1. Heat therapy provides vasodilation, increased blood circulation, and relaxation of muscle spasm and tension with relief of pain.

2. Physiological reactions to heat causes a decrease in muscle spasm and spasticity and an increase in various metabolites at the side of the heat application; a soothing effect can be obtained. However, the relief of pain from heat application may be experienced for only a few hours.

3. The selection of various heat modalities is governed by the location of the pain, whether the pain is deep or superficial, and so forth.

4. Short wave and microwave diathermy penetrate deeper into the body than hot packs or infrared therapy, which have a more superficial heating effect. Each modality may be applied from 20 to 40 minutes daily.

5. Clinical indications for use of short wave diathermy and microwave modalities are bursitis, frozen shoulder syndrome, fractures (those without a cast), arthritis, tenosynovitis, strains, sprains, dislocations, traumatic injuries (after initial application of cold), fibrositis, and myositis and so on.

6. Indications for use of hot packs and infrared therapy are arthritis, infections, tenosynovitis, contusions, painful back conditions, sinusitis, neuritis, neuralgia, and so on.

7. Extreme caution should be exercised when utilizing short wave diathermy and microwave diathermy because of their deep-heating effects and their electromagnetic waves, which may be detrimental to patients who have metalic implantations in the area to which these modalities are applied. Such metalic objects are nails and plates for internal fixation and prosthetic devices or cups used for arthroplasty. If a patient has an implanted pacemaker, these treatments should not be given.

8. The application of some form of heat therapy prior to gentle exercises tends to diminish the degree of pain experienced on mobilization of the extremity. Rigorous exercises are not recommended until pain has subsided significantly.

## Paraffin

1. Paraffin mixed with mineral oil applied to a body part at temperatures from 118° F to 126° F is another effective form of heat therapy.

2. It is useful for heat therapy to the hands, forearms, knees, and ankles because of the ease with which it can be applied. It is painted on the skin or the part is dipped into the liquefied paraffin sev-

eral times (six or more) and wrapped with a towel or plastic bag. Paraffin should be left on the body part for at least 20 minutes.

3. Prior to application, all parts should be examined for any skin opening, cuts, or rashes. If present, paraffin should not be applied.

4. Mobilization of painful or stiff joints preceded by the application of paraffin is less difficult and less painful to the patient.

5. Paraffin can be used in rheumatoid arthritis, in limited joint range of motion when there are skin contractures, or after traumatic hand injuries.

### Ultrasound Therapy

1. The use of ultrasound is indicated when it is determined that localized deep penetrating heat therapy is needed.

2. Ultrasound may be applied using a stroking technique, which is a circular overlapping motion of back-and-forth overlapping strokes, or may be applied in a stationary position, for treatment of the nerve roots. The amount of time for the latter must be indicated by the physician.

3. The duration of treatment varies from 3 to 10 minutes per field; the intensity varies from less than 1 W per sq cm to 2.5 W per sq cm. This is prescribed by a physician.

4. If the patient complains of pain during the application of ultrasound, the amount of intensity should be reduced or the sound head of the ultrasound machine should be moved a bit faster during this treatment.

5. Some conditions in which ultrasound therapy can be applied are calcified bursitis and tendinitis, neuromuscular and muscloskeletal diseases, and arthritic conditions. It is also used for relief of pain from postoperative neuroma following amputation.

### Traction

1. Depending upon the cause and location of the pain, cervical or lumbar traction is often prescribed.

2. The application of some form of heat modality prior to traction increases the effectiveness of treatment.

3. Cervical traction is usually applied in the sitting position. A head halter is applied to fit snugly under the chin and base of the skull and is attached to the crossbar of the traction unit (Fig. 9–5). The patient should be positioned in the traction unit so that the head is in 10 to 15 degrees of flexion during traction (Fig. 9–6). (See also Figure 13–2).

4. Lumbar traction is usually applied in the supine position with the hips flexed to 80 to 85 degrees and 10 to 15 degrees of external rotation and knees flexed to 85 to 90 degrees (Fig. 9–7). This positoin provides for good alignment during traction and prevents extreme lordosis. A traction belt

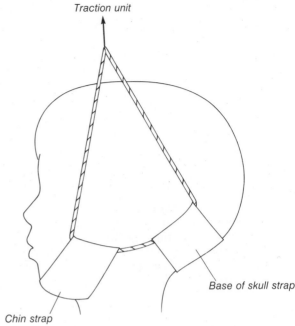

**Figure 9–5.** Cervical traction halter.

is placed around the waist at the lumbosacral level.

5. Traction can be applied intermittently or continuously for 20 to 25 minutes daily or as prescribed.

6. Traction is indicated for whiplash injuries, arthritis of spine, pinched nerves, herniated discs, cervical radiculoneuropathy, and so forth.

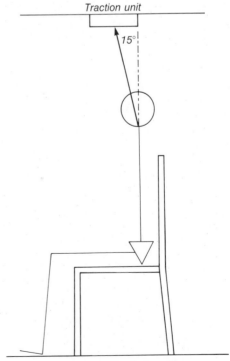

**Figure 9–6.** Cervical traction.

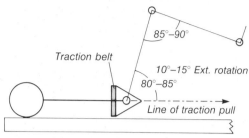

**Figure 9–7.** Lumbar traction.

### Electrical Stimulation

1. The effect of electrical stimulation on denervated muscle is to retard the progression of atrophy, improve blood circulation and nutrition, and assist movement of lymph out of the muscle.

2. The electrical stimulation of innervated muscle produces relaxation of muscles in spasm, prevents muscle atrophy, re-educates muscles, reduces spasticity, and sometimes prevents phlebothrombosis (see Chapter 10).

3. This treatment is often applied to various post-traumatic conditions associated with chronic pain.

### Muscle Re-education Exercises

1. When pain exists in a part of the body, muscles surrounding this area tend to increase their tone, sometimes to the point of spasms. This is perhaps a part of the body's defense mechanism. Nevertheless, such increased muscle tone itself often causes chronic pain or discomfort.

2. In such cases, mild muscle re-education exercises can relax muscles. This exercise is often more effective if it is preceded by heat therapy or hydrotherapy.

3. The purpose of this exercise is not to increase muscle power but to increase blood flow in affected muscles and aid relaxation. Therefore, there is no need to provide resistance.

4. The patient can be taught to perform this method of excercise on his own as often as he would like to.

5. Massage, Hydrotherapy and TENS are discussed under acute pain.

### Acupuncture Therapy

Historically, acupuncture first came to the United States in the early 19th century via an article translated into English and published in Philadelphia in 1825 by Benjamin Franklin Bache. Interest in its use declined by the 1860's, mainly because of infections caused by the absence of aseptic techniques. By the end of the 19th century, Sir William Osler became an advocate and mentioned its therapeutic efficacy for "lumbago."

Within this decade, the concept of acupuncture has burst upon the Western mind as a potential therapeutic tool that must be taken seriously. This development has brought with it the suggestion that perhaps there are other dimensions to health care than had previously been realized. Professionals and the lay public alike find this idea both exciting and vaguely unsettling to their accustomed way of thinking.

As so often happens in history, political developments and the opening of new channels of communication between cultures result in serendipitous rewards that are totally unexpected. The recent rapprochement of the People's Republic of China and the United States is a prime example of this kind of interrelatedness between international politics and cultural interchange. Because of this development, Western medicine has begun to examine seriously the potentials of acupuncture as a mode of therapy.

The gate control theory of pain and the discovery that acupuncture causes the release of beta-endorphin and ACTH in the ventricular cerebrospinal fluid offer the beginnings of a scientific basis for this form of therapy.

The patient whose pain is not relieved by conventional treatment seeks other methods for relief. Physicians should be familiar with acupuncture as another mode of therapy, whether for their own use or for patient referral. In addition, the physician needs to know some details concerning hazards, precautions, and criteria for efficacy.

Patients with osteoarthritis, rheumatoid arthritis, cephalalgia, low back syndrome, cervical radiculopathy, and various dental and orofacial pain problems may be helped by acupuncture when conventional therapy fails. Patients with pain problems complicated by allergic reactions to cortisone, aspirin, or other medications, as well as patients suffering from bursitis with associated peptic or gastric ulcers, or in whom certain medications are contraindicated because of the presence of an ulcer, might all be considered candidates for acupuncture therapy.

**Therapeutic Trial.** An initial course of acupuncture therapy should consist of six treatments given initially biweekly and later weekly. If the patient does not improve, therapy is discontinued. The consensus is that 50 per cent of patients responding favorably to acupuncture will do so within three treatments and 90 to 95 per cent within six.

**Acupuncture Response.** Hyperemia at the site of needle insertion is frequently noted, probably resulting from release of histamine-like substances. Response time can be immediate, hours later, or perhaps not initially but following a course of therapy, when gradual cumulative relief may be observed.

Duration of pain relief may vary. For example, in low back syndrome, some patients following a course of acupuncture therapy may not require further treatment for over a year, while others may need periodic booster therapy. Criteria for efficacy include functional improvement in performing daily tasks, increased joint mobility (range of motion) and muscle strength, and reduction in necessity for pain medication. Having the patient chart time on a horizontal axis and a scale response of pain (0 to 10) on a vertical axis can give both physician and patient a visual record of progress. Inserting time of medication and major events that might affect the painful condition positively or negatively, such as changes in weather, adds further information concerning etiologic factors that might be significant.

**Hazards and Precautions.** Syncope, hematoma, pneumothorax, and sepsis have been observed following therapy. Appropriate knowledge of neuroanatomy and basic anatomical structures, including organ location, is essential to avoid harm. Caution is advised in treating patients who are epileptics. It is prudent not to treat patients equipped with cardiac or diaphramatic pacemakers with electroacupuncture.

Pregnancy is not an absolute contraindication for therapy, although strong stimulation may result in uterine contractions.

## Psychosocial Treatment

There are many psychosocial treatment techniques applicable to chronic pain. However, no single therapeutic technique is effective in all situations for all patients. We suggest providing a treatment package that combines various specific treatment methods. This combination allows for variability to meet the needs of the specific individual in the specific situation. A particular feature of the combination allows the patient to receive the alternative that is most appropriate for him in the given situation. If treatment is to be successful, it must match the patient's understanding of the nature of his problem. Therapeutic intervention is presented to the chronic pain patient in a manner conforming to his expectations with an emphasis on psychological arousal.

## Cognitive Coping Strategy Technique

The aim of this technique is to change the patient's understanding of his pain and enable him to adjust to the pain experience. It provides the patient with a sense of control over his thoughts and feelings and makes him aware of his pain, engendering verbalization. The patient is trained in awareness of his thoughts and in self-expression before or during pain experience.

In order to utilize coping techniques for best advantage, patients may engage in role playing, relating the content of instruction technique to one another. They are encouraged to verbally reinforce themselves each time they use the procedure.

There are various types of cognitive strategies, such as reinterpreting pain stimuli, diverting one's attention from it, and concentrating on the sensation itself. Reinterpreting the pain stimuli is a procedure in which the experience of pain is changed by means of a fantasy that entails interpreting the sensation as something other than pain, i.e., imagining the arm as only cold or numb and not painful. Diverting one's attention involves ignoring the pain by engaging in goal-directed fantasies such as thinking about pleasant events. Concentrating on pain itself means that the patient himself analyzes the pain sensation, its origin, and its consequences, such as anxiety and tension. In addition, in a group setting, the patient can express his own feeling toward the pain problem in general and reinforce the coping skills in which he has been instructed. These techniques may be taught in four to six sessions spaced over three to five weeks.

## Relaxation Training

This training is one of the techniques that distracts the patient's attention from the pain itself. The main focus of this training is to direct attention to the muscle that is to be relaxed. The net result is to reduce any pain from muscle tension or anxiety or both. There are many techniques to reduce muscle tension, including hypnosis, self-induced relaxation, and biofeedback.

## Biofeedback Procedures

This is one of the distractive techniques in which the patient concentrates on physiological sensations (see Chapter 4). The electromyography apparatus is connected to muscles surrounding the point where the patient is experiencing pain. An audiovisual attachment to the apparatus can be regulated so that an audiovisual signal is activated when muscle activity is reduced to a lower level. The patient is instructed to relax his muscle(s) until the signal is activated. By activation of the signal, the patient recognizes that relaxation took place. Almost all patients can achieve such relaxation. If the pain originated from muscle spasm, a great relief of pain may be observed after several sessions. Through this procedure, the patient will learn how to relax his muscles.

## Team Approach

Chronic pain syndrome is very complex; therefore, no single medical or paramedical discipline can successfully control it. In a rehabilitation setting, the team approach is a common daily practice that utilizes expertise of various professional disciplines. In management of chronic pain, one of the most important aspects is teaching the patient. The physician is responsible for determining the cause of pain, establishing a treatment plan, directing appropriate paramedical professionals, explaining the cause, mechanism, and treatment plan to the patient as clearly as possible, and prescribing a minimum amount of medication. The physical therapist provides the patient with exercise and physical modalities that will reduce pain and maximize flexibility, strength, and mobility. The vocational counselor provides assistance in pursuing vocational and educational goals. The social worker determines the patient's coping skills and secondary gains from chronic pain and provides, whenever possible, support, clarification, the opportunity for expression of feelings, and insight. The psychologist explores the patient's personality, coping pattern, and emotional and psychological attitude and administers various behavior modification treatments and supportive therapies. The patient is the central member in this team approach. In order to guide and teach the patient coping skills, the professional members of the team should not give conflicting information to the patient. Thus, close communication among them is fundamental to effective management.

# 10

# Electrotherapy

*by W. T. Liberson, M.D., Ph.D.*

Electrotherapy has always been a cornerstone of physical medicine, to the point that at times these two terms were interchangeable. In a larger sense it included deep heat therapy modalities such as diathermy that involve effects of electromagnetic waves on human tissues. However, classical electrotherapy was limited to galvanic and "progressive" currents, stimulating denervated muscles, and to the use of iontophoresis applied to scar tissues, for example. *Classical electrotherapy has rarely been applied to normal nerves or totally innervated muscles, even if the latter were paralyzed as a result of a CNS lesion.* Two reasons were given for this neglect: (1) If muscles can be activated voluntarily, there is no rationale behind applying electric currents that may be resented by the patient. (2) If muscles are paralyzed by a central nervous system lesion, no therapeutic effect can be expected from peripheral stimulation.

Both of these statements have been proved wrong during the past 20 years. Relevant to the first statement, voluntary muscle exercises are subject to "psychological" fatigue due to shifting attention and motivation. When the therapist provides electrical stimulation maintained for a prolonged time with electronically controlled interruption (i.e., every two to ten seconds) and the subject is asked to "help the current," the normal muscle may be activated for hours if there is no additional load except the distal part of the extremity. Indeed, electrical stimulation may constitute the best "pacemaker" for voluntary contractions.

About the second point, peripheral electrical stimulation was found to produce several effects, even in centrally paralyzed muscles.

1. It contracts the corresponding innervated muscle through its nerves or directly.

2. It increases the strength of muscles as well as their endurance.

3. It maintains the vitality and strength of *denervated* muscles in compound lesions.

4. It pulls and therefore stretches antagonistic retracted muscles or adhesions or both as well as overcomes joint stiffness.

5. It elicits inhibition of pain, spasms, and spasticity in the corresponding extremity.

6. It permits, when properly programmed, an electrically induced functional performance.

7. It integrates elicited contractions with the functionally reconstructed voluntary movements using additional occupational and physical therapy facilitation techniques.

8. It produces milking effects in the extremities of patients with vascular deficiency.

9. It contributes to the prevention and cure of decubitus and other ulcers.

10. It contributes to respiratory therapy.

These additional effects of electric currents have been dramatized by several developments in the past 20 years.

(1) "Functional electrotherapy" emerged from the work done in my laboratory since 1961. It is now generally called *functional electrical stimulation* and has been extensively investigated by Yugoslavian workers (Vodovnik et al., 1982).

(2) Electrotherapy for pain was commonly introduced after Melzak and Wall formulated their celebrated "gate theory" of pain in the mid-1960s. It results from induced inhibitory processes known since Beritoff's work in the 1940s.

(3) Electrotherapy for spasticity also was used in my laboratory in 1961, but more recently this ther-

Drawings by Kevin Earls, M.S., O.T.R.

**161**

apy was extended by me and my colleagues to other "spasms" and joint stiffness. It was also derived from the classical work of Setchenoff and Beritoff on widespread inhibition of reflexes by electrical stimulation of the skin, nerves, viscera, and spinal cord.

(4) Electrical stimulation induces facilitation of voluntary movements in hemiplegics as I reported in 1977.

(5) Electrical stimulation may be used for "reflex walking." (Liberson, 1973).

(6) Differential electrical stimulation in lower extremities (for example, for vastus medialis in chondromalacia patellae according to the Russian technique, Johnson et al., 1977) or in upper extremities (after hand surgery, for example, according to Thomas, 1979).

(7) Treatment of surgical scars with resulting analgesic effects.

(8) Stimulation of the spinal cord and cerebellum to treat pain, spasticity, seizures, and incoordination.

These various newer developments constitute the main subject of this chapter. Electrotherapy of denervated muscles is considered in many classical textbooks and will only be mentioned here. Furthermore, it has become controversial inasmuch as it has been recently claimed that such therapy may delay the healing process by inhibition of intramuscular sprouting. Previously used in facial palsies, it is now obsolete in view of the effectiveness of biofeedback therapy applied to these patients (see Chapter 4). However, in partially denervated muscles of the extremities, electrical stimulation of the remaining nerve fibers retains its full justification, although here again biofeedback therapy should also be used. Electrotherapy of fractures will be only mentioned here; it is still in its infancy.

We shall not consider here electroshock for mental illness, electrosleep, or electroanesthesia, as these topics are not related to physical medicine. Only brief reference will be given to electrotherapy of the cord and cerebellum because this is also a therapeutic modality that has not been universally accepted.

One cannot, obviously, effectively administer electrotherapy to muscles and nerves without a knowledge of the effects of the electric current on these structures. In order to understand the physiological aspects of modern electrotherapy, used primarily for pain, stiffness, spasms, and spasticity as well as for exercising innervated muscles or eliciting their functional activities, the operator must be familiar with the effects of electrical stimulation on myelinated nerves and muscles free of any peripheral nerve damage. For this purpose the effects of electrical stimulation with and without denervation will be briefly reviewed. Following the discussion of related electrophysiology, other neurophysiological effects of electrostimulation will be considered.

# PHYSIOLOGICAL ACTION OF ELECTRIC CURRENT ON NERVE AND MUSCLE FIBERS

## ELECTROPHYSIOLOGY OF NERVE AND MUSCLE STIMULATION

The essentials of the subject will be briefly discussed; the reader is advised to refer elsewhere for a more penetrating review of electrophysiology.

### Effects of Electrical Stimulation on Nerves and Innervated Muscle Fibers

**Immediate Effects.** The immediate result of electrical stimulation is a depolarization of the excitable membrane of nerve and muscle fibers that initiates a traveling nerve or muscle impulse. Normally, the "inside" of the nerve and muscle fibers contains more positively charged potassium ions and less positively charged sodium ions than the fluid outside the membrane. The ionic distribution of the electrolytes on either side of the excitable membrane that envelops a nerve or muscle fiber requires a sodium pump to expel the sodium ions from inside the fibers. In addition, this membrane has to maintain, inside the fiber, a high concentration of negatively charged large organic molecules that are unable to cross it. The net result of this ionic distribution is the presence of a positive polarization of the outer surface of the membrane. The cathode of the stimulating current depolarizes this positivity (excitation being always initiated from the negative pole) and causes a breakdown of the sodium pump. As a result of this breakdown, sodium rushes inside the fiber while potassium leaks out more slowly. Because of a momentary negative polarization of the membrane at one point, the positive ions crowding the outer surface of the neighboring segment of the nerve or muscle fiber "sink" into the point of depolarization (Fig. 10–1A). This, in turn, depolarizes the neighboring points of the fiber with a resulting breakdown of the local sodium pump. This process repeats itself from point to point so that the excitation spreads in both directions from the stimulated nerve point. In the case of myelinated nerve fibers this propagation of the action potential takes place by depolarization "jumping" from one to the other Ranvier node, thus ensuring a rapid nerve conduction velocity. In the case of nonmyelinated nerve fibers, free of Ranvier nodes, or in the case of muscle fibers, the excitatory process spreads at a considerably slower pace.

The process of excitation, or depolarization, at one point of the nerve is very fast; however, it is not instantaneous. Its rapidity determines the time characteristics of an effective stimulus. Figures 10–2 and 10–3 show schematically the process of depolarization during the application of the cathodal

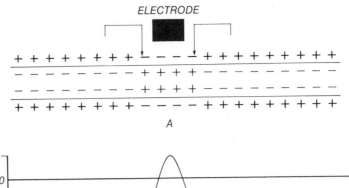

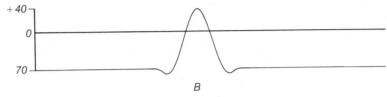

**Figure 10–1.** *A,* Black rectangle: stimulating electrode ( − ), causing a "sink." The arrows on both sides represent this sink. *B,* Action current, that propagates in both directions from the stimulated point.

current to an excitable point. The *critical level T* (threshold) is not reached instantaneously. The process of depolarization takes a certain time, being fast at the beginning, then developing slowly "in search of the asymptote," when it stops. This time course is analogous if not identical to that of charging a condenser. If the stimulating current is not strong enough, the threshold is never reached; therefore, the nerve or muscle impulse is never elicited. In addition, an antagonistic process sets up, analogous to that taking place in a leaking condenser, and the level of the induced depolarization slowly decreases until a certain equilibrium is reached, indicated by a *plateau.* This is the model for the process of *accommodation.*

If the current is strong enough, the threshold is reached, and the involved membrane point sends out a traveling wave of excitation according to the mechanism just described and recorded as an action current (see Fig. 10–1*B*). Moreover, at each point of application of the cathodal current, a momentary *refractory period* sets up, during which the membrane is at first incapable of generating a traveling impulse (absolute refractory period) and then generates it with progressively decreasing difficulty (relative refractory period). These periods of absolute and relative refractoriness occur even in cases when the stimulating current is turned off at the time the nerve discharges a traveling *action cur-*

*rent.* However, if the current continues to flow, the aforementioned process of accommodation, slower than the decay of the refractory period, sets up and interferes with the excitability of the membrane for some time.

Figure 10–3*A* clearly shows that when one uses progressively increasing strength during *successive trials* with the stimulating current, the threshold is reached after decreasing periods of time. On the other hand, the plateau of accommodation may become high enough to be above the threshold; therefore the accommodation breaks down for very strong currents, depolarization remaining continuously above the threshold. This results in a persistent "galvanotonic" or, really, "galvanotetanic" contraction (Liberson, 1932). This discussion permits understanding of the shape of the resulting fundamental law of electrical stimulation, expressed by the *strength duration curve* as well as the effects of progressive currents (see later discussion.)

**Strength Duration Curve.** Let us assume, in order to simplify the explanation of the nature of the strength duration curve, that the level of depolarization is proportional to the strength of the stimulating current. In other words, assume that when the current is doubled or tripled, the level of depolarization is also doubled or tripled. Then we may simply transpose the depolarization time curve into a strength duration curve (Fig. 10–3*B*). The current that is just sufficient to reach the threshold is called *rheobasic current,* or simply a *rheobase.* Figure 10–2 shows that for this minimally effective intensity of stimulation the current may be turned off at the time when the threshold is reached without affecting the generation of the nerve discharge. If the current is prolonged beyond this duration, no advantage is achieved. This is why this time is called *utilization time* (UT). In other words, no current below this intensity is able to induce a single traveling action current, even if its duration is infinitely long. On the contrary, the

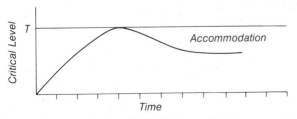

**Figure 10–2.** This figure schematically represents a process of polarization reaching the critical level T, followed by an antagonistic process due to "accommodation."

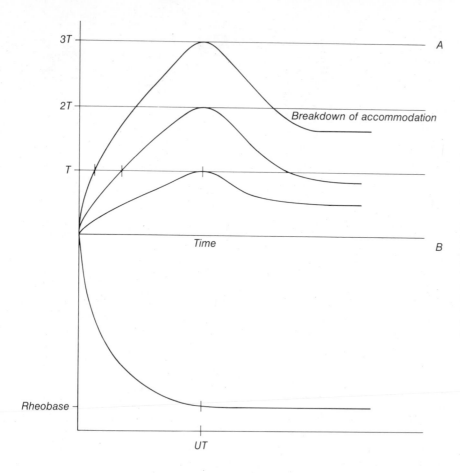

**Figure 10–3.** *A,* Schematic representation of the depolarization of the nerve axon membrane during successive trials with the stimulating current first with a threshold intensity, then two thresholds intensity, then three thresholds intensity. One can see that threshold T is reached after successively shorter periods of time. On the other hand, the plateau of accommodation remains continuously above the threshold when the strongest current is used, resulting in repetitive stimulation by a single strong stimulus. *B,* Visualization of reconstruction of the strength duration curve by reversing the polarization curves. UT: utilization time.

process of accommodation will reduce its effectiveness. These terms were discussed early in this century by Lapicque, who introduced another term: *chronaxy.* Lapicque defined chronaxy as the minimal duration of an electrical pulse with intensity equal to two rheobases (Lapicque, 1938).

If the intensity of the stimulation is doubled, then the stimulating current can be turned off and the critical depolarization level is achieved after a significantly shorter period of time. If the stimulating current is turned off after the threshold of effective depolarization is reached using the intensity equal to three rheobases, the effective duration of the stimulating current will be still shorter. The meaning of the strength duration curve is to show this physiological reality (Fig. 10–3B).

To recapitulate: there is an electric pulse duration corresponding to the minimal possible intensity of the stimulating current capable of inducing a single traveling nerve impulse. An increase of this pulse duration does not bring any further reduction in the strength of the effective stimulating current. If this pulse duration is decreased, the strength of the stimulating current has to be increased in order to reach the threshold of effective stimulation. The pulse duration corresponding to the lowest possible effective stimulating current is called utilization time and the corresponding current strength is called rheobase.

When the pulse duration is relatively shorter, the threshold intensity of the stimulating current must be increased in order to be effective. This increase of strength of the threshold current is gradually more pronounced when the pulse duration is progressively decreased. When one considers the curve expressing the strength-duration law above the level of the rheobase, it resembles a hyperbole without being identical to it. It is known from elementary mathematics that a hyperbole may be expressed by the simple equation: $y = \dfrac{a}{x}$, *a* being a constant. In this case, *y* is the threshold strength of the stimulating current minus the *rheobase* and *x* is the pulse duration (t). One may, therefore, view this equation as follows:

*(1)*
$$I - r = \frac{a}{t} \text{ or}$$

*(2)*
$$I = r + \frac{a}{t}$$

*I* being the threshold current and
*r* being equal to the rheobasic current.

**Quantity of Electricity.** If the terms on each side of equation (2) are multiplied by *t*:

(3) $$It = rt + a \text{ or}$$

(4) $$It = a + rt$$

It is a mathematical expression of the *quantity of electricity*. Equation (4) is a familiar mathematical expression of a straight line originating above the point 0 of rectangular coordinates (at a constant point *a*, above the zero point of the axis of ordinates) and *r* is a slope of the line. We called *r* a rheobase, which is a constant independent of either the duration of a given stimulus or its instantaneous intensity. Since for a time equal to a chronaxy, *I* must be equal to 2r, one may write *for that duration* of the stimulus equation (4) as follows:

(5) $$2r(\text{chronaxy}) = a + r(\text{chronaxy}) \text{ or}$$

(6) $$2r(\text{chronaxy}) - r(\text{chronaxy}) = a \text{ or}$$

(7) $$r(\text{chronaxy}) = a \text{ or}$$

(8) $$(\text{chronaxy}) = \frac{a}{r}$$

In other words, the chronaxy of Lapicque represents a ratio of two constants, *a* and rheobase, *a* being a constant in itself. Figure 4 helps to visualize the constant *a*. For each individual value of pulse duration, the threshold quantity of electricity used is made of two parts: one equal to *a* and remaining always the same and the other equal to the product of the rheobase by the actual pulse duration. Figure 10–4 shows quite convincingly that the minimal threshold quantity of electricity is used when the pulse durations are very brief. However, then the threshold intensity becomes exceedingly high and therefore electrical energy increases, since it is proportional to the square of current intensity.

This consideration of the quantity of electricity is also of interest because it shows that the chronaxy corresponding to two rheobases is not as arbitrary a notion as it might seem at first.

**Energy.** The quantity of electricity is directly related to the process of depolarization involved in excitation. The preceding discussion shows that in order to elicit an effective depolarization with a low threshold quantity of electricity, brief stimuli must be used. However, when one considers the energy or power involved in electrical stimulation, the situation becomes slightly different. We showed experimentally that this parameter of stimulation becomes of great significance when electrical stimulation of the brain is used for electroshock therapy, for example, in order to reduce possible damage to the brain tissue (Liberson, 1949). It was shown that the use of excessive energy increased the incidence and the extent of memory disorders and EEG changes (Liberson, 1948, 1952, 1953, 1956). In light of this demonstration the therapist should not accept the risk of damaging nerve fibers during therapeutic stimulation. Considerations of energy also became crucial with the development of portable stimulators carried by patients. Indeed, the batteries used have only limited amounts of energy to be spent. Any reduction of energy of the stimulating current becomes an important practical consideration, inasmuch as the life of a battery may be correspondingly increased. Energy is proportional to the square of the current intensity (with resistance remaining constant).

Experimental studies of Lapicque showed that the minimal threshold energy corresponds roughly to the pulse duration equal to one chronaxy. When the pulse durations are significantly shorter or longer than one chronaxy, the energy expenditure is increased. Thus it is desirable to use brief dura-

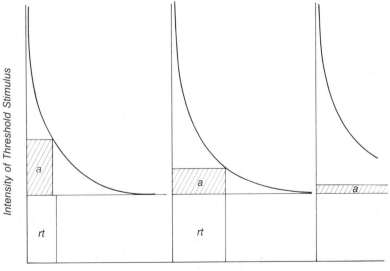

**Figure 10–4.** This figure represents three identical strength duration curves to visualize how the quantity of electricity is composed of two squares: one constant area *a* (threshold intensity minus the rheobase times corresponding pulse duration, increasing from left to right). This area is striped. The other portion is represented by an increased area (rt) due to an increased pulse duration. Indeed, quantity of electricity may be represented by an area of a rectangle corresponding to intensity times pulse duration.

*Intensity of Threshold Stimulus*

*Pulse Duration*

tion of stimuli near the value of the chronaxy of the stimulated nerve or the stimulated muscle in order to elicit single traveling impulses for each stimulating pulse with the least energy expenditure.

Bourguignon in 1920 determined the normal chronaxies of nerves and muscles in men and found them to be from 30 to 200 microseconds according to different nerves and different skeletal muscles. The muscle chronaxy proper in the innervated muscle is difficult to determine (and is of controversial value) because the intramuscular nerve fibers are more sensitive to stimulation than the muscles (Bonnardel and Liberson, 1934); therefore, in practice, the intramuscular nerve fibers become stimulated first, at the *motor point* where they are the closest to the electrodes. For both elicited sensory messages and muscle twitches it is advantageous to use pulse durations on the order of 50 to 100 microseconds. During therapeutic stimulation of mixed nerves the sensory fibers carry the stimuli toward the spinal cord and elicit there the process of temporal and spatial summation, which leads to perception in the brain and/or to reflex activation or inhibition of moto- or interneurons.

Another justification for using brief pulse duration is related to the perception of pain. Bourguignon showed that when extra brief stimuli are applied to the skin, particularly near the threshold value, a feeling of brief tactile shock is perceived; when long stimuli with the same intensity of the stimulating current are used the feeling or perception is painful. Whenever stimulation is used for more or less prolonged periods of time, stimuli must be brief.

**Frequency of Stimuli.** The simplest way to increase the effect of stimulation is to use trains of stimuli instead of a single stimulus. If we wish to produce a tetanic contraction of a muscle, frequencies of 30 to 50 stimuli per second may be used. However, it was recently demonstrated that 10 c/s stimulation may be advantageous for selective stimulation of "slow" muscle fibers. Repetitive stimulation is also more effective when applied to the sensory nerve fibers, as it produces temporal summation effects in the corresponding postsynaptic areas. Again a view was recently expressed that two different optimal frequencies may be used for pain-reducing electrical stimulation: (1) either low frequency, about 1 to 10 c/s with very strong stimuli, (analogous of the techniques of electroacupuncture) or (2) frequency of 50 to 100 c/s with lower intensity stimulation. Very strong stimuli of relatively prolonged duration each elicit, in fact, brief trains of very high frequency discharges (see later discussion). An opinion was expressed that these two modes of stimulation correspond to two different physiological mechanisms of pain inhibition; this hypothesis has not yet been proved. (See Cheng and Pomeranz, 1979, and Vrbova et al., 1980).

In most cases, my colleagues and I use a technique involving interrupted trains of high-intensity brief stimuli delivered at a rate of 40 c/s but interrupted every 2½ seconds. It is possible that this technique affects both mechanisms of pain reduction.

Sometimes experience shows that better therapeutic results are obtained by using stimuli prolonged beyond the duration necessary to elicit a single action potential. Such single stimulus may elicit a series of very rapidly succeeding stimuli—several hundred per second. This is achieved only by using currents higher than two or three rheobases, when as Figure 10–3 shows the level of depolarization is not affected by accommodation. The frequency is determined by the successive refractory states and may produce effective summation in reflex activities.

Such high levels of stimuli cannot be used for prolonged periods of time or by the patient himself because of the pain involved in stimulation. However, the patient may accept such stimulation when the physician administers it and produces tangible therapeutic results in a matter of seconds.

**Progressive Currents.** If prolonged stimulating pulses below the intensity of the two rheobases are used, their effects can be suppressed by progressively establishing their full strength. There is a critical "slope" of the current below which the currents of low intensities are not effective. Yet this progressively established current is fully effective on denervated muscle fibers. It was shown, however (Liberson, 1934, 1962), that lack of effectiveness of the progressive currents on the normal innervated fibers is not observed on human muscles and nerves with the currents above two rheobases. With relatively low-intensity currents, progressive onset may be slower than the antagonistic progress of accommodation. Stimulation can never "catch up" with the "leak" in the membrane. However, there is always intensity of the stimulating current that is higher than the plateau of accommodation. For such current intensity, depolarization repeatedly reaches the threshold level as soon as the refractory period is over, resulting in rapidly succeeding discharges.

## EFFECTS OF ELECTRICAL STIMULATION ON DENERVATED MUSCLES

It is well known that a denervated muscle has a chronaxy 10 to 100 times longer than the innervated one. Electrotherapists have attempted to stimulate such a muscle to maintain its vitality for many decades. This procedure is facilitated by the findings of a considerably lower rheobase in recently denervated muscles, such as facial muscles, for example. Simple battery-powered portable stimulators were developed for patients with recent complete facial palsy. It can be easily shown, however, that biofeedback therapy of Bell's palsy is much more effective than electrical stimulation. Because of the low threshold of denervated muscles, this current is not too painful. On the other hand, since the denervated muscle does not accommodate to the stimulation with low intensity of current, a sinusoidal current of relatively low frequency may be used, in which each pulse shows a progressively rising and decreasing current. The question arises whether a short period of stimulation, say one half hour per day, is sufficient to preserve the vitality of the muscle during a period of months prior to the reinnervation of the muscle. There are experimental animal data suggesting that stimulation for a few seconds of every minute around the clock may retard deterioration of the denervated muscle. Therefore, it would seem desirable to implement the same techniques for patients. However, recently this technique has become controversial. In a normal muscle there are acetylcholine-sensitive receptive areas around the nerve terminations of the motor fibers in the muscle. When wallerian degeneration takes place, other acetylcholine receptor sites may appear in the muscle. Their presence is believed to play a part in the process of "sprouting" in the reinnervation of the muscle that follows. Because it was recently suggested that electrical stimulation may inhibit the formation of these secondary additional receptive sites, the wisdom of electrical stimulation of denervated muscles has been questioned.

The whole problem needs additional research, both empirical and neurophysiological. This is why in this chapter we will concentrate on the effects of electrotherapy on still-innervated muscles, either in a neurologically intact individual or in patients suffering from central nervous system (upper motor neuron) disease or pain and spasms. The possibility must be considered of a therapeutic effect of stimulation on the demyelinated fibers of the autonomic nervous system. Such fibers may have a prolonged chronaxy; they require both prolonged stimuli and high current for their activation. Inasmuch as it is difficult to use such stimuli in practice primarily because of the produced pain, reflex activation of the autonomic nervous system is the only practical possibility. As mentioned previously and discussed later, prolonged stimuli prove at times to be more effective than brief stimuli, provided that they are used by the physician during relatively short periods of time.

## REFLEX INHIBITIORY ACTION OF ELECTRIC CURRENT

The history of the discovery of a reflex inhibitory action of currents upon skin sensibility is more than a hundred years old. Indeed, it was in the sixties of the last century that the Russian physiologist Setchenoff, working in the laboratory of the celebrated French physiologist Claude Bernard, discovered reflex inhibition in the central nervous system. Prior to this discovery, the only process of inhibition known to physiologists was the inhibition of heart activity following stimulation of the vagus nerve. Setchenoff placed small crystals of salt on minute areas of sections of the brain stem of decerebrated frog while spinal cord reflexes were elicited from the animal (Setchenoff, 1963).

At that time the experimental reflex model was devised by a physiologist named Türk (Fig. 10–5). One leg of the frog was placed in a glass containing a weak solution of sulphuric acid. After a few seconds, the decerebrated frog withdrew its leg from the solution. This withdrawal is abolished by destruction of the spinal cord. Setchenoff showed that when he irritated a particular small region of the brain stem, the latency time for such a withdrawal was shortened. Yet if the irritation was made in another area of the brain stem, the latency of the reflex time was prolonged. Setchenoff concluded that there are areas of the brain stem that facilitate the elicitation of reflexes and other areas that inhibit these reflexes, producing corresponding changes of the reflex latency. We now know that in this experiment Setchenoff discovered both facilitating and inhibiting areas of the reticular for-

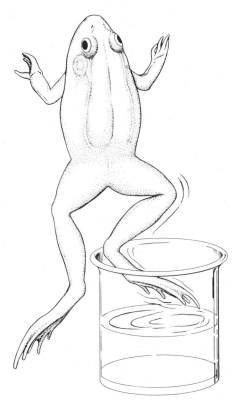

**Figure 10–5.** Schematic representation of Türk reflex.

mation of the brain stem that were rediscovered in this country by Morruzi and Magoun (see Magoun, 1958).

Shortly after it was demonstrated that irritation of certain regions of the brain stem may inhibit reflexes, a student named Herzen attending Setchenoff's courses challenged the professor, according to a story reported from generation to generation of Russian physiologists. Herzen claimed that he could prolong the latency reflexes of Türk under the same experimental conditions by simply pricking different areas of the skin of the frog. Setchenoff, although being sure of his experimental results, became interested in the report of his challenger. He suggested with tongue-in-cheek that the student repeat his experiment in humans. Herzen recruited a few volunteers for his study. While they courageously kept their fingers in a weak solution of the sulphuric acid, he pinched different areas of their skin. Sure enough, the skin stimulation succeeded in inhibiting the reflexes of the finger withdrawal, as its latency time was prolonged during stimulation. Thus the notion of peripheral inhibition was born in that laboratory.

Obviously, one could not ascertain from this experiment whether it was the motor reflexes that were inhibited by skin stimulation or whether the perception of pain was inhibited. It was much later, in the 1940s, that another Russian physiologist, Beritoff, and his coworkers repeated this experiment involving pain alone. They assembled a group of patients suffering from causalgia of the median nerve, a very painful condition. A mechanical stimulation of the skin of the same extremity markedly decreased pain perception in these patients. In 1948 Livingston independently confirmed these findings and showed that causalgia could be relieved by hydrotherapy of the arm and by massage. Beritoff attributed this remarkable effect to the process of widespread inhibition that involved not only pain but also motor reflexes. He believed that this inhibition took place in the substantia gelatinosa, the neuronal formation of the dorsal cord (see Beritoff, 1965).

Melzak and Wall postulated the role of this formation in pain suppression a quarter of a century later, in 1965, in their famous paper on gate theory. According to Melzak and Wall, the substantia gelatinosa, receiving both large cutaneous fibers (touch) and thin fibers (pain), modulates pain perception. If large nerve fiber input dominates thin fiber input, the chances for pain perception are decreased. The opposite is true when the reverse takes place—for instance, after degeneration of large fibers by neuropathy.

Beritoff and his associates carried out a greal deal of research on "widespread inhibition." For example, in Figure 10–6, extracted from Beritoff's book, reflexes of leg withdrawal following electrical stimulation of the appropriate nerves may systematically be suppressed or inhibited by cold water applied to the animal's back. Incidentally, this experiment shows that the concept of Melzak and Wall was incorrect, the sense of temperature being transmitted by thin nerve fibers. There could not be a better demonstration of inhibition than the one that we physiatrists induce in our patients by using cooling sprays. Indeed, cooling sprays do decrease pain (Dzidzishvili, 1940).

The figure was extracted from an abbreviated

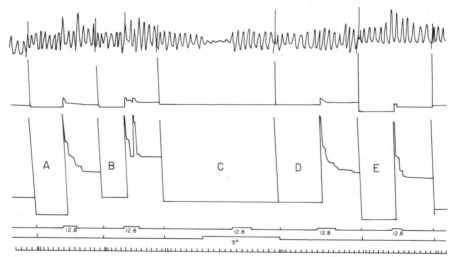

**Figure 10–6.** Diffuse inhibition from application of cold water in normal rabbit. Upper record, respiration; middle record, left hindleg; lower record, right hindleg stimulated by a faradic current (upper signal). General movements occur during stimulation (experiments A, B, D, and E). Cold circulating water (3°C) is applied to the back (lower signal). This stimulation does not elicit any movement, but suspends respiration as well as the reflex reaction elicited by the electrical stimulus (experiment C). Lowest trace, time in seconds (Dzidzishvili, 1940). (From Beritoff, I. S.: Neural Mechanisms of Higher Vertebrate Behavior. Boston, Little, Brown & Co., 1965.)

version of Beritoff's book that I published in English in 1965. This partial failure of the "gate theory" anticipated by the work of Beritoff was demonstrated by Gregor and Zimmerman (1973), as in their studies stimulation of thin fibers also produced inhibition in the posterior cord (Zimmerman, 1979). As Nathan remarked in this connection, "Ideas need to be fruitful; they do not have to be right." The truth of the matter is that Beritoff's idea was both fruitful and right. Yet he too had to miss a great deal of information that followed (Nathan, 1976).

Inasmuch as Beritoff placed the focus of such inhibition in the posterior horn of the spinal cord, he successfully stimulated the posterior aspect of the spinal cord in order to induce inhibition of spinal reflexes. This, of course, anteceded the disclosure of American neurosurgeons who inhibited pain by dorsal column stimulation (Shealy, 1969). Beritoff also produced reflex inhibition by stimulating visceral structures that could affect the central nervous system via autonomic nervous structures involving thin fibers.

Beritoff's notion that the same widespread inhibition may be responsible for both inhibition of reflexes and inhibition of pain became helpful in developing a system of functional electrical stimulation: functional activation of desirable muscle contractions and functional inhibition of undesirable contractions, spasticity, pain, and spasms. In addition, direct intermittent activation of weak voluntary muscles associated with concomitant voluntary contractions of the patient provided another aspect of this therapy. Indeed, without an electrical "pacemaker" resulting from this technique, the subject is unable to steadily exercise his muscles by pure voluntary contractions because of inattention, distraction, and fatigue. Moreover, electrically contracted muscles provide an effective repeated traction on shortened antagonistic muscles or adhesions. Recently discovered brain stem mechanisms in pain inhibition showed also that the neurotransmitter mechanisms may be effective in inhibition of flexor reflexes.

Inhibition as a major factor in therapy of pain and spasms has been considered in another area. Robert Maigne (1979), introduced in the field of manipulation the notion that a forced *nonpainful* stretch of the involved segment in a free direction is more effective than manipulation in the opposite direction. I suggested in 1972 that this maneuver may produce a stretch reflex with a concomitant reciprocal inhibition of the antagonists leading to the suppressing of the muscle spasm (see my preface to Maigne's book).

As a result of all these considerations, my colleagues and I developed a new form of electrotherapy, not only for relief of pain but also for relief of spasms and spasticity. I shall describe later this technique and its uses.

## ROLE OF NEUROTRANSMITTERS

During the past decade a series of completely new developments showed that all of the previous investigators of basic neurophysiological mechanisms of pain reduction (and in some cases, reflex inhibition) were only partially right. They missed an important ingredient of the neurophysiological mechanisms, although the previously outlined scenario including the brain stem, the substantia gelatinosa, and the inhibition resulting from the competitive stimulation remained valid. This new factor consists of pain suppression by endogenously manufactured neurotransmitters. The new information, gathered by new methods of exploration of nervous system mechanisms, microscopic autoradiography, and immunohistochemical methodology, is summarized in the following paragraphs.

1. It was discovered by several investigators (see Kukar, 1980 for the history of their discoveries) that the receptors that constitute the site of the initial action of morphine, a well-known and powerful analgesic, are located mostly in the brain stem reticular formation, particularly near the midline raphé of the pons and in the substantia gelatinosa in the spinal cord.

2. There are endogenous substances (*peptides*) manufactured by the body that have analogous analgesic properties. They are called *enkephalins*. They also predominate in the area of raphé in the brain stem and in the substantia gelatinosa.

3. Stimulation of these brain stem areas produces activation of the nervous pathways that are located in the lateral funiculi of the spinal cord and terminate in the substantia gelatinosa, where they influence modulation of the incoming pain-producing nerve discharges (transmitted by P substance, constituting another neurotransmitter). The analgesic mechanism can be inhibited by an injection of naloxone hydrochloride, which also antagonizes the action of morphine, possibly acting upon the same neurophysiological mechanisms.

4. Another pain-inhibiting mechanism involves another neurotransmitter, *serotonin*, concentrated in other areas of the brain stem but also acting through the connecting tracts upon the substantia gelatinosa. Some monoamines of the sympathetic nervous sytem are synergistic with serotonin; others are antagonistic to its action.

5. Acupuncture may be associated with release of enkephalin mechanism, while the electrical stimulation of the afferent nerves may be effective not only by the spinal but also supraspinal mechanisms (Zimmerman, 1979).

And so the roles of the brain stem (discovered by Setchenoff) and of the substantia gelatinosa, proposed first by Beritoff in pain and reflex inhibition, are found now to be implicated by the discovery of new neurotransmitters and of their predominent locations—what remarkably slow but inexorable progress in scientific discovery! Already, electrical stimulation of the brain stem has been tried in human stereotactic surgery with partial success. Peripheral electrical stimulation is now receiving additional support for its use.

Let us consider now the difficulty in explaining the mechanisms of therapeutic inhibition by classical processes. Indeed, inhibition as seen in classical experiments repeated by Beritoff, or for that matter seen in electromyographic studies carried out in my laboratory, subsides shortly after the cessation of stimulation. There may be an "afterdischarge" of inhibitory effects resulting from the multiplicity of involved neurons, but everything returns to normal within a fraction of a second (a few seconds at most). In contradiction to this, inhibition of pain and spasms may be observed for minutes following the end of the stimulation, sometimes even longer. In order to obviate this difficulty, we considered additional hypotheses. One may postulate that a short-term inhibition of spasm may re-establish blood and lymph circulation that removes substances causing pain and spasm. We also postulated that production of pain and spasm is a result of a progressive, time consuming summation in the net of reverberating neuronal circuits. Inhibition only *seems* to be prolonged, but it may not be: it takes time to re-establish previously built-up reverberating summation processes to again bring about spasms, spasticity, or pain. Zimmerman (1979) discussed pertinent new experiments relevant to this problem (Carsten, Yokata and Zimmerman, unpublished data). They stimulated periaqueductal gray (PAG), inducing inhibition of pain-producing discharges in the spinal cord. Stimulation lasted for 10 seconds and no aftereffects were noted. However, Dickhaus et al. (1976 and 1978) stimulated peripheral A fibers for ten minutes or more; inhibition persisted for almost one half hour, being only partially dissipated. Zimmerman (1979) hypothesized that such prolonged stimulation induces alteration of the extra- and intracellular ionic compositions (eg of K+).

## ROLE OF THE AUTONOMIC NERVOUS SYSTEM

Inibition of both spasms and pain implicates not only large fibers but also thin fibers that carry temperature sensation and sensation of the autonomic nervous system arising from viscera. Recently we observed a curious phenomenon that occurs during therapeutic stimulation leading to decrease of pain, spasm, or spasticity. This phenomenon, which lasted for a relatively long period of time, appeared to be a concomitant activation of autonomic nervous system reflexes. Figure 10–7 shows the result of a one- to nine-minute stimulation of the median nerve, while a thermogram of the hand was intermittently recorded. During and following stimulation, the temperature of different hand areas showed a marked decrease, suggesting either a vasoconstriction or an increase of evaporation, or both. This persisted in one subject for several minutes. In another subject it slowly returned to the original values over a period of several minutes. In a third, it reversed itself so that both hands (only one was stimulated) became warmer than originally and remained warm for at least 15 minutes. Moreover, in two of these subjects we could document reflex temperature changes on the nonstim-

BACKGROUND PLETHYSMOGRAM

MEDIAN NERVE STIMULATION

4 MINUTES AFTER STIMULATION

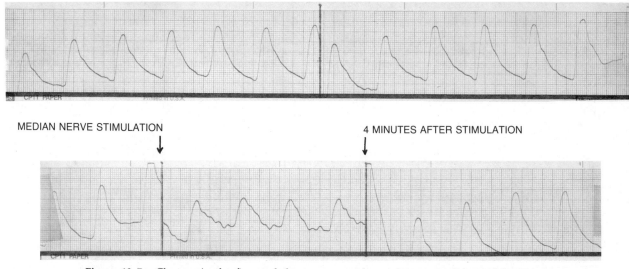

**Figure 10–7.** Changes in the finger plethysmogram under analogous conditions. (Liberson, reported at the International Meeting of EEG and Clinical Neurophysiology, Kyoto, Japan, 1981.)

*Illustration continued on opposite page*

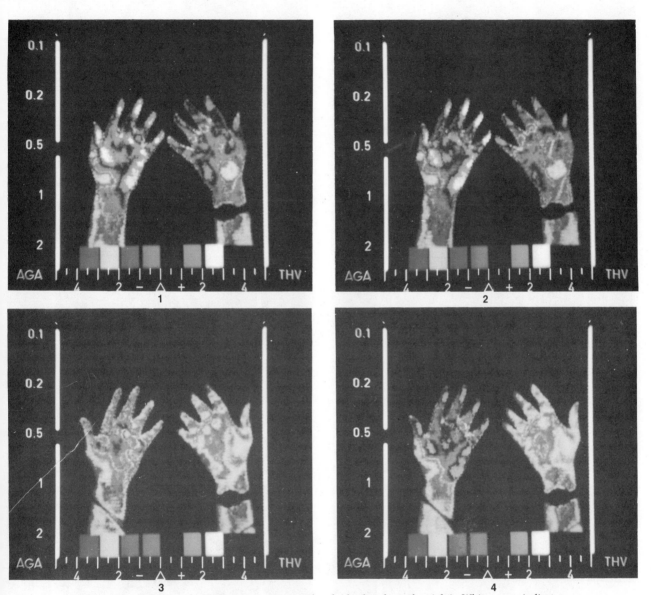

**Figure 10–7** *Continued* Median nerve is stimulated (the hand on the right). White areas indicate cooling.1–2: Prestimulation resting condition. Most of the hand's surface shows gray areas; 3–4: beginning of nine minutes of stimulation. Note pallor, particularly of the stimulated hand (on the right); 5–6: stimulation continued. White area is predominant on the right with some pallor on the left also; 7–8: stimulation stopped. The grey areas reappear on the nonstimulated side (left) while white area still predominates over the right side (12 minutes after the end of stimulation).

*Illustration continued on following page*

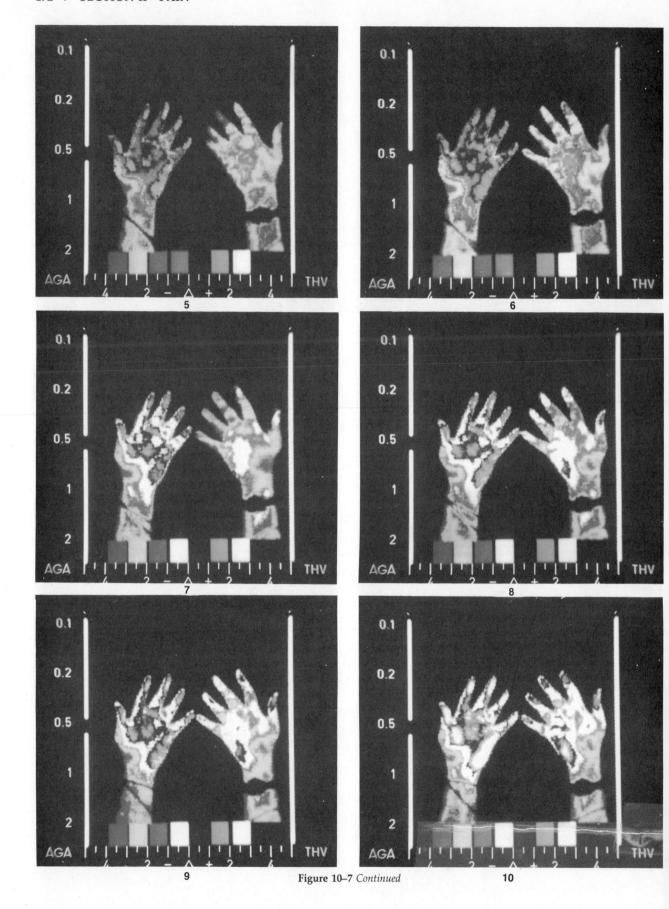

**Figure 10–7** *Continued*

ulated hand, also lasting several minutes. These phenomena should be investigated in greater detail. The fact remains that they indicate a major activation of the autonomic nervous sytem by stimulation of the peripheral nerves lasting for minutes after the end of the stimulation.

Further investigation is needed to understand the part played by the autonomic nervous sytem in the decrease of pain, spasms, and spasticity. Several notions come to mind: (1) In contradistinction to the "somatic" nervous system, the "autonomic" system is notoriously slow, showing prolonged afterdischarges. (2) It is known (see Chapter 7) that an intranasal application of cocaine to the splenopalatine ganglions may decrease pain and spasms in patients with low back pain; this application is associated with activation of the sympathetic nervous system. (3) Maigne describes many patients who submitted to manipulations and afterward described true autonomic system crises.* (4) In Beritoff's experiment, inhibition of reflexes could be produced by distentions of viscera, an action that could have been conducted to the spinal cord by the thin, unmyelinated autonomic fibers. This also seems to contradict the "gate theory" insofar as the latter postulated that only fast-conducting fibers transmit impulses that close the "gate" to painful stimuli. (5) We saw that the activation of the autonomic nervous system may participate in pain-reducing mechanisms. For all these reasons, the role of the autonomic nervous sytem for the decrease of pain, spasm, and spasticity should be investigated along with cases of true somatic "inhibition" and the action of pain-reducing transmitters.

## CLINICAL EFFECTS OF ELECTRIC CURRENTS

### FUNCTIONAL ELECTRICAL STIMULATION

**Principle of Substitution.** In the late 1950s and early 1960s, I began experimenting with what I initially called *functional electrotherapy* and that was later—less adequately—called *functional electrical stimulation* (FES). The latter term is less adequate because electrical currents may cause not only direct stimulation but also indirect inhibition. However, since the term functional electrical stimulation (FES) has become accepted in current terminology, it will be discussed under this designation.

FES is based on a principle of substitution that I discussed exhaustively in a previous paper. Suppose I wish to touch a certain point in space. I can reach it with my finger, or if necessary with a stick or a pencil. In the latter case I can "feel" a distant object through the pencil as if my sensory receptors were not in the skin that is in contact with the pencil but as if they were located at the tip of the pencil. I can vividly "feel" the object that I touch with the pencil even with my eyes closed, and "perceive" its texture. In other words, my brain substitues for the skin perception a feeling projected to the tip of the pencil. In reverse, when I rotate the steering wheel of my car, I do not think to rotate it either clockwise or counter-clockwise, but rather to move the front of my car in different directions and along different paths. In this case not only do I substitute the movement of the car for the movements of the steering wheel but I actually feel the front end of my car as if it had sensory receptors at its front bumper.

This remarkable capacity of the brain may be put to use for rehabilitation of the disabled. Indeed, if every time an artificial hand (prosthesis) touches an object, an electrical stimulus is applied to a nerve of the upper arm, the patient must identify these artificial sensations with the encountering of resistance by his artificial fingers. If a patient's contraction of a shoulder muscle closes the switch of a motor that mobilizes the artificial fingers, then after a period of training or conditioning, the patient automatically contracts shoulder muscles each time he wishes to grasp an object with his artificial hand. These are the principles of functional orthoses or prostheses. This is also the principle of a tenodesis splint when the patient dorsiflexes his wrist in order to grasp an object with the fingers (Fields, 1973; Beeker et al., 1967; Alles, 1968, Kawamura and Sueda, 1969).

Now consider, instead of orthoses or prostheses, centrally paralyzed legs or arms with muscles preserving their electrical excitability. In such patients, utilization of either a sensory or a motor signal can electrically induce a function by muscle contraction; this is another example of "substitution." Thus an artificial sensor in the guise of a switch in the shoe may close an electric circuit that stimulates an appropriate muscle: at the time of heel strike, the gluteus maximus and medius as well as the quadriceps; at the time of toe-on, the gastrocnemius; at the time of toe-off, the dorsiflexors and evertors of the foot. A knowledge of the precise timing of the "reciprocal contractions" of the leg muscles in a paraplegic patient may help in programming appropriate signals coming from one or both feet so that appropriate muscles of both lower extremities and of the erector spinae can be stimulated in functional sequence. Indeed, such stimuli should be able to be applied at the appropriate time with appropriate intensities, frequencies, and pulse durations and cause no pain or appreciable

---

*A recently treated patient, following a transrectal maneuver (see Maigne) to reduce her lower back pain, had repeated autonomic crises.

discomfort. In the case of deep-seated muscles, such as flexors, extensors, and abductors of the hips, the electrodes must be introduced surgically. Instead of being transcutaneous (applied to motor or nerve points on the skin) or percutaneous (piercing the skin), they should be implanted in the same way as a cardiac pacemaker, activated from a distance.

In the case of upper extremities, it is obvious that functional electrical stimulation must be much more diversified than in the case of lower extremities. One may reproduce an artificial reflex by this method. For example, a centrally paralyzed child may have a thermosensitive sensor fixed at his hand so that whenever the latter approaches a hot object, the biceps and the posterior deltoid may be electrically stimulated with a resulting backward jerk of the hand. This is a contemporary model of the reflex action that Descartes introduced to illustrate the notion of a reflex, centuries ago.

In other cases the muscles may be activated by substitution of muscles. For example, a voluntary contraction of the left suprascapular muscle may close the switch that activates an electric current applied to finger flexors, and voluntary contraction of the right suprascapular muscle may close the switch that activates the circuit that stimulates finger extensors through the appropriately located electrodes. The biceps, deltoid, and triceps may be stimulated by similar schemes in a programmed sequence. Corresponding switches may be activated mechanically—for example, by voluntary shoulder elevation or voluntary rotation of the head—or they may be activated using myoelectric integrated signals now commercially available. These switches may either be closed or opened, resulting in movements having maximal amplitude and strength, or the stimulation may be made progressively stronger with variable strength, the latter being proportioned to the strength of the contractions of the substituted muscles.

It is obvious that the voluntarily contracted substituted muscles should not be used at the same time for their natural purposes; for example, the subject should not turn his head to look around if the head rotation is used to activate finger flexors to produce a grasping movement. There are a few "indifferent" muscles that may be made avilable for such purposes without any significant interference at the time of the substituted use—for example, the rectal sphincter, the abductor of the big toe, or even the bulbocavernosus muscle.

In 1959 when we started to study functional electrical stimulation, it was only a dream. Now at least two major applications of this methodology are available.

**Peroneal Electrophysiological Brace for Hemiplegic Patients.** This was introduced in 1961. A switch located in the shoe is activated each time the patient lifts his involved leg. The switch is open when the foot is on the floor. When the foot is off the floor, the switch is "on" and it "commands" a stimulator to activate the peroneal nerve at the knee and the tibialis anticus. Peroneus longus indirectly activated by the peroneal nerve produces dorsiflexion and eversion of the foot; tibialis anticus elicits dorsiflexion and inversion of the foot. Because eversion and inversion compensate each other, a "pure" dorsiflexion results from this electrical stimulation. We called this device an *electrophysiological brace* (Fig. 10–8). Transcutaneous electrical stimulation has not been used in all cases. Surgical implantation of electrodes was tried but has not been universally successful (Liberson et al., 1961; Liberson, 1962a, 1966, 1972, 1973; Offner and Liberson, 1967).

This simple and effective device was used in our laboratory on more than 100 hemiplegics. According to a recent review, more than 3000 Yugoslavian peroneal braces have been used in Europe and the United States on hemiplegic patients. The parameters of stimulation used by us were as follows: (1) pulse duration below 1 millisecond, ideally 60 microseconds to 200 microseconds; (2) pulse frequency at least 40 c/s, no more than 100 c/s; (3) voltage sufficient to activate the corresponding muscles, at least 60 volts, generally not exceeding 150 to 200 volts. Functional electrical stimulation correcting foot drop was well tolerated by the subjects.

The fact that a relatively small number of patients have used this brace can be explained primarily because simple mechanical and therefore therapeutically "neutral" devices are considerably cheaper and do not require a relatively sophisticated approach by patients and their families for

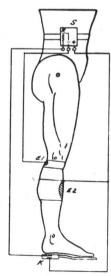

**Figure 10–8.** Electrophysiological brace. S, stimulator; E1, E2, electrodes; K, switch. (From Liberson, W. T. et al.: Functional Electrotherapy. Stimulation of the Peroneal nerve synchronized with the swing phase of the grit of hemiplegic patients. Arch. Phys. Med. Rehab. 42:101, 1961.)

correct placement of electrodes and maintenance and recharge of batteries. Also, proper evaluation of a patient's progress by a competent medical and paramedical team is less important in the case of a neutral device than it is in the case of an electrophysiologic brace. At present a two-channel stimulator is available. With it a second pair of electrodes, significantly larger in size, may be placed either on the quadriceps or, in the case of hyperextended knee, on the gastrocnemius. In both these cases the second channel is activated through a second switch at the time that the weight of the standing leg presses it toward the floor. Multichannel systems (up to eight channels) were also developed with programmable controls. Yugoslavian workers proved that this device could be used by young children with cerebral palsy (Vodovnick et al., 1981).

**Upper Extremity Functional Splints.** The second successful application of FES is the functional splint that has been developed for opening and closing the centrally paralyzed hand. First we applied this splint to hemiplegic patients who had hypertonic finger flexors, which usually is the case. An extension of the wrist and fingers is easily accomplished by electrical stimulation of the corresponding muscles. Such stimulation is universally tolerated by the patient with a simple orthosis immobilizing one finger. The finger flexion is accomplished by the hypertonicity of the flexors, thus maintaining a grasping movement interrupted by the stimulation of extensors (Fig. 10–9). The switch is activated by shoulder movements. It was found later that repeated electrical stimulation decreases spasticity of the flexors, thus decreasing their effectiveness. A tenodesis splint was then activated by the electrically induced wrist extension. (The stimulation should be limited in this case to the extensors of the wrist, leaving extensors of the fingers inactivated.) More recently the possibility of producing a "lateral pinch" by combined stimulation of the median and ulnar nerves has been under investigation. All of these systems may be quite successful; however, most hemiplegic patients are satisfied with having only one active hand and prefer to use electrical stimulation for other purposes (see later discussion) (See also Long and Macersalli, 1963; Hines, 1966; Baker et al., 1979; Liberson, 1975).

In patients with quadriplegia having at least partially innervated distal muscles of the upper extremities, these applications may prove to be most useful. In these patients electrical stimulation of lower extremity muscles has been successful in improving standing and at times locomotion unless the patient's spasms prevent the use of these devices.

**Additional Benefits of Research on Functional Electrotherapy.** Although the dream of "functional electrotherapy" has been only partially ful-

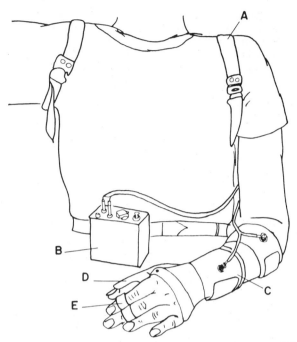

**Figure 10–9.** This figure shows a general arrangement of the initial version of the functional splint. *A*, shoulder switch; *B*, stimulator; *C*, electrodes; *D*, C bar; *E*, Velcro bands. (From Hines, T. F.: Indications and Principles. In S. Licht (ed.): Orthotics. Elizabeth Licht, Publisher, 1966.)

filled so far, an important fallout of newer information has considerably increased our knowledge of these patients and of the effects of electrical stimulation. This may benefit many other patients using electrical stimulation and may give rise to unexpected developments and new techniques.

I) FUNCTIONAL INHIBITION. As mentioned before, the term functional electrical stimulation may give the impression that the latter may only induce activation of the muscles. Nothing is farther from the truth insofar as functional electrotherapy is concerned. Indeed, the success of such therapy is due as much to muscle activation as to muscle inhibition.

Earlier I published an experiment that showed (Liberson, 1965) that the principle of reciprocal inhibition is true not only for voluntary movements in man but also for those that are induced electrically. Moreover, I published (1971) a note describing "widespread inhibition" in man (Fig. 10–10). In the early days of development of the peroneal electrophysiological brace, during a demonstration of a patient in whom the correction of foot drop by stimulation was quite effective, I was embarrassed in front of the audience to observe that the patient continued to manifest a corrected foot drop for a few more minutes after the current was turned off. My initial embarrassment was relieved by a successful analysis of the situation. The stimulation of the peroneal nerve apparently produced for a few minutes not only a reflex activation of dorsiflexion

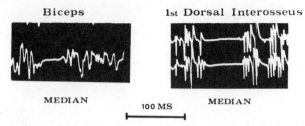

**Figure 10–10.** "Widespread inhibition" in man. Stimulation applied to the median nerve at the wrist is followed by inhibition of muscles of the hand and the arm during voluntary contractions of these muscles. (After Liberson, W. T.).

but also an inhibition of spasticity of the muscle that interfered with the dorsiflex ion, namely the gastrocnemius. The latter exhibited a temporary aftereffect. The presence of concomitant inhibition of the antagonists was not only easily explained but also directly proved by experimentation. Thus, a prolonged stimulation of the extensor communis is followed by a temporary disappearance of spasticity of the upper extremity flexors in hemiplegic patients (Liberson, 1975). Recently, Schneider and I (unpublished observations) documented our findings in hemiplegics over a one-month period by measuring active and passive motion of the wrist extension (Figs. 10–11 and 10–12) (see also Kabat, 1961; Liberson, 1962; Chase et al., 1972).

II) MUSCLE EXERCISE. Experimentation with functional electrical stimulation demonstrated that repeated stimulation of the same muscle leads to an increase of its bulk and strength. As mentioned before, a normal muscle may be electrically activated without any apparent fatigue almost indefinitely when no additional load is moved against gravity other than the weight of the distal segment of the extremity.

It was found, however, earlier in this work, that large muscles of the body were quite fatiguable in hemiplegics and particularly in paraplegics. In the latter, a type of vermicular contraction was elicited in the quadriceps after a few minutes of stimulation. At first this observation was quite puzzling, inasmuch as this muscle was fully peripherally innervated. However, following the publication of Goldcamp, it became apparent that the muscles of these patients, although showing no Wallerian degeneration, suffer from what we have called *functional neuropathy*. Indeed, the motor axons not only transmit the action current traveling with great velocity from the anterior horn cell to the muscles, they also transmit considerably more slowly moving protoplasmic chemicals that maintain the muscle fibers in a state of readiness. As Weiss in 1948 showed, if their flow is arrested by a ligature applied to a nerve trunk, the protoplasmic fluid accumulates above the ligature. It was shown that fibrillations and positive sharp waves occur in the

muscles of hemiplegics (Goldcamp, 1967; Zalis et al., 1976) and paraplegics. A deficiency of this flow appeared responsible for this (Zalis et al., 1976) as Liberson and Yhu (1977) showed that proximal muscles are less involved than distal ones, which was consistent with previous findings. Apparently the anterior horn cells that manufacture these chemicals are less proficient in this function when they themselves receive a lesser supraspinal influence from the brain. Lapicque anticipated these changes when he wrote of "subordination." Only several decades later was the reality of this influence experimentally demonstrated. However, fortunately for the patients, the deficiency observed in an excessively fatiguable muscle at least partially subsides as a result of repeated stimulation. This improvement was demonstrated by Kralj and colleagues on patients with lesions above T12. They found that muscle strength was restored after three weeks of stimulation. More recently Kralj et al., 1980, showed that rising from a sitting to the standing position can be performed by such patients with electrical stimulation of the hip and knee extensors and ankle plantar flexors using a three-channel muscle stimulator. The fatigue time was increased by Wilemon et al., 1970. In a T5 paraplegic (implanted electrodes) with stimulation frequency of 20 to 25 c/s, 0.3 ms pulse duration. A 12-hour stimulation progressively increased fatigue time from 15 seconds to 2 hours sustained muscle contraction. Analogous results may be achieved by one-hour stimulation of the quadriceps for three months.

III) FES DURING GAIT TRAINING. Functional electrical stimulation is helpful when applied during the acute rehabilitation process in hemiplegics. It is directed to individual muscles of the lower extremities, different in different hemiplegics. They may be selected by gait analysis of individual patients.

We reported a most remarkable finding of facilitation of the voluntary movements of the fingers in hemiplegic patients by concommitent stimulation of the extensors of the forearm and the wrist. As soon as stimulation is discontinued, voluntary movements of finger flexion subside. This remarkable observation suggests that some of the pathways remaining blocked at rest in these patients are "deblocked" by facilitation resulting from the stimulation (Fig. 10–13).

REFLEX WALKING. Activation of the triple flexion reflex at the hip, knee, and ankle may be elicited with relatively low intensity of stimulation in certain hemiplegics and paraplegics by stimulation of the posterior tibial nerve. When such stimulation is synchronized with the swing phase of the gait by a shoe switch, the locomotion of the patient may be improved.

ASSOCIATION WITH BIOFEEDBACK. FES may be successfully combined with biofeedback or condi-

Figure 10–11

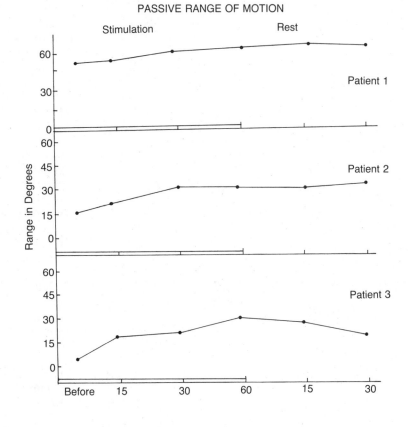

**Figure 10–11 and 12.** Progressive reduction of spasticity in hemiplegic patients by repeated sessions of electrical stimulation of extensor mass of the forearm. Three different patients (1, 2, and 3). Passive (Fig. 10–11) and active (Fig. 10–12) range of motion. Wrist extension. Note the increase of the range during stimulation. (After Liberson and Shneider, unpublished.)

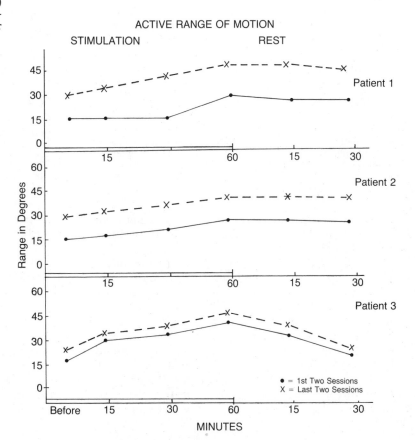

Figure 10–12

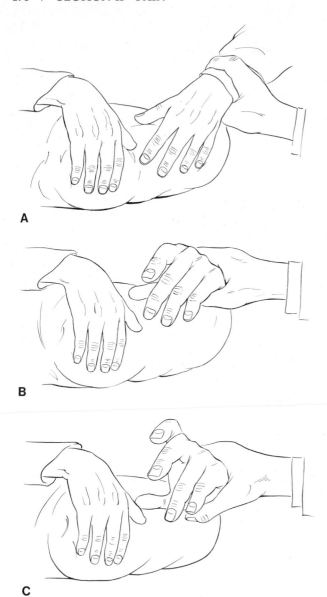

A

B

C

**Figure 10–13.** Example of facilitation, *A*, left-sided, hemiplegic with no voluntary movement at rest. *B*, Electrical stimulation of extensors. *C*, 15 minutes later, moves hand up. (Liberson, reported at the International Meeting of EEG and Clinical Neurophysiology, Kyoto, Japan, 1981.)

tioning procedures in hemiplegics. Movements of the wrist could be improved by such procedures (Bowen et al., 1979) (see Chapter 4).

**Further Possibilities For Improving Peroneal Brace.** Clearly a final judgment concerning these techniques cannot yet be made because they are still being developed. It is legitimate, however, to wonder why, with different equipment now available in France, Italy, Belgium, Germany, Yugoslavia, Scandinavian countries, and the United States, only limited numbers of hemiplegics are walking with the help of FES in this country. We have already mentioned some of the technical problems. The shoe switches may deteriorate in

the midst of walking in a hemiplegic patient; this may constitute a frightening experience. This should never happen if the patient is given shoe switches in both shoes. Then the switches placed in the shoe of the involved leg would be operational at the time of heel-off and the one in the shoe on the normal side at the time of heel-on. Batteries contribute another source of concern. However, it seems that the recent review of Vodovnick et al. gives the correct answer: "The large majority of neurologists, orthopedic surgeons, and physiatrists remain uninformed about the potential benefit their patients could obtain from FES. FES definitely requires a minimum of familiarity with electronic systems. . . . Since in general medical doctors and physiatrists have no engineering background, it is quite understandable that they might consider FES systems a rather exotic gadget." May I add that not only an engineering background but also knowledge of electrophysiology may be of great importance.

Currently we have in mind several schemes for simplification of these systems. These are: (1) A peroneal-quadriceps brace may be included within a light plastic brace, making the heel switches and wires more secure. (2) The power supply may be separated from the rest of the stimulator and may be worn on the chest or waist, for example. This will contribute to the miniaturization of the stimulator proper. (3) The switch may be discarded altogether, with electrical stimulation being used for positioning of the foot and inhibition of spasticity. (4) Instead of determining the timing of stimulation and release by the switches, the patient may be taught to follow the gait progress by a properly preprogrammed stimulator.

All this makes the author of these lines remain optimistic about the future of electrophysiological bracing. After all, 20 years compared to hundreds of years caring for hemiplegics is only a fleeting moment in the history of medicine. We are all the more optimistic because FES and transcutaneous nerve stimulation for pain have been the precursors for electrotherapy of painful spasms and other deficiencies that have already helped hundreds of patients during the last few years of practice, to the joy of both sufferers and healers.

## TRANSCUTANEOUS ELECTRICAL STIMULUS FOR PAIN

The aforementioned paper by Melzak and Wall (1965) had a remarkable effect on electrotherapy. This paper suggested that peripheral pain-eliciting nerve impulses, traveling in the slow-conducting nonmyelinated pain fibers, may be stopped at a "gate" in the posterior cord by rapidly conducted nerve discharges elicited by electrical stimulation of he skin or peripheral nerve; thus the "gate" may be closed. What a century of research on reflex inhibition and even direct demonstrations by Beritoff and Livingston on patients affected by causalgia could not achieve, this image of a "gate," now greatly in doubt, produced, by initiating the whole new field of transcutaneous electrical stimulation (TNS)! Obviously, all preceding electrotherapy done by transcutaneous electrical stimulation has been disregarded. Such is the power of words in our culture; in this case we must be grateful to Melzak and Wall for coining such powerful terminology.

Another major factor in the development of TNS is the building of portable transistorized stimulators that Offner and I introduced around 1960, following my research on brief stimulus therapy (1944).

I shall not describe here the portable stimulators now used for FES and TNS. It must be realized that the so-called TNS and muscle stimulators essentially involve the same type of current, either unidirectional or bidirectional, but with pulses of very short duration (below 1 millisecond). Usually the muscle stimulators offer a higher amplitude current and the secondary interruption of tetanizing current (10 to 100 c/s). The electrodes used in both cases are generally made of conductive rubber. The reader is referred to the excellent review of Vodovnick et al. for further information.

At first, practitioners of TNS placed electrodes on the painful skin areas. Maps of the locations of the electrodes were published, inspired by acupuncture literature but having very limited scientific basis. Later experience showed that stimulation of nerve trunks, such as the ulnar nerve in the upper extremity, was more effective.

**Postherpetic Neuralgia.** Some studies in well-defined clinical conditions were conducted. For example, Nathan and Wall (1974) treated 30 patients with postherpetic neuralgia by prolonged electrical stimulation using portable stimulators. In 11 patients they reported good results; in 8, there was an improvement in the course of the neuralgia. The improvement was not observed in patients with the most severe cases of neuralgia; in some cases the pain was made worse with stimulation.

**Other Painful Syndromes.** An indiscriminately chosen pool of patients suffering from chronic pain became the clientele of the so-called "pain clinics." In these clinics patients with well-defined syndromes such as median nerve causalgia or pain produced by growing neoplasms were treated along with patients having neck and back pain of different etiologies. In some of these patients drug addiction and psychological pressures of litigation and secondary gains interfered with the therapy.

In cases of acute pain related to injury or wounds less than a week old, 80 per cent of patients had their pain controlled (Shealy and Mauer 1974). However, in patients with chronic pain (cancers, bursitis, phantom limb, causalgia, herpes zoster, and chronic neuralgia) only 25 per cent showed satisfactory results. In a group of 198 consecutive patients with chronic pain (Loeser et al., 1975), 63 had no relief and 25 had long-term improvement. According to Picaza et al., (1975), 55 per cent of 100 patients with chronic pain obtained effective relief. Patients with organic spinal cord disease and peripheral nerve damage were most particularly improved. However, according to Loeser et al. (1975), patients with central pain and severe peripheral neuropathies were rarely helped.

The statistics show almost invariably that the initial success in a great proportion of patients was progressively diminished and, in this population of pain sufferers, dwindled to something like 30 per cent after months of application of TNS.

## ELECTROTHERAPY OF PAINFUL SPASMS AND STIFFNESS

In contradiction to the indiscriminate application of TNS in most of these publications, I selected patients with conditions characterized by mixtures of pain and spasms, that seemed to be more amenable to modified TNS therapy than those with cases of pure pain, so often complicated by drug addiction. The technique and preliminary results of such application are now described (See also Liberson, 1972).

### TECHNIQUES

Two major treatment patterns should be distinguished: (1) treatment in relatively short sessions in which the physician is actively treating the patient, who remains essentially passive, and (2) treatment that is directed or may be supervised by the physician but that is essentially self-administered by the patients themselves, aides, or families, and does not require the constant presence of a physician.*

### Treatment Entirely Conducted by Physician

In such cases stationary equipment may be used, such as the chronaxy machine, as well as portable stimulators. At times, for this kind of short session, long stimuli on the order of 10 milliseconds or

---

*Inasmuch as these techniques have been devised, developed and constantly modified in my service, their efficiency cannot be scientifically and objectively proved without repeated controlled studies by other practitioners.

more may be more effective than brief stimuli. A large "diffuse" reference electrode (positive) is used, attached to the shoulder, chest, back, or leg, according to different stimulation strategies, and one small electrode with a handle that the physician applies to the motor or nerve points that he chooses to stimulate. Saline solution is used as a conductor. At times, the physician, properly insulated, uses his fingers or thumb with an attached electrode as an active mobile electrode. In such cases, he should avoid placing his other hand on the body of the patient.

Four different categories of conditions emerged from our clinical practice as suitable for application of this type of treatment.

**Acute Torticollis.** These are patients who wake up one morning unable to turn their heads in one direction, the opposite rotation movement being free. In such cases a small electrode is applied to the motor point of the sternocleidomastoideus *on the side to which the patient is unable to turn*. Using a frequency of 1c/s and pulse duration of 15 ms or more, the physician produces three or four powerful "jerking" rotations to the side of the free movements. This maneuver is somewhat painful and at times frightening, bringing tears to the eyes of some patients (autonomic system excitation?), but invariably rewarding, with instantaneous recovery of the lost movement at times. Sometimes this stimulation is repeated two or three times during the same session and supplemented by the stimulation of cervical trapezius. This "electromanipulation" is indeed nearly 100 per cent successful, leaving only moderate soreness that may be then treated by physical therapy modalities: heat, massage, and electrical stimulation using brief stimuli.

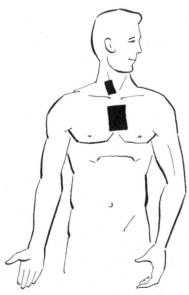

**Figure 10–14.** Position of electrodes for brief session of stimulation of cleidomastoid with long stimuli (by the physician).

Obviously this technique should not be used in patients suspected of vertebral artery involvement.

**Limitation of Straight Leg Raising.** This is a familiar sign of low back pain syndrome. In such patients, the hip range of motion is limited in flexion, the knee being fully extended. The patient's usual complaint during this diagnostic maneuver is pain in the posterior thigh (case of sciatica, or true sign of Lasègue) or in their habitual painful area of the back. In either case, the physician applies the small electrode to the peroneal nerve behind the fibula head, the large reference electrode being bandaged to the lower leg. Strong currents with relatively long stimuli (10 ms), frequency of about 4 c/s may be used with extreme caution, as the stimulation is painful and the patient may pay for its effectiveness by a sleepless night afterward. However, brief stimuli may be just as effective and less painful (40 c/s, 60 microseconds). The physician stimulates the leg while he slowly and progressively raises the leg beyond the previous limit. The patient may still complain of pain in the back or in the thigh but, overwhelmed by the electrical stimulation, allows the physician to slowly move the leg up.

After a few maneuvers of this kind the patient (now raising his leg himself) and the doctor are often pleasantly surprised at having broken the previous limit of the straight leg raising, sometimes to an amazing degree. Obviously this therapeutic success does not mean a cure of lumbago or of discogenic disease (in which case the physician should obviously be much more cautious and perform an initial electromyography test). However, it may be of decisive help for the former and a contribution to the treatment of the latter.

**Painful Back or Neck.** Electromassage with a small electrode or with a finger or thumb is a very useful technique in cases of painful back or neck. Again, one easily observes the resulting redness of the skin, indicating a concomitant activation of the autonomic nervous system. Electromassage is helpful, even though it contributes only symptomatic relief in difficult cases. Brief stimuli at 40 c/s frequency should be used in this technique (Figs. 10–15 and 10–16.) Stimulation of the thoracic and lumbar erector spinae, as well as of the gluteus maximus, is facilitated if the indifferent (large) electrode is applied to the abdomen.

**Referred Pain.** Electrical stimulation of individual muscles in the areas of referred pain is often amazingly effective. With a trial-and-error method, in each individual case a strategically placed muscle should be chosen, the stimulation of which is followed by a suppression of pain. As is well known, painful muscles contain nodosities that can be rolled under the fingers (see Chapter 6). We observed that initially electrical stimulation contributes to the increase of their number, but afterward deep manual massage may reduce their size or sensibility.

*Treatment with a Portable Stimulator with
Brief Stimuli by the Patient without Constant
Physician Presence*

A few principles have emerged from our experience on patients.

(1) The most success in therapy occurs when stimulation is associated with voluntary movements by the patients, stretching contractured muscles and "helping the current."

(2) Stimulation must be applied to large bundles of nerve fibers, such as brachial plexus in the axilla, nerves in the popliteal fossa, or at least single peripheral nerves of extremities.

(3) Stimulation supervised by the physician involving sessions of at least one to two hours should be repeated either daily or three times a week. At home twice-daily sessions may be recommended.

(4) Stimulation should be done to the same extremity as that involved with pain and spasms. Exceptions to this rule are associations of axilla (brachial plexus) stimulation in back and neck pain.

(5) Stimulation should be carried out with maximally tolerated currents.

(6) Stimulation should most often involve direct activation of the weak muscles, inhibition of spasms of the antagonists, and traction of the shortened muscles.

(7) Stimulation may be associated with other forms of therapy.

Let us consider more specific conditions, leaving aside for the moment back and neck pain.

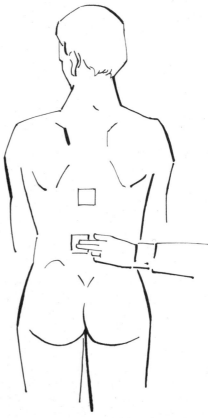

**Figure 10–16.** Electromassage of the back muscles. A large indifferent abdominal electrode may also be used.

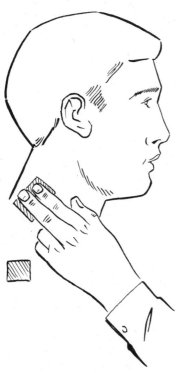

**Figure 10–15.** Electromassage of the neck muscles.

**Partially Frozen Shoulders.** Consistently favorable results are obtained in patients who have suffered for a few weeks or months from a partially frozen shoulder. These are the patients who for obscure reasons have developed pain in one shoulder and a spasm primarily involving the pectoralis major, among other muscles. These spasms considerably restrict the shoulder's range of motion. Clinical diagnosis of bicipital tendinitis, deltoid bursitis, or periarthritis is made. The patient usually comes to a physiatrist after treatments involving muscle relaxants, heat, and cortisone that have been either mostly or totally, ineffective.

On examination, the patient is unable to abduct the arm for more than 40 to 70 degrees, experiencing pain at the end or in the middle of the range of motion. External and particularly internal rotation of the shoulder is more involved than its abduction. The patients are handicapped in self-care as well as in occupational activities.

They complain also of pain at night.

An active electrode (negative) is placed at the tip of the axilla and maintained there by dry cotton and bandages. The second electrode is slipped under the bandages on top of the shoulder or over the deltoid. The patient is led to a wall and asked

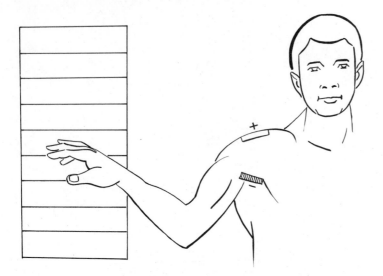

**Figure 10–17.** Patient with restricted shoulder abduction using finger ladder at the beginning of the treatment. Note that the negative electrode is placed at the tip of the axilla, while the positive electrode is applied over the deltoid. These electrodes have to be firmly attached by a bandage.

to place his fingers on its surface. The current is turned on to a point at which the patient feels pins and needles in the hand, resulting from the brachial plexus stimulation through the axilla; the therapist should also observe an actual curling of the patient's fingers. Then the patient is asked to finger-walk up the wall as he is moved closer and closer to the wall, tending to apply the corresponding side of the body to the wall. The patient "walks" the wall up and sidewise for one hour or more (Figs. 10–17—10–22). Invariably, improvement is noted during the first session. During the following sessions, three times a week, two hours at a time the patient is asked, in addition, to successively place the hand over the head and to reach the opposite ear from behind the head (external rotation) or to bring the fingers from behind

the back (internal rotation) while the normal hand pulls the involved hand backward and upward. The sessions may last several weeks or more, depending on how complete a recovery is desired and how advanced the initial handicap was. Ordinary heat or cold therapy may be associated with this therapy, as well as massage or electromassage.

The therapist should not expect to see the contracture of the pectoralis muscle "melting" before

**Figure 10–18.** Limitation of the range of motion of the shoulder in external rotation: the patient cannot touch his ear on the normal side by moving his hand behind his head.

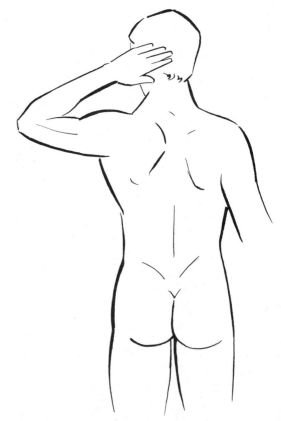

**Figure 10–19.** The same patient showing an improvement.

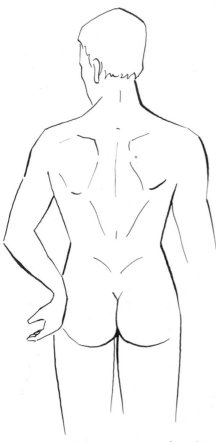

**Figure 10–20.** Limitation of the range of motion in internal rotation.

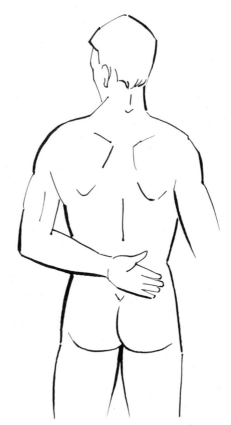

**Figure 10–21.** The same patient at the end of treatment.

his eyes. Improvement is due to increase of the range of motion of the glenoid joint and of the movements of the scapula over the thoracic cage. The initial success continues to be appreciated by patients, who can now shave, comb their hair, and fasten clothing. In more recalcitrant cases "walking up the wall" is alternated with using pulleys during the stimulation; the noninvolved hand only minimally helps the involved shoulder. In other cases, the patients hang over a bar. In all these cases the patient tolerates a degree of stretching that he would not be able to tolerate without the concomitant excitation of the plexus. In all cases the range of motion improves before the decrease of pain. In cases of peripheral nerve involvement, biofeedback should also be used. It has been observed that the patient should not have the same stretching exercises without electricity at home because it appears that he develops additional defense spasms when electrical stimulation is not used at the same time.

An analogous technique is used in hemiplegics with painful restriction of the involved shoulder movement. In such cases the therapist uses pulleys to produce a forceful pull on the contractured muscles by the noninvolved hand during electrical stimulation of the plexus.

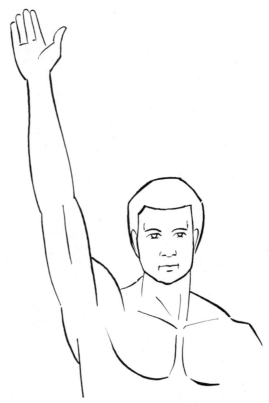

**Figure 10–22.** The patient after a successful treatment.

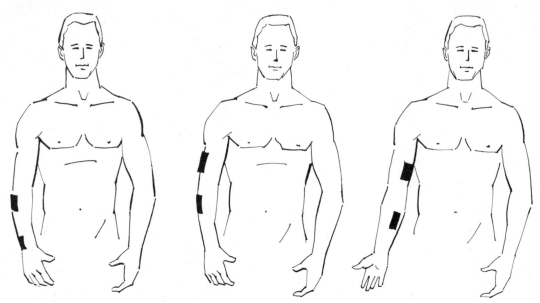

**Figure 10–23.** Summary of electrode placement for upper extremities: *Left,* limitation of wrist and fingers in extension; *center,* limitation of elbow extension; *right,* limitation of wrist and finger in flexion.

**Limitation of Elbow Movements.** Satisfactory results are obtained in patients with limitations of 10 to 20 degrees in elbow extension following fractures of the upper extremity. A negative electrode is placed over the triceps and a positive one over the extensor mass of the forearm or vice versa. It is essential to stimulate these points intermittently, once every three to six seconds, for about three seconds at a time. Each time the muscle is stimulated, the patient is asked to forcibly extend the elbow voluntarily. A reduction of the limitation of the range of motion is obtained in most cases. Limitations of supination are more difficult to treat. The patient is placed in front of an apparatus that permits him to rotate a handle while he supinates his hand. At the same time the extensors of the wrist and fingers are stimulated, although stimulation may be applied selectively to the supinator's motor point. Our stimulator, in addition to the delivery of 40 c/s pulses, has an automatic interrupter that suspends the tetanizing current for periods of two to six seconds following the stimulation of two to three seconds; otherwise the voluntary participation of the patient in therapy cannot be assured (Fig. 10–23).

**Tennis Elbow.** Tennis elbow is treated in about the same way. One electrode (negative) is applied over the motor points of the extensor mass of the forearm and the other over the lateral epicondyle, while the patient supinates his hand. Although on the whole these patients are improved, improvement is not as dramatic as in the previously discussed conditions and the trouble recurs, since most of the patients will not give up playing tennis or participating in the other activities that led to the trouble.

**Post-traumatic Syndrome Following Applications of Casts.** The physiatrist must distinguish cases in which electromyography has showed evidence of partial denervation. Prognosis then, of course, is guarded and therapy only partially effective. (However, biofeedback therapy is quite effective in cases of partial denervation.) In cases in which there is no denervation, the therapy that I apply always brings about some improvement in the range of motion and in some cases a complete recovery. In no case has this therapy made the situation worse. Of course, more documentation is needed to compare different therapies. Yet, nothing seems to contraindicate the association of this therapy with such other classical therapies as whirlpool, diathermy, massage, and manual stretching.

In the case of limitation of wrist or finger extension, the extensor mass of the forearm is stimulated; the deficit in flexion is treated by stimulating the median nerve of the arm and the flexor mass of the forearm, or an individual muscle stimulation can be used (see later discussion) (Figs. 10–23, 24, and 25).

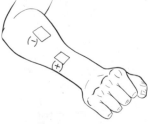

**Figure 10–24.** Electrical stimulation of the extensor mass of the forearm elicits a predominent extension of the wrist.

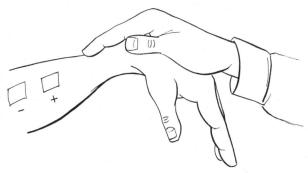

**Figure 10–25.** Same stimulation as in Figure 10–24 with forced flexion of the wrist results in extension of fingers.

**Painful Limitation of the Knee.** These are cases of knee restriction in which surgery is not indicated. In most of our patients, surgery was performed beforehand and was followed by restriction of motion. In case of limitation of extension of the knee, the stimulation is applied intermittently to the quadriceps through very large electrodes, while the patient helps the current by voluntary extensions of the knee (Fig. 10–26). In cases of limitation of flexion the same technique is applied by placing large electrodes over the hamstrings.

For flexion contracture of the knee due to prolonged faulty positioning of the patient, persistent quasicontinuous daily stimulation of the quadriceps while mechanical traction was applied to the lower leg, proved to be successful in some cases.

**Painful Limitation of the Ankle.** Essentially the same techniques are applied to post-traumatic

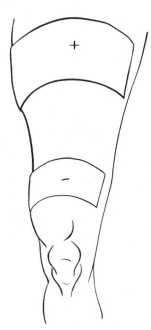

**Figure 10–26.** Application of large electrodes over the quadriceps in cases of limitation of the range of motion in extension.

cases in which there is limitation of dorsiflexion of the foot without denervation. Peroneal and tibialis anticus are stimulated intermittently, the patient helping the current. The treatment, always helpful, can be used in conjunction with other therapies. Such therapy always shortens time of recovery from a sprained ankle (Fig. 10–27C).

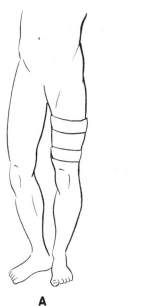

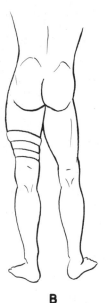

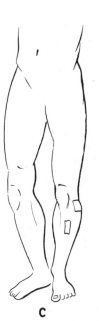

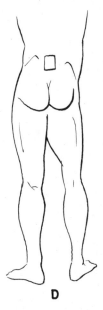

A  B  C  D

**Figure 10–27.** Summary of electrode positions in the lower extremities.

**Neuropathies (Excluding Sciatica).** As we saw before, median nerve causalgia is helped by stimulation in most cases, but the patient should realize that this treatment is a palliation. Of course, when the patient is suffering greatly, his attitude toward palliation and various inconveniences is a function of his mental make-up. Almost invariably, he will reject it if there is a case of litigation, and may revert to drugs. It may be the same when there is increasing pressure on the nerves from metastatic lesions; the physician would have difficulty arguing in favor of reducing sedation. Moreover, the use of electrical stimulators at home is associated with many inconveniences: care of the batteries and of electrodes, perception of the electrical stimulation, correct placement and maintenance of the electrodes, in addition to expense of the equipment, batteries, electrodes, gel, and bandages. However, we did have some success in patients with distal neuropathies of diabetic etiology (Figs. 10–28 and 10–29). Some reasonable patients accept trading their sensation of pins-and-needles of the foot (which continually suggests to them that their diabetes is getting out of control) for the perception of electrical current. In these cases, I place the negative electrode over the posterior tibial nerve at the ankle, the other electrode over the plantar region, the peroneal nerve, or the sural nerve. Obviously, in all cases the patient, after a period of trial, must purchase the stimulator and must sleep with it, if necessary. In case of pain, the patient turns on the stimulator; when the pain subsides, the stimulator is turned off. It has been my repeated experience that patients with finger deformities in rheumatoid arthritis may temporarily regain an increased range of motion of several fingers after a short session of electrical stimulation that reduces the spasms of the corresponding muscles and the stiffness of corresponding joints, while pain subsides.

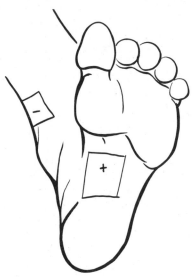

**Figure 10–29.** Another position of electrodes in diabetic patients.

**Neck Pain.** With the exception of an acute torticolis, TNS alone does not seem to provide the entire answer for patients with neck pain, even when patients with discogenic disease are excluded. Yet I systematically use this therapy on patients with this problem, placing the negative electrode in the axilla and the positive on the painful area, even though in cases with litigation one almost invariably has no success (Fig. 10–30). Electromassage as described earlier is particularly appreciated by the suffering patient. I always associate electrical stimulation with cooling sprays and reciprocal resisted mobilization and massage (Fig. 10–31).

Resistive mobilization of the neck, first to the nonpainful direction but covering all the movements of the neck at different degrees of flexion

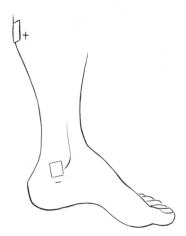

**Figure 10–28.** Position of electrodes in some patients with diabetic neuropathy.

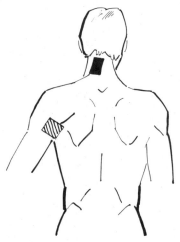

**Figure 10–30.** Position of electrodes for prolonged stimulation of patients with painful neck.

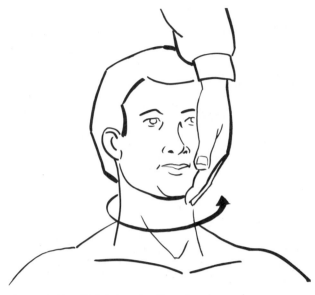

**Figure 10–31.** Resisted contraction of neck muscles.

and extension, seems to me a more acceptable technique than manipulations that appear entirely safe only in the hands of a trained and skilled physician (Fig. 10–31). I believe that they both act mainly by inhibiting spasms and pain. A brief sequence of long stimuli applied to the sternomastoid may be used in some patients after ruling out vertebral artery involvement. In such trials the same technique as described for the acute torticolis is used at the beginning of each session of a more prolonged electrotherapy. During this prolonged stage of the therapeutic session the patient is asked to turn the head to different positions, trying to reach the extreme of the range of motion.

**Low Back Pain.** Here again medicolegal, occupational, and psychological factors interfere with the outcome. In patients in whom there is evidence of disc pathology by electromyography, I prescribe all classical therapies with the electrical stimulation: bed rest, injection in triggerpoints, continuous pelvic traction (15 lbs) and sessions of more intense traction (50 to 70 lbs) for one half hour each; massage with Ger-O-Foam; diathermy to the back, or hot packs, cooling sprays, and a high corset. As stated earlier, limitation of straight leg raising may be treated by brief stimuli. When the patient is ready to walk, he is given a portable stimulator with peroneal-tibialis anticus electrode and asked to walk in the clinic for increased periods of time. If pain recurs, the patient is put back on a continuous bed program. I am extremely cautious about resuming exercises too early (abdominal exercises first under supervision of physician and therapist). Swimming may be permitted early in those patients who are expert swimmers. Electrical therapy alone rarely controls low back syndrome.

During electrical stimulation the electrodes are applied to the popliteal fossa and the back or to the popliteal fossa and axilla (except in cardiac patients). The patient flexes his extended leg from time to time. Electromassage is applied by the physician to the contracted erector spinae using a large abdominal indifferent electrode.

## DIFFERENTIAL MUSCLE STIMULATION

**Chondromalacia Patellae.** As mentioned before, differential muscle stimulation may be used by selective activation of individual muscle points. This was done in a case of chondromalacia patellae, for which Russian physicians applied faradic currents to the motor point of the vastus medialis with great success. Our technique can be used just as effectively to produce selective strengthening of this muscle.

**Contribution to Hand Surgery and Burn Treatment.** The principles of electrical stimulation for muscle strengthening, inhibition of spasms, increase in joint range of motion, decrease in stiffness, and release of adhesions described in the previous chapters may be successfully used after hand or burn surgery. Thomas et al. (1979) have contributed to the development of techniques applied in this area. He has verified the location of some classical "motor points" and added a few additional ones (Figs. 10–32 and 10–33). He uses either monopolar technique (with a larger electrode attached above the elbow either over the anterior or posterior aspects of the arm) or bipolar technique. He showed that by placing an active electrode over the thenar eminence pronation of the

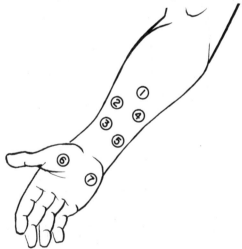

**Figure 10–32.** Position of motor points on the anterior aspect of the forearm. 1, Flexor sublimus digitorum, third, fourth, and fifth fingers; 2, Flexor sublimus second and third fingers; 3, Flexor longus pollicis; 4 and 5, Wrist flexors; 6, Abductor pollicis and pronators; 7, Interossei and flexor digitorum minimi. (Modified from Thomas, D. et Frere, G.: Le Point sur L'Electrostimulation Selective dans la Reeducation de la Main Traumatique Innervee. Cahiers de Kinesitherapie. No. 76, 1979.)

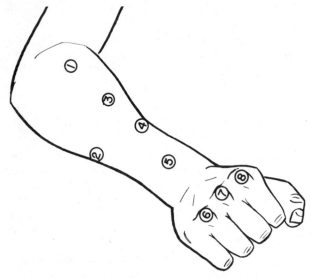

**Figure 10–33.** Position of motor points on the posterior aspect of the forearm. 1, Supinator; 2, Flexor profundus digitorum, medial half; 3, Extensor digitorum; 4, Extensor and abductor pollicis; 5, Flexor profundus digitorum, lateral half; 6, Interosseous muscles. (Modified from Thomas, by permission.)

forearm is produced. He also demonstrated that stimulation of the medial half of the posterior aspect of the forearm about half way between the elbow and the wrist elicits contraction of the lateral half of the flexor profoundus, a paradoxical finding that I verified. Any change of the position of the forearm shifts the projection of "motor points" on the skin. Therefore, the forearm should be immobilized by appropriate measures.

Thomas combines such selective stimulation of specific muscles for their individual re-education with classical facilitation techniques. He confirmed my contention that electrical stimulation is much more effective when used in conjunction with voluntary movements of the patient for a relatively long time, not less than one hour per session. He also stressed the importance of the sensory feedback produced by this combined activation of muscles, helping the patient to re-learn a "forgotten" motor pattern.

One should be careful not to apply a strong electrical stimulation to muscles with recently transplanted tendons. A period of about two months should elapse after surgery before such application. The patient himself may be taught to use the potentiometer of the stimulator, so that the current remains within safe limits.

The same technique of electrical stimulation may be used for breaking adhesions. In the case of skin adhesions, such as in burns, the therapist may hold and pull the adhesion by one hand while applying the stimulating electrode with the other to the appropriate muscle.

**Hand and Arm.** Another technique of the combination of voluntary contraction with electrical

stimulation may be used for hemiplegic patients. A minimal voluntary wrist extension may close a switch initiating a strong electrically induced contraction of the same extensor of the wrist.

In hemiplegic patients with subluxation of the involved shoulder, continuous stimulation of the deltoid invariably reduces the subluxation. Unfortunately, it recurs after cessation of stimulation. In a recently treated patient, I reduced the flexion of a "trigger finger" by stimulating its long extensor and simultaneously spraying its palmar aspect with a cooling spray. One wonders whether electrical stimulation of the appropriate muscle may facilitate reduction of some fractures.

**Incontinence.** Electrical stimulation acts like a sphincter.

## ELECTRICAL STIMULATION IN OTHER CONDITIONS

**Decubitus Ulcers.** A few decades ago claims were made that a special current wave configuration when applied to ulcers has a positive therapeutic effect. We checked the claim and confirmed that electrical stimulation contributed to the treatment of decubitus ulcers. However, when treating large decubitus ulcers, we divided the ulcer into halves. One half was treated by this special type of current while the other received ordinary house AC current, appropriately reduced in intensity. No difference in the speed of recovery of the two halves of the ulcers was noted on comparison.

More recently, I made the observation that if electrical stimulation is applied to a mixed nerve corresponding to the area involved in the ulcer, the speed of recovery appears to be accelerated. I learned from Thomas that he successfully uses currents analogous to those used in our service for treatment of ulcers. However, his approach has been somewhat different from ours, as he actually elicits contractions of the muscles in the neighborhood of the ulcer (for instance, that of the gluteus maximus) (Fig. 10–34). In this case a mobilization of the corresponding body region may contribute significantly to the therapeutic effect. These attempts at using electrical stimulation for ulcers are therefore still in a preliminary phase. We believe, however, that the results are sufficiently encouraging to be reported here.

Recently we observed that if we apply a surface electrode to the gluteal area (positive) and an intramuscular needle electrode, insulated to its tip (negative), introduced into erector spinae, the contraction of the gluteal muscle may be significantly increased. The same technique may be used for the stimulation of erector spinae. However, essentially the same results are obtained using a large indifferent abdominal electrode.

**Surgical Scars.** New observations have been

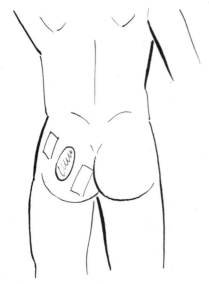

**Figure 10–34.** Position of the electrodes for treatment of decubitus ulcer of the left buttock. Our technique involves a large indifferent abdominal electrode. (After Thomas, D. et Frere, G.: Le Point sur L'Electrostimulation Selective dans la Reeducation de la Main Traumatique Innervee. Cahiers de Kinesitherapie No. 76, 1979.)

reported concerning benefits of TNS applied along healing surgical incisions using sterile electrodes. The resulting decrease of pain is documented by a decrease in the amount of antalgic medication needed by the patient.

**Respiratory Function.** Stimulation of the phrenic nerve in order to activate the diaphragm in patients in need of artificial respiration using implanted electrodes has been done for a number of years. The obvious prerequisite is the functional integrity of this nerve.

Stimulation of the abdominal expiratory muscles has a still longer history. It is quite easy to implement, two electrodes being placed on the recti, shifting polarity from side to side during consecutive sessions. These muscles have been stimulated for either cosmetic reasons or to improve the abdominal support in patients prone to exaggerated lordosis or low back pain. However, because these muscles have a powerful expiratory function, their stimulation may be of functional help for patients suffering from chronic pulmonary disease with emphysema. According to Thomas, in such cases stimulation of the lateral areas of the abdomen is more effective than that of the medial ones.

**Chronic Carotid Sinus Nerve Stimulation in Hypertension.** Techniques with implanted electrodes were successfully used for carotid nerve stimulation effecting reversal of systemic arterial hypertension.

**Cardiac Function.** The possibility of using skeletal muscles to form an adjunct to the deficient heart muscle has been the subject of a research

proposal by me to the Veterans Administration. An analogous study has been recently published by Italian investigators. All that can be stated now is that the results are encouraging.

**Spinal Cord.** As stated in a previous section, Beritoff was the first to apply electric stimulation in animals to the posterior aspects of the spinal cord in order to elicit widespread inhibition of reflexes and pain. Shealy et al. (1970) applied an analogous technique in humans with intractable pain by subdural placement of electrodes over the thoracic spinal cord following laminectomy. Cook et al., (1979) applied such stimulation to patients with multiple sclerosis and reported not only relief from pain but also a decrease of incoordination. In other words, he confirmed the idea of Beritoff that the same process of widespread inhibition affects both pain and spacticity, which may cause incoordination together with deficiency of cerebellar function. Cook's technique has been simplified by introducing electrodes through the epidural space and using transmitter antennae over the skin.

Some but not all patients studied with other neurological disorders such as cerebral palsy, dystonia muscularum deformans, and spasmodic torticollis were helped by this technique. Dimitrijevic and Sherwood (1980) assume that such improvement, also observed in spinal cord injury patients, is due to the supraspinal mechanisms, an opinion not shared entirely by Illis et al. Livshitz delivers subthreshold stimuli (1 to 5 ma, 20 c/s, .1 to .5 ms pulse duration) through implanted electrodes placed above and below traumatic lesions of the spinal cord, using radio frequency control. He claims faster recovery after treatment effected in the acute state. Nashold (1971) used electrical stimulation of the sacral spinal cord in some patients with bladder disorders (see also Bradley (1963) and Susset (1969). (See for the above and below Fields, 1973).

**Cerebellum.** Cooper introduced cerebellar stimulation for treatment of spasticity, rigidity, and epilepsy in 1973. At present there are more than 700 cerebellar implants (see Bensman and Szegho, 1978).

**Sensory Disabilities.** Electrical stimulation for deaf or blind patients is being considered by several researchers.

## NEW PERSPECTIVES

Therapeutic applications of electrical stimulation are now being considerably expanded in comparison to classical electrotherapy. Reports have reached me suggesting that electrical stimulation has been used by some obstetricians during labor to decrease pain during delivery. Some of the claims will no doubt be abandoned as more information is gathered, but it appears to me that most of the new developments will remain in the armamentarium of future physiatrists.

It may well be that the importance of functional nerve stimulation of the peroneal nerve in hemiplegics will be overshadowed by other applications of the stimulating of nerves and muscles in patients who do not exhibit Wallerian degeneration of muscles. The introduction of the peroneal electrophysiological brace, the first application of FES, may prove to have been merely a catalyst for further and more fruitful applications in the continuously expanding field of modern electrotherapy.

# REFERENCES

Alles, D. S.: Kinesthetic feedback system for amputees via the tactile sense. Presented at 2nd Canadian Medical and Biological Engineering Conference. Toronto, Canada, Sept. 1968.

Beeker, T. W., During J. and Den Hertog, A.: Artificial touch in a hand prosthesis. Med. Biol. Eng. 5:47–49, 1967.

Bensman, A. S. and Szegho: Cerebellar electrical stimulation. Arch. Phy. Med. Rehab. 59:458, 1978.

Beritoff, I. S.: Neural Mechanisms of Higher Vertebrate Behavior. Translated and edited by W. T. Liberson. Boston, Little, Brown & Co., 1965.

Bourguignon, G.: La Chronaxie Chez l'Homme. Paris, Masson, 1923.

Bowman, B. R., Baker, L. L. and Waters, R. L.: Positional feedback and electrical stimulation; an automated treatment for the hemiplegic wrist. Arch. Phys. Med. Rehab. 60:497, 1979.

Chase, J. L., Pollack, S. F. and Morris, L.: Inhibition of human muscle by stimulation of cutaneous nerves. In Functional Neuromuscular Stimulation. Washington, D. C., National Academy of Sciences, 1972.

Cheng, R. S. S. and Pomeranz, B.: Electro-acupuncture analgesia could be mediated by at least two pain-relieving mechanisms: endorphin and nonendorphin systems. Life Sciences 25:957, 1962.

Cook, A. W., Taylor, J. K. and Nidzgorski, F.: Functional stimulation of the spinal cord in multiple sclerosis. J. Med. Eng. Technol. 3:18, 1979.

Dickhaus, H., Pauser, G. and Zimmerman, M.: Hemmung im Ruckenmark, ein Neurophysiologischer Wirkungs mechanismam beider hypalgesie durch stimulation sakupankfur. Wien. Klin. Wochenschr. 90:59–64, 1978.

Dickhaus, H., Zimmerman, M. and Zotterman, Y.: The development in regenerating cutaneous nerves of C-fibre receptors responding to noxious heating of the skin. In Sensory Functions of the Skin in Primates, Edited by Zotterman, pp. 415–425. Oxford, New Jersey, Pergamon Press, 1976.

Dimitrijevic, M. R. and Sherwood, A. M.: Spasticity: Medical and surgical treatment. Neurology 30:19–27, 1980.

Dzidzishvili, N.: On the general inhibition and facilitation caused by thermal stimulation of the skin. Mitt. Akad. Wiss. Georg. S.S.R. 1, 217–224, 1940.

Fields, W. S. (ed.): Neural Organization and its Relevance to Prosthetics. New York, Intercontinental Med. Book Corp., 1973.

Goldcamp, O.: Electromyography and nerve conduction studies in 116 patients with hemiplegia. Arch. Phys. Med. Rehab. 46:59–63, 1967.

Gregor and Zimmerman, M. J.: Physiol. (Lond) 232:413–425, 1973.

Herzen, A.: Experiences sur les Centres Moderateurs de l'Action Reflexe. Turin, 1864.

Hines, T. F.: Indications and principles of bracing. In S. Licht, Orthotics. Elizabeth Licht, Publisher, 1966.

Illis, L. S., Sedgwick, E. M. and Tallis, R. C.: Evaluation of possible mechanisms of action of spinal cord stimulation. In Proc. Internatl. Symp. External Control Human Extremities Dubrovnik, 1978, 647.

Kabat, H.: In Therapeutic Exercise. S. Licht, editor. New Haven

Kawamura, Z. and Sueda, O.: Sensory feedback device for the artificial arm. Monograph Presented at 4th Pan-Pacific Rehabilitation Conference, 1969.

Kralj, A., Grobelhik, S. and Vodovnik, D.: Electrical stimulation of paraplegic patients. Proc. Int. Symp. External Control o Human Extremities, Dubrovnik, 1973.

Kralj, A., Bajd, T. and Türk, R.: Functional electrical stimulation providing functional use of paraplegic patient muscles. Med Prog. Technol. 1:3, 1980.

Kukar, M. J.: Opioid peptides and receptors in the rat brain stem. In Reticular Formation Revisited. J. A. Hobson and M. A. B. Brazier, eds. New York, Raven Press, 1980.

Lapicque, L.: La Chronaxie et ses Applications Physiologiques In Physiologie Generale due Systeme Nerveux. Vol. 5, p. 23, Paris, 1938.

Liberson, W. T.: Brief stimulus therapy. Physiological and clinical observations. Am. J. Psychiat. 105:28, 1948.

Liberson, W. T. et al: Functional electrotherapy. Stimulation of the peroneal nerve synchronized with the swing phase of the gait of hemiplegic patients. Arch. Phys. Med. Rehab. 42:101, 1961.

Liberson, W. T.: Some applications of electronics in rehabilitation. In Gerjucy, H., ed. Proc. First Natl. Rehab. Workshop, Toledo, 1962.

Liberson, W. T.: Monosynaptic reflexes and their clinical significance. Suppl. 22, EEG Clin. Neurophysiol. 1962.

Liberson, W. T.: Experiment concerning reciprocal inhibition of antagonists elicited by electrical stimulation of agonists in a normal individual. Am. J. Phys. Med. 44:6,006, 1965.

Liberson, W. T.: Application of computer techniques to electromyography and related problems. Proc. Caribbean Cong. Phy. Med. Rehab. San Juan, 1966.

Liberson, W. T.: Introduction. In Maigne, R.: Orthopedic Medicine, Translated and edited by W. T. Liberson. Springfield, Charles C Thomas, 1971.

Liberson, W. T.: Silent periods and widespread inhibition in man. Abstracts Fourth Internatl. Cong. EMG, Brussels, 1971.

Liberson, W. T.: New developments in electrotherapy. Proceedings of the Internatl. Meeting of Phys. Med. and Rehab. Barcelona, Spain, 1972.

Liberson, W. T.: Functional neuromuscular stimulation, historical background and personal experience. In Functional Neuromuscular Stimulation. Washington, D.C., Natl. Acad. of Sciences, 1972.

Liberson, W. T.: Discussion of gait mechanisms. Medicine and Sport, Biomechanics III, 8:288–293, Basel, 1973.

Liberson, W. T.: Functional electrical stimulation and reflex walking. Arch. Phys. Med. Rehab. 54:588, 1973.

Liberson, W. T.: Discussion in "Neural Organization," New York, 1973.

Liberson, W. T.: Electric aids in hemiplegia. In Stroke and its Rehabilitation. Licht, ed. Baltimore, Waverly Press, 1975.

Liberson, W. T.: Electrically induced facilitation of upper extremity voluntary movements in hemiplegic patients. Proceedings of the Int. Meeting on Motor Control, Dubrovnic, 1978.

Liberson, W. T., Holmquest, H., Scott, R. and Dow, A.: The peroneal nerve synchronized with the swing phase of the gait of hemiplegic patients. Arch. Phys. Med. Rehab. 42:101, 1961.

Liberson, W. T. and Halls, A.: Accelerographic study of gait. Arch. Phy. Med. Rehab. 43:547, 1962.

Liberson, W. T. and Yhu, H. L.: Proximal-distal gradient in the involvement of the peripheral neurons in the upper extremities of hemiplegics. EMG Clin. Neurophysiol. 17:281–284, 1977.

Livingston, W. K.: The vicious circle in causalgia. N.Y. Acad. Sci. 50:247, 1948.

Livshitz, A. V.: Radiofrequency electrostimulation of the spinal cord in acute and chronic phases of traumatic spinal cord lesions. *In* Proc. 2nd all Soviet Conference, Electrostimulation of Organs and Tissues, Kiev, 1979.

Loeser, J. D., Black, R. G. and Christman, R. N.: Relief of pain by transcutaneous stimulation. J. Neurosurg. 42:308–313, 1975.

Long, C. H. and Macersalli, V. D.: An electrophysiologic splint of the hand. Arch. Phys. Med. Rehab. 44:499, 1963.

Maigne, R.: Orthopedic Medicine, Translated and edited by W. T. Liberson. Springfield, Charles C Thomas, 1979.

Magoun, H. W.: The Waking Brain. Springfield, Charles C Thomas, 1958.

Melzack, H. and Wall, P. D. Pain mechanisms: A new theory. Science 150:971, 1965.

Nathan, P. W.: The gate control theory of pain. Brain, 99:123–158, 1976.

Nathan, P. W. and Wall, P. P.: Treatment of postherpetic neuralgia by prolonged electric stimulation. Br. Med. J. 3:645–647, 1974.

Offner, F. F. and Liberson, W. T.: Method of muscular stimulation in human beings to aid in walking. U.S. Pat. 3,344,792. Washington, D.C., 1967.

Pfeiffer, E. A., Rhode, C. M. and Fabric, S.: An experimental device to provide substitute tactile sensation from the anesthetic hand. Med. Biol. Eng. 7:191–199, 1969.

Picaza, J. A., Cannon, B. W., Hunter, S. E., Boyd, A. S., Guma, J. and Mauren, D.: Pain suppression by peripheral stimulation, Part I. Observation with transcutaneous stimuli. Surg. Neurol. 4:105–114, 1975.

Setschenow, J.: Physiologishe studien uber die Hemmungmechanismen fur die reflex thatigkeit des Ruckenmarks in Gehirne des Frosches. Berlin, 1863.

Shealy, C. N. and Mauer, P.: Transcutaneous nerve stimulation for the control of pain. Surg. Neurol. 2:45–47, 1974.

Shealy, C. N., Mortimer, J. T. and Hagfors, N. R.: Dorsal column electroanalgesia. J. Neurosurg. 32:560, 1970.

Thomas, D. et Frere, G.: Le Point sur L'Electrostimulation Selective dans la Reeducation de la Main Traumatique Innervee. Cahiers de Kinesitherapie No. 76, 1979.

Vodovnik, L., Bajd, T., Kralj, A., Gracanin, F. and Strojnik, P.: Functional electrical stimulation for control of locomotor systems. CRC Critical Reviews of Bioengineering. Sept. 1981, Preprint, pp. 63–131.

Vrbova, G., Gordon, T. and Jones, R.: Nerve-Muscle Interaction, London Chapman and Hall, New York, John Wiley and Sons, 1981.

Weiss, P. and Hiscoe, H. B.: Experiments on the mechanism of nerve growth. J. Exper. Zool. 107:315–395, 1948.

Wilemon, W. K., Mooney, V., McNeal, D. and Reswick, J.: Surgically implanted peripheral neuroelectric stimulation. Report, Los Amigos Hospital, Los Angeles, 1970.

Zimmerman, M.: Peripheral and Central Nervous Mechanisms of Nociception, Pain and Pain Therapy: Facts and Hypotheses Advances in Pain Research and Therapies. Vol. 3. J. Bonica, et al. eds. New York, Raven Press, 1979.

Zalis, A. W., Lafratta, C. W., Fauls, L. B. and Oester, Y. T.: Electrophysiological studies in hemiplegia: Lower motor neuron findings and correlates. EMG Clin. Neurophysiol. 16:2–3, 1976.

# Section III

# EXTREMITIES

# 11

# Disabling Peripheral Vascular Disease

*by Heinz I. Lippman, M.D., F.A.C.P., F.A.C.A.*

## Occlusive Arterial Disease

With increasing longevity, occlusive arterial diseases (OAD) have become our number one health problem. They account for heart attacks, strokes, uremia, and sundry complications, which kill more people than all other causes combined, or they may disable the survivor. Chronic arteriosclerosis obliterans (ASO) of the extremities is a common affliction of old and middle age. It causes chronic ischemia and its most feared outcome is the loss of a limb.

Other more acute and less common causes of such conditions as ischemia of the extremities, embolization, industrial and other accidents, and Buerger's disease will not be considered here.

Chronic ASO is statistically highly correlated with coronary artery disease. In a diabetic, ASO appears at a somewhat younger age, runs a slightly faster course, and shows an even higher association with coronary artery disease than in a nondiabetic. Persistence of the risk factors (smoking, hypertension, low-density lipidemia, diabetes, and inheritance), some additional factors ("Type A" personality, viral infections) and perhaps some as yet vaguely defined influences accelerate the disabling course of ASO. Nevertheless, ASO progresses slowly, and while it runs its course, collaterals develop, retarding its incapacitating sequelae.

Fontaine's classification of ASO, which is popular among angiologists, describes four natural stages: the early asymptomatic stage, intermittent claudication, and the two advanced stages of rest pain and necrobiosis (gangrene). The experience of the past 20 years, however, suggests that gangrene is the result of complications rather than manifestations of ASO, while the several kinds of rest pain appearing in chronic ASO carry no certain prognostic implication. The downhill course terminating in an amputation almost always starts with trophic damage to the skin caused by injury or infection. Preventive habits can avert such extrinsic causes, and increased awareness of danger signs facilitates successful early treatment. Good preventive habits include skin care that aims at keeping vital tissue demands for blood at a minimum while vascular reserve is curtailed in the presence of ASO. The smallest skin break opens the door to bacterial invasion and triggers a steep rise in demand for blood by the inflamed open areas, easily leading to more extensive breakdown. Moreover, in diabetics more than in nondiabetics, when neuropathy is present, foot deformities resulting from muscle weakness, desensitization, and autonomic denervation producing dry, fissuring skin render such an extremity highly vulnerable to injury. Such predisposing conditions appear early enough to enable a compliant educated patient to develop effective hygiene habits. Such a patient has practically no chance of losing a limb, even in the presence of advanced chronic ASO and severe claudication.

This statement is supported by my experience in a prospective study on the natural course of ASO.

The study included 506 middle-aged and older ambulating workers, members of the Sidney Hillman Health Center in New York, and extended over a period of 16 years, with a 100 per cent follow-up and an individual observation time of $6.3 \pm 4.6$ years. All were afflicted with ASO, 50 per cent were diabetics, and the majority were men. The only "therapeutic" measure was a well-supervised foot care program in addition to general care of the individual cardiac, diabetic, or hypertensive status. In this group four major amputations, all of which were necessitated by major injury, were performed in three individuals.

In the Workmen's Circle Home for the Aged (a 500-bed institution, residents' mean age 86) the foot clinic serving 15 to 25 patients a day was started 18 years ago. Prior to the program 8 to 15 residents had to undergo major leg amputations every year. No resident on foot care has had an amputation since. Obviously, loss of limb is not part of the natural course of chronic ASO in the presence of good foot care and in the absence of injuries or infections.

The described examples prove that amputation can be prevented in an aging, well-supervised, compliant ambulatory or residential group of people suffering from ASO, obviously a statistically biased group. This experience can hardly be extrapolated to the majority of individuals with an ischemic limb, who are exposed to trauma and to physical encounters with the environment, and who are unaware of the need for preventive habits or of ways to implement them.

The emergence of reconstructive surgery nearly three decades ago seemed to hold a promise of permanent revascularization. Bypass procedures have in fact become the treatment of choice for the salvage of limbs in cases of *immediate danger of loss* when conservative treatment has failed. When, however, bypass procedures are carried out as preventive measures, the long-term results become questionable if compared with good foot care alone. In practice, vascular surgeons and medical angiologists are not always in agreement as to what constitutes an immediate danger of loss to a limb, even though it appears that such opinion gaps tend to close with growing experience of both parties. Such arguments usually center on the prognostic significance of severe claudication, rest pain, rubor on dependency, the drop in distal arterial pressure, and localized trophic lesions.

## PROGNOSTIC SIGNIFICANCE FACTORS

**Intermittent Claudication.** This may or may not incapacitate, which strangely enough is often unrelated to its severity but depends more on the patient's first contact with a physician. If the patient is told that his walking problem may lead to loss of limb and that it might be cured by implanting a bypass (made of vein, umbilical cord, or plastic), he will be disabled as long as he must stop during walking. If he learns the supplemental truth early, that good foot care rather than a bypass operation will always protect him from losing his limb while his walking capacity will improve little if at all, he nevertheless often accepts this handicap as merely a nuisance. The readiness with which such a hindrance is accepted is influenced by the patient's personality traits, his educational and religious background, and his relationship with the physician as well as the latter's persuasiveness and perseverance.

It is a fact that in our society intermittent claudication is compatible with almost any occupation in industry, in the professions, in business, in administration, and in farming. I know letter carriers who have severe claudication but who manage to continue working.

**Rest Pain.** Leg, foot, or thigh pain at rest may have diverse causes, requiring specific therapeutic approaches. One uncommon kind of rest pain carrying a serious prognosis occurs in the pregangrenous state. This typically happens soon after a major arterial occlusion in a previously normal extremity. In such cases, local anesthesia and motor paralysis, as well as livid or mottled discoloration and coldness, are also present. This situation calls for an emergency surgical intervention, embolectomy, bypass, other constructive surgery, or amputation. In the patient with chronic ASO this contingency used to be extremely rare, but in the past few years unhappily such disastrous events have occurred months or years after bypass revascularization for intermittent claudication only.

More frequently, rest pain is caused by an ischemic or diabetic neuropathy. The symptom is usually reversible only after weeks or months have passed, during which difficulties in management can arise. Percutaneous cordotomy, which controls all pain and abolishes perception for hot or cold but leaves all other sensory modalities intact, is a risky but effective procedure available to specially trained neurosurgeons. Intra-arterial injection of small amounts of a concentrated procaine solution (0.2 to 0.5 ml of 20 per cent procaine) may at times be effective for hours or days after injection. It does not produce systemic or other undesirable effects. Simple analgesics (ASA, Tylenol, oral alcoholic drinks) or transcutaneous nerve stimulation should be tried first. A diabetic neuropathy occasionally responds to oral pyridoxine (50 mg daily) or thiamine chloride (100 mg bid), or, strictly on empirical grounds, to a 4- to 6-week series of daily injections of 500 μg vitamin B12; no rationale is available for this last form of treatment. Narcotics are not more helpful than aspirin and should be withheld. In most cases, the pain gradually subsides after several months, often spontaneously. Recent trials with myoinositol (500 mg twice a day by mouth) or, if not available, inositol (same dose), are based upon good rationale but are as yet inconclusive.

The most common cause of rest pain is tissue ischemia, caused by a combination of advanced ASO and extrinsic complications. This typically happens in ischemic legs in dependency when edema develops. A weak or inactive muscle pump may be responsible: hence leg dependency during sleep, arthritis, stroke, neuropathy, or congestive heart failure may cause it. Elevation to level may empty edema, but it also reduces arterial inflow and is not always tolerated. As a compromise, tilting of the bed by inserting an eight-inch block under its head may suffice. With this method better arterial perfusion is secured while part of the edema is emptied. The patient can alleviate this pain by walking about for one or two minutes. In borderline cases we find Benadryl, 25 mg orally, effective in helping the patient to sleep through the night. Oral diuretics are of only minor help for edematous extremities in an ambulating patient.

Other less frequent causes of rest pain are anemia (drop in tissue $Po_2$), drop in systemic blood pressure (excessive treatment with hypotensives), and hyperthyroidism (relative oxygen deficiency). Local pathology and changes in bone and soft tissue are to be ruled out.

In summary, rest pain is managed according to its pathogenesis, but dependent edema combined with advanced ASO is the most common cause. Serious prognostic implications are attached to rest pain only when it develops in pregangrene due to a major arterial occlusion in a previously normal leg, an event of extreme rarity in chronic ASO and one that mandates emergency surgical intervention.

**Rubor of Dependency.** This indicates long-standing anoxic damage to precapillary sphincters interfering with normal constriction to the stimulus of gravity. It consists of dusky-red discoloration in a cold foot or lower leg in dependency. Pallor on elevation is usually present. True rubor that indicates ischemia of many months' duration carries no prognostic significance. A prognostically ominous diagnosis of a first-degree burn that is often missed results from exposure to warm baths or soaks. (Temperatures of 95°F may be "hot" to the ischemic foot.) It resembles in appearance the rubor of dependency; in burns of ischemic feet, red discoloration does not pale on elevation to level or higher, and occasionally small telangiectases can be discerned.

"Pseudorubor" on dependency may appear after long bed rest when a local gravity-induced constriction becomes inefficient. A few days after resumption of ambulation this reaction gradually abates. Buerger's positional exercises accelerate the return to normal. Pseudorubor is seen in nonischemic legs as well.

**Drop in Distal Arterial Pressure.** Distal pressure drop in OAD is grossly evidenced by pallor on elevation. It can be measured by identifying the pressure in an arterial cuff applied just above the ankle, at which pulsatile blood flow, as evidenced by the ultrasonic Doppler effect, disappears or reappears when the cuff is inflated or deflated. The method is not applicable when Mönckeberg's arteriosclerosis (media calcification) interferes with the arterial collapse induced by the compressing cuff.

While the method of measurement with the help of ultrasound is straightforward, the clinical prognostic meaning of a lowered systolic pressure continues to be under debate. A commonly held opinion states that a distal pressure above 50 per cent of systemic systolic pressure (over the arm) indicates that the patient can be managed conservatively. A recent paper will have the safety level raised to 70 mm Hg, which has boosted the number of bypass procedures below that level, the rationale being danger of loss of limb. I have seen permanent viability in cases in which only 40 mm Hg was obtainable in the one pulsating distal artery.

A more convincing way to be guided by systolic pressures was developed by Swedish investigators. If arterial pressures do not exceed 20 mm Hg in the big toe, chances for survival without surgical revascularization are slim. In this meticulous study actual capillary pressures were measured by identifying the counter pressure, that just abolishes the absorption of locally injected radionuclear-tagged substances.

## DIAGNOSTIC TESTS FOR OCCLUSIVE ARTERIAL DISEASE

A comprehensive diagnosis should establish the presence of arterial occlusion, the degree of vasoconstriction, the presence of vasospasm, the site(s) of occlusion, the nature of collaterals and the vascular reserve, and an etiology. For all these objectives, numerous instrumental methods are available to the specialist, but an adequate functional and prognostic assessment can be obtained with little instrumentation and with judicious use of the senses. In venous diseases, more instrumentation is needed.

**History and Postural Tests.** Intermittent claudication is an inability to walk more than a short distance without stopping because of pain, weakness, numbness, stiffness, or cramp in foot, calf, thigh, or buttock. The symptoms subside in seconds on standing still and recur on walking. Intermittent claudication is often unilateral and may shift sides later (Fig. 11–1).

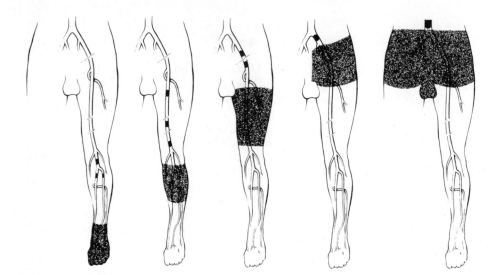

**Figure 11–1.** Intermittent claudication (black shaded) and site of arterial occlusion.

In postural tests, blanching is seen on elevation of the foot by 50 to 60 cm above level with the patient supine, the sole pressing against the observer's palm for 20 seconds. Flush appears within 9 seconds in normal persons. Delay indicates proximal occlusion or stenosis. The test grossly assesses arterial pressure (Fig. 11–2).

In rubor of dependency, dusky-red discoloration in a dependent cold foot appears within one to two minutes. The positive test indicates that OAD has been present for months. On elevation the color vanishes.

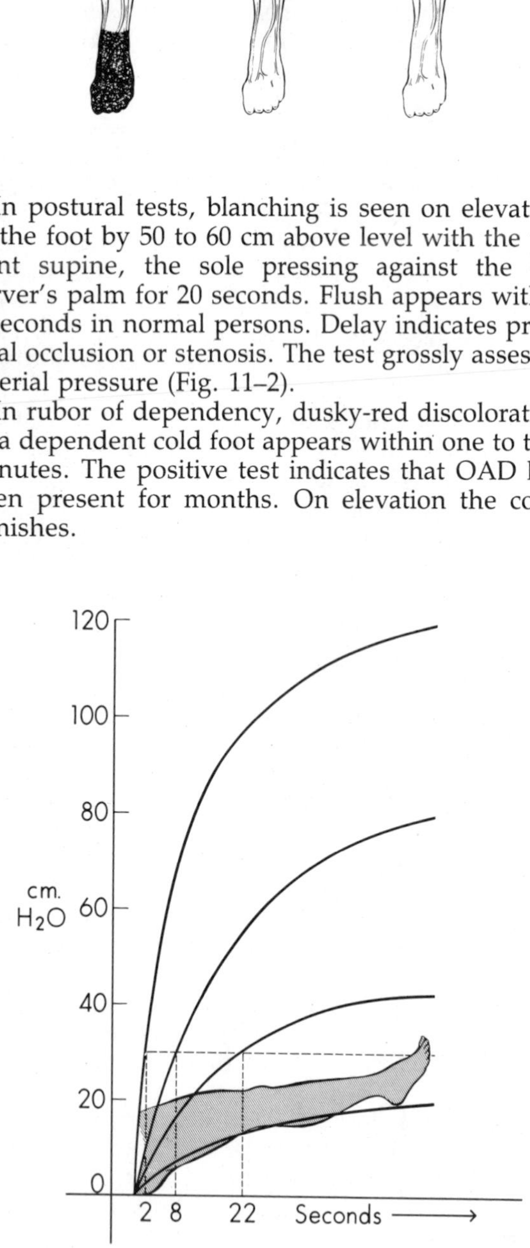

**Ankle Pulses and Oscillometric Readings.** Posterior and anterior tibial pulses are present in the normal person. The dorsalis pedis pulse is absent in 20 per cent and the perforating peroneal pulse in 30 per cent of normal persons. Popliteal, femoral, and external iliac pulses are identified. By tracing the pulse from the groin down to the foot it is often possible to pinpoint segmental occlusions in the artery's course; in the obese or muscular patient this is not possible (Fig. 11–3).

Oscillometric readings (Fig. 11–3) confirm the pulse findings; a large cuff is used for thighs with circumferences in excess of 16 inches. Readings are taken at ankle, high calf, and low thigh level.

**Reactive Hyperemia Tests for Gross Assessment of Total Flow.** LEWIS-PICKERING TEST FOR LEGS. An arterial cuff high on calf is inflated to 20 mm Hg above systolic pressure for 5 minutes and suddenly released; in the normal state, full reactive hyperemia of the sole is present within 12 seconds. Delayed inflow pinpoints ischemic areas, severity in proportion to delay.

ALLEN TEST 1 (FOR HANDS). The patient tightens his fist for 20 seconds while the physician compresses the ulnar and radial arteries at the wrist for 3 minutes. Release of pressure over one of the arteries in the normal person is followed by flush into the hand. Absence of reactive hyperemia indicates closure of the respective artery.

ALLEN TEST 2 (FOR DIGITS OR LOCAL ISCHEMIA). The same test procedure applies as for Allen test 1, with both arteries released after two minutes. Ischemic areas (e.g., digits) are recognized by delay in inflow.

For testing the degree of vasoconstriction, vasospasm, or blood distribution into peripheral tissues, consult textbooks on peripheral vascular disease. They are unnecessary for ordinary purposes.

**Ultrasonic Doppler Effect.** The method that

**Figure 11–2.** Postural test: Delay in inflow and blanching on elevation as function of pressure drop (in cm water) in occlusive arterial disease.

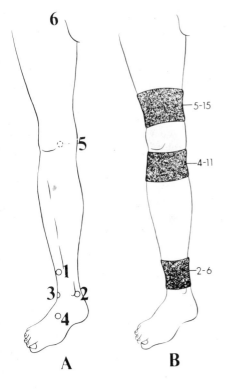

A. Leg Pulses     B. Oscillometric Indices

1. Anterior Tibial
2. Posterior Tibial
3. Peroneal
4. Dorsalis Pedis
5. Popliteal
6. Femoral

**Figure 11–3.** Leg pulses and oscillometric indices in clinical examination for OAD.

measures blood flow velocity is used as an indicator for pulsatile flow resumption while a proximally placed blood pressure cuff is deflated, measuring systolic pressure. In the presence of arterial media calcification (often seen in diabetics), the method cannot be used. The method can be used with some practice to trace collateral flow; concomittant use of an anatomical text is advised.

Skin temperature, because of its sympathetic regulation and because of low correlation with large blood shifts, does not serve well, unless sympathetic tone is under control (sympathetic block, temperature-controlled room). Hair growth is of no practical value because of large individual and local inconsistencies.

Arteriography is needed in preparation for reconstructive or other surgical procedures but is not used as routine procedure for work-up. It is not discussed here.

**The Vanishing Exercise Pulse (Fig. 11–4).** Oscillometric readings are recorded at the ankle of the resting supine patient. The patient, with the instrument in place, plantar-dorsiflexes the ankle against a mild (about 30 inch lbs) resistance, for 25 seconds at a rate of one completed extreme plantar-dorsiflexion per two seconds. Oscillometric readings are recorded immediately after cessation of the ankle movements. Any drop compared to pre-exercise values or drop of mean pressure (where readings are maximal) indicates a proximal segmental occlusion or significant (more than 75 per cent reduced cross section) stenosis.

The time to full recovery of pressure and oscillometric index furnishes a good estimate of the severity of the occlusion.

If a segmental occlusion is suspected proximally to the femoral bifurcation, the test is repeated with the instrument placed to the calf just below the knee joint. The knee is stretched and bent against resistance to extension, and the whole procedure is repeated as described previously with the instrument at the higher site and the exercise being continued to 40 seconds. If immediately after cessation of exercise the oscillometric readings drop, the occlusion is located proximally to the femoral bifurcation.

**Figure 11–4.** The vanishing exercise pulse—drop in pressure and oscillometric indices immediately after ankle exercise. This patient had a segmental occlusion in the superficial femoral artery, with fair collaterals. See text.

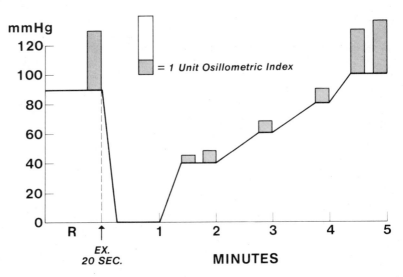

In lieu of oscillometry, ultrasonic Doppler procedure can be used to trace the blood pressures in this test, which correlate well with the oscillometric indices.

## MANAGEMENT OF PATIENTS WITH OCCLUSIVE ARTERIAL DISEASE: (OAD)

Treatment aims at providing optimal control of the patient's general condition and the cardiac and metabolic status and at treating anemia, renal and respiratory malfunctions, and hormonal and electrolyte imbalances. For the ischemic state, two basic therapeutic goals can be pursued: the increase of arterial blood flow and the diminution of the demand for blood of the peripheral tissues, mainly skin (Table 11–1).

**Walking.** Active muscle contraction increases collateral flow. Walking up to the onset of claudication enhances collateral formation. The subsidence of all symptoms by walking can be accomplished only in the earliest stages of OAD, but the habit of regular walking should be considered "therapeutic" for the maintenance of function. Passive (Buerger's) positional exercises are of no value for the opening of collaterals.

**Vasodilators.** Oral vasodilators that increase arterial flow in the normal person are ineffective when blood flow is through collaterals, as in advanced OAD. Injected intra-arterially, such agents accelerate collateral formation, help in separating gangrene, and aid in revascularizing tissues. This is proved by the resumption of normal nail growth, which follows the initiation of intra-arterial therapy. Proper treatment, however, is cumbersome

**TABLE 11–1.** MANAGEMENT OF PATIENTS WITH OCCLUSIVE ARTERIAL DISEASES (OAD) AND NO TROPHIC CHANGES

INCREASE IN BLOOD FLOW

Exercise—walking, swimming, bicycling, etc.

Vasodilators—oral, parenteral, intravenous (ineffective in practice), intra-arterial

Avoidance of vasoconstriction—tobacco, cold, etc.

Sympathetic denervation—chemical blocking, regional blocks, lumbar sympathectomy, stellate ganglionectomy, reflex heating

Reduction of blood viscosity—Arvin

Transcutaneous vasoplastic procedures—Dotter, Gruentzig, Zeitler

Reconstructive surgical procedures—bypass (vein, umbilical cord, plastic materials); endarterectomy, grafts

DECREASE IN TISSUE DEMANDS FOR BLOOD

Foot care, skin care

Patient education—self-observation, healthy habits, protection from trauma, detection of incipient trouble; proper shoes, avoidance of heat

and requires three to four injections daily for one week and two to three per day for the ensuing several weeks. This requires hospitalization and close follow-up. That is why this form of therapy is not used much today; however, it may remain the only choice in desperate situations when surgical reconstruction is technically impossible. If a sufficiently small dose is chosen, systemic effects can be avoided. Substances proved reliable are papaverine hydrochloride, Priscoline, dihydroergocornine, and histamine. For proper technique use reference 2.

**Transcutaneous Transluminal Vasoplasty.** Dotter's procedure has proved to be safe and effective in selected cases defined by the authors.[3] The procedure requires intensifier screen guidance and a good arteriographic technique. Dotter's probes or Gruentzig's modified ones are used. Segmental occlusions can be re-opened. European investigators have demonstrated that long-term results, as well as the number of complications, are almost identical with those obtained after autogenous vein bypass procedures. Follow-up has been up to 8½ years.[4] The procedure can be carried out in forward or in retrograde fashion and involves no anesthesia or operating room. It costs less than bypass procedures. Back-up surgical facilities should be available, however, for the few complications that may occur during the procedure.

**Other Helps.** Purified Malayan Pit Viper venom administered by injection reduces circulating fibrinogen proteolytically, thereby increasing the fluidity of the blood (decreasing the viscosity), allegedly increasing peripheral tissue blood flow. I have no experience with this method, which is said to increase walking tolerance in ASO.[5]

Cessation of smoking and of other vasoconstrictor agents will often help a better flow to develop.

Use of surgical revascularization procedures is mandatory when possible, when the limb is an immediate danger to survival. However, they should not be used otherwise.

**Techniques to Reduce Tissue Demands for Blood.** Normal skin at an ambient temperature of 70 to 75° F needs 0.4 to 0.5 ml/100 g/min of blood to survive. Such small amounts are available to healthy cool skin even in the presence of advanced OAD. Skin heated to 104° F needs 11 ml/100 g/min. Skin inflamed from whatever cause needs 25 to 35 ml/100 g/min just to survive. For comparison, resting muscle needs 2 to 3 ml/100 g/min, vigorously contracting muscle needs 40 to 60 ml/100 g/min; ganglionic cells need 46 ml/100 g/min. The need to reduce the demand for blood in advanced OAD when vascular reserve is low mandates foot care. Heat must be avoided beyond the safe temperature of 92° F. Higher temperatures may be too "hot" for ischemic tissue. Mechanical injury must be avoided. Skin must stay pliable and should be greased every day; however, maceration must be avoided. The procedure is carried out by washing the foot, the area between the toes, and the heel and sole in lukewarm water for not more than a few minutes. The foot is dried and lanolin (or Eucerin, olive oil, mink oil) is applied between toes and around nails, soles, and heels and removed with a dry cloth after 20 to 30 minutes every night before retiring. Patients must learn to inspect their feet every day and to recognize danger signs (ingrowing or infested nails, infected calluses, red or hot spots, small ulcerations).

Proper shoes must be worn. Shoes should distribute body weight evenly over the sole, protect against injury, and prevent edema. A comfortable oxford shoe with strong medial counter fulfills this task for a normally shaped foot.

In the deformed foot of the arthritic patient or the neuropathic foot of the diabetic, selection of proper shoes can prevent skin breakdown (see Chapter 15). The foot in the diabetic is often deformed because of intrinsic muscle weakness, hammering of toes, and shifting of the fat pad under the metatarsophalangeal area, resulting in overloading of the ball of the foot.

**Shoes.** Because of the reduced resiliency of such a foot, the configuration of which changes in stance and swing phase, typical molded shoes (space shoes) should not be prescribed. Shoes to be used should contain a molded insole made of one of the newer plastics or of leather-latex, with a soft leather top and good medial support. Often, in severe deformity, such shoes must be fabricated individually by an expert shoemaker because mass-manufactured shoes are risky. In early stages, adjusted oxford shoes with Denver heels, metatarsal bars, or rocker bottoms are usable. Shoe prescription is a complicated art and requires close collaboration of physician and shoemaker. Deformed feet often change shape and shoes must be adjusted accordingly (Lippman and Farrar).

**Nail Care.** Nails are best cared for by a podiatrist. Subungual infections in dystrophic nails that are often fungus-infested should be drained by cutting a wedge-shaped piece into the nailplate.

Trimming of normal nails is usually done straight across; I believe, however, that corners which often harbor detritus and keratinized skin can be dug into. The shibboleth that nail will grow into corners thereafter is unsupported by long follow-up experience. Nails severely infested with fungus may occasionally require systemic treatment with griseofulvin. Toenails are the principal troublemakers in advanced OAD and must be given careful sustained attention.

**Treatment of Trophic Lesions.** When trophic lesions (fissures, ulcerations, abscesses, osteomyelitis, phlegmones, necrosis, gangrene) develop in advanced OAD the questions always arise as to when conservative therapy is justified and when surgical intervention is indicated. Most abscesses or phlegmones necessitate surgical intervention. An exceptional situation may arise if conservative measures ensure adequate drainage, e.g., when a loose callus is unroofed and an abscess opens widely, or when a wide wedge in a toenail provides adequate drainage for pus from a subungual abscess.

The radical attitude of former generations of health workers in the presence of local gangrene must be revised. Gangrenous toes or more proximal necrotic lesions that show even minimal tendency to demarcate call for patience in treatment and for use of all available measures that will enhance separation from viable tissue. In toe gangrene this may sometimes take several months, while the patient continues to be ambulatory. Development of local edema is a contraindication. It sets the stage for the extension of gangrene and for the development of infection and for lymphangitic spread: the dreaded "wet" gangrene threatens; in such case the patient must stay off his feet.

**Heels.** Special attention is to be paid to heel protection overnight or for patients forced to bed in day time. The Foot cradle,* the Spanco Protector,† and the Span-Aid‡ are effective. The traditional sheepskin posey is inadequate.

An unusual situation may arise with the appearance of an arteriolosclerotic lateral leg ulcer that is painful and has little tendency to heal. The use of collagenase ointment, which in this case works as an anti-inflammatory agent, can accelerate healing.

The osteomyelitic changes in the foot of a diabetic that may lead to Charcot's foot rarely require emergency measures. They may seal off by themselves or slowly sequestrate out, especially if they involve a toe end or middle phalanx of a bunion or a malleolus. A sinogram may trace the involved bone. A slow drip with Elase or with a specific antibiotic-saline solution through a small catheter may then facilitate cleaning the area and separating the dead bone. Patience and close observation for spreading are needed to justify conservative management. In "kissing" toe ulcers in an ambulatory patient that may involve a middle phalanx, it may take months for the dead bone to sequester out. Good judgment is imperative in timing the removal of sequesters, guided by the expectation that natural sequestration is near complete. Conservative intervention then is limited to aiding the separation of attached tendon or other soft tissue remnants with strict avoidance of traumatizing viable tissue. The same is true for the ablation of gangrenous phalanges, a toe, several toes, or occasionally the whole forefoot.

---

*Med. Plastics Laboratory, Gatesville, TX 75828.
†P.O. Box 32, Brookfield, IL 60513.
‡Span-America, Inc., Box 5231, Greenville, SC 29606.

Collagenase ointment, if applied sparingly to avoid skin maceration, exerts an anti-inflammatory effect that becomes apparent after four to five days of use. Therefore, it may be useful for the treatment of any trophic lesion. By reducing the inflammatory response it may lead to an adequate blood supply in the presence of reduced vascular reserve.[6]

Antibiotics are given systematically; local antibiotics do not reach infected tissues and may cause sensitizing effects or bacterial resistance.

Whenever trophic lesions spread or when signs of healing or demarcation, no matter how subtle or slow, are not clearly evident, surgical help is needed. This often applies to a patient who cannot be permitted to ambulate because of uncontrollable leg or foot edema. Such situations imply an immediate danger of loss of limb. Surgical intervention in chronic OAD for any reason other than salvaging the limb, in my opinion, is not acceptable.

Necessary surgical intervention, however, should not be delayed. Unnecessary bed rest, pain, and the administration of analgesics and narcotics drain the patient of courage, health, and money, and may turn out to be less conservative than surgery. Prolonged indigency in bed with all its deleterious effects is weighed initially against the expected duration of recovery by conservative management. Changing treatment in view of changing developments (diabetic control, fluctuations of the cardiac status, onset or subsidence of renal complications, changes in bacterial resistance) is part of the management of often uncertain and unpredictable situations that call for clinical judgment and experience.

## REFERENCES

Lippmann, H. I. and Farrar, R.: Prevention of amputation in diabetics. Angiology, 30:649, 1979.

Lippmann, H. I.: Intraarterial Priscoline therapy for peripheral vascular disturbances. Angiology 3:69, 1952.

Dotter, C. T. and Judkins, M. P.: Percutaneous transluminal treatment of arteriosclerotic obstruction. Radiology 84:631, 1965 and Dotter, C. T. et al: J.A.M.A. 230:117, 1974.

Schmidtke, I., Zeitler, E. and Schoop, W.: Late results (5–8 years) of transluminal dilatation-recanalization (Dotter's technique) in femoropopliteal occlusions of stage II. Vasa 7:4, 1978 and Denk et al.: Vasa 7:16, 1978.

Ehrly, A. M. and Koehler, H. J.: Modifiziertes Dosisschema fuer die subcutane Anwendung von Arwin bei Patienten mit chronischen arteriellen Durchblutungsstoerungen. Vasa 5:155, 1976.

Lippmann, H. I.: Medical management of "trophic" ulcers in chronic arterial occlusive disease. Angiology 29:683, 1979.

# Disabling Diseases of the Venous System

## VARICOSE VEINS

Varicose veins have stimulated the inventiveness of creative surgeons since time immemorial. With the inheritance of a leaking valve at the saphenofemoral junction, one distal valve after another follows suit, including those of the perforators. This leads to unsightly legs with minimal symptoms. The inevitable accumulation of blood during dependency, however, may cause heaviness but no functional impairment. Impaired cosmesis with extensive varicosities may in some individuals become a source of psychogenic disability, justifying removal of the offending varices. If complaints include "excruciating" pain at the site of a varix, another cause should be looked for (radiculopathy, bursitis, bone pathology, arthritis), or else the suffering may be psychogenic. Neither sclerotherapy, stripping, nor surgical removal, all of which leave visible scars, discoloration, or are followed by recurrences, will satisfy the patient in search of cosmetic perfection. Therefore, knowledge of the patient's personality is often crucial in advising appropriate treatment.

Uncomplicated varicose veins do not cause physical disability. Superficial thrombophlebitis is a fairly common complication in extensive varicosis of the greater saphena. Pulmonary embolism is a rare complication that may occur when the greater saphena is inflamed near the foramen ovale and a thrombus protrudes into the femoral vein. I refer a patient to a vascular surgeon for a high saphenous vein ligation if a thrombus can be palpated $2\frac{1}{2}$ inches distally or less from the fossa ovalis.

Superficial thrombophlebitis requires no bed rest or anticoagulants; occasionally, simple analgesics (acetaminophen or salicylates) are needed; the common use of such anti-inflammatory drugs as phenylbutazone should be discouraged, since clot adherence to the vein intima is desirable. Antibiotics are needed only in the case of infected thrombophlebitis, a form of sepsis.

# DEEP VEIN THROMBOSIS (DVT)

This condition and associated pulmonary embolism represent a major health problem causing more than 60,000 yearly deaths in the United States, and afflicting an unknown additional number of survivors. DVT is common in all surgical procedures, in normal childbirth, and in a variety of acute and chronic diseases. The presence of DVT is often missed on clinical examination without the aid of more sophisticated instrumental methods.

# CHRONIC VENOUS INSUFFICIENCY (CVI)

CVI is a prime cause of invalidism; it does not shorten life expectancy in contrast to ASO, in which coronary artery disease takes its toll. It has not received the attention it deserves by the health care professions or the national census. It probably affects more than 4 million people in the United States and ranks second only to arthritis as cause of disability.

CVI is defined as damage to skin, subcutis and deep tissues, mostly of the lower extremities, resulting from an increase in local venous pressure. It interferes with normal walking because of cellulitis and periphlebitis, which develop as a result of a combination of edema and mechanical injury. An etiologic association with bacterial invasion or fungous infestation is also conjectured. Edema, without which CVI neither develops nor progresses, may have manifold causes (Table 11–2). It may present without primary venous disease. Prolonged leg dependency or any morbid condition that interferes with the leg muscle pump may cause it. Valvular insufficiency in perforators secondary to DVT, or rarely extensive varicosis, may predispose to CVI. The patient in congestive cardiac failure is less subject to CVI in spite of elevated peripheral venous pressures, perhaps because he is less exposed to trauma.

The visible or palpable manifestations of CVI are edema, induration, discoloration, fibrosis, sclerosis, patchy or confluent subcutaneous ossification,[1] ulcerations, and dermatitis ("venous" eczema or "stasis dermatitis"). CVI is often misdiagnosed as active DVT, whereas in fact it involves fat and other periphlebic tissues. Remissions and exacerbations are common, depending on the degree of recurrent edema or trauma.

## MANAGEMENT

Edema control is the paramount goal in the management of CVI and in the treatment of venous leg ulcers. Edema is difficult to control in the presence of subcutaneous ossification, and ulcerations recur easily. In some cases they do not heal until the underlying subcutaneous bone has been removed and the defect covered with a skin graft.

Apart from diuretics, which are of limited value, edema control is based on creating pressure gradients that enhance reabsorption of tissue fluid into venous and lymphatic channels in the Frank-Starling equilibrium process. Traditionally this has been accomplished by rest and leg elevation, by elastic or nonelastic compression, or by pumps. Of these approaches the ones compatible with normal daily activities are those provided for by elastic or nonelastic compression.

**TABLE 11–2.** COMMON CONDITIONS CAUSING CHRONIC VENOUS INSUFFICIENCY

| DISEASE | ADDITIONAL FACTORS | | |
|---|---|---|---|
| Varicose veins (greater saphenous system) | ? A-V fistulas (Piulachs) | | Edema |
| Varicose veins (greater saphenous system) | Trauma | | Edema |
| Deep venous valvular insufficiency | Trauma (occas.) | | Edema—Infection (occas.) |
| Deep vein obstruction or compression | | | Edema—Infection (occas.) |
| No disease—dependency | Trauma | | Edema |
| Congestive heart failure | Trauma | | Edema |
| Poliomyelitis<br>Stroke<br>Neuropathy<br><br>Arthritis (knee, ankle)<br>Rheumatoid arthritis<br>Systemic lupus erythematosus | Muscle weakness<br>Immobility<br>Dependency | | Edema |
| Sickle cell disease | Local venule obstruction | trauma (occas.) | Edema—Infection (occas.) |

By far the most effective and least incapacitating method is the application of the nonelastic Unna's boot (described in 1885).* It consists of a non-stretchable, pliable, porous, stickable, nonsensitizing mold applied with even pressure along the involved leg, from toe base to just below the knee. Normal ankle movements, regardless of whether active or passive or up or down, cause shifts in segmental leg volumes. When the leg is harnessed in the nonstretchable envelope of the boot, volume changes are converted into pressure changes instantaneously as in a pump across the leg circumference, most in distal and least in proximal segments. The degree of compression depends on the force and actual range of the ankle movement. In the "neutral" position (at which the bandage is applied) compression values immediately return to base, even during fast transition from dorisflexion to plantar flexion and vice versa. Isometric muscle contraction in any position is ineffective. The boot therefore functions similarly to the muscle fascia, which converts muscular contractions into a compartmental pump. The "ankle pump" set up by the boot is mediated by compressive and by shearing forces.[2] Similar joint pumps can be created by applying Unna's boots to other accessible joints, e.g., the knee in below-knee amputations or the finger-knuckle-wrist-elbow in postmastectomy lymphedema.

The technique of applying an Unna's boot requires special training and continued practice. The physician accustomed to handling plaster will have to unlearn these techniques before learning de novo. The bandage is not manually directed in any but a straight line. It is cut and not folded if a change in direction is desired, lest an undesirable tourniquet effect result. The bandage does not shrink with the leg. A new boot must take up the slack; three or four such bandages usually suffice to reduce any leg volume to a minimum. We change the bandage each one to six weeks for expediency's sake. (It could well be changed every day, since in an ambulating individual maximum shrinkage takes place after a few hours.) The Unna's boot is applied in direct contact with an ulcer. Interposing any material would interfere with obtaining the proper pressure gradients. Simple calculation establishes that interference with compression by a 1.3 mm stretch without increase in resistance around the ankle circumference in an average adult would reduce the pumping effect of the ankle movement by reversing pressure into volume change. The usefulness of the boot depends on the patient's cooperation in walking; it is useless if the ankle is ankylosed. Ankle excursions of ±5 degrees suffice for setting up the pump.

Gelatin, which gives the boot its consistence, is water-soluble. In summer, or when the patient tends to perspire, an Ace bandage cover helps to absorb fluid. The Elastoplast cover that some physicians prefer creates a wet-chamber effect that causes skin maceration, which in some cases expedites epithelialization but enhances development of infection. Normally, a Surgitube (tube gauze) No. 3 cover suffices.

The Unna's boot is indicated solely for edema control. It is contraindicated in several situations, including wetting dermatitis, which calls for moist saline or aluminum acetate dressings. It should not be used in severe contact dermatitis or fungous infestation or in the arteriolosclerotic ulcer of hypertension or diabetes, which is located anterolaterally in the leg, over the tips of the toes or the back of the heel. Also contraindicated is use in ischemic lesions without edema and in the presence of extensive cellulitis (e.g., in erysipelas).

While bacterial cultures will grow from almost any leg ulcer, a distinction between contamination and infection is essential. In a contaminated ulcer the adjacent tissues are not invaded, and good granulation will control bacterial growth. In infection, specific systemic antibiotics are given before or during boot treatment. Local antibiotics are avoided because of the danger of skin sensitization, which in the presence of ASO may result in necrosis and loss of limb.

Scabs should be removed gently (with the aid of mineral oil) and necrotic tissue should be removed only after spontaneous separation is adequately advanced. The leg is washed with tincture of green soap, particularly between Unna's boot applications.

Local cleansing of the ulceration can be expedited by cleansing agents (Debrisan) or chemical debriders (collagenase ointment). Both aid in obtaining a well-granulating base and stimulate epithelialization to some extent. Debrisan is useful in cleansing and drying an ulcer, but if tight necrotic sloughs are present, thinly applied collagenase ointment becomes the best choice. Other chemical debriders such as Ananase and Ribonuclease-varidase aid in cleaning fibrinous sloughs. Topical treatment of any kind is discontinued with Unna's boot compression treatment.

The ubiquitous uncritical use of cleansing agents on any ulcer and the rationale that enthusiastic uncontrolled reports has advanced must be viewed with caution. A variety of local treatments has been proposed at one time or another, from powdered sugar, gold leaf, gelfoam-serum mixture, powdered blood cells, and honey to Debrisan. This indicates that empiricism rules the subject of leg ulcer therapy. Under these circumstances the choice of an appropriate form of management must take into account the patient's total problems, of which CVI and leg ulceration can only be part. Thus,

---

*A roller bandage impregnated with a combination of water, glycerin, gelatin, and zinc oxide.

from the points of view of comfort and cost efficiency, a three-month healing period with two Unna's boot applications a month to a patient who continues to work through this period might be more acceptable than an 18-day course with Debrisan in a hospital bed.

Occasionally, when a leg perspires excessively, the glue in the Unna's boot will dissolve, no matter what is done to prevent this. A dry compression bandage must then be substituted. It is applied over a thin layer of cotton gauze over the ulcer and a three- to four-inch roller bandage is snugly applied over it with an Ace bandage and criss-cross adhesive covered to stay in place. The roller bandage provides the nonelastic cover that sets up the pump effect, albeit at considerably less efficiency than the Unna's boot. It compares in effect with an Elastoplast bandage without the latter's hazard in causing skin maceration.

Ulcer healing proceeds in three noninterrelated visible steps: granulation, epithelialization, and contraction. Edema, which is controlled with Unna's boots, seems to interfere principally with epithelialization. Some observers believe that the zinc content of the boot contributes to healing. The rate of healing under an Unna's boot depends on size and location of the ulcer, the technique of application, and the patient's cooperation in walking. The larger the ulcer, the more proximal its location, and the less vigorous the patient's walking, the longer it will take for the ulcer to heal.

The patient's general condition has relatively little impact on the healing of a venous ulcer under an Unna's boot. The presence of OAD, diabetes, sickle cell disease, and collagen disorders does not delay healing. Extensive subcutaneous ossification or simultaneous steroid therapy may retard it. Skin or muscle grafting may acclerate healing, but the associated forced rest makes such a gain in time often illusory, while with Unna's boot treatment activities can continue.

After the venous ulcer is healed, edema control is needed to prevent recurrences. Self-application of a nonelastic mold is well-nigh impossible; an elastic cover of sufficient strength is an adequate compromise. In severely indurated legs, a one-way stretch, woven to measure, heel-covered, cotton and elastic, heavy or medium heavy seamless stocking of garter length (below the knee) is needed. Measurements are best taken when the leg is edema-free, immediately after removal of the boot. Help is often needed by aged patients to apply these tough stockings. Elasticity is usually lost after four to eight months of wear. Another stocking must then be made after measurements are taken.

Recurrences of venous ulcers are most unusual under this regimen. Groups evaluating compensation claims and insurance companies often have difficulties in grasping the need for the continued leg compression in CVI that safeguards the patient from suffering another relapse into painful and costly temporary disability. The reward of such a patient's continued fitness makes the exasperating struggles against penny wise–pound foolish policies worthwhile.

Occasionally, in less indurated legs, or indeed in conditions like varicosities when counterpressures needed do not exceed hydrostatic pressure, two-way stretch stockings will do. In milder cases of CVI a SigVaris stocking of garter length is acceptable, while in even less involved cases, a Parke-Davis or Bauer & Black stocking is effective. Hose made of less resistant material (Supphose, Jobst stockings) we find of no value.

## REFERENCES

Lippmann, H. I. and Goldin, R. R.: Subcutaneous ossification of the legs in chronic venous insufficiency. Radiology 74:279, 1960.

Lippmann, H. I. and Brière, J-P.: Physical basis of external supports in chronic venous insufficiency. Arch. Phys. Med. Rehabil. 52:555, 1971 and Arch. Phys. Med. Rehabil. 56:224, 1975.

# Functional Vascular Diseases

## VASOSPASTIC DISEASE

An arterial spasm is an abnormal event that may close a structurally normal artery. Vasoconstriction is the physiologic mechanism operative in the distribution of blood and in the regulation of body temperature. It is governed by sympathetic activity. It reduces but does not stop blood flow, unless the vascular lumen is narrowed by disease. In vasospasm, as Lewis has demonstrated, the fault lies in the arterial wall. Recent work revealed ultrastructural alterations in digital capillaries that may be secondary, as well as in glomus bodies through which 80 per cent of all digital blood flows. The latter changes may represent the primary lesion in Raynaud's attacks.[1]

In clinical practice, spastic occlusion is observed in three situations: in Raynaud's attacks, in embolic arterial occlusion, on which arterial spasm may be superimposed, and in trauma consisting of high-energy vibration, caused by one of many occupational tools or by projectiles penetrating a member at high velocity in the vicinity of a major or middle-sized artery.

**Raynaud's attacks (Raynaud's phenomenon, Raynaud's disease, Primary and Secondary Attacks).** Raynaud in his original report described digital discoloration and gangrene, which he considered one disease of a malfunctioning vasomotor center causing vasoconstriction. His view might have been inspired by Claude Bernard's exciting discoveries of the functions of a vasomotor center. Today we know that Raynaud's attacks may present in various diseases with diverse prognostic implications. The clinician who encounters an individual with Raynaud's attacks must search for an underlying condition.

Raynaud's attacks may involve any protruding body part, nose, ears, penis, breasts, and any one of all four extremities. Mostly, however, its appearance is limited to the digits of hand and foot. It is usually elicited by exposure to cold but may in some cases start with excitement or psychologically unsettling experiences. Immersing a hand in cold water, taking a dip in a cool pool, or going outdoors in winter are the most common immediate causes of an attack. Ice-cold water elicits a different response.

The attack, regardless of etiology, begins at the fingertip. This blanches, shutting off all blood flow; puncturing a blanched finger will produce no blood. The attack may start with a livid-blue discoloration representing trapping of some blood; puncturing such a finger produces only a drop of blood. The blanching progresses proximally to the finger base. If the blood is squeezed out, the blanching process is accelerated. A pale gray color may follow and indicates that stagnating blood has given up oxygen, and the color becomes waxen. All this may be asymptomatic. When a digit is deprived of blood for 30 minutes or so it will become numb, finally calling the patient's attention to the attack. With recovery, after warming of body or hand, the digit reddens from the base distally and a border cyanotic region can be discerned when blood stagnates. Redness may then alternate with cyanosis before reactive hyperemia pervades the whole digit. After the attack, digital circulation reverts to normal, and arteries subject to spastic occlusion studied histologically by light microscopy appear normal.

PRIMARY RAYNAUD'S ATTACKS (RAYNAUD'S DISEASE). Such attacks may present symmetrically in all digits with or without thumb participation in youngsters around puberty, with a female-to-male preponderance at 10:1. The attacks are precipitated by exposure to cold; in severe cases a slight cooling

of the body or a hand may bring on an attack even in summer. Trophic changes are generally not observed in this benign form. The toes may be involved in winter. Infrequently, blanching involves the whole hand or foot. Evolution and resolution of a typical attack follow the description given earlier. The attacks cease usually after a few years or in middle age, possibly correlating with the concomitant increase in systemic blood pressure. The attacks are termed a "primary disease" because the etiology is unknown and no underlying disease has as yet been discovered.

Raynaud's disease can often be controlled by keeping body or extremity warm, by a high-vitamin diet, by some oral vasodilators, by oral reserpine 0.1 or 0.25 mg twice or three times a day, or by intra-arterial injection of tolazoline or reserpine in this order of increasing effectiveness. Biofeedback methods that enable the patient to increase body temperature may in some cases prevent the onset of an attack. Spontaneous subsidence often precedes iatrogenic relief.

SECONDARY RAYNAUD'S ATTACKS (RAYNAUD'S PHENOMENA). The denomination "secondary" is given vasospastic episodes that occur symptomatically in various conditions that differ widely in severity and prognostic implication. Secondary attacks occur more frequently in males and include pathogenetically different forms of vasospastic occlusion. They are encountered most often in trauma, occlusive arterial disease, collagen disease, cold agglutinins, thoracic outlet syndromes, cryoproteinemia, cold injury, hypothyroidism, and the toxic effect of beta blockers, as well as conditions of unclear etiology. Conditions causally related and mentioned in the literature but seldom seen are thromboangiitis obliterans (Buerger) and ergot poisoning.

Vibrating tools are used in a number of occupations. The high-energy vibration developed by pneumatic hammers, chain saws, swaging tools (which bend metals), tools for caulking (used in boiler making), and others, predispose to Raynaud's attacks after some use. Powerful shaking seems to interfere with the contractile mechanism of smooth muscle rather than with the chemistry of muscle activity. Longitudinal vibration reduces the twitch force of smooth muscle while blood flow and energy consumption are being maintained unchanged, thus suggesting interference with the cross-linking of actin and myosin. A compensatory hypertrophy of the artery media is said to result; this makes the vessel prone to close.

Disabling high-powered vibration presents problems with workmen's compensation. Objective tests for evaluation include measuring finger circumference, and digital vibrotactile threshold, assessing thresholds for hot and cold in digits, and looking for osteoporosis in terminal phalanges and for bony cysts in hands. Also used are depth anesthesiometry, two-point discrimination, and thermography. The patient's history is given great importance. Compensation awards depend on. the condition of involved digits and on job interference. Work load and exposure time to vibration usually correlate with the severity of the digital blanching (vibration-induced white finger syndrome or VWS). A worker with established VWS must be taken off the job and must find another occupation. None of the drugs used in Raynaud's attacks helps to overcome the noxious effects of vibration.

Digital arteries narrowed by intimal thickening in occlusive arterial disease (OAD) may temporarily close upon normal vasocontrictor response to cold, excitement, pain, or anger. This mechanism is suspected when one or several digits blanche without symmetric involvement of both hands.

A positive Allen test 2 corroborates the diagnosis. It is performed by a three-minute compression of both radial and ulnar arteries at wrist level. Sudden release is followed within nine seconds by full reactive hyperemia of the hand in normal ambient temperature. Any delay pinpoints the site of an occlusion or narrowing. In the corresponding test in the foot (Lewis-Pickering test) a calf cuff is inflated at suprasystolic level for five minutes and released suddenly. In the normal individual, a reactive hyperemia is complete within 12 seconds.

Additional tests available to the specialist include plethysmography, arteriography, fluorescein studies, and ultrasonic Doppler effect in toes, requiring special small digital cuffs and radionuclear clearance studies. All of these can indicate the site of abnormal arterial narrowing with greater precision.

Collagen disorders may be heralded by Raynaud's attacks before presenting other clinical problems. This is true for scleroderma, systemic lupus erythematosus (SLE), and arteritic processes such as periarteritis nodosa). When fingers blanche without exposure to cold in a young person, a collagen disorder must be suspected. Skin alterations in fingers, forearms, chest, and lower extremities are looked for, esophageal changes are explored by x-ray examination, antinuclear antibodies are searched for, renal function is studied, and the patient is followed regularly. Steroid treatment may have to be initiated and skin hygiene is enforced.

Raynaud's attacks, especially in sclerodactyly and in SLE, often result in trophic damage (necrosis of fingertips and shafts). In scleroderma painful small ulcerations may develop at the site of breakthrough of calcific concretions. They usually heal with a scar. Paronychial infections are common and painful. Roentgenographic films may disclose soft-tissue calcification in the digits of hands or feet. Frequent washings of hands and feet with Betadine soap minimizes the development of the infections, and greasing of the skin with water-soluble fats (mink oil, lanolin, olive oil, Eucerin) adds to the protection. Careful handling of mechanical tasks and protection with gloves are mandatory in these cases.

Thoracic outlet syndromes (see p. 210) are frequently associated with Raynaud's attacks. Subclavian artery stenosis causes a drop in distal arterial pressure that may be reduced to the level of the tone of the arterial wall, which equals the arterial closing pressure. In addition, microembolism from diseased subclavian intima has been cited in accounting for digital artery occlusion. This is an attractive hypothesis because long-term anticoagulation has in some cases reduced the incidence of Raynaud's attacks in thoracic outlet syndromes. Diagnostic tests for thoracic outlet syndromes are described on page 210.

A diagnostic survey in a patient presenting with a history of Raynaud's attacks will gather all pertinent data on age, sex, medications (including drugs containing ergot derivatives and beta blockers, which may precipitate or aggravate spastic arterial closure), occupation and length of exposure on the job, onset, frequency and duration of attacks, and possible eliciting events. Digital pulses and prevailing pressures should be assessed by the Allen test 2 and the Lewis-Pickering test for hand and foot, respectively. Laboratory tests include a complete blood count, red cell sedimentation rate, Fluorescent Antinuclear Antibody reaction, cryoproteins, cold agglutinins, x-ray of the involved member, chest film, blood fibrinogen, and electrophoresis. Special investigations available to the specialist include arteriograms, digital plethysmograms, provocative tests after heat and cold exposure, thermograms, functional oscillometry during Adson and other outlet maneuvers, pulsewave studies, and others.

**Management.** Protection from cold and oral vasodilators are of value in Raynaud's disease but of little help in secondary Raynaud's attacks. Beta-blockers are contraindicated and use of oral or systemic vasodilators is based on questionable rationale; if effective, they would cause an undesirable shift of blood from high-toned vessels into normal vessels in which peripheral resistance would be reduced. In practice, oral vasodilators lack this effect in secondary Raynaud's attacks and are at best innocuous.

An unorthodox reasonable therapeutic approach is the subcutaneous administration of the purified venom of the Malayan pit viper, which reduces blood viscosity by proteolytic fibrinogen reduction and an apparent decrease of red blood cell aggregation. Good results in pain relief and healing of vasospastic digital necrosis are claimed.[2] We have as yet no experience with this method. Nitroglycerine-containing ointment (Nitrol ointment) may protect the digits from attacks. Some drugs seem to prevent Raynaud's attacks; they all enhance vaso-dilatation in response to warmth. This is true for methyldopa (1.5 gm/day for several weeks), prazo-sin (1 mg/day for 7 to 10 days), guanethidine (10 mg/day), reserpine (0.25 twice or three times a day after an initial period with 0.1 mg/day), tola-zoline (5 to 7.5 mg intra-arterially once a day for 1 week) or reserpine hydrochloride (0.05 mg intra-arterially once every 4 to 12 weeks) in this order of increasing effectiveness. Each one these medica-tions may produce undesirable effects. The patient with an attack in outside cold who enters a warm room will have warm fingers in a few minutes if treated, after more than 30 minutes if untreated. Recently, biofeedback methods have been used successfully; they require long training periods. The treatment is aimed at enabling the patient to control body temperature; the resting patient must learn how to raise his body temperature 2.8° F above baseline by concentrated thinking.

**Secondary Arterial Spasm.** Emboli tend to lodge at arterial bifurcations and often elicit a proximal, distal, and collateral intense spasm that adds to the ischemia. Sympathetic blockade or intra-arterial di-lators are rarely helpful; surgical intervention is called for. The same is true for post-traumatic va-sospasm induced by fractures or by projectiles. It is unwise to wait for spontaneous subsiding of the spasm that can be expected, since ischemic damage may then be irreparable. Thus, after a shotgun wound in the arm followed by ischemia of the hand, a differential diagnosis of arterial spasm or compression by hematoma can most safely be made by surgical exposure of the artery.

An arterial spasm was occasionally observed when a catheter made of nylon was made indwell-ing into the femoral artery during a course of intra-arterial dilator therapy. The spasm subsided shortly after catheter removal. Injection of vasoactive sub-stances such as norepinephrine does not produce arterial spasm in my experience, but I have seen addicts with severe ischemic damage after acciden-tal injection of narcotics into an artery.

## ABNORMAL VASOCONSTRICTION

Acrocyanosis is a persistent blue discoloration of a cold hand, sometimes extending to the forearm, usually in young women. The hand will become red if exposed to icy or to warm temperatures; palms often perspire. The coldness suggests a high arteriolar tone. While the condition is cosmetically disturbing, it is asymptomatic except for an occa-sional swelling of the hands. One investigator sug-gested that the arterioles in this condition were sensitive to cold, and they constricted while the cu-taneous capillary network remained open.

Treatment is unrewarding, but keeping body and hands warm helps. Iontophoresis with dilators occasionally works. Sympathetic ganglionectomy, claimed to be a remedy, is usually ineffective.

**Livedo Reticularis (Cutis Marmorata, Livedo Annularis).** This is reticular mottling of the skin with bluish-red color involving the skin in legs and forearms and occasionally upper arms, thighs, and trunk. It is caused by constriction or occlusion of the peripheral portions of the arborizing arterioles piercing the cutis. The discoloration becomes visi-ble in the lax peripheral capillary arborizations in which blood is slowed down and hemoglobin is re-duced. Exposure to cold accentuates it.

The condition is idiopathic and symptomatic, with the prognosis varying according to the under-lying disease. The closure may be functional and temporary or organic and permanent. It may be caused, in the latter category, by arteritides (periar-teriitis nodosa) or by compression as in the bacter-emic phase of meningococcal meningitis or in peri-arteriolar leukemic infiltration. Occasionally, even in the usually benign idiopathic form, leg ulcera-tions may be associated. They are painful and slow in healing. Lumbar sympathectomy has accelerated healing in several cases known to me. In the ma-jority of cases livedo reticularis remains a cosmetic problem that can be temporarily controlled by warming of the body, by lumbar or peripheral sympathetic blocking with procaine, or by oral treatment with alpha-adrenergic blocking agents. Oral vasodilators are usually of no help. Biofeed-back methods, with which I have no experience, may be worth a trial.

## COLD DAMAGE

*Cold hypersensitivity* may be manifested in urti-caria of body parts exposed to cold, associated oc-casionally with facial flush, tachycardia, and a drop in systemic blood pressure. Whether or not this ab-normal reaction can be considered truly allergic is uncertain; intradermal serum injection can occa-sionally transfer hypersensitivity to another per-son. An individual unaware of cold sensitivity may plunge into danger by diving into a swimming pool; drowning has been reported in such cases. Body parts touching a cold object may itch and a wheal may be formed. A cold shower may result in shock. Eating ice cream or drinking ice water may be followed by hives, nausea, and vomiting.

Treatment is not too effective. One might expect some tolerance to develop upon exposure to grad-ually lowered temperature. Injections of small amounts of histamine hydrochloride (0.1 ml of a 1:1000 solution biw, gradually increasing to 1.0 ml) or Benadryl (50 mg or 25 mg three times a day) have been tried with some success. Use of steroids is not recommended for this purpose.

*Frostbite* is produced by exposure of body parts to temperatures of 28.4 to 32° F (−2 to 0° C), the true range in which skin removed from the body would freeze. Living skin freezes at a somewhat lower temperature 14 to 24.8° F (−10 to −4° C) because of a "supercooling" effect that prevents the formation of ice crystals immediately below the freezing point of water. Some climatic factors may aggravate frost damage to the skin. Wind dissipates a layer of radiant warmth surrounding the body surface; blood stasis reduces the resistance to local frost damage, as does a lowered oxygen tissue tension, occlusive arterial disease, or Raynaud's attacks.

Frostbite can be classified in four stages.[3] The first degree consists of white or yellow skin discoloration that may be associated with numbness or paresthesias, such as of the cheek. Upon return to a warm environment full recovery is the rule, but the exposed area may remain sensitive to cold for periods from days to years. The second degree produces blistering and skin peeling, involving superficial cutaneous layers. Tissue becomes indurated and digits grow stiff. On thawing, a painful reactive hyperemia spreads from the periphery of the exposed area to its center. Blisters may dry out and peel off, with normal skin forming the base. In third degree frostbite, deep tissues may be involved; digits or parts of limbs may be lost. In fourth degree frostbite gangrene of digits or extremities may result in massive limb loss after demarcation. In all stages cold sensitivity outlasts the frostbite episode for long periods.

Prevention by wearing warm clothing and insulated shoes is obviously the best form of management. If true freezing with the formation of ice crystals has taken place, cellular membranes have been destroyed and thawing must proceed slowly, best at room temperature without the application of external heat in any form. Friction (as with snow) should be avoided to prevent destruction by shearing stresses. Measures to protect the involved skin against bacterial invasion should be taken early, such as moist Betadine dressings.

*Trench foot* and *immersion foot* are complicated forms of frostbite, of special pertinence to war conditions, when soldiers or sailors are exposed to cold and moisture for long periods without being able to change clothes or shoes. Skin maceration, necrosis, and infection are complications and may cause long-term damage.[3]

*Acute pernio (acute chilblains)* is encountered in the damp and cold northern United States in fall and winter. It symmetrically involves inadequately protected legs. The exposed skin is red, cyanotic, edematous, and covered with small blebs or purpuric spots. Burning and itching are aggravated by rubbing or heat application. Contact dermatitis must be ruled out.

Treatment includes protection against repeat exposure to cold. Scratching is avoided. No application of heat beyond 85° F (29.4° C) is permitted. Blebs are treated sterilely; ointments are not used. Repeat exposure may result in chronic pernio, a disabling condition.

*Chronic pernio (chronic chilblains, erythrocyanosis)* is not uncommon among susceptible young women living in cold climates and venturing into the cold without leg protection. The nature of susceptibility is not known. The lesion is an ugly, indurated, erythematous, painful, occasionally hemorrhagic area that may ulcerate in winter and close in spring or early summer. During fall, small indurated lesions may appear over the legs. When the disease has been present for years, ulcerations may fail to heal during the warm season and ambulation is severely curtailed because of pain and ulceration—a truly incapacitating condition. Vasoconstriction may involve the whole extremity, leading to coldness and cyanosis. Pathologically, periarterial round cell infiltration and angiitis may be present, the panniculus adiposus may atrophy, and subcutaneous giant cell inflammation may be present. Vasospasm, vasoconstriction, and intimal damage may be part of the pathogenesis. At the site of healed lesions, brown discoloration is quite characteristic.

The differential diagnosis includes erythema induratum, which occasionally hides cutaneous tuberculosis, and which presents with more nodular and deeper ulcerations. It resembles erythema nodosum, which often presents with sarcoidosis. Arthralgias and nodular vasculitis accompanying periarteritis must also be ruled out.

Again, proper protection against the cold is the best form of management. No specific therapy exists for chronic pernio. Symptomatically, pain relief may require strong analgesia; broad-spectrum antibiotics may have to be given systemically. In case of complicating lower extremity edema, compression with Unna's boot may be required. In the rare case of a grossly contaminated and draining ulcer, Debrisan is useful. Topical medication is useless. Sensitizing substances should be avoided as topical medication. Silver sulfadiazine cream can be useful; skin sensitization is exceedingly rare but should be watched for.

## REFERENCES

Burch, G. E., Harb, J. M. and Sun, C. S.: Fine structure of digital vascular lesions in Raynaud's phenomenon and disease. Angiology 30:361, 1979.

Ehrly, A. M.: Treatment of patients with secondary Raynaud's syndrome. In Gjores, J. E. and Thulesius, O. (eds.): Primary and Secondary Raynaud phenomena. Acta Chir. Scand. Suppl. 465, pp. 92–5, 1975.

Wright, I. S.: Vascular Diseases in clinical practice. Chicago, Year Book Medical Publishers, 1948.

# Thoracic Outlet Syndromes

Thoracic outlet syndromes are caused by compression of the neurovascular bundle (brachial plexus and subclavian vessels), which on its way to the upper extremity traverses three areas of potential narrowing. Local compressive damage to the bundle may cause alterations of vascular or neurologic nature to the upper extremity.

## ANATOMY (Fig. 11–5)

The brachial plexus contains the intertwining and ramifying axons coming down via the cervical roots 4, 5, 6, 7, and 8 and thoracic root 1. Together with the subclavian artery it passes between the anterior and middle scalenus muscles that form the roof of a narrow space, with the first rib and the pleura forming the base. During deep inhalation the pleura rises and further restricts the space. The subclavian artery lies in close approximation to the anterior scalenus muscle. The artery and its tendinous attachment to the first rib and the lowermost segments of the plexus, that is, fibers derived from C7 and 8 as well as T1, are most exposed to compression damage. At this level, the subclavian vein passes outside the space, between first rib and clavicle.

Somewhat more distally, the bundle and the subclavian vessels, after exiting the thoracic cavity, are vulnerable to compression between first rib and clavicle.

At the third potential compression site, when the neural bundle and the subclavian vessels enter the axilla, they are confined anteriorly by the pectoralis minor muscle, which inserts with a tight fascia to the coracoid process, often forming a sharp edge around which the subclavian vein and some elements of the plexus wind when the arm is elevated or angulated in adduction.

## GENERAL SYMPTOMS AND SIGNS

Thoracic outlet syndromes can produce pain, numbness, paresthesias or dysesthesias, weakness, atrophy, discoloration, edema, ulcerations, and gangrene in the upper extremity, as well as Raynaud's attacks. Pain may be hardly perceptible or excruciating, not interfering with ADL or truly incapacitating, intermittent or continuous; it may be burning, aching, lancinating, stabbing, or dull. Regardless of site, symptoms and signs present with a wide range of severity. Special tests are applied to define the site and degree of compression; they reproduce the narrowing at each of the potential sites of compression. In addition, root compression at the neural foramina must be ruled out to arrive at a useful clinical diagnosis.

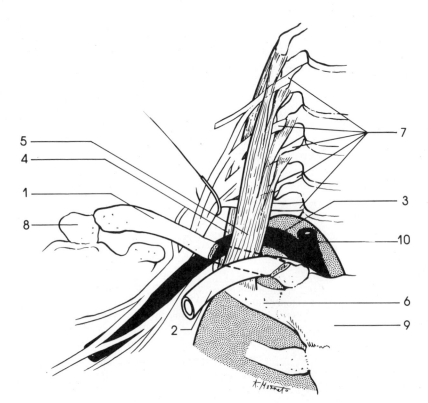

**Figure 11–5.** 1, Clavicle; 2, Subclavian vein; 3, Subclavian artery; 4, Scalenus medius muscle; 5, Scalenus anterior muscle; 6, First rib; 7, Cervical Roots 4, 5, 6, 7, 8; 8, Acromion; 9, Sternum; 10, Common carotid artery. Grey background is the pleura.

## SCALENUS ANTICUS AND CERVICAL RIB SYNDROMES

A cervical rib runs through the center of the narrow interscalene space and inserts behind the anterior scalenus muscle at the first rib, potentially causing compression of the C7 and 8 and the T1 elements of the plexus. Minor accidents such as falls on the outstretched arm may seriously damage these fibers or the subclavian artery.

A cervical rib can be demonstrated by x-ray, but a tight band occasionally transects the interscalene space in lieu of a cervical rib and is difficult to find. The neural elements are elevated by rib or band, angulated, and easily damaged. Compression of the neurovascular bundle in the interscalene space is diagnosed by the Adson maneuver.

With the arm abducted 70 to 80 degrees in the frontal plane, the head is turned maximally to the side to be examined (and to the opposite side at second attempt), the chin is lifted up maximally, and a deep breath is taken and held. The test is positive if radial and ulnar wrist pulses disappear, easily demonstrated by the disappearance of oscillometric readings over the forearm.

Cervical ribs or bands, or a tough, broad tendinous attachment of the anterior scalenus muscle, may cause a local subclavian artery stenosis, which in turn may be the source of emboli causing digital ischemia or Raynaud's attacks. Poststenotic subclavian aneurysms occasionally develop at the site.

When ischemia threatens the viability of parts of the upper limb, surgical intervention is usually indicated to relieve interscalene space narrowing by resection of parts of the first rib involving separation of anterior scalene muscle attachment, and occasionally reconstruction of the subclavian artery. An upper thoracic sympathectomy is often done at the same time.

If compression damage and ischemia are less threatening, conservative management may be adequate. It consists of scrupulous skin care and the avoidance of daily activities that entail extreme arm motions. Patients who may have to change their jobs include house painters, electricians, automobile mechanics, plumbers, tree surgeons, orchestral conductors, baseball pitchers, and other athletes. Sleeping posture in bed should be given particular attention. Hyperabduction or sleeping on one side should be avoided; a supine position with shoulder and neck support is best and can be learned by a willing individual within a few weeks. Occupations requiring vibrating tools may have to be given up.

## COSTOCLAVICULAR SYNDROMES

These were first described in people carrying heavy shoulder packs exerting downward and backward pull for long periods. Compression takes place in a space confined by clavicle and subclavian muscle, which inserts at the first rib cartilage and costocoracoid ligament, posteromedially and the anterior third of the 1st rib, and posterolaterally at the superior scapular border. The subclavian vein passes through the median angle of this space, between the clavicle and the anterior scalenus muscle insertion. Clavicular fractures may compress this space; abnormal first rib shapes or an exaggerated lordosis of the cervical spine may aggravate the narrowing.

Testing is done by pulling the arm downward and backward; this narrows the space. The test is positive if radial and ulnar wrist pulses disappear with the arm held in a dependent position. If trophic changes threaten the survival of parts of the upper extremity or if ischemia is severe, resection of the middle portion of the first rib may be needed, or else removal of compressing exostoses or calluses from a previously fractured clavicle. Section of the scalenus muscle insertion may bring relief, but scar formation may cause recurrences.

If the symptoms are less disabling, conservative treatment may be adequate. The shoulder elevators are strengthened through progressive resistive exercises; the patient is instructed to avoid carrying heavy objects in one hand, under one arm, or over the shoulder; a heavy bra should be supported by a broad band rather than by a narrow strap, which cuts into the shoulder.

## HYPERABDUCTION SYNDROMES (WRIGHT)

Compression of the neurovascular structures caused by a 180-degree abduction of the arm for extended periods (e.g., during sleep) are described. Indeed, numbness of forearms and hands after a night's rest is a common symptom in middle-aged and older people. The most common site of compression is near the coracoid process where the bundle passes around the sharp edge of the pectoralis minor fascia. Wright describes a second narrowing between clavicle and first rib in which the bundle may be pinched on arm abduction.

The test is positive if ulnar and radial arteries stop pulsating with the arm hyperabducted at 180 degrees and bent over the head in a frontal plane. We find this test positive in many asymptomatic individuals; perhaps such persons rarely assume a posture of hyperabduction for long periods. Hyperabduction is not a natural position in adults; and it is usually not difficult to dishabituate the asymptomatic patient of the posture; this usually results in abatement of the symptoms. In other cases an axillary vein obstruction may necessitate the division of the pectoralis minor insertion, or, if trophic changes threaten digits or the hand, more radical surgery has to remedy the narrowing of the second or third site of compression.

Distal nerve entrapment syndromes are common in thoracic outlet syndromes at the sites of the carpal or cubital tunnel. They are discussed in Chapter 17.

# 12

# Management of the Amputee

by Victor Cummings, M.D., Justin Alexander, Ph.D. RPT, and Susan O. Gans, M.A., OTR

Total management of the amputee should be a team effort led by the physician, with input and consultation from other specialized disciplines. The physical therapist, occupational therapist, nurse, social worker, psychologist, vocational counselor, and prosthetist all play important parts in the comprehensive approach to the physical, emotional, social, and financial implications of limb amputation. Amputation should not be considered an admission of failure, but another option of treatment open to the physician to convert a painful nonfunctional body part into a limb that will allow the patient to resume a life of relative independence and comfort. Whereas bypass grafts may be indicated in some situations, unless there is adequate distal arterial runoff, they usually fail. It also appears to be foolish to gamble with microsurgery reimplantation techniques in the hope of salvaging a limb, especially if the salvage means many months or even years of hospitalization and repeated surgical procedures. This is especially true because it has yet to be proved that limb reimplantation provides a functional body part. Thus far, the best results have been seen with simple digit reimplantations. Reasonable and practical medical and surgical management, including the art of modern prosthetics, should enable the patient to resume a productive and meaningful life in as short a time as three to four weeks after amputation.

Amputee or prosthetic clinics are common. The steps generally involve referral and preadmission evaluation; evaluation in the clinic, where the pre-scription is written after surgical, medical, physical, and prosthetic factors are considered; pre-prosthetic training; prosthetic fabrication; initial check-out of the prosthesis; prosthetic training; and a final check-out to ensure that the patient is using the prosthesis satisfactorily. All patients should be followed up routinely in the prosthetic clinic once training is completed.

## FABRICATION OF PROSTHESIS

The prosthetist is responsible for fabricating the prosthesis prescribed by the physician. Fabrication begins with the socket, which must be fitted to the stump accurately to provide stability yet also to distribute pressure widely over the stump for comfort. The proper anatomical landmarks, bony prominences, and tender areas are marked and measurements are recorded of various girth measurements and the length of the stump and the intact limb for guidance in shaping and sizing the prosthesis.

Next, a primary stump cast is made with plaster of Paris bandage, and the master mold is made by pouring plaster into the hollow primary stump cast. Any corrections can be made on the master mold. In many cases a wax check socket is then made so that the prosthetist can locate trim lines for comfort, purchase, and mobility and can accommodate for any pressure-sensitive areas. The final socket is made of a plastic laminate (polyester resin) and component parts are added. Cuffs, hinges, harnessing, and control systems are all fitted to the individual amputee.

On the average it takes two to three weeks to fabricate a below-knee prosthesis, three to four weeks for an above-knee, four to five weeks for a below-elbow, and five to eight weeks for an above-elbow. Generally, an amputee must make two visits to the prosthetist for fittings.

Cost of prosthetic devices can be high; therefore ways of financing them must be considered, but never at the expense of essential features for the safety of the patient. It is the obligation of the physician to discuss payment with the patient or family or both. In many instances a third party will be the payee, either through private insurance or Medicare/Medicaid. If coverage has not been determined early, it may lead to unnecessary delay in obtaining a prosthesis.

## PROBLEMS OF THE AMPUTEE

### PHANTOM LIMB

The entity of the phantom limb is not well understood and little has been done to shed scientific light on this interesting phenomenon. Phantom sensation following removal of a limb or part of a limb is almost universal. Phantom pain is not at all universal, and the two terms should not be considered as synonymous. It must be remembered that the etiology of the phantom is primarily central in origin. It is in the sensory homunculus of the brain that distal body parts are sensorily represented. Even though the body part has been removed, its representation in the brain continues to be present. With sensory input from elsewhere in the body, external or internal and not necessarily from the amputation site, the phantom can be triggered or reinforced. Phantom limb should be discussed with the patient very early in the postoperative period. A patient who knows that he has lost a limb, but who still feels that the limb remains a part of him, may worry that he has lost his mental faculties in addition to his limb. Some patients, through confusion or repression of the fact of the amputation, may "forget" that they have had a limb removed, may feel the phantom, and may try to walk on it; this could lead to serious injury.

### PAIN

Pain in the stump can develop soon after amputation. This pain may be due to local conditions in the stump itself that are not related to the phantom phenomenon. Infection, neuroma, and edema are common causes of stump pain and can be treated appropriately. Infection, if superficial along the suture line, usually responds to frequent saline irrigation. If the wound is badly infected with a pocket of slough and pus, it will have to be opened and drained. Painful neuromas usually respond to injection of procaine directly into the painful area. This treatment may maintain comfort for varying periods of time and may have to be repeated. If the response to procaine injection is good but short-lived, the neuroma should be surgically resected. Edema of the stump is best treated by proper positioning, compressive bandaging, or application of an Unna boot. True phantom pain is a most fearsome and challenging situation. The painful phantom is usually described as burning, aching, itching, or cramping, and the pain may be located in or at the end of the stump or some distance from the stump. Phantom pain is not a common occurrence following amputation. It occurs more frequently in the patient whose body part was chronically painful prior to amputation. Unfortunately, there is no specific treatment for the painful phantom. Analgesics, especially narcotics, are of no real value. The patient may demand increases in dosages, and addiction is a real danger. Local surgery for any reason or even revision to a higher level of amputation usually has no effect on the pain and may even make it worse. Acupuncture, transcutaneous nerve stimulation, nerve blocks, and hypnosis are of little value.

It is important that the members of the treatment team be sympathetic and understanding and that they make it clear to the patient that the pain is real and not imagined. Positive reassurance that as time goes by the pain will decrease or disappear is the best approach.

### REACTION TO AMPUTATION

The wishes of the individual amputee should always be considered, because without cooperation and motivation there can be no successful prosthetic use. It is imperative that the patient and family be oriented to the prosthetic training program as soon as possible. They must understand what is available, the advantages and disadvantages of a prosthesis for that individual patient, and all implications of the training program.

The patient's reaction to the loss of a limb and the success of the prosthetic program depend on many variables: age when amputation occurs, sex, intelligence, physical development, level of amputation, social and economic status, motivation, vocational and avocational interests, and quality of the surgical and prosthetic management. The rehabilitation program starts with the decision to amputate a limb and ends once the patient has successfully completed the training program and utilizes the prosthesis as functionally as possible. It is essential that the patient have all questions answered carefully and honestly by all members of the team.

## LOWER EXTREMITY AMPUTATION

Rehabilitation must begin prior to amputation while medical and surgical work-up is in progress. The physical therapist plays a decisive role during the preoperative period by initiating a treatment program designed to reduce the effects of inactivity and deconditioning. The nurses and the patient are instructed in a program of resistive exercises to all major muscle groups. Resistance can be provided manually or with weights. The arms should be especially strengthened to prepare the patient for crutch walking. During this time the patient should be taught a non-weight-bearing gait so that he can resume ambulation soon after surgery. The muscles that will remain in the limb to be amputated must not be neglected because they will act as the motor to propel a prosthetic device. Passive range of motion and stretching of tight muscles are essential to prevent limitation of joint motion. A flexion contracture of a hip or knee will delay or may prohibit prosthetic fitting.

### LEVEL OF AMPUTATION

Prediction of the level at which wound healing occurs may be the determining factor in the level of amputation. Whenever possible the knee joint must be preserved. The energy demands of ambulating with an above-knee prosthesis are so much higher than with a below-knee prosthesis that the older infirm patient may never be able to use a prosthesis if the knee is sacrificed. Even if blood flow studies demonstrate little flow below the upper thigh, it is really only at operation that a true determination can be made as to the probability of healing. If the incision is made below the knee and if the posterior skin flap is viable as evidenced by bleeding, a below-knee amputation should heal per primum. However, if infection with cellulitis and lymphangitis is present above the level of contemplated amputation, two procedures are called for. First is immediate removal of the infected distal part by guillotine or ankle disarticulation with the wound left open. This is followed in five to seven days by standard below-knee amputation after the infection has subsided.

Discussion of surgical technique is beyond the scope of this chapter, but it will be assumed that scrupulous attention to tissues is given, and tension on suture lines avoided by proper handling of skin edges. The application of a rigid or semirigid dressing to the amputation stump at operation merits serious consideration if someone is available at all times to remove it and reapply it quickly whenever indicated. There is good evidence that a plaster or Unna paste dressing controls edema immediately after surgery; this in turn promotes wound healing.

### STUMP LENGTH

Stump length is of considerable importance because it affects prosthetic design and fit. The old rule to save all possible bone length no longer applies to lower extremity amputation. The ideal length of an above-knee amputation is eight inches as measured from the inner groin to the end of the healed padded stump. If the femur is too long there may not be enough room for an internal knee joint in the prosthesis. An internal knee joint usually requires two or three inches of space at the knee joint. Failure to take this into account might result in the placement of the artificial knee lower than the knee of the intact extremity. The ideal length of a below-knee stump is six inches as measured from the tibial plateau to the end of the healed padded stump. A stump longer than this would require a bulky prosthesis because it would have to be larger in circumference around the calf area than the intact leg.

Partial foot amputation and Syme's amputation, although advantageous for function because they are weight-bearing amputations, may be indicated in younger patients with adequate blood supply distally, but usually fail in older patients with arteriosclerotic distal vessels. Unless healing is assured, these amputations are risky. Knee disarticulation, which is also an end-bearing amputation, requires an external prosthetic knee joint that may adversely affect gait.

### POSTOPERATIVE CARE

Following the amputation, care must be taken to guard against complications that can endanger the amputation stump or the intact foot and leg. Hip and knee flexion contractures have been previously mentioned. It is essential that stretching of joints is carried out at least once daily, either by a physical therapist or by the nursing staff after proper instruction. A well-padded splint placed behind the knee of the amputation stump is a simple way to assure that the knee is maintained in extension. This also indirectly maintains the hip joint in extension in the supine position. A simple way to strech the hip of the above-knee amputee is to place the patient in the prone position and press down on the buttocks while pulling the stump into hyperextension.

Skin breakdown of the intact heel can be disastrous and often leads to the amputation of the remaining limb. An amputee lying supine in bed tends to change position by pushing down with the remaining foot. This often leads to a sheet burn followed by a blister and subsequent skin necrosis. The heel must be protected, either by carefully padding it or by using a commercially available heel protector. Providing a trapeze bar hanging over the bed enables the patient to use his arms to change position. The patient must be instructed in its purpose and use by the physical therapist or the nursing staff. Ambulation with crutches or a walker

as soon as the patient's condition permits not only promotes the reconditioning process but is of enormous psychological help to the patient and family.

At this stage of the patient's progress, the aim must be toward prosthetic rehabilitation. Toward this aim, muscle strengthening must be carried out by repetitive resistive exercises to increase strength and also endurance. While the patient is ambulating on one foot, that limb accepts all the weight-bearing; thus, greater muscle power is needed. Prosthetic ambulation requires some modification in the biomechanics and kinesiology of normal

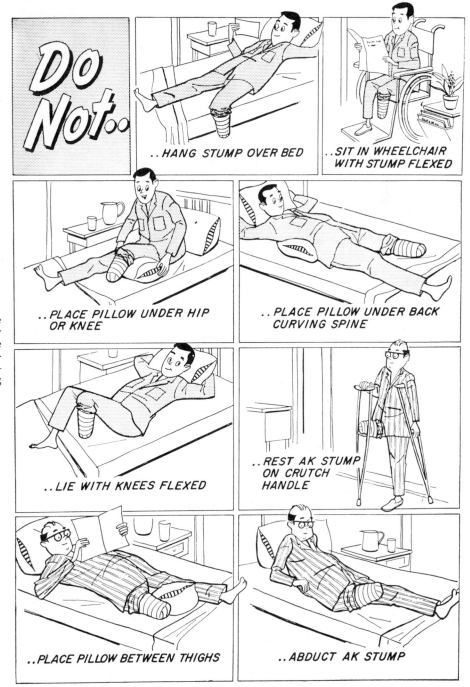

**Figure 12–1.** Actions to be avoided by the lower extremity amputee during the immediate postoperative period. (From Wilson, A. B., Jr.: Limb prosthesics—1970. Artif. Limbs 14:1, Spring 1970.)

gait. The hip muscles, particularly the glutei, are of great importance. The gluteus medius muscle stabilizes the pelvis on one side when the opposite leg is off the ground, and the gluteus maximus maintains the trunk erect at the hip and also serves as the motor that extends and locks the prosthetic knee (in the above-knee prosthesis) when the prosthetic foot is on the floor. These muscles must receive special attention under the supervision of a physical therapist.

The majority of amputations are performed because of irreversible arteriosclerotic peripheral vascular disease with or without diabetes. Almost always both legs are involved in the process. In many instances the remaining limb may also be in jeopardy. It makes little sense to prohibit ambulation to save the intact limb, since the arteriosclerotic process is progressive. However, the remaining leg and foot must be protected from trauma and infection. Careful cutting of toenails, paring of callosities, treatment of fungus infection, application of lanolin or other skin softeners to dry skin to prevent fissures, and placement of wedges of absorbent cotton between the toes to keep them separated and dry will protect the foot. Shoes should be modified to ensure the best possible distribution of weight-bearing. This is especially necessary when dealing with the diabetic patient, who may have a deformed or insensate foot. When all has been done to protect the foot, in the absence of frank gangrene or necrosis on weight-bearing surfaces of the foot, the patient should be encouraged to walk.

### Stump Preparation

The immediate postoperative period is the time when stump shrinkage and shaping may be started. All prosthetic devices require close, intimate fit between the stump and the prosthetic socket. The stump must be conical in shape, firm in consistency, and nonadherent to underlying bone. There should be no redundant tissue at the end of the stump. Circumference must be smaller distally than proximally.

To shrink and shape the amputation stump, no matter what the level, it must be compressed with a good grade of elastic bandage. The bandage must be ample in size to exert even pressure around the stump. Different techniques of applying bandages have been advocated. Generally, the best technique is the one in which a spiral or figure 8 configuration is used, with greater tightness and pressure distally. In the above-knee amputation the elastic bandage must be applied very close to the perineum to prevent adductor roll. Taking a few turns of the bandage above the waist will keep it from slipping off the stump. Molded elastic stump shrinkers are commercially available, but they do

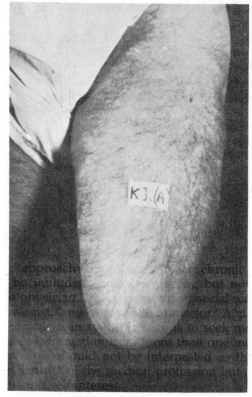

**Figure 12–2.** A well-formed above-knee stump. (From Wilson A. B., Jr.: Limb prosthesics—1970. Artif. Limbs 14:1, Spring 1970.)

not work as well as correct bandaging. The shrinker can be worn over the bandage to increase the compressive force on the stump.

An Unna paste dressing applied directly to the stump is another effective method to shrink and shape the stump. Using this method, care must be taken to cut out the area over the patella to avoid friction and pressure on the bony prominence.

The most effective means of providing shrinkage and shaping of the stump is ambulation with a temporary walking device or pylon. A pylon is a temporary socket that is molded and fitted to the stump and then attached to a shank portion (hollow aluminum tube, discarded prosthesis, or wooden crutch length) with a foot at the end. The socket may be fabricated out of plaster of Paris or other suitable material by a physical therapist, or it may be a plastic laminated socket fabricated by a prosthetist. The socket must be very carefully constructed so as not to cause undue pressure or trauma to those points which are prone to breakdown. The pylon is also valuable because it indicates how well the patient may use a finished permanent prosthesis. When a pylon is to be used for preliminary training, a very important series of exercises to be included are those that enable the patient to shift weight from one stance leg to the other. This will increase the patient's confidence in his ability to bear weight on a permanent prosthesis. These balancing exercises can be started within parallel bars, and the patient can progress to crutches, canes, or a walker. A standard nonflexible walker might interfere with the development of a reciprocal gait pattern and therefore, if indicated, a reciprocal flexible walker might be more useful.

## PROSTHETIC REHABILITATION

Successful prosthetic rehabilitation depends on many factors. As previously stated, one of the most important, and often overlooked, is the patient's honest desire and motivation to function with a prosthetic device. It makes no difference how simple or sophisticated the prosthesis is if the patient will not make the effort to use it. A large majority of patients initially appear eager to wear a prosthesis after amputation; however, once they have actually seen and touched one and felt its weight, they may be less enthusiastic. It is for this reason that all amputees should be given an opportunity to closely inspect the type of prosthesis they might need or talk to a patient who wears one. If, after this has been done, they remain honestly motivated toward prosthetic rehabilitation, all other factors must be considered. These include cardiovascular reserve, vascular problems in the remaining leg, cerebrovascular deficits, and problems with sensation, vision, or hearing. With regard to the patient's actual physiological response to the energy costs of prosthetic use, it is necessary to measure vital signs, heart rate, and the EKG during and after exercise on a bicycle or treadmill and to collect expired air to be immediately analyzed. If this is not possible, at the very least it is incumbent upon the physician to instruct the physical therapists and nurses to monitor blood pressure and heart rate before and after exercise and inform them which clinical signs and symptoms to regard with alarm.

The problems of using an above-knee prosthesis far outweigh those of using the below-knee prosthesis. It is the rare patient with the below-knee amputation who cannot use a below-knee prosthesis, as long as the functional goals are practical and reasonable. Goals should be assessed in terms of simple everyday activities, from homemaking to vocation. Successful rehabilitation depends on the patient's ability to reach the goals set for him with his cooperation by those who treat him, not goals set independently by the patient or family, which may be unrealistic.

The decision to order a prosthesis is the responsibility of the physician, but whenever possible that decision should be with input from a team of health professionals whose expertise can be most helpful in reaching the decision. If it has been decided to go ahead and order a prosthesis, a precise prescription must be written so there can be no mistake or misunderstanding about what is or-

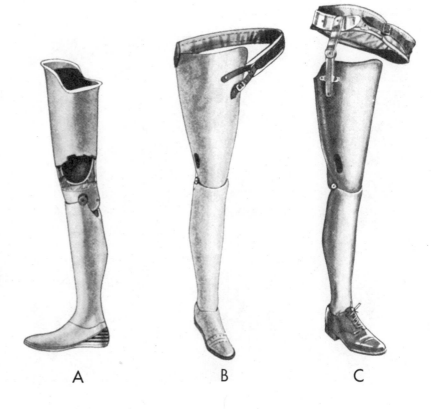

**Figure 12–3.** Above-knee sockets and suspension methods. *A,* total-contact suction socket; *B,* above-knee leg with Silesian bandage for suspension; *C,* above-knee leg with pelvic belt for suspension. (From Wilson, A. B., Jr.: Limb prosthesics—1970. Artif. Limbs 14:1, Spring 1970.)

A                    B                    C

dered. The detailed written prescription must list all components, including material used in fabrication, shape of sockets, method of suspension, type of knee mechanisms (in above-knee prostheses), molded inserts, and ankle-foot assembly. Components for lower extremity prostheses are numerous and varied.

Above-knee suspension can be obtained by means of a pelvic band or a strap to control rotation of the prosthesis (Silesian belt). In younger patients with a well-shaped, firm, nonpainful stump, suction alone can suspend the prosthesis. This is accomplished by placing a one-way valve in the socket that allows for air to be pumped out. A vacuum is created that holds the prosthesis on if it is fitted to total, intimate skin contact. In special cases any or all types of suspension can be used, including over-the-shoulder straps. Below-knee suspension can be by way of steel side joints attached to a leather thigh corset or by a leather or canvas strap over the patella. Numerous variations of this type of suspension are available. There are many types of knee joints for the above-knee prosthesis. Some use friction to maintain the knee in extension, some can be manually locked, and some are hydraulically operated.

The prosthetic foot can be of the single-axis type, the multi-axis type, or the cushion heel type. Suffice it to say, the prosthesis must meet the needs of the individual patient. It does not serve the patient's best interests to simply send him to the nearest prosthetic shop for an "artificial leg." The patient's physician must bear the ethical and legal responsibility of ordering the device.

A mention should be made about cosmesis at this point. There are some patients who cannot use a functional prosthesis but who cannot face the world sitting in a wheelchair, hopelessly disabled and crippled in appearance. Most often, they are bilateral amputees. They should have cosmetic prostheses fabricated out of lightweight polyester laminate with no functional components and very simple strap suspension. It must be made clear to the patient that he cannot stand or walk with these devices and that they are purely for cosmesis.

Prosthetic training should be carried out under the supervision of a physical therapist who is skilled in gait training, balancing, strengthening, and the use of assistive devices. Perfection of gait is almost never reached, especially in elderly patients, so practicality must rule. Once a patient can walk safely, with or without assistive devices, minor or even major gait abnormalities might have to be overlooked. For most patients no amount of training will produce a textbook gait. Safe ambulation is the most important goal of prosthetic training, but some gait deviations might be avoided with training. The patient should be taught to take steps of equal length, to spend the same time on each foot, and to have equal arm swing. Gait deviations can best be observed when attention is given to each separate phase of the gait cycle: heel strike, foot flat, toe off, and leg swing. There are also abnormalities of gait that result from a faulty prosthesis. These must be identified and adjusted. It is reasonable to wait about two weeks into the training period before prosthetic adjustments are ordered to evaluate the prosthesis as a whole

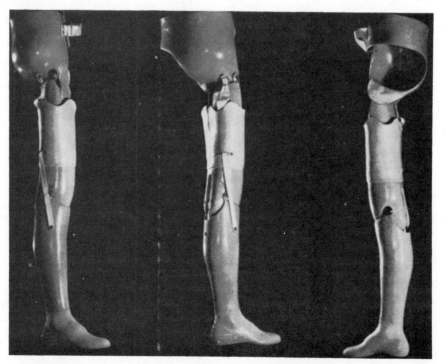

Figure 12–4. Hip disarticulation prosthesis. (From Wilson, A. B., Jr.: Limb prosthesics—1970. Artif. Limbs 14:1, Spring 1970.)

VARIATIONS OF THE PATELLAR-TENDON-BEARING (PTB) PROSTHESIS

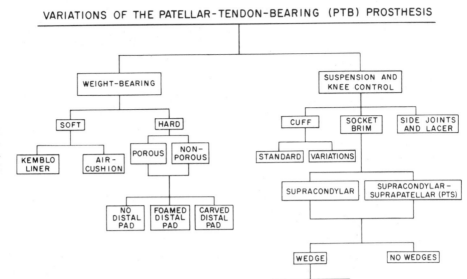

**Figure 12–5.** Cutaway schematic of a PTB prosthesis. (From Wilson, A. B., Jr.: Limb prosthesics—1970. Artif. Limbs 14:1, Spring 1970.)

rather than adjust each difficulty individually. The patient must be taught to don the prosthesis correctly, to walk on level and irregular terrains, to use public transportation, to climb and descend stairs, and to negotiate curbs. He should be taught how to fall and get up from the floor.

Care of the stump and stump hygiene should be stressed and the patient should learn to maintain the prosthetic device in good order. In light of the fact that a prosthetic socket is a rigid container surrounding a stump that is constantly changing in volume and size, the patient must learn to compensate for this by varying the number of stump socks worn. He should be cautioned to change socks frequently in summer so that the stump does not become macerated by a damp sweaty sock. Above all, he should be instructed not to wait if he develops any problem with the stump. A small area of redness, some soreness or friction, or a tiny blister often lead to major difficulties if not attended to promptly. Most often all that is needed is a minor prosthetic adjustment which can be attended to immediately.

Consideration should also be given to making the home safe. The installation of grab bars in the tub or shower area, the use of a tub bench, safety bars at the toilet, and removal of architectural barriers should be suggested when indicated. While the goal of prosthetic rehabilitation is to enable the patient to ambulate and not depend on a wheelchair, it might be desirable to have one available for emergencies, such as going to the bathroom at night. It might also be useful if a problem develops with the stump that would contraindicate the use of the prosthesis or in the event that the prosthesis needs to be returned to the shop for repairs.

## UPPER EXTREMITY AMPUTATIONS

In contrast to lower extremity amputations in adults, in which well over 50 per cent are the result of vascular disease or its complications, 70 per cent of all amputations of the upper extremities are the result of trauma. Accidents involving industrial or farm machinery account for the greatest number, followed by accidents involving automobiles, boats, motorcycles, firearms, and burns. Infection and tumors account for the rest. Amputation of the upper extremity due to vascular disease is very rare. Elective operations are done rarely and they usually involve only the hand.

Surgical management of the upper extremity amputation differs from that of the lower extremity primarily with respect to stump length. As previously stated, there are ideal stump lengths for above-knee and below-knee amputations so that prosthetic management are facilitated. This is not the case in below-elbow and above-elbow upper-extremity amputations. The cardinal rule must be to save all possible bone length, soft tissue, and skin. The lower the amputation, the better is the function with a prosthesis because a lower amputation may preserve the ability to pronate and supinate the forearm (in below-elbow amputations) in order that the terminal device may be pre-positioned. In a wrist disarticulation procedure, the radial and ulnar styloid should be resected so that their bony prominences are not a problem and attention must be given to overall forearm-to-hand length so that the prosthetic device is not longer than the intact arm. Of equal importance, the lower the level of amputation, the more sensation is preserved to provide the sensory feedback that is so necessary for arm and hand function. The loss of sensation in an upper limb by amputation is the greatest factor limiting effective use of a prosthesis. A blind person cannot use an upper extremity functional prosthesis because he must rely on sensory feedback to use the hand. A prosthetic device covers the stump so there is no longer sensory feedback. The patient will need to rely on visual cues to know if he is holding an object in the terminal device. The patient must also adjust to the pressure of the socket on the stump, the tightness of the harness that holds the prosthesis on, and the weight of the prosthetic device.

Once the decision is made to operate, it is up to the physician to be sure that the patient understands why the operation is necessary. The patient should also know the level of amputation selected and reasons for this decision. The step-by-step plan for postoperative care of the stump and the pre-prosthetic exercise program should be explained. The patient should know what he will most likely be able to do with the prosthesis, and social, psychological, and economic adjustments that he may have to face.

## PREPARATION BEFORE AMPUTATION

The rehabilitation program should begin prior to amputation, if there is time. Strength and range of joint motion proximal to the anticipated level of amputation should be maintained by an exercise program, performed by an occupational therapist or by a nurse who is supervised by an occupational therapist. The exercises are designed to maintain adequate range of motion of both shoulders and to strengthen those muscles that forward flex the humerus at the glenoid and abduct the scapula. If the elbow joint is to be preserved, range of flexion, extension, and rotation of the forearm (if 55 per cent or more of bone length is to remain) must be maintained and the biceps and triceps strengthened. If the amputation will be above elbow, the patient also must strengthen his shoulder extensors and scapula depressors on the side where the amputation will be because these muscles are used to operate the elbow lock.

## OPERATION AND AFTER

At surgery, the same consideration should be given to the application of a rigid or semirigid dressing as discussed with the lower extremity amputation. The aim of surgery is to produce a firm, tapered, cylindrical stump, free of sensitive scars with the bone well padded along the length and covered at the tip. It is important for the surgeon to save as much healthy tissue as possible. As stated before, the higher the level of amputation, the less functional the patient will be with the prosthesis. Skin coverage, stump sensitivity, and padding are important considerations so that there will be no pain when the prosthesis is used.

Amputations in the hand may be transcarpal, transmetacarpal, or of any digit. Amputations through a joint are generally at the wrist, elbow, or shoulder. Amputations between the elbow and wrist are below elbow (BE) and between the elbow and humeral neck are above elbow (AE). A forequarter amputation is of the entire upper extremity, including the scapula and clavicle and is generally performed because of malignancy. There are generally prostheses for each level of amputation, but each individual must be evaluated so that the prostheses prescribed meets each patient's needs (Figs. 12–6, 7, and 8).

A major difference between upper and lower extremity amputees is their expectation of prosthetic function and prosthetic goals. The lower extremity amputee will almost always use a prosthesis to function, no matter how limited his walking may be. Without it, he must be relegated to a wheelchair. In truth, the unilateral upper limb amputee becomes one-handed with or without a prosthesis. With an amputation above the hand, all function is usually performed with the remaining upper extremity. The prosthesis will be used only as an assistive device. Many times the patient will discard the prosthesis and use the bare stump as the assistive device because the stump has sensation and the prosthesis does not. It is the rare amputee who bothers to wear a prosthetic device in the privacy of his home. The question to be asked then is: Should a patient with a unilateral arm amputation be provided with a prosthesis? The answer is yes, but with limited functional expectations. Cosmesis is usually the greatest benefit.

Following surgery, joint range of motion must be maintained, hemorrhage and edema minimized, and stump shrinkage and shaping started if a rigid dressing is not used. The stump should be bandaged with a compression wrap of elastic bandage applied tightly at the distal and snugly at the proximal end to ensure a cone-shaped stump (Figs. 12–9 and 10). Wrapping should continue until a prosthesis is fitted. To prevent contractures, all joints proximal to the amputation should be moved passively and actively through their full range of motion each day by the nursing staff. Even though there is some pain associated with motion, the exercises must be encouraged. If full range of motion is not achieved with exercises once a day, they should be done more often. Since both shoulders are important for operating the prosthesis, one to drive the prosthesis and one to stabilize the harnessing, they must both be included in the exercises. The exercises provided by an occupational therapist should involve vigorous muscle contractions to assist in circulation, thereby reducing

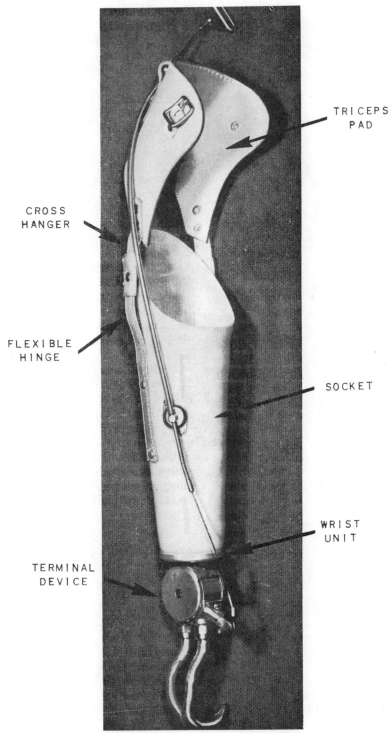

TRICEPS
PAD

CROSS
HANGER

FLEXIBLE
HINGE

SOCKET

WRIST
UNIT

TERMINAL
DEVICE

**Figure 12–6.** Standard below-elbow prosthesis. (From Stoner, E. K.: Care of the Amputee. *In* Krusen, F. H. (ed.): Handbook of Physical Medicine and Rehabilitation. Philadelphia, W. B. Saunders Co., 1971.)

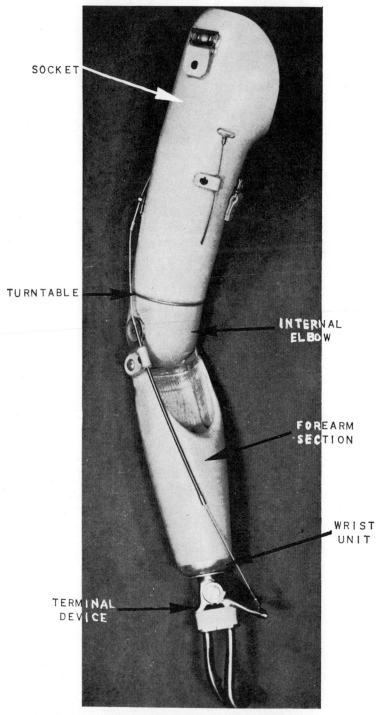

SOCKET

TURNTABLE

INTERNAL ELBOW

FOREARM SECTION

WRIST UNIT

TERMINAL DEVICE

**Figure 12–7.** Standard above-elbow prosthesis. (From Stoner, E. K.: Care of the Amputee. *In* Krusen, F. H. (ed.): Handbook of Physical Medicine and Rehabilitation. Philadelphia, W. B. Saunders Co., 1971.)

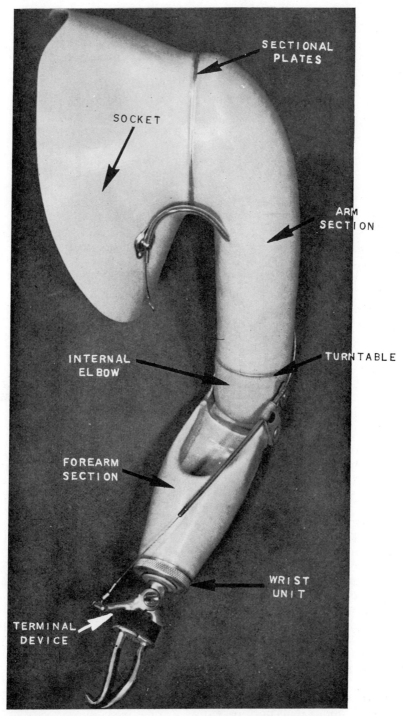

**Figure 12–8.** Shoulder disarticulation prosthesis. (From Stoner, E. K.: Care of the Amputee. *In* Krusen, F. H. (ed.): Handbook of Physical Medicine and Rehabilitation. Philadelphia, W. B. Saunders Co., 1971.)

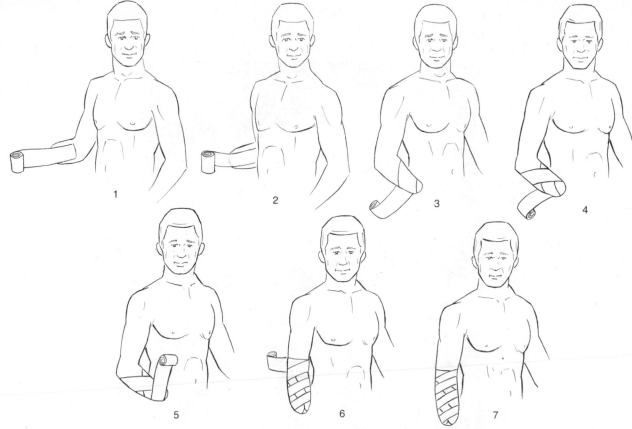

**Figure 12–9.** Wrapping a below-elbow stump. (From Wellerson, T. L.: A Manual for Occupational Therapists on the Rehabilitation of Upper Extremity Amputees. Dubuque, Iowa, William C. Brown Co., 1958.)

edema, and to prevent adhesion of soft tissue and muscle to bone. Progressive resistance exercises should also be started to strengthen muscles needed to operate the prosthesis.

For the above-elbow amputee, exercises to mobilize the shoulder are essential. These involve elevation of both shoulders and abduction/adduction of the scapulae. Flexion of the humerus is a source of power for flexion of the prosthetic forearm and operation of the terminal device in standard dual control systems. Extension of the humerus is used to lock the elbow. Thus, all of these motions must be full and as strong as possible. Exercises should be done each day, without resistance for joint range of motion and against resistance for muscle strengthening, to prepare the patient for using the prosthesis.

For the below-elbow amputee, the important motions are forearm flexion, extension, pronation, and supination. If forearm motion is limited, functional use of the prosthesis at the mouth or chest will be limited. Exercises to develop full range of motion and normal strength of forearm flexion should be done each day.

The stump should be washed daily and dried thoroughly. Gentle massage of the stump and rubbing or tapping the stump at the same time tends to desensitize it and decrease the patient's fears of having it moved and handled. Before prosthetic fitting the patient must be encouraged to use the stump as much as possible in daily activities. Compensatory one-handed activities should be stressed, especially if the remaining extremity is the nondominant one. A temporary prosthesis might be fabricated by an occupational therapist or prosthetist in order to incorporate the stump in a socket to further toughen it and to teach use of movements needed to control the cables. It might also lend guidelines for prescription of prosthetic components.

## DECISION ON PROSTHESIS

Patient motivation to use an upper extremity prosthesis plays a very important part in the overall decision to order a prosthesis, probably more so that in the case of the lower extremity amputee. There are three reasons for this. First, it is easier to use a prosthetic leg than a prosthetic arm. Second, if the amputation is unilateral, the patient will probably not use the prosthesis functionally, and

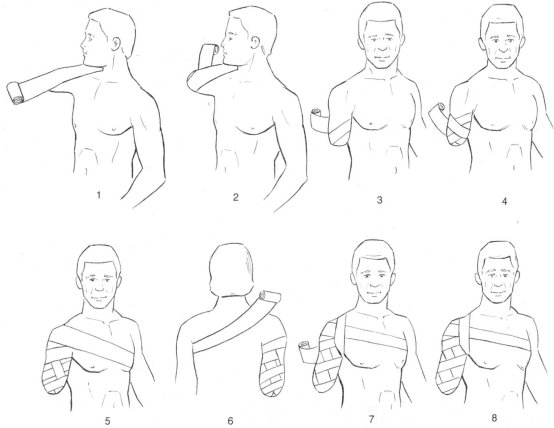

**Figure 12–10.** Wrapping an above-elbow stump. (From Wellerson, T. L.: A Manual for Occupational Therapists on the Rehabilitation of Upper Extremity Amputees. Dubuque, Iowa, William C. Brown Co., 1958.)

third, the appearance of a prosthetic upper extremity is less appealing than a lower extremity device. Many unilateral amputees opt for a purely nonfunctional cosmetic prosthesis with a passive hand.

The energy costs of upper extremity prosthetic use are of little or no consequence and should not enter into the decision regarding prosthetic prescription. This is because most upper extremity amutations are traumatic and are seen in otherwise healthy young people.

As in the case of the lower extremity amputee, the decision to order a prosthesis is the responsibility of the physician with input from the multidisciplinary team. The written prescription must be precise and detailed, listing all types of sockets, harnessing, components, and terminal devices. If the patient is not expected to use a prosthetic device functionally in bimanual activities, then a passive arm with only a cosmetic hand and glove should be ordered. If both function and cosmesis are important, a functional terminal device that can be interchanged with a hand and cosmetic glove should be prescribed. The patient's home life, vocation, hobbies, and social life must all be considered when the prescription is written.

## PROSTHETIC DEVICES

Two types of terminal devices are generally used. They are the prosthetic hand and the split hook. Prosthetic hands can be nonfunctional cosmetic devices covered with a skin-colored glove, or functional hands designed so that the index and middle fingers oppose the thumb, allowing for pinch by activation of the control mechanism. Hooks are preferable for function. They provide a more precise pinch and are lighter, durable, and easily cleaned. They allow the patient to more readily see objects to be picked up. Appearance is the major disadvantage of the hook. Many amputees use the hand for social occasions and the hook for daily activities.

**Dorrance Hooks.** The most frequently prescribed hooks are the Dorrance utility-shaped hooks. They come in various sizes in either stainless steel or lightweight aluminum (Fig. 12–11). The Dorrance hook is also made as a farmer's hook, allowing handling of tools. These hooks are voluntary opening. Rubber bands keep the hook closed and a force from the control cable opens the hook. An increased number of rubber bands means

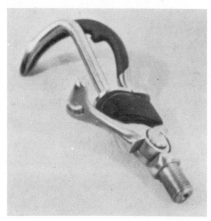

**Figure 12–11.** The Dorrance 5X hook. (From Trombly, C. A. and Scott, A.D.: Occupational Therapy for Physical Disabilities. Baltimore, Williams and Wilkins Co., 1977.)

a stronger pinch force and more strength needed to open the hook.

**APRL Hook.** There are also voluntary closing hooks such as the Army Prosthetics Research Laboratory (APRL) hook. It closes by a force on the control cable and then locks into position. A

slightly stronger force is then required to release the pinch. The voluntary opening hook is generally preferred, but both should be explored for each patient.

**APRL Hand.** The APRL hand is the most often presribed functional hand. It is voluntary closing and has a two-position thumb that can be adjusted for large or small objects. The index and middle fingers move together to meet the thumb while the ring and little fingers are nonfunctional. The hand is not recommended for hard manual labor (Fig. 12–12).

## REHABILITATION

Stump socks are worn by amputees to absorb perspiration, to provide warmth, and as a padding for comfort and fit of the socket. A T-shirt sleeve can be used in place of the stump sock by patients with short above-elbow amputations.

Checking of the completed upper extremity prosthesis is generally the responsibility of an experienced occupational therapist. This is done prior to presentation at a prosthetic clinic, and the findings and recommendations are then shared with the team.

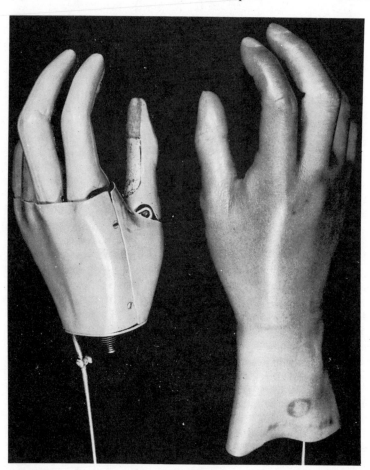

**Figure 12–12.** APRL No. 4C hand. (From Stoner, E. K.: Care of the Amputee. *In* Krusen, F. H. (ed.): Handbook of Physical Medicine and Rehabilitation. Philadelphia, W. B. Saunders Co., 1971.)

Change of hand dominance to the remaining extremity begins postoperatively during pre-prosthetic training. If the dominant extremity was amputated, activites to increase fine coordination will be indicated for the remaining nondominant extremity. If the nondominant extremity is lost, patients will usually use the remaining dominant extremity for most activities, relying very little on the prosthesis.

In most cases the amputee will be discharged from the hospital prior to obtaining the prosthetic device so that all prosthetic training is provided on an outpatient basis. All training should be carried out under the supervision of an occupational therapist with prosthetic expertise. The first thing to be learned is to don and remove the prosthesis. Training to operate the controls comes next. It is important that cable control movement be minimal to conserve energy and strength so that the patient can wear the prosthesis for extended periods without tiring. The amputee must be taught to operate the terminal devices: first the hook and then the hand. The below-elbow prosthesis has a single control system in which one cable operates the terminal device. The above-elbow prosthesis has a dual control system; one cable operates the terminal device and flexes the elbow unit while the second cable operates the locking mechanism at the elbow. Thus the above-elbow amputee must learn to flex the prosthetic elbow to position the forearm, maintain tension on the cable while locking the elbow, and then he can open and close the terminal device. The amputee must learn to control the prosthesis while working with objects of varying size, shape, consistency, and weight. He must learn to operate the terminal device in different planes, such as at the waist, mouth, and side.

The patient must be trained in daily living skills with the prosthesis. The hook is used for the static part of the activity and the sound hand for the active part. For example, to cut meat, the fork should be positioned in the hook and the knife is used in the sound hand. There are many things that the patient will do at home that cannot be simulated in the clinic, so the patient should be encouraged to try new things at home and to report successes or difficulties with new tasks. In this way the therapist is able to assist the patient not only in controls, training drills, and activities, but also in tasks and responsibilities in his daily routine. This makes the program more relevant to the amputee's needs. Recreational activities will also provide general body conditioning and development of a new image for the amputee.

Vocational training should be considered and included in the training program if indicated so that the amputee can recognize his capabilities using a prosthesis. Work tolerance can be assessed by the use of timed job-simulated tasks. Specific tasks related to the individual's type of work should be included to assess his safe and efficient handling of tools, power equipment, and various materials.

Homemakers should have training in various household activities such as meal preparation, cleaning, and household repairs. Child care should be included in the program if indicated. Each patient should be trained for his individual needs.

The average number of hours necessary to complete upper extremity amputee training depends on many factors such as age, intelligence, and level of amputation. Generally, an amputee with a standard below-elbow prosthesis with a voluntary opening terminal device needs about five hours. An amputee with a standard above-elbow prosthesis with a voluntary opening terminal device needs about ten hours. Learning to use a cosmetic passive hand requires about one to two hours, whereas a functional hand takes longer. Because expectations are less for a patient with a shoulder disarticulation, about 7.5 hours of training are needed; however, if the patient is trained to use the functional device with voluntary opening terminal device and nudge or waist band control, the time would be about 15 hours.

Care of the upper extremity prosthesis is of utmost importance. The amputee should be taught the correct terminology of all components of the prosthesis so he can report any difficulties to the professional team. He should replace weakened rubber bands to ensure terminal device pinch strength. One rubber band is equivalent to about a pound of pressure. Most patients wear two or three but can wear more if they are needed.

The hook should be kept clean and free from dirt and the socket should be washed weekly with mild soap and water. The amputee should be sure to put the harness back together correctly to ensure proper fit. The glove should be washed daily with a wash cloth, soap, and lukewarm water, with care taken not to allow any water to get into the mechanism of the hand. The hand should be stored in its plastic bag in a dark place when not being used, as the glove will darken slightly with exposure to light and with age. Grease, ink, and some foods will stain the glove and should be washed off immediately. Alcohol should be used to gently rub out stains. Newsprint, carbon paper, lipstick, tobacco stains, mustard, ketchup, graphite, shoe polish, and egg yolk will stain the glove permanently. Gasoline, benzene, kerosene, turpentine, shellac, and lacquer will weaken the glove if they are not removed quickly. Stump socks should be washed daily with a mild soap and water, squeezed gently to get out the water, and dried on a flat surface. Each amputee should be provided with at least six stump socks.

# 13

# Office and Home Rehabilitation in Arthritis

*by Kurt G. Leichtentritt, M. D.*

Rehabilitation in arthritis has run the gamut from overenthusiasm with active therapy to defeatism with a nihilistic approach. While some treatment methods have not stood up to our expectations and have had to be discarded, many procedures have empirically or rationally become valuable in our management of the arthritic patient. Many different forms of arthritis have been recognized, but only patients with osteoarthritis and rheumatoid arthritis are suitable for office and home rehabilitation. This is done by applying established and rational therapeutic procedures.

## CERVICAL TRACTION

Patients with osteoarthritis of the cervical spine with cervical spondylosis deformans plus discogenic disease may have root compression by bony spurs encroaching on the intervertebral foramina. They suffer from posterior neck pain and pain in the occipital area, and shoulders (also radiating into the arms), plus sensory and motor disturbances with electromyographic findings. They are usually given a soft foam rubber collar or a plastic rubber-lined cervical collar (Fig. 13–1).

These collars give very little protection, but will remind the patient to hold his neck still and will thereby decrease the pain produced by excessive motion, especially by nodding of the head. One has to make sure that the collars are not too wide and that they are long enough to comfortably encircle the neck. A sturdier collar will usually be re-

jected by the patient. The patient should be encouraged to wear his collar most of the day but instructed to remove it when lying down. During resting hours, a turkish towel rolled in the shape of a cylinder should be placed under the patient's neck, on top of his pillow.

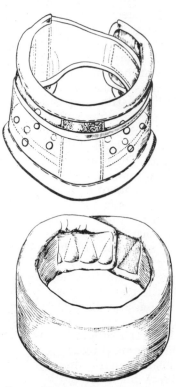

**Figure 13–1.** Foam rubber and plastic collars.

In rheumatoid arthritis of the cervical spine the facet joints may become affected. A dreaded complication is atlantoaxial subluxation by erosion of the dens of the axis or attenuation atrophy with unseating of the transverse, and alar ligaments of the atlas. The condition calls for a four-poster Somi cervical brace for complete immobilization. This will eventually require surgical stabilization.

For advanced cases of osteoarthritis of the cervical spine with persisting pain, continuous cervical traction should be prescribed for either office or home treatment. The traction equipment has been quite simplified, and can be applied to almost any door (Fig. 13–2).

It is advisable to explain and start the whole procedure in the office. Traction to the head halter should be in about 30 degrees of forward flexion. Either weights are attached or a bag is filled with the proper amount of water. The patient should sit on a sturdy chair. The chin and occiput are padded with gauze, and each procedure should last for about 25 minutes. Eventually the patient must buy the apparatus for home care. Treatments should be given daily for at least half a year. The patient can apply the traction in such a way that he will be able to read or watch television.

Controversy exists as to the amount of traction that should be applied. Theoretically, at least 30 to 35 lbs of traction will be needed to overcome the weight of the head and to produce cervical distraction. Empirically, it has been found that enlargement of the intervertebral foramina is not necessary for therapeutic results. All that is needed is relief of enough pressure so that the perineural root edema can diminish. In practice one may start with 7-lb weight pull and increase this by adding 1 lb a week. The average patient tolerates between 13 to 15 lbs of pull. Others may require much more or will only accept less weight. Some nervous patients compare cervical traction with a form of hanging. They will complain of nausea, dizziness, or faint feeling, and may never be able to tolerate it.

Motorized or intermittent traction is best used in a hospital setting.

## USES OF HEAT

The application of heat to painful joints, tendons, and muscles in arthritis has recently produced much controversy. Heat increases collagenous activity and therefore may destroy already compromised articular cartilage. This especially applies to rheumatoid arthritis. Nevertheless, heat has a temporary soothing and pain-relieving effect. Many patients suffering from rheumatoid arthritis automatically let hot water run over their hands to alleviate morning stiffness and pain. Melted paraffin with its low specific heat can be used as home treatment for prolonged warming of the arthritic hand. A double boiler, a candy thermometer, and a paint brush are needed. Thirty gm of mineral oil are added to 2 lbs of paraffin, depending on the size of the boiler. The mixture is heated to 130° F, then allowed to cool to the point when a thin coat of paraffin forms on the top. The paint brush is then used to coat the hand completely with a fine layer of paraffin. The hand is wrapped in wax paper and covered with a turkish towel. The paraffin wrap will stay warm for about 30 minutes. It should then be peeled off and placed into the double boiler for further use.

Moist heat in the form of hot wet towels or commercial hot packs (e.g., Hydrocollator) is preferred in rheumatoid arthritis. Hot packs have the advantage of molding to the part being treated. These should be wrapped in either one or two towels.

For deep heating, shortwave diathermy will be the method of choice in the office. A dry turkish towel is placed over the part to be treated and the drum placed over it. The dial setting should be between 15 and 20; some machines vary. Treatment should last for about 20 minutes. The back and hips in the prone position, the knees and ankles in the supine position, and the shoulders, elbows, and hands in the sitting position are suitable for diathermy therapy. The knees, ankles, and hands should not touch each other. The hands are best placed on a pillow on the lap. No metal should be in the field of diathermy, especially no metal hip implant, cardiac pacemaker, or hearing aid. No

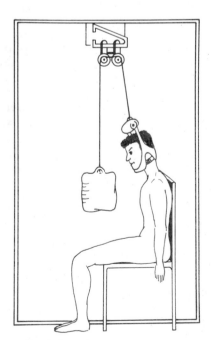

**Figure 13–2.** Cervical traction.

form of heat should be given to the low back of a menstruating woman. Heat should not be applied to any area suspected of harboring tumor, because heat will induce mestastatic spread.

Ultrasound is most effective in acute or chronic bursitis, especially in subdeltoid and subtrochanteric bursitis. This helps to break up calcium deposits. It is usually given at a setting of 1.5 watts per square centimeter for 3 to 10 minutes. The transducer is coupled to the skin by a mineral oil agent, using a continuous stroking motion on the part to be treated. It will not heat metal and can be used over a metallic prosthetic implant. Because of its power of distraction, it should not be used over any part of the central or peripheral nervous system.

### EXERCISE

Exercises in arthritis are needed to keep the patient limbered up. To prevent ulnar deviation of

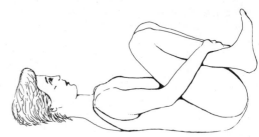

**Figure 13–4.** Bilateral knee-chest exercise.

the fingers in rheumatoid arthritis, the patient should sit with arms folded in front of him. He may also at times sit on both hands with the palms down on a chair and the fingers of each hand facing each other. Ulnar deviation of the metacarpophalangeal joints is most likely due to faulty stresses in grasping on the inflamed flexor tendons, causing them to slip in an ulnar direction. Finger flexion exercises should be avoided. The fingers should be kept in extension as much as possible. Typing and piano playing are desirable activities.

Ulnar deviation combined with wrist-stabilizing splints may be worn during the day, but mainly at night (Fig. 13–3 and Fig. 14–10).

The patient wears his splint on different hands alternately, as he needs one hand free to maneuver.

For back problems, back-strengthening exercises should be prescribed together with a lumbosacral corset. The ligaments and muscles of the knee can be strengthened by DeLorme's progressive resistive exercises. A simple method for home use is a woman's pocketbook filled with weights of 5 to 10 lbs. Bricks or some grocery cans will do. The patient should place the handle of the pocketbook over the ankle and lift the foot straight up from the floor in the sitting position, 10 times twice daily. The pocketbook has to clear the floor completely each time.

There are many back flexion and strengthening exercises. I prefer the supine bilateral knee-chest

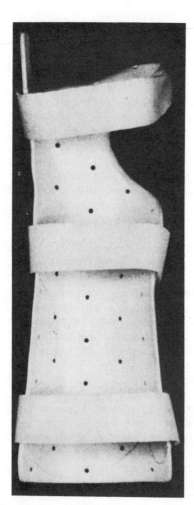

**Figure 13–3.** An ulnar deviation splint.

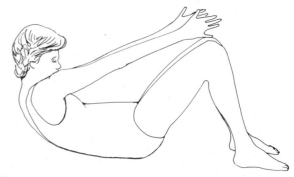

**Figure 13–5.** Strengthening exercise for abdominal muscles.

exercises that stretch and strengthen the lumbo-sacral fascia (Fig. 13–4).

The patient is also taught strengthening exercises for his abdominal muscles. He extends, from the supine position, the arms and raises the upper torso (Fig. 13–5). He may remain in this position for several seconds for isometric strengthening of the abdominal musculature, or he may perform repeated up-and-down movements.

## THE LUMBOSACRAL CORSET

A lumbosacral corset cannot completely immobilize the spine, but it will restrict some spinal movements. In addition, by compression of the abdominal muscles, it relieves local load stresses on the lumbosacral spine.

A lumbosacral corset can be prescribed for persistent low back pain, with or without shoulder straps. The corset should extend from the lower ribs to the lower buttocks but should not impinge on the groin. Most of these corsets have side lacing; steel stays are incorporated for better support.

The best way of donning and removing these corsets is in the supine position.

Two of the most often prescribed back supports are illustrated. They are the lumbosacral corset (Fig. 13–6) and the thoracolumbar corset (Fig. 13–7).

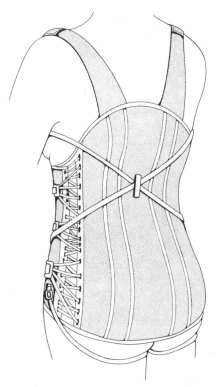

**Figure 13–7.** Thoracolumbar corset.

## CANES

Walking exercises are still the best means to strengthen the muscles of the body and maintain their coordination. If the hips, knees, or ankles are involved by the arthritic process, a cane may be used in the opposite hand from the affected joint. The length of the cane should be from the handle held in the hand with the elbow flexed to 45 degrees, with the tip placed 2 inches in front of and 2 inches laterally to the toes.

The patient should be sure that the ringed grooves of the rubber tip are not worn out. A smooth rubber tip will slip on wet pavement and is more hazardous than not carrying a cane at all. Platform canes are available for deformed and weakened hands. Patients with stiff backs may use a long-handed shoe horn and a reacher to supply the required length. A wall-attached wheel and a finger ladder will help improve range of motion of the shoulder. For weak fingers, thick-handled utensils will provide a better grasp.

## SPECIAL SHOES

Foot problems (see Chapter 15) will require special shoes in patients suffering from rheumatoid ar-

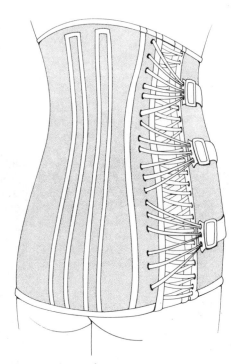

**Figure 13–6.** Lumbosacral corset.

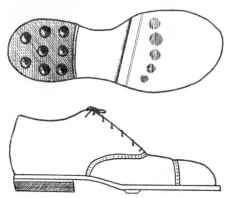

**Figure 13–8.** Orthopedic shoe.

thritis consisting of metatarsalgia with dropped, painful metatarsal heads, cocked toes, painful calluses, bunions, Achilles tendinitis, calcaneal bursitis, spurs, and plantar fasciitis (Fig. 13–8). These shoes should have a firm medial counter, a soft top with a high toe box, spot stretching over deformed toes, a leather sole, a molded insole, a low rubber heel, and, if required for painful metatarsal heads, a leather metatarsal bar under the sole of the shoe ⅛ inch in height. The shoes are prescribed for patients with moderately advanced rheumatoid arthritis. I also recommend the wearing of a Whitman special arch support, molded to the contour of the transverse and longitudinal arches of the patient's foot (Fig. 13–9).

These arch supports are removable and can be worn in any shoe. They should be covered with soft leather, otherwise they will be too hot in summer and too cold in winter. For the rheumatoid foot with advanced deformity, special molded space shoes will become a necessity (Fig. 13–10).

Heel spurs are treated by means of a foam rubber cushion with a hole cut out combined with steroid injections and ultrasound therapy. Some heel spurs completely disappear with time or their point becomes blunt and glued to the calcaneous with subsidence of the plantar fasciitis.

## ARTHRITIS TREATMENTS

Steroid injections can be given into joints or periarticularly and are part of the medical treatment of arthritis. They should also be the first ther-

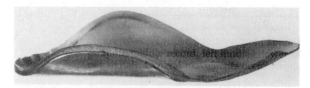

**Figure 13–9.** Whitman arch support.

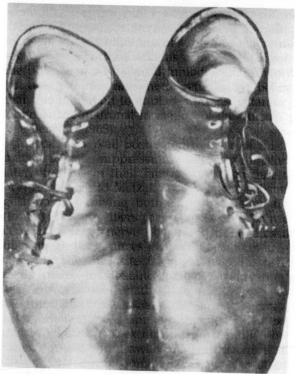

**Figure 13–10.** Molded space shoes.

apeutic approach in the carpal tunnel syndrome. Should this fail, surgery will become necessary. Triggerpoint injections of long-acting local anesthetic solutions are invaluable in the treatment of myofasciitis. In addition, vaporized coolant sprays may be applied. Electric stimulation, acupuncture, biofeedback, operant conditioning, and transcutaneous nerve stimulation are all being used in the treatment of arthritis. They do not seem to give the expected lasting results because of the progressive disabling nature of arthritis.

### TREATMENT RESULTS

How effective is rehabilitation in arthritis? This question can be answered only by comparing the results of treated and untreated patients with corresponding age, sex, and disease stage distributions. The results of the use of wrist-hand splints, worn mostly at night, to prevent ulnar deviation of the wrist and fingers in 48 women between the ages 20 to 55 suffering from active rheumatoid arthritis were compared with the results in 48 women with active rheumatoid arthritis of the same age group and disease activity who refused to wear such splints. The treated and untreated groups both had minimal ulnar deviation when first observed (Table 13–1).

After a period of one year, 27 of the untreated women had progressed to an ulnar deviation of the fifth fingers of 20 degrees or more. Only three patients who had worn their splints regularly had

**TABLE 13–1.** EFFECT OF SPLINTING ON ULNAR DEVIATION OF THE FIFTH FINGER IN WOMEN WITH RHEUMATOID ARTHRITIS

| Modality Hand Splint | No. of Patients | At Start of Observation | ULNAR DEVIATION | |
|---|---|---|---|---|
| | | | 20°+ After 1 Year | 20°+ After 5 Years |
| NON WEARERS | 48 | MINIMAL | 27 (56%) | 37 (77%) |
| WEARERS | 48 | MINIMAL | 3 (6.3%) regular wearers 8 (16.6%) irregular wearers | 36 (75%) |

this degree of ulnar deviation. Eight additional women who had worn their splints haphazardly also had 20 degrees or more of ulnar deviation.

Five years later, both groups had about the same degree of ulnar deviation. This leads to the conclusion that ulnar deviation splints will delay the progress of ulnar deviation. However, the natural progression of the rheumatoid disease will inevitably even out the score, regardless of whether the patient wears the splint or not.

Similar studies were made in women with rheumatoid arthritis between the ages of 20 and 45 who suffered from early foot problems (Table 13–2). Forty-three women who accepted the previously described special shoes and wore them according to instructions were compared with 43 women of same age and severity of illness who either refused special shoes or accepted and did not wear them.

After one year, 19 of the untreated women had moderate to severe progression of their foot problems. The remaining 25 untreated women had the same complaints relating to their feet as at the start of the observation period. Twelve women who wore their shoes were completely free of discomfort. Only four had progressive deformity and pain. The feet of the remaining 27 women remained unchanged.

Re-examination after 5 years of 41 women who had worn their shoes and of 42 nonwearers (3 patients could not be located) revealed no fundamental differences in their foot complaints and deformities. Almost two thirds of both groups (26 wearers and 27 nonwearers) had progressive and severe foot deformities. Here again, one can conclude that short-term results in the rehabilitation of such a rapidly progressive disease as rheumatoid arthritis

are good but that long-term results leave much to be desired.

In another study, the results of the alleviation of pain in osteoarthritis of the cervical spine were evaluated. Ninety-seven patients treated by means of cervical traction were compared with 97 other patients of similar age and disease activity who either refused cervical traction or were unable to tolerate traction after a trial period. The distribution of sexes was about equal, with 51 females and 46 males in the treated group and 49 female and 48 male untreated patients. All patients suffered from moderately severe to severe pain in the back of the neck, occipital region, and one or both shoulders with radiation into one or both arms. In addition, they were suffering from various degrees of motor and sensory disturbances. Only their symptoms of pain were considered, as pain was the only symptom that allowed a somewhat reliable comparison with the pretreatment state.

The treated group was instructed to apply with weekly increments 13 to 20 lbs of continuous cervical traction for one half hour daily, for at least 6 months (Table 13–3). After this period, 86 per cent of the untreated group had progressively severe pain. Only 3 per cent had spontaneous remission of their symptoms, and 11 per cent were unimproved. After 5 years, an additional 12 per cent had spontaneous remissions, bringing the total spontaneous remissions to 4 men and 11 women. This shows a certain number of spontaneous remissions with a female preponderance.

In the other group of 97 patients who applied cervical traction and continued their therapy as instructed, 46 per cent had complete subsidence of all pain after 6 months of therapy. The remaining

**TABLE 13–2.** EFFECT ON FOOT DEFORMITIES IN RHEUMATOID ARTHRITIS

| Modality Special Shoes | No. of Patients | AFTER 1 YEAR | | | AFTER 5 YEARS* | | |
|---|---|---|---|---|---|---|---|
| | | No Deformity | No Change | Increased Deformity | No Deformity | No Change | Increased Deformity |
| WEARERS | 43 WOMEN | 12 (27.8%) | 27 (62.8%) | 4 (9.3%) | 4 | 11 (26.8%) | 26 (63.5%) |
| NON WEARERS | 43 WOMEN | 0 | 25 (58.19%) | 19 (41.9%) | 0 | 15 (35.7%) | 27 (64.3%) |

*41 wearers; 42 non wearers.

**TABLE 13–3.** RESULTS OF CERVICAL TRACTION*

| No. of Patients | | | After ½ Year | | After 1 Year & up to 5 Years | | |
|---|---|---|---|---|---|---|---|
| | | Worse | Unimproved | Improved | Worse | Unimproved | Improved |
| | | | TREATED CASES | | | | |
| | | 0 | 55 (54%) | 42 (46%) | 0 | 44 (45.4%) | 53 (54.6%) |
| WOMEN | 51 | 0 | 27 | 24 | 0 | 19 | 32 |
| MEN | 46 | 0 | 28 | 18 | 0 | 25 | 21 |
| | | | UNTREATED CASES | | | | |
| | | 83 (86%) | 11 (11%) | 3 (3%) | 78 (81%) | 4 (4%) | 15 (15%) |
| WOMEN | 49 | 38 | 9 | 2 | 35 | 3 | 11 |
| MEN | 48 | 45 | 2 | 1 | 43 | 1 | 4 |

*97 treated, 97 untreated.

54 per cent were advised to continue traction for another 6 months. The result was more patients free of all complaints relative to their cervical arthritis at the end of a year.

The 53 patients who were free of symptoms after a year were instructed to resume traction at the slightest recurrence of their pain (Table 13–4). They were to continue their traction from one to three months or until they were completely free of discomfort for three weeks. This was required in 17 patients. Three of these 17 needed one course of treatment averaging one and one half month, five required two additional courses of traction of about two months' duration, and nine patients had more than two courses of traction of varying intervals and duration.

After 5 years, 53 improved patients (a preponderance of 32 women over 21 men) of the group of 97 with cervical spondylitis who had been treated with cervical traction were still completely free of discomfort relative to their cervical spine. Others had minimal discomfort that did not interfere with activities of daily living. At times, additional cervical traction or the wearing of a foam rubber collar was necessary.

Finally, 100 patients (52 men and 48 women) with moderately advanced rheumatoid and osteoarthritis were asked which modality in their rehabilitation treatment had been most important to them (Table 13–5). They all had received at least three months or longer of intensive rehabilitation treatment in the office or at home, consisting of all modalities applicable to their individual case. A total

**TABLE 13–4.** CERVICAL TRACTION AFTER 5 YEARS*

| | No. of Treatments Required | | | |
|---|---|---|---|---|
| | | 1 | 2 | Several |
| NO. OF PATIENTS | 17 | 3 | 5 | 9 |
| MEN | 6 | 1 | 2 | 3 |
| WOMEN | 11 | 2 | 3 | 6 |

*17 Patients of 53 required further traction.

of 69 per cent of these patients stated that the prescribed exercises kept them active, gave them something to do, and limbered them up; 9 per cent were most grateful for the help they had received from social service, 8 per cent for their vocational training, and 7 per cent for all instructions and training to cope with activities of daily living. Four per cent were most grateful for their self-help devices, and 3 per cent for their braces and splints.

Five years later, 68 of the 100 patients who could be contacted were again asked what had been most valuable to them in their rehabilitation treatment. Some of the 68 patients still received office rehabilitation therapy; others continued to exercise at home. The majority had stopped their rehabilitation efforts. They were not reminded of their original answers and most likely did not remember them. Therefore, it was quite surprising that their answers were almost identical to their previous statements. Namely, 66 per cent valued their prescribed exercises, 11 per cent their instructions in activities of daily living, 10 per cent the social service, 6 per cent the vocational training received, 5 per cent their self-help devices, and only 1 woman (2 per cent) her splint. It appears that a patient's evaluation of his rehabilitation modalities remains unchanged throughout the years.

It is well known that how a patient will accept rehabilitation efforts depends on the kind of individual he is. The patient, in addition to adequate ego strength and body image, needs real guts to live with his disability. We all see severely affected arthritic cripples who push themselves on canes, walkers, or crutches and continue working with minimal loss of time resulting from their disability. Some even continue to work up to their normal retirement age—one wonders how they were able to accomplish this. Others whine and wince with every little pain, sit almost completely immobile in their chairs, and develop deformities, contractures, and muscle wasting at a rapid pace.

Most of our arthritic patients fall in between these two extremes, managing to carry on their ac-

**TABLE 13–5.**    100 PATIENTS' OPINION OF THE MOST VALUABLE PART OF THEIR REHABILITATION*

| | Exercises | Self-Help Devices | Braces and Splints | Social Service | Vocational Rehab. | ADL |
|---|---|---|---|---|---|---|
| | QUESTIONED 5 YEARS AGO | | | | | |
| % | 69 | 4 | 3 | 9 | 8 | 7 |
| WOMEN | 33 | 3 | 2 | 5 | 5 | 4 |
| MEN | 36 | 1 | 1 | 4 | 3 | 3 |
| | QUESTIONED SEVERAL MONTHS AGO† | | | | | |
| % | 66 | 5 | 2 | 10 | 6 | 11 |
| WOMEN | 25 | 2 | 1 | 4 | 3 | 4 |
| MEN | 22 | 1 | 0 | 2 | 2 | 2 |

*52 women, 48 men.
†68 of patients questioned 5 years ago (39 women, 29 men).

tivities within the limits of their tolerance. It is in this large group that our rehabilitation efforts will continue to give some measure of relief from pain and disability. This can extend the period in which they are able to live a richer and more productive life. Unfortunately, even with our present methods of treating our arthritic patients, we are still unable to evaluate in detail and percentage every effort invested in rehabilitation.

## REHABILITATION AFTER JOINT SURGERY

The most important role that rehabilitation plays in arthritis is rehabilitation of the arthritic patient after specific joint surgery. This is done for the correction of joint pain and deformity, especially by means of total joint replacement. The rehabilitation effort in patients after orthopedic correction has almost become standardized as to modality, sequence, and duration, and results of therapy can almost be accurately predicted. Without any question, this is the greatest contribution rehabilitation has made for the previously disabled arthritic patient. The second most important role of rehabilitation in arthritis is the prevention of effects of im-

mobilization by the prescribing of strengthening and corrective exercises.

Physical therapy after total hip replacement can be summarized as follows: On the first and second days postoperatively, isometric gluteal and quadriceps sitting exercises are performed. On the third day gentle passive and active assisted range of motion exercises are given to the hip by the physical therapist. On the fourth day the patient may stand at his bedside with assistance from the therapist. He starts from touch-down weight bearing to as much weight as he can tolerate on the affected leg. From the fifth day on, gait training is being taught with the help of a walker. The leg should be in slight abduction after hip surgery. From days 6 to 12 gait training continues at progressive speed and dexterity, with the addition of stair climbing and descending.

After total knee replacement isometric quadriceps exercises are started as soon as permitted by the patient's tolerance to pain, which is usually on the third day postoperatively. Passive exercises are not given. The patient is encouraged to perform active range of motion exercises from day 6 postoperatively. Standing on the affected leg is usually started after 14 days, followed by progressive ambulation therapy.

# The Arthritic Patient and Recreation

*by Robert Frazer, M.A.*

One of the primary roles of the recreation therapist is to ensure the patient's success in rehabilitation. Individuals with physical or psychological impairments or both often have experienced a whole series of disappointments, failures, and frustrations. Medical and other therapeutic disciplines focus on and even exaggerate these impairments. In contrast, the field of recreation therapy deals with the healthy part of the patient: the strengths of the patient and less often the weaknesses.

During a group therapy session conducted by a psychologist at the David Menkin Rehabilitation Institute in Brooklyn, New York, a patient expressed the philosophy that he had adopted through his own experience with a condition involving multiple handicaps. It was clear that this patient had learned to concentrate on his strong points. He expressed his feelings through a comic story, which he told to the other patients in the group.

A man entered a pet shop seeking the best type of pet for his needs. The store owner, an elderly Jewish man, suggested a small yellow canary. "They're very nice, very entertaining, and have a wonderful song," he said. The customer agreed, and bought the bird and all the accessories needed for a happy pet. Once the pet was home and placed in its new cage, the owner realized that the bird repeatedly fell off his perch. Upon further examination the owner realized that the bird had a broken leg. Infuriated, the customer brought the bird back to the store and angrily explained about the broken leg. The store owner looked at the customer and exclaimed, "You vanted a singer, or a dancer?" The patient who told the story summarized, "I might not be good at everything these days, but there are still some things I can do well."

Extensive information has been documented on the rehabilitation and adjustment of the arthritic patient. Almost all areas have been touched and heavily researched. The areas of vocational readjustment, family and sexual adjustments, as well as early retirement and economic factors, have been explored. However, almost nothing has been written on the arthritic patient's leisure and recreation needs.

Unfortunately, recreation for patients in general is often taken for granted or given low priority. Our culture strongly emphasizes the work ethic and de-emphasizes the importance of the recreational process and experience. All individuals need recreation, yet some of us feel impelled to rename the process in order to lessen our guilt for "just having fun." Asked about previous recreational endeavors, patients will often insist that they never had recreational pursuits. "When I was done with my work, I had to visit my family, or knit, or bake, or read." Often these individuals disguise their fun and do not recognize that they are in fact participating in recreation.

Recreation allows us to express emotions and energies that have no outlets in our daily routines. In our systemized, mechanized world, creativity becomes stifled. Recreation, however, encourages healthy outlets for creativity, such as painting, drawing, and making music. Sports and exercise are healthy outlets for dispelling anger, frustration, depression, and anxiety.

The need for companionship and sharing, and giving and receiving of affection may be expressed through social and leisure activities.

The physician who counsels his arthritic patient on medical, physical, vocational, and family adjustment must also counsel the patient on his leisure and recreation needs, since this area is too often neglected and the patient fails to make a healthy adjustment. The recreation process, so important to all individuals, becomes increasingly important to the patient who faces the complex changes associated with arthritis.

## PSYCHOLOGICAL FACTORS

What do we know about the psychological needs of the arthritic patient? Many investigators concerned with these patients have reported similar results. Rheumatoid arthritis patients tend to be self-sacrificing, masochistic, conforming, self-conscious, shy, inhibited, perfectionistic, and, on another level, interested in sports and games. They also tend to overreact to their illness.

There are several common psychological responses that patients have to arthritis.

1. Denial. The patient may tell himself, "This is a temporary problem and will go away." The patient will find fuel for this belief expressly during remissions and when swelling is not apparent.

2. Anxiety. The patient worries about what is going to happen to him and his family.

3. Anger. Often the anger is a defense against a greater depression.

4. General depression. Sometimes this interferes with the patient's functioning more than the condition itself.

5. Dependency. The patient might enjoy the secondary gains of the attention of others yet feel increasingly helpless and anxious.

6. Negative self-image. The patient asks, "How can I face others now that I am so ugly and disformed?"

In general, the arthritic patient exhibits personality traits characterized by depression, rigidity, and great concern for his physical functioning. Actually, these feelings of frustration and helplessness are characteristic points of any disabling disease.

## PHYSICAL PROBLEMS THAT ALTER THE RECREATION PROCESS

**Fatigue.** Because the arthritic patient tires easily, former recreational outlets must often be readjusted to this situation. The former sports-oriented patient might be urged to divide the time between active and spectator involvement. Less active sports can be suggested. The tennis player might discover that golf is really enjoyable. The individual who enjoyed knitting might find that hook- or latch-rug making is more comfortable.

The patient will be able to accomplish more if he paces himself properly. If reading and needlework are of major interest, alternating the two will increase the success of both. Rather than aiming to complete a piece of needlepoint in three weeks and read a book the fourth, alternating periods of both will make the patient more comfortable and successful. If the patient feels that he has more energy in the morning, more active endeavors should be scheduled during those hours.

Rest periods can become recreative. Perhaps one of the most frustrating aspects of arthritis is the patient's need for prolonged and frequent periods of rest. The patient should be encouraged during these blocks of time to pursue reading, listening to radio, writing, and even watching television.

The physician should set guidelines for his patient, depending on how much physical resistance is constructive and at what point it becomes counterproductive. The physician will probably suggest that the patient should rest affected joints during periods of swelling.

## ADAPTING ACTIVITIES AND FINDING NEW ONES

The patient should be encouraged to adapt activities that have given pleasure in the past but bring discomfort now. The individual who enjoys painting could use a smaller canvas, placing it on a flat surface. Building up a brush with padding can create a much more acceptable situation. Sitting down for a former stand-up activity might help. The arthritic painter can sit by his easel and the gourmet cook can prepare almost everything while seated without spoiling the picture or the stew.

Test batteries such as the Mirende Leisure Interest Finder reveal that individuals enjoy activities that fall into major categories such as competitive or noncompetitive sports, appreciate or expressive arts, and so forth. If the arthritic patient can no longer actively participate in a specific activity, substitutions can easily be made. If a patient can no longer sculpt, learning about architecture or taking walking tours, for example, might meet the same psychological and creative needs. The qualified recreation therapist is quite familiar with these test batteries and has counseling skills; however, many of these tests, as well as a general self-evaluation, can often be done by the patient on his own.

These tests are part of a longer process used in leisure counseling. There are recreation therapists who specialize in this and have helped many patients readjust to a modified yet rewarding leisure-recreative life style.

## SOCIALIZATION AS OPPOSED TO ISOLATION

Because of the disabling process of arthritis, the patient tends to spend more and more time alone. He might feel that too much effort is needed to travel and socialize. The arthritic patient may fear being a burden to others, and he may become extremely self-conscious and embarrassed by physical deformities. Aloneness may trigger loneliness and isolation. The patient should be encouraged and perhaps persuaded to continue normal socialization.

Some patients feel more comfortable with peers who are similarly handicapped. In these cases, the patient should be encouraged to start his socialization with other arthritics. However, some patients often say that they can forget their problems more easily if they are with "healthy individuals" who do not reflect their own ills. Any of these options is acceptable as long as the patient continues socialization.

In an institutional setting, the qualified recreation therapist will be fully aware of each patient's social needs and will help develop individual therapeutic goals. Music, arts and crafts, and movement and dance are launching points for resocialization. With progress, the patient will start to accept himself as an individual with certain impairments and will recognize that he can still relate to others. Support systems can be set up by the recreation therapist to allow for one-to-one therapy when the patient finds the socialization process difficult.

For the arthritic outpatient without the support

of the recreation therapist, socialization can become more of a problem. However, community recreation centers for the physically disabled and the aged are more and more available nationwide. Often the local chapter of the Arthritis Foundation can aid in locating these resources. Many recreation organizations encourage the mainstreaming of the disabled into nondisabled programs. Others have special programs for the various disabled groups.

As mentioned earlier, many individuals are not comfortable with recreation for its own sake. These individuals might feel that they must accomplish something concrete. Others believe that leisure time should be spent helping others. Actually, supporting others who are considered less fortunate goes a long way in decreasing self-pity and self-absorption. There are many programs that the physically handicapped can utilize. Peter Verhoven, in a chapter on "Recreation and the Ageing," has discussed programs that the elderly could tap.* He believes that such programs would be quite constructive for the arthritic patient who has been forced into early retirement or who has excessive leisure time on his hands. Some of these are Head Start, Foster Grandparents, Home Health Aides, and sheltered workshops.

Whatever the individual's interests, a course can be found dealing with that subject. Public schools now offer a wide range of adult evening courses, and community centers as well as private organizations offer inexpensive classes. The courses run the gamut from trigonometry to cooking. Many people indicate that they feel more comfortable meeting others in settings where socialization is a secondary process.

## RECREATION ACTIVITIES ESPECIALLY SUITABLE

**Painting.** Painting is an extremely adaptable leisure endeavor and can be quite suitable for the arthritic patient. While adjusting to a disabling arthritic condition the individual experiences a multitude of emotions. These feelings need healthy and constructive outlets. Painting, for example, offers the patient a nonverbal, nonthreatening means of expression. Some of the necessary adaptions for the medium are quite easy. In general, the rule in painting is the larger the canvas, the easier the painting, since details are easier to paint on a large scale. However, the rule is often the reverse for the patient with limited range of motion in the upper extremities. For him, a small canvas is easier to handle.

---

*Stein, T. A. and Sessones, H. D.: Recreation and Special Population. Holbrook Press, Boston, 1973.

Newly developed acrylic paint is a real plus to handicapped artists. Watercolor requires a great deal of coordination and might prove to be frustrating, as can oil paint with its prolonged drying period. Acrylic dries quickly and mistakes can be covered 15 minutes later.

Some common adaptive devices for those with limited movements or severe pain include mouth sticks, cuffs, and headbands that can hold brushes and can actually be used to create fine works.

For the patient who lacks fine motor coordination, rag painting is often successful. Crumpled cotton rags are dipped into acrylic paint and then dabbed on the canvas, eliminating the need to hold a brush. This method can create beautiful scenes that seem impressionistic in style. Some patients find it more comfortable to work with a flat canvas while others prefer an easel angled at 45 or 80 degrees. Acrylic paint will work either way.

**Pottery.** Working with clay usually involves all the joints of the hands and is a very complete exercise. It is often the perfect medium for the angry and depressed to vent their frustrations. With craft shows and sales so popular today, the pottery hobbyist can find his leisure pursuit financially rewarding as well.

Pottery has many methods and styles to accommodate special physical limitations, preferences, and aesthetic ideas. Use of a pottery wheel is a very sophisticated method that requires much concentration and coordination. The manual wheel offers exercise for the lower extremities as well. The coil method can be used to make a variety of cylindrical objects. Pouring guarantees success. Slip (liquid clay) is poured into plaster of Paris molds. Many pottery classes are available from studios and in community centers throughout the country.

**Mosaic Designing.** Everyone enjoys working with mosaic tiles, and who can't use an extra ashtray? Mosaic tile work has built-in success and offers little frustration for the individual seeking a new hobby. Individuals can work with aluminum forms and create ashtrays, serving dishes, and so on. All this can lead to creating large mosaic designs on wood suitable for framing. This can be created with special equipment, and the possibilities of arrangement of these pieces in a mosaic are endless. Mosaic art is one of the chief forms of expression is Israel, where priceless pieces hang in museums.

## EXERCISE AS RECREATION

Exercise is often prescribed by the physician and dreaded by the arthritic patient. General exercise can be boring, but movement, dance, and exercise programs are very popular in community recreation facilities. Almost every "Y" and commercial health club offers some type of exercise program in a class atmosphere. The patient with a mild arthritic condition can easily fit into such programs and enjoy the social aspects of the activities. For the individual with a more disabling condition, many senior citizen centers have exercise programs specially adopted for the arthritic individual.

Perhaps swimming, the best form of exercise discovered, can be constructive for the arthritic patient. Heated pools can be especially comfortable and floats can be used to lessen strain and provide rest periods. The buoyancy of the body in water often allows the arthritic greater freedom and less painful movement. The psychological benefit of increased mobility, even if temporary, is very therapeutic.

## VACATION TRAVEL AND THE ARTHRITIC PATIENT

A question frequently asked by the arthritic patient of the leisure-recreational counselor is "Can I travel?" The answer is yes. The arthritic patient needing the use of a cane, walker, or wheelchair will face many unique problems in travel. However, with some ingenuity, adaptability, resourcefulness—and, unfortunately, a few extra dollars—the physically disabled can travel.

The United States leads the world in the development of technological advances in the area of mobility and travel for the handicapped. It is therefore suggested that severely or even mildly handicapped persons restrict their travel to the continental United States until they become more seasoned travelers.

**By Car.** Automobiles are, of course, the most convenient way of travel for the handicapped. Cars can be fitted with hand controls for those without use of the legs. Using such vehicles obviously requires special training. However, many individuals say that this relearning is not as difficult as one might think. Individuals who need hand controls for travel find that many of the major car rental companies offer equipped cars for no additional charge.

When traveling by car, wheelchair-bound patients can find many barrier-free restaurants, hotels, and rest areas. Organizations such as the American Automobile Association (AAA) can be helpful in planning such travel. The handicapped vacationer, especially wheelchair-bound individuals, will always be on the lookout for the barrier-free emblem.

The disabled driver should place his own sign on his front windshield or obtain a special license plate, alerting others that he is a "Physically Disabled Driver." It is often surprising how many courtesies will be extended and how flexible rules can be.

Of course, luxury can be bought for the disabled driver who can afford it. Vans, trucks, and campers especially designed for the handicapped with hydrolic lifts, wide-sliding doors, and so forth, are now on the market. Many of these designs are standard options and, for a price, the adaptions that can be obtained are endless.

**Other Transportation Modes.** Planning ahead is the key for the handicapped traveler riding buses and trains. Many trains and stations are especially equipped, and the Red Caps are cooperative and helpful. When reservations are made in advance, a seat will be reserved and space is often provided for the wheelchair right behind the passenger. Crutches, canes, and folding wheelchairs can be carried free of charge in the luggage compartment.

A most exciting advantage for disabled bus riders is offered by the two major bus lines, Greyhound and Trailways. A disabled rider who needs assistance in travel may bring a companion-helper *free*.

For air travelers, the number of handicapped or nonambulatory passengers is restricted to a certain maximum for each plane. Passengers cannot remain in wheelchairs during flight. Some airlines ask disabled passengers to sign a waiver of their rights, allowing the airlines to waive their responsibility in the event of an accident. This, however, is not the case for domestic airlines or flights that originate in the United States.

Many handicapped travelers prefer ocean cruises, since most of the trip is planned out and there is less to fear regarding accessibility and other special needs. For further information it is suggested that the reader consult *Travel Ability* by Lois Reamy, Macmillan Publishing Co., 1978.

# Appendix

## Dressing Techniques and Adaptations for Patients with Rheumatoid Arthritis

*by Pauline P. Tan, O.T.R.*

### GENERAL PRINCIPLES

1. Give minimal amount of equipment; if possible, give one versatile, durable piece of equipment that is within the patient's financial capabilities

2. Keep equipment simple so it is easily repairable and easily set up by the family or attendant.

3. Have patient and therapist evaluate the effectiveness of equipment while in the hospital; if the patient does not use it consistently while in the hospital or if family cooperation after discharge is doubtful, the equipment will probably not be used at home.

4. See that equipment is not:
a. Eliminating or decreasing the patient's use of his active range of motion (ROM).
b. Encouraging deformities.

5. Evaluate the feasibility of dressing, considering time, consumption of energy, and priority in patient's activities.

| ACTIVITY | TECHNIQUES AND ADAPTATIONS | DIAGRAM |
|---|---|---|
| I. Dressing<br>  A. Putting on and removing cardigan | 1. *Dressing stick*–severe involvement (shoulder weakness, limited ROM and pain). Use shortest stick possible to encourage use of available ROM. (See Procedure for putting on a Cardigan with a Stocking Device.)<br><br>2. Insert extremity with the more limited ROM or with the more pain into sleeve first. | <br>*Dressing stick* |
|   B. Putting on and removing pullover garment | 1. If shoulders are severely involved (limited ROM, weakness, pain), with patient uunable to manage pullovers, recommend cardigans.<br><br>2. *U-shirts*–easier to manage than T-shirts.<br><br>3. *Front openings*–slit T-shirt or U-shirt in front and put in fastenings (velcro easiest). | *Velcro*<br>*Front openings* |
|   C. Putting on and removing bra | 1. Fasten back fastenings of bra in front and turn around (stretch bras are easiest to manage). Bra extensions can be added to allow more room for turning bra. | *Bra extension* |

240

2. *Front-fastening bras*–available commercially in department stores and Fashion-able catalog.

3. Velcro and D-ring front fastening.

4. Dressing stick can be used to push straps over shoulders.

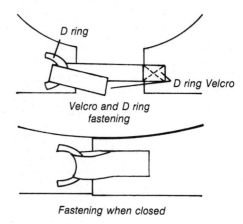

*Velcro and D ring fastening*

*Fastening when closed*

**. Putting on and removing slip**

1. Pull over feet while sitting in wheel chair (w/c), then stand to pull up or remain seated and lean from side to side and pull over hips.

2. Pull over feet when sitting in bed; pull up to buttocks, then lie down and roll from side to side and pull over hips.

3. *Slips with front zippers*–available commercially (Fashion-able catalog)

**. Putting on and removing dress**

1. *Dresses with front opening*–easiest to manage; recommend purchase of this type of dress to patients with severe involvement in upper extremities.

2. *Zipper pull*–assists in managing back or side zippers or fly.

3. *Velcro closings*–replaces buttons, but difficult to align so garment looks neat.

4. *Button hook*–assists patients with very severe hand deformities in managing buttons. Enlarged handle makes grasp easier.

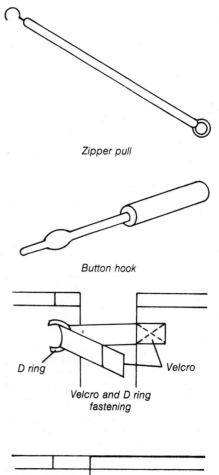

*Zipper pull*

*Button hook*

**. Putting on and removing trousers or slacks, skirts, and panties**

1. Pull over feet while sitting in bed. Using dressing stick, pull up to buttocks, then lie down and roll from side to side while pulling garment over hips.

2. Pull over feet while sitting in w/c, then stand to pull up or remain seated and lean from side to side and pull over hips.

3. *Fastenings–zipper pull* aids in zipping fly or other zippers. Elastic tops are easier for women. *Velcro* and a small D-ring may be used to replace hooks or top buttons on men's fly or shirt.

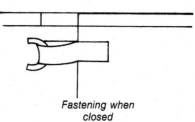

*Velcro and D ring fastening*

*Fastening when closed*

G. Putting on and re-
moving girdle

1. Difficult to manage if patient has pain, weakness, or deformities in hands.

2. Pantyhose are easiest to manage.

3. Garter belts are easier to manage if hand problems do not hinder fastening garters. Velcro fastenings can replace hook and eye fastenings.

4. Girdles without garters are easier to manage than those with garters but would still be difficult if hands are weak.

H. Putting on socks

*(See procedure for putting on a stocking with a sock cone)*

1. *Sock cone*—assists in putting on socks when hip and knee are painful or with limited ROM. Easiest to manage cone if patient can place cone on foot and then pull cone on with ropes. (Instead of placing cone on foot, patient can drop cone with ropes and maneuver cone over toes; however, this is more time consuming and often very frustrating.) Requires some grasp to pull ropes while putting sock on.

2. *Stocking device*—assists in putting on socks in patients with severe hip and knee ROM limitations who can only reach to knee. Requires good grasp and some ankle motion. (See Procedure For Using Stocking Device.)

I. Putting on shoes

1. *Long shoehorn*—assists in sliding foot into shoe when patient has difficulty or is unable to reach foot.

2. *Elastic shoelace*—eliminates need to tie shoe when patient is unable to reach foot; adjustable. Elasticity allows some give for edema; cuts down on opening of sore.
    (A shoeshop should sew corner of tongue to shoe to prevent it from sliding down in shoe.)

3. *Zipper shoelaces*—use if patient is unable to reach foot to tie shoe. Allows for wide opening. (Fasten zipper shoelace by punching 2 holes at bottom of tongue and lace zipper into shoe.)

4. If unable to reach zipper to zip, tie loop on zipper and zip with dressing stick.

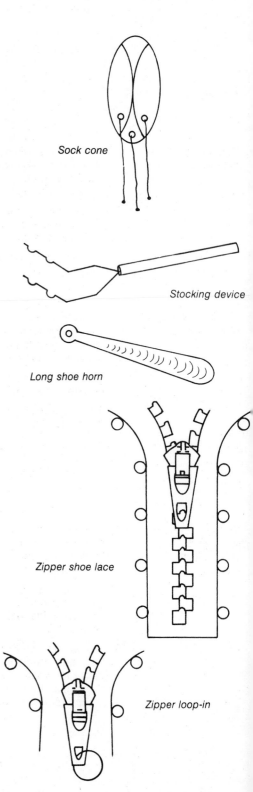

Sock cone

Stocking device

Long shoe horn

Zipper shoe lace

Zipper loop-in

# EQUIPMENT

| EQUIPMENT | DIAGRAM | USES |
|---|---|---|
| . Dressing stick | | Versatile, durable, inexpensive, and one of most valuable pieces of equipment for arthritic. Uses: reacher (pulling up pedals on w/c, getting clothes out of closet), assists in dressing (putting on and removing cardigan, pullover, trousers, socks and shoes). Construction: ½″ doweling to desired length, cup hook inserted in one end and coat hook inserted into opposite end. Portion of the hook that is parallel to dowel is bent to a 90° angle so it is then perpendicular to the dowel. (Bend before inserting hook in dowel.) |
| ². Zipperpull | | Substitutes for reaching back of dress, side or back of skirt, or fly of men's trousers. Requires some prehension to insert and remove hook. Advantage: can be put in before putting on garment. Disadvantages: must remove from zipper; particularly difficult to reach back of dress. Commercially available. |
| ³. Button hook | | Assists in buttoning buttons when prehension is severely limited. Handle can be enlarged to allow gross grasp. Commercially available. |
| ⁴. Sock cone | | Assists in putting on socks and nylons when hip and knee are painful or limited in ROM. Easiest to manage if patient can reach foot to place cone on toes and then pull on with ropes; otherwise, can drop cone with ropes and maneuver cone over toes with rope. Requires some grasp to pull sock cone on with ropes. Construction: See "How to Make a Sock Cone from Naugahyde." |
| ⁵. Stocking device | | Assists in putting on socks and nylons for those with severe hip and knee ROM limitations that limit reach to the knee. Requires good grasp and some ankle motion. Commercially available. |
| ⁶. Long shoehorn | | Assists in sliding foot into shoe when patient has difficulty or is unable to reach foot to put on shoe. Commercially available. |
| ⁷. Elastic shoelaces | | Similar to shoelace but elastic. Allows patient to slide foot into shoe and eliminates need to tie shoes. Opening of shoe somewhat restricted unless he can reach down to adjust the metal stop on the shoe lace. May allow too much motion of foot in shoe. Commercially available. |
| ⁸. Zipper shoelace | | (Zipper laces lace into 5 and 6 hole shoes). Allows a wide opening to insert foot. Patient can zip shoe using dressing stick if unable to reach foot. Eliminates need to tie shoes, at same time allows full shoe opening, but shoe will also fit snugly when zipped. Commercially available. |

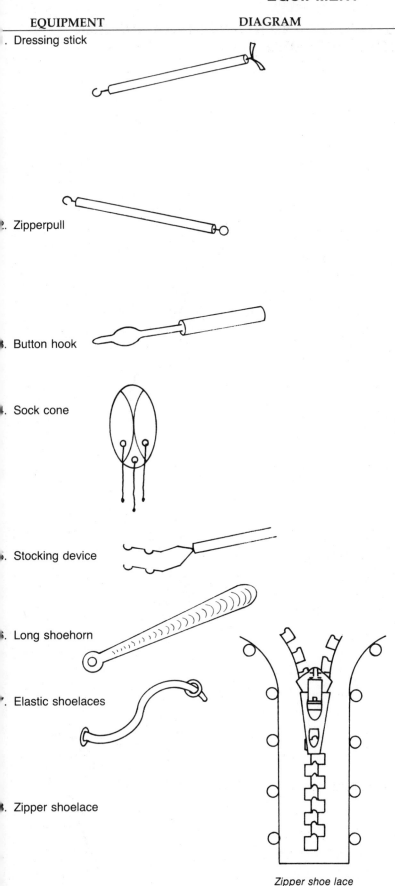

*Zipper shoe lace*

## PROCEDURE FOR PUTTING ON AND REMOVING A CARDIGAN WITH A DRESSING STICK

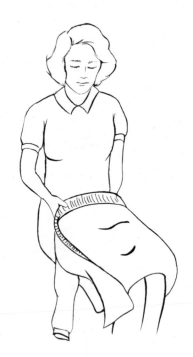

*(Person should be sitting or standing.)*
1. Position the cardigan on your lap with the *back* of the cardigan *up* and the collar toward you. The label is facing down.

2. Put your left arm in the left sleeve and pull the sleeve up so it is above your elbow. (For a shirt, start with the right arm and reverse the procedure. This is necessary to use the buttonholes, which are opposite for men.)

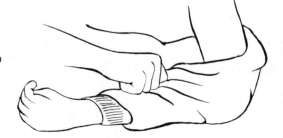

3. Place the hook of the dressing stick in the top buttonhole of the cardigan.

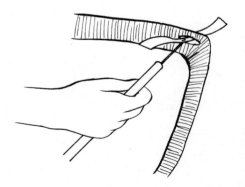

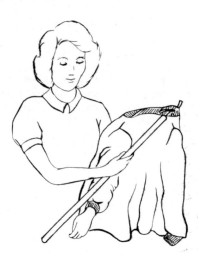

4. Maintain the hook of the dressing stick in the button hole and hang onto the opposite end of the stick.

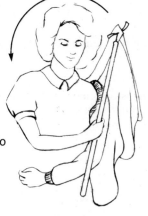
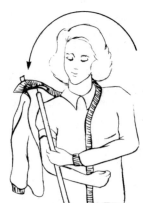

5. A. Circle the stick over your head and around behind you to the right.

   B. This will bring the right sleeve around toward the right shoulder.

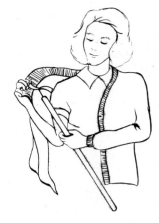

6. Remove the dressing stick from the buttonhole.

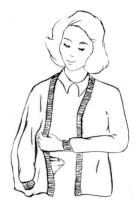

7. Pull the remainder of the cardigan around to the front.

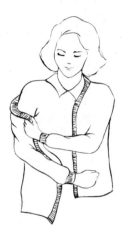

8. Put your arm in the right armhole. (If the cardigan is restricting this step, push the cardigan off the right shoulder to get the armhole low enough to insert your arm. If necessary, use the dressing stick to push the cardigan off the shoulder.)

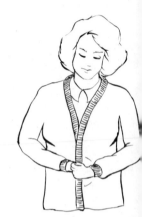

9. Pull the sleeve up on your right arm and pull the cardigan around to the front.

10. If the back of the cardigan is up, slide forward in the chair and either push it down with the dressing stick or wiggle to make it fall down in place.

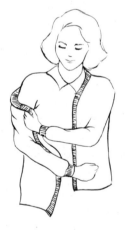

11. To *remove* the cardigan, slide it off the right shoulder. (Reverse the procedure for shirts because buttonholes are on the opposite side.) Use the dressing stick for this step if necessary.

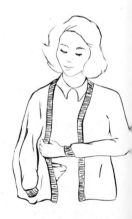

12. Slide the right sleeve off the right arm.

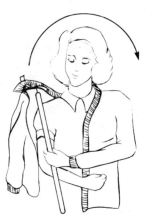

13. Place the hook of the dressing stick in the top buttonhole of the cardigan. Maintain the hook of the dressing stick in the buttonhole and hang onto the opposite end of the stick.

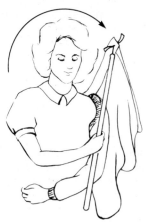

14. Circle the stick over your head and around behind you to the left to remove the cardigan.

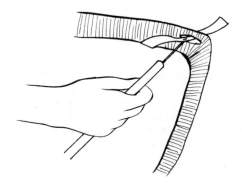

15. Remove the dressing stick from the buttonhole.

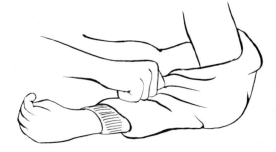

16. Slide the cardigan off the left arm and remove the cardigan.

# PROCEDURE FOR USING STOCKING DEVICE

*(Person should be sitting.)*

1. Tightly roll the top of the sock down to the heel *(A)*.

2. Turn the sock inside out, leaving the top of the sock rolled down.

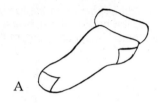

A

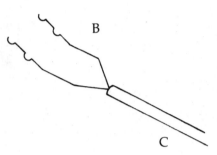

B

C

3. Lay the stocking device in your lap with the wire end away from you. Turn the stocking device so that the wire part comes up as shown in the illustration.

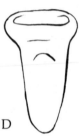

4. Keep the sock inside out. Position the sock so the toe is down and the heel is up and toward you *(D)*. It is critical that the heel is in this position when putting the sock on the device.

D

5. Place the sock on the wires so the rolled part of the sock fits in the "U-shaped" grooves. Push the wires together while putting on the sock. Begin by putting the rolled part of the sock on the two grooves nearest the handle *(E)*. Continue to push the top of the sock over the wire until the sock slips into the other two grooves *(F)*.

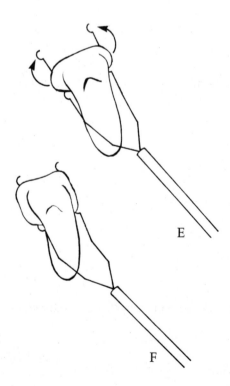

E

F

6. Turn the stocking device over so the angle is now down *(G)*.

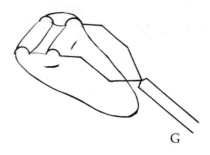

7. Leaving sock on the stocking device and holding the stocking device with the angle still downward, push the toe of the sock through so the sock is right side out *(H)*.

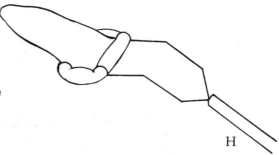

8. Holding onto wooden handle, lower the sock with the angle still downward and insert foot in the opening of the sock. If you have ankle motion, move your ankle up and down as you push your foot in the sock *(I)*.

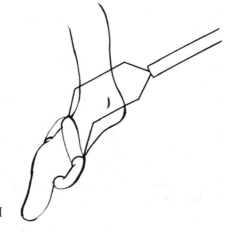

9. Pull the sock up over heel. If you have difficulty getting the sock over the heel of your foot, push the handle forward and scoop the end of the sock under the heel, pushing down and forward on the handle *(J)*.

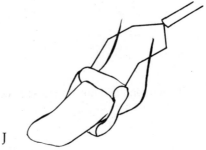

10. Pull up on the handle to pull the top of the sock up. Pull the sock off the stocking device. If you are unable to get the sock off the stocking device, use a dressing stick. Let go of the stocking device handle and use the dressing stick to slide the sock off the stocking device *(L)*.

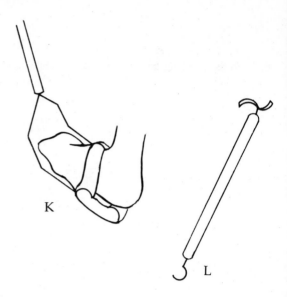

## PUTTING ON A STOCKING WITH A SOCK CONE

1. Roll the sock cone.

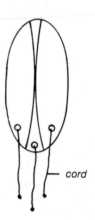

2. Powder the inside of the rolled cone so the cone will slide on the foot. Keep the cone rolled.

3. Gather the stocking and pull on the sock cone. The heel should be toward the floor.

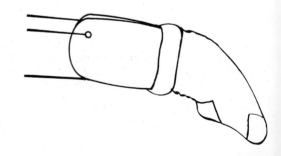

4. Pull the stocking on so the toe of the stocking is onto the tip of the sock cone. The cuff of the stocking should only be up to 2/3 the sock cone.

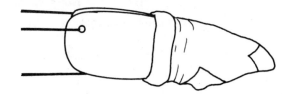

5. Grasp the toe of the stocking and sock cone so the heel of the stocking is toward the floor and place the sock cone under your foot.

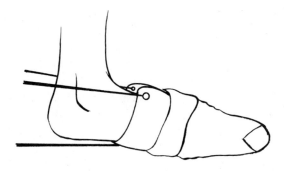

6. Grasp the three cords in both hands and pull the sock cone on with the cords. If possible, move your ankle up and down to help get the sock cone on. (If the sock cone should come out of the stocking before you have the stocking on, start over and try not pulling so hard on the cords and holding your ankle down and wiggling it in that position.)

7. Once the stocking is over your heel, pull the sock cone out slowly; this should pull the stocking top up.

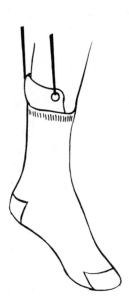

# HOW TO MAKE A SOCK CONE FROM NAUGAHYDE

A. Materials needed
1. Naugahyde

2. Grommet setter

3. Grommet posts and washers

4. 1/8″ clothesline rope

5. Hammer

6. Scissors

> If you do not have grommets available, stitch around the holes several times with a sewing machine to reinforce the holes.

7. Punch

8. Pencil

9. Pattern

B. Procedure
1. Trace around the pattern onto the naugahyde twice so the two wrong sides will fit together.

2. Cut out pattern.

3. Stitch the two pieces together with the right sides out. If you wish, you may bind the edges with tape.

4. Mark three holes for grommets: one at the top (wide end) about 3/4″ down from edge and one on each side (3/4″ from edge).

5. Place the post of the grommet in the hole.

6. Turn the sock cone over to the other side.

7. Check the grommet washer—one side of center is slightly raised. This raised side should be up (facing you) as you place it on top of the grommet post.

8. Hold grommet parts together and place the sock cone on the grommet base.

9. Take the other part of the grommet set and place inside post; hit with a hammer several times until post and washer are secure.

10. Cut three pieces of rope or heavy yarn to desired length. (It depends on how far the patient can reach.)

11. Insert rope or yarn through the grommet holes and tie or put a knot on the end.

12. Make loops on other end for the patient to hold and pull on while putting on the sock.

# SPECIAL CONSIDERATIONS FOR ARTHRITIC HOMEMAKERS

Homemaking activities of the arthritic can be an excellent medium for continuing therapy in the home situation. The therapist attempts to maintain joint motion, prevent fixation of joints, relieve pain, and maintain muscle strength. Flexion contractures are typical of patients who have hand involvement. Increased trauma on joints results from weight bearing and pushing on knuckles.

The following suggestions can be introduced in the homemaking training program:

### Avoid Overweight

Knees and ankles are particularly affected by excess weight. Attention to diet and means of maintaining good nutrition is a specific need. The physician's recommendations for any diet restrictions should be followed.

### Avoid Fatigue

Simplified methods of work and good work schedules will help, but work should not be minimized to the point where the necessary exercise is not possible. The degree to which this is emphasized should be considered in relation to the age and responsibilities of the arthritic. Many older arthritics need encouragement to do more.

In general, the arthritic should be encouraged to change position frequently, to change chairs, and to alternate sitting with standing.

*Avoid Increasing Flexion Deformities in the Hands*

Work with fingers extended in pushing up from a chair, pushing drawers shut, using a sponge, using dusting mitts, using a rolling pin.

To overcome the typical ulnar deviation (hand turned toward the little finger side), screw tops off with the right hand, on with the left, and turn rotary egg beater backward, beating counterclockwise.

*Include Exercise*

Be guided by physician's recommendations, not the complaints of the patient. If increased pain continues for 24 hours or if swelling is markedly increased, check with the physician. Remember that the arthritic has "good" and "bad" days, which may occur whether or not there has been more exercise than usual.

Reaching is helpful to encourage shoulder flexion and elbow extension. Bending encourages flexion and extension of the knees, hips, and back.

Kitchen arrangements can be planned to encourage these types of exercise but natural limits must also be considered.

*Adjustment to Limitations*

Select chairs that are slightly higher and firmer.
Select devices that will increase reaching distance.
Use wheeled vehicles to avoid the necessity of lifting and carrying.
Minimize fine finger motions.
Adjust the size of handles on utensils for a safe, comfortable grip.
Adjust the angle of the grip to accommodate to any fixed position of the hand.

# ARTHRITIS CLINIC CLASS

There are basic principles of motion that, if you use them consistently, will help control some of the changes caused by arthritis. These principles are listed, and underneath each are a few examples, showing how they can be applied to your daily life. Try to keep the idea of correct motion in mind as you work during the day and use these motions in as many situations as you can.

I. To help control outward turning of wrist and fingers (ulnar deviation):

A. *When using a twisting motion always turn hand toward thumb.* Examples: Turning doorknobs, keys in locks, screwing jar lids on and off, wringing clothes.

B. When lifting objects, place side of hand on table as object is grasped. Example: Lifting glass or dish.

II. To help control bending (flexion) of finger joints:
*Place fingers flat against surface.* Examples: Washing dishes, dusting, wiping table, cleaning sink or tub.

III. To help maintain or increase motion of shoulder, elbow, and wrist:
*Use long, smooth strokes.* Examples: Ironing, dusting, or polishing furniture, using push broom or vacuum cleaner, washing windows, painting.

IV. To conserve your strength:

A. *Push or roll heavy objects when possible, rather than lifting them.*
Casters added to a small table will help you save many steps as well as decrease the amount of lifting or carrying.

B. *Sit rather than stand when possible.*
During meal preparation, peeling, mixing, and other procedures can be done while sitting. When ironing, lower board to a height that is comfortable for sitting; have a chair or table nearby on which to hang or stack ironed clothes.

C. *Use lightweight kitchen equipment* (aluminum or plastic). *Stack only those things that are the same size.*

D. *Place kitchen equipment at the place where it is first used.* Examples: Pans for cooking vegetables near water. Baking utensils (bowls, measuring cups, spoons) near flour, sugar.

E. *Reduce the amount of bending you must do.*
Use long-handled brushes, dustpan.

# 14

# The Hand

## Evaluation of the Hand and Its Function

*by Dora A. Sorell, M.D.*

The hand is an intricate instrument of grasp and expression, capable of perceiving the most subtle stimuli of various kinds. Adequate evaluation of hand function is complex and multifaceted. A systematic didactic approach is presented.

### INSPECTION

Alteration in the contours and form of bony and muscular tissue is readily identifiable. Some aspects of hand problems are so obvious that diagnosis can be easily made by inspection only, e.g., atrophy, wrist drop, edema, rheumatoid deformities, and color changes. Other changes in the appearance of the hand are more subtle and reflect specific nerve involvement (e.g., "simian hand" and "guttering") and only familiarity with nerve injuries will permit us to recognize them.

### RANGE OF MOTION

Restoration of the range of motion of the hand is one of the more common problems in rehabilitation. Range of motion of finger joints may be limited or even lost after injury because of edema, hematoma, ecchymosis, infection, or immobilization. Weakness, pain, causalgia, and impaired blood supply are additional causes and are very effective in producing contractures.

Each joint must be examined separately. The combined range of motion of multiple joints is then determined, first with full wrist flexion, then with full wrist extension. The difference between these two measurements of each joint defines the amount of joint limitation caused by tendon shortening or scarring.

The range of motion may be estimated with the practiced eye or measured with a goniometer. Pain, edema, or spasticity will cause *limitation of motion*, which can vary from day to day or from one examiner to another, and therefore should be mentioned in the patient's chart. *Contractures*, however, can be measured with greater accuracy and recorded periodically.

After measuring the range of motion of individual joints, more functional assessments should then be made, such as combined finger and metacarpophalangeal joint (MCP) extension, pulp-to-pulp pinch, and total flexion of fingers, the measurement being the distance from fingertips to palmar surface.

If the hand has to be immobilized for any reason in plaster, splint, or bandage, it is imperative that one know the *position of function* of the hand, since contracture in that position will be least detrimental to function. This position is 20 degrees of wrist dorsiflexion, 45 degrees of metaphalangeal flexion, 30 degrees of proximal interphalangeal (PIP) flexion, and 20 degrees of distal interphalangeal (DIP) flexion. The thumb should oppose the index and third finger with a few degrees of interphalangeal flexion. The elbow should be in 90 degrees of flexion and midposition between pronation and supination.

254

## STRENGTH

Function of the hand can be divided into prehensile and nonprehensile. The prehensile activities (grip) are the most important and are of infinite variety, but they can be grouped into a relatively small number of functional types. Napier has stressed stability as the fundamental requisite of prehension because the objects being held should be held securely. Stability combined with prehension gives two types of grip—power and precision—and this classification has been universally accepted.

*Power grip* is exemplified by holding a hammer. The strength of power grip is measured by dynamometer or by special grasp meters. The difference between the normal hand and the affected hand is of significance. A normal grip is 30 to 60 pounds, and it varies with age, occupation, and handedness.

*Precision grip,* exemplified by holding a needle, is measured by pinch meter, and the normal range is 12 to 18 pounds. Very broadly speaking, the median nerve is most important for precision, and the ulnar nerve for power.

Other patterns of grip have been described. They are palmar grasp, lateral grasp, fingertip pinch, three-jaw chuck, hook grasp, and cylindrical grasp. Most of them are actually variations of the power and the precision grips. Exceptions to this are lateral pinch and hook grip.

*Lateral pinch,* or *lateral grasp,* as in holding a key, requires the use of adductor pollicis and first dorsal interosseous muscles with assistance from the long flexor and extensors of the thumb and flexor digi-

**TABLE 14–1.** NERVE SUPPLY OF HAND

| NERVES | MOTIONS | MUSCLES |
|---|---|---|
| Median Nerve | Flexors (most) of wrist | Flexor carpi radialis<br>Palmaris longus |
| | of fingers | Flexor digitorum superficialis<br>Flexor digitorum profoundus ½<br>Flexor pollicis longus |
| | Thenar eminence | Abductor pollicis brevis<br>Opponens pollicis<br>Flexor pollicis brevis |
| | Pronators | Pronator teres<br>Pronator quadratus |
| Ulnar Nerve | Ulnar flexors of wrist<br>of fingers | Flexor carpi ulnaris<br>Flexor digitorum profundus ½ |
| | Hypothenar eminence | Abductor digiti minimi<br>Opponens digiti minimi<br>Flexor digiti minimi |
| | Intrinsic muscles of palm | Dorsal interossei<br>Palmar interossei<br>Lumbricals ½ |
| Radial Nerve | Extensors of elbow | Triceps |
| | of wrist | Extensor carpi radialis longus<br>Extensor carpi radialis brevis<br>Extensor carpi ulnaris |
| | of fingers | Extensor digitorum communis<br>Extensor indicis proprius<br>Extensor digiti minimi proprius |
| | of thumb | Extensor pollicis longus<br>Extensor pollicis brevis<br>Abductor pollicis longus |
| | Supinator | Supinator |

torum profundus. This grip is primarily a function of the ulnar nerve, and it is the only grip that is left in median nerve deficit. This grip is also present late in rheumatoid arthritis, even in the presence of severe ulnar drift and destruction of the metaphalangeal joint.

*Hook grip,* as in carrying a suitcase, requires the use of either or both long flexors of the four lesser digits. Therefore, in the absence of all of the hand intrinsic muscles, this function may be preserved. Interestingly enough, contracture of the same muscles, even in the absence of active motor power of both, may still allow this grip.

The nonprehensile functions of the hand are push, lift, and club use, which require no active motor power in the hand per se.

Independent free motion of each digit, as in typing and playing a musical instrument, depends upon integrated use of intrinsic muscles as well as extrinsic muscles of the hand; therefore, deficit of either group will compromise these skilled functions.

Strength of a given muscle or group of muscles is determined by the manual muscle test (MMT). The system used is a set of grades from 0 to 5; or O, T(race), P(oor), F(air), G(ood), and N(ormal). When the distribution of weakness is evaluated in any hand, the importance of grading each muscle becomes clear (see Table 14–1 on innervation of muscles and motions).

## JOINT STABILITY

The ligamentous and tendinous structures maintain the integrity of a given joint. In the absence of adequate support, the joint may become unstable and subluxed or even dislocated. This occurs in rheumatoid arthritis, in which weakening and stretching of the volar plate results in subluxation of the head of the metacarpal volarly, with subsequent dislocation of the proximal phalanx on the metacarpal bone. In this position, the cumulative forces of the long extensors and long flexors and gravity result in ulnar displacement of the distal ray, producing so-called *ulnar drift.*

Any weakening of supporting structures, whether by disease or by trauma, may result in a malposition of that joint, such that the forces exerted on that joint will result in deformity.

*Trigger finger* is a particular variety of tendon lesion. In this condition, because of rupture, tear, or swelling of the encasing external sheath, the normally fluid movements of the internal tendon are episodically limited.

## SENSORY EXAMINATION

Examination of sensibility requires an evaluation of the primary modes of sensation, which are touch, pain, and temperature, and two-point discrimination, which is the most sensitive of these, and it is altered first. The distribution of loss or deficit leads one to deduce the localization of lesion—whether affecting a single peripheral nerve or several, whether proximal or diffuse.

In recovery from nerve injury, the classical Tinel's sign is a reliable and helpful test to assess nerve regeneration.

## FUNCTION

The motor performance, the ability to carry out motor tasks, depends on several factors, some of which are highly individualized. They are motor power, integrity of sensory mechanism, and skill and psychological considerations such as learning capacity, reaction to pain, memory, and motivation. It is often surprising to see how patients with severely affected and deformed hands, as in rheumatoid arthritis, are still able to perform a wide range of functional activities.

There are specific functional deficits with involvement of each of the peripheral nerves (Table 14–2). Absence of the median nerve causes the

**TABLE 14–2.** FUNCTIONAL DISABILITY IN SPECIFIC NERVE LESIONS

| | |
|---|---|
| Median | Interference with precision grip (loss of pinch) |
| | Weakness of powergrip (loss of stabilizing action of thumb) |
| | Clumsiness (loss of sensation) |
| Ulnar | Power grip is most affected (inability to wrap fingers around an object, failure of elevation of hypothenar eminence, ineffective clamping action of the thumb—loss of adductor) |
| | Pinch is poor (instability of MP joint of thumb, loss of adductor) |
| | Writing is difficult (loss of sensation) |
| | Holding a knife is difficult (loss of adductor of thumb and of first degree dorsal interosseous) |
| | Difficulty with skilled movement, playing instruments (loss of intrinsics) |
| Radial | Grip is poor (lack of stabilization at the wrist) |
| | Difficulty with most functional activities (because of wrist drop) |

greatest functional impairment because grasp, pinch, and opposition capabilities depend on this nerve. Loss of the ulnar nerve precludes finely coordinated activities because the intrinsic muscles supply joint stability. There are, however, substitutions or "trick movements" available when one nerve only is damaged that will result in function, however altered.

The mechanism of these substitutions varies; ulnar nerve paralysis gives one of the best known "trick motions," which is called Froment's sign. To compensate for the inability to adduct the thumb and abduct the index finger, as in holding a newspaper, the patient substitutes with the long flexor of the thumb.

In radial nerve paralysis, using the rebound effect of the wrist and finger flexors will simulate extensor action. Also, the effect of gravity can simulate wrist extension. Pinch that is lost in median nerve injury at the wrist can be substituted for by lateral pinch. In high median nerve injury with loss of long flexors, if the tendons become shortened through the process of constant length phenomenon, wrist extension will result in increased finger flexion.

## DEXTERITY

This is the ability to perform skillful motion needed at work, in activities of daily living, or in hobbies. Dexterity is impaired in the presence of weakness, pain, incoordination from any neurological disease, sensory deficit, or even as a result of disuse.

The patient is tested in special activities or with standardized dexterity tests (pegboard test), the measure of dexterity being the time in seconds it takes the subject to complete the task.

## REST OF UPPER EXTREMITY

The hand is directed to its destination for function by shoulder and elbow motions. Thus, any disease or traumatic condition that limits the ability of the shoulder or elbow to deliver the hand appropriately will interfere with hand function. The shoulder can also become secondarily involved in many hand and forearm conditions that require immobilization for healing (fracture) or for relief of pain (rheumatoid arthritis). Frozen shoulder may develop, and prevention of it is paramount.

## SYSTEMIC MANIFESTATION

Some systemic conditions may produce primary manifestations in the hand. There are others (rheumatoid arthritis, systemic lupus erythematosus) in which many systems are involved simultaneously. They should be recognized because of their influence on the management and outcome of the hand problem.

## PSYCHOSOCIAL IMPLICATIONS

A hand injury does more than interfere with hand function—it affects the personality. The total patient must be evaluated and treated, with his complex needs and expectation recognized. Additionally, the long-term effects of the hand dysfunction on the patient and his family, along with its effect on his ability to earn a living, must be considered at the initial evaluation.

Occasionally, the hand problem results from a maladjusted behavior pattern such as drug abuse, depression, or destructive behavior. In these instances, inclusion of these issues as well is part of the rehabilitation program.

Contrariwise, the person who has already been victimized by chronic and increasingly debilitating insults may be psychologically unable to deal with just one small additional insult.

Industrial accidents are a particular problem because of their frequency, severity, and implications. The loss of earning capacity, the degree of impairment, the remaining skills and abilities, as well as vocational needs, should be recognized as early as possible.

Adequate documentation of present status and of progress made is essential. The records of range of motion, manual muscle test, grip strength, functional attainment, and activities of daily living, when accurate and consistent, give a quantitative estimate of the progress and are most helpful to the examiner and encouraging to the patient.

# Rehabilitation of the Burned Hand

*by Joji Sakuma, M.D.*

The rehabilitation objective of the burned hand is to restore optimal hand function as rapidly as possible and to prevent fixed deformities from developing.

All patients with hand burns except minor superficial burns should be admitted to a hospital so that they can receive comprehensive rehabilitation by a team of health professionals from the day of the injury. Even when the patient is critically ill, the initiation of rehabilitation care of the hand should not be delayed.

## PROGNOSTIC FACTORS FOR FUNCTION

**Depth of the Burn.** All superficial partial-thickness burns heal with good quality of skin, but deep partial- and full-thickness burns heal with poor quality of skin and frequent hypertrophic scar, resulting in poor appearance and function and deformities unless early excision and grafting are done.

**Location of the Burn.** The most commonly burned area is the dorsum of the hand. Because the dorsal skin is thin, extensor tendons and periarticular structure are more susceptible to injury with subsequent deformities. Deep burn on the palm is less common but can cause a palmar contracture.

**Cooperation of the Patient.** The functional outcome may be unsatisfactory in young children and in elderly and very ill patients who cannot cooperate in an active program and must be treated by passive measures.

## RESIDUAL HAND DEFORMITIES

The specific exercise and splinting should be based on an understanding of the mechanism of different deformities that may develop without proper rehabilitation care.

*Claw deformity* consists of metacarpophalangeal extension and proximal interphalangeal flexion, and is most common after a dorsal hand burn. Metacarpophalangeal hyperextension is caused by wrist flexion as a result of pain, distention of dorsal skin by edema, rigid eschar, and contraction of granulation tissue. This in turn leads to interphalangeal flexion without destruction of the central slip by tightening of transverse lamina.

*Boutonnière deformity* consists of proximal interphalangeal flexion with distal interphalangeal extension and is caused by destruction of the central slip over the proximal interphalangeal joint either directly by the burn or by secondary infection. It is usually combined with claw deformity.

*Web space adduction deformity* may be due to contracture of the skin only or additional muscle contracture. Digits may be fused.

*Palmar contracture* results from deep palmar burn and may be combined with *flexion deformities of all three finger joints* by the wound contraction and pull of the flexor tendon.

*Hypertrophic scar* usually results from deeper burns that are left to heal spontaneously. Its contraction causes adduction deformities and reversal of transverse arch when the scar is in the dorsum of the hand.

## BASIC METHODS OF REHABILITATION MANAGEMENT

**Early Motion.** To reduce edema and maintain mobility and function, active motion of the hand and proximal joints of the upper extremity should start as soon as the patient can cooperate after the burn and as soon as allowed after the skin grafting and other surgical procedures. Whenever active motion is indicated, the patient should be encouraged to use the hand in daily activities with the splint removed. When the skin or tendon is weakened by burn, possibly harmful passive motion and overstretching should be avoided.

To protect weakened extensor tendons over proximal interphalangeal joints from rupture, the simultaneous flexion of all finger joints as in making a full fist or on passive stretching should be avoided in deep partial- and full-thickness burns.

**Elevation.** To reduce edema the hand should be elevated for the first few days after the burn and as long as the edema remains after the surgical procedures. The splinted hand can be elevated by pillows or by a stockinette attached to an intravenous pole.

**Splinting.** To prevent fixed deformities, joints should be positioned by the splint in the opposite direction of the anticipated deformities, namely in the so-called "antideformity" position and not in the classical "functional" position. However, this exaggerated preventive positioning may have to be compromised in severe hand burn because of restricted mobility caused by edema and unyielding tissue. Frequent adjustment may be necessary as the edema subsides. It should be removed as soon as the patient can perform active exercise adequately.

The basic splint for a dorsal hand burn is a static palmar splint, made of thermoplastic material such as Orthoplast, that maintains the wrist in 30 to 40 degrees extension, metacarpophalangeal joints in 70 to 90 degrees flexion, proximal interphalangeal and distal interphalangeal joints in extension, and the thumb in opposition with a large web space.

**Hydrotherapy.** Whirlpool or Hubbard tank baths may be useful in wound cleansing, debridement, and underwater exercise. Bath water should be mixed with a bactericidal agent such as household bleach (5.25 per cent sodium hypochlorite) in 1:60 dilution, or in 1:120 dilution if too painful. After the bath the hand should be thoroughly rinsed. The temperature of the bath should be 38 to 41° C (100 to 105° F) for whirlpool, and 35 to 37° C (95 to 98° F) for Hubbard tank; the duration of the bath is 15 to 20 minutes. A lower temperature and shorter duration should be used when the new graft develops venous congestion.

**Compression Garment.** To reduce hypertrophic scar in deeper burns an elastic glove is beneficial for the hand and fingers and a gauntlet for the hand and wrist. They should be fitted with 35 mm Hg of compressive pressure as soon as a good dry skin develops. They should be worn continuously except when bathing for at least six months or more until the scar tissue or graft matures.

## REHABILITATION PROGRAM OF DORSAL HAND BURN

### Very Superficial (First-Degree) and Superficial Partial-Thickness (Superficial Second-Degree) Burn

Except for small first-degree burn with minimal pain and edema with which the patient can perform adequate active exercise, the hand should be positioned in a basic dorsal burn splint, elevated, and actively exercised in combinations of all joint motions from the day of admission.

### Deep Partial Thickness (Deep Second-Degree) and Full-Thickness (Third-Degree) Burn

Early surgical excision and immediate or delayed grafting is the treatment of choice. During the preoperative period, the hand should be splinted and elevated. In exercising the fingers, only one joint should be flexed at a time while two other joints of the same finger are kept extended.

In the immediate postoperative period the hand should be rigidly immobilized for seven to ten days either by a new paddle-shaped splint or by a modified basic splint with an added platform for the fingers and extension for the thumb. The tips of fingers and thumb are attached to the splint by rubber bands through dress hooks glued to nails or by stainless steel suture wires passed through the tips of the distal phalanx. The splint is wrapped only on the forearm with gauze bandage.

In the later postoperative period after the splint is removed, active exercise is resumed. Before discharge from the hospital the patient and family should be instructed in a long-term home program. Continued follow-up care by the team is essential after discharge to help the patient regain optimal hand function and return to as normal a life as before.

# Hand Orthoses

*by P. Mukkamala, M.D.*

The indications for the use of an orthosis are: (1) Relief of pain by providing rest to the part by support of the joints, by limitation of motion and by elimination of unwanted motion. (2) Prevention and correction of a deformity caused by muscle imbalance, spasticity, arthritis (see chapter 13), infection, and injury. (3) Protection of healing tissues such as after tendon surgery. (4) Substitution or addition of function by assisting weak muscles.

## TYPES OF ORTHOSES

There are static and dynamic orthoses.

A static orthosis does not permit any motion and basically serves the purpose of supporting the anatomical part. Figure 14–1 shows a static splint with the wrist and hand in a functional position.

A dynamic or functional orthosis permits or facilitates motion and may have powered compo-

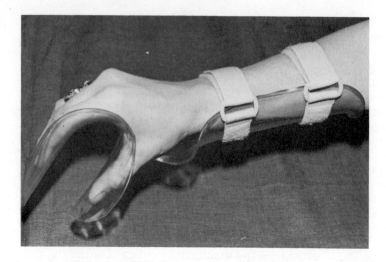

Figure 14–1. Static splint.

nents. The functions of static and dynamic orthoses overlap, and a given orthosis may serve as a static orthosis at one joint and a dynamic one at another.

### Wrist Orthoses

The wrist should be splinted in functional position, which is partial dorsiflexion, to facilitate optimal function of the finger flexors. This is the position of choice when the finger flexors are weak. However, if the finger extensors are weak, the wrist should be splinted in a neutral position or slight flexion to put the finger extensors under slight stretch. A volar splint is more commonly used than a dorsal one. However, if flexor spasticity is severe and if there is concern that a volar splint will aggravate the spasticity, a dorsal splint may be preferable. If an outrigger is needed, its position determines whether the orthosis should be volar or dorsal.

**Bunnel Cock-up Wrist Splint.** This consists of a forearm trough that is bound to the forearm by straps. From the forearm trough a spring metal extends into the palm to support the hand and an outrigger can be attached to the forearm trough. The hand support should not extend beyond the distal palmar crease so as not to obstruct the motion of metacarpophalangeal joints. A Bunnel-Oppenheimer variety with knuckle bender splint is shown in Figure 14–2.

**Long Opponens Orthosis.** This is essentially similar to the short opponens orthosis described in the following discussion with a forearm extension to stabilize the wrist (Fig. 14–3).

### Hand Orthoses

**Short Opponens Orthosis.** The opponens orthosis is designed to maintain stability, assist function, or provide opposition by stabilizing the fingers in a functional position. The patient is then able to use active muscle power to grasp objects in the three-jaw chuck prehension pattern. It can be used as a basic splint to which activities of daily living adaptive pockets, outriggers, and assistive

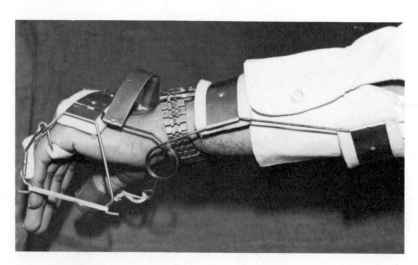

Figure 14–2. Bunnel-Oppenheimer wrist splint.

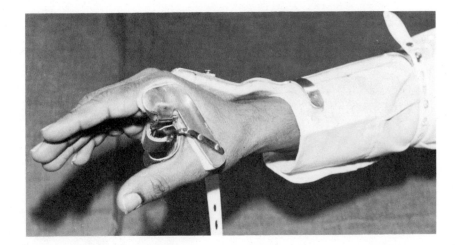

**Figure 14–3.** Long opponens orthosis.

devices may be added. It can be custom made of aluminum or plastic and consists of dorsal, palmar, opponens, and "C" bars. The dorsal and palmar bar is designed to support the palmar arch and should not extend beyond the metacarpophalangeal joints. The opponens bar formed by a radial extension to the dorsal and palmar bar applies forces to the ulnar side directed over the first metacarpal, thereby maintaining the thumb in a preset opposition position to the index and middle fingers. It serves as a first metacarpal extension stop.

The "C" bar maintains the web space between the thumb and the palm and stabilizes the thumb. The "C" bar is set with the thumb in minus 35 degrees adduction stop. A wrist strap holds the orthosis on the hand. A lumbrical bar can be attached to the orthosis, which pre-positions the fingers in 30-degree flexion at the metacarpophalangeal joints and serves as metacarpophalangeal extension stop (Fig. 14–4). In intrinsic muscle weakness, there is metacarpophalangeal hyperextension and interphalangeal flexion on attempting prehension. The lumbrical bar places the long finger flexors in a mechanical advantage. If there is weakness of long extensors, metacarpophalangeal extension assist can be provided by suspending proximal phalanges of fingers with rubber bands from an outrigger attached to the orthosis. If there is weakness of intrinsic muscles and long extensors, metacarpophalangeal extension stop can be used with interphalangeal extension assist by suspending distal phalanges of fingers with rubber bands from an outrigger.

**Knuckle Bender Splint.** The splint is used to stretch extension contractures at the metacarpophalangeal joints. It is formed by joining one plate over the dorsum of the hand and another over the dorsum of the fingers through linked wires to a palmar bar. The stretching force is provided by rubber bands, which can be varied by changing their size and strength. The joints being stretched should be set in a position of approximately 5 degrees less than that which causes pain. As the tissues yield, the position should be adjusted. The

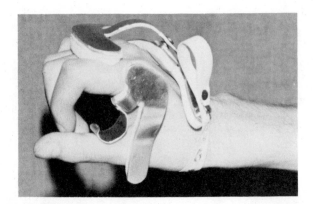

**Figure 14–4.** Short opponens orthosis.

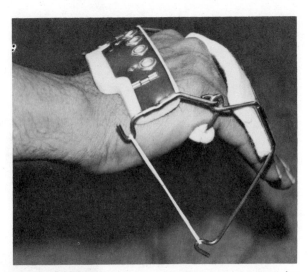

**Figure 14–5.** Knuckle bender splint allowing contraction of antagonistic muscles.

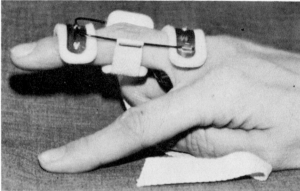

**Figure 14–6.** Finger bender splint.

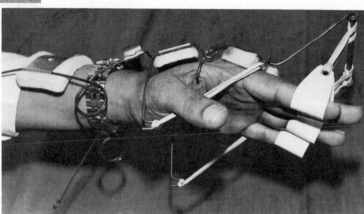

**Figure 14–7.** Outrigger with finger loops.

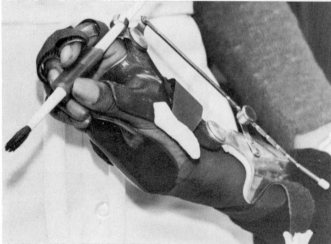

**Figure 14–8.** Wrist extensor tenodesis orthosis.

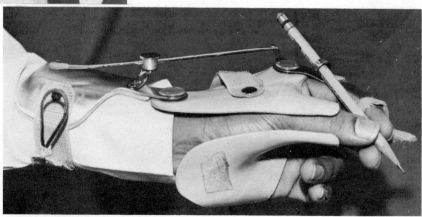

Figure 14–9.

antagonist muscles should be strong enough so that when the stretch becomes uncomfortable the patient can get relief by contracting the antagonistic muscles (Fig. 14–5). In flexion contracture of metacarpophalangeal joints, a reverse knuckle bender splint can be used. The design is the same as the knuckle bender splint, except the tractive force is reversed. Based on the same principle, a finger bender splint can be used to stretch interphalangeal joints (Fig. 14–6). When individual finger traction is needed, an outrigger with finger loops suspended with rubber bands can be attached to any basic splint (Fig. 14–7).

**Flexor Hinge Orthosis.** This orthosis is useful for paralysis of all finger flexor muscles but may also be used in the presence of paralysis of both flexors and extensors. It is a hinge orthosis that aligns the thumb in opposition to the index and middle fingers in a three-jaw chuck pattern. The placement of the finger flexor hinge at the level of the second metacarpophalangeal joint is very critical to avoid riding up and down of the digital component as the fingers open and close. The digital unit is connected to the forearm through a palmar segment with a hinge placed at the level of the second metacarpophalangeal joint and another placed at the level of the wrist.

The following are examples of this type of orthosis. *The elastic flexor assist* is the simplest of all in this category in which a flexor force is provided by the use of rubber bands. It is essential that the opposing extensors should have adequate strength to oppose the flexor power of the rubber bands in order to open the pinch pattern of the orthosis.

*The wrist extensor tenodesis orthosis* is based on the principles of surgical tenodesis in which the finger flexor muscles are surgically attached to the radius and thereby active wrist extension causes the fingers to close. The forearm component is connected to a digital component by a bar linkage through the palmar component. Active wrist extension opposes the thumb to the fingers. If the wrist flexors are effective, release of grasp can be achieved by wrist flexion, otherwise relaxation of the wrist extensors with the help of gravity will release the grasp. The wrist extensors must have better than fair muscle power to achieve a useful pinch by this orthosis. C6-spared quadriplegic patients can use this type of orthosis with great benefit (Figs. 14–8 and 9). High-level quadriparetic patients with severe weakness of the wrist extensors have to derive power from external sources to activate the digital components of this orthosis. The external power can be electric or pneumatic, or the patient's own proximal muscle power can be harnessed and transmitted through a cable.

# Management of Shoulder-Hand Syndrome

*by Catherine Hinterbuchner, M.D.*

The shoulder-hand syndrome is frequently encountered in physiatric practice associated with stroke, fractures of the upper extremity, and other major or minor trauma to the upper extremity. Approximately 20 to 30 per cent of hemiplegic patients may develop shoulder-hand syndrome in the ipsilateral extremity. Occasionally, there is no recognizable precipitating factor or associated disorder (see Chapters 2 and 4).

## DIAGNOSIS

Early diagnosis offers the best opportunity for successful management. Awareness of the existence of this syndrome and the frequency of its occurrence, particularly in strokes, may lead to early diagnosis. It should be suspected immediately upon the appearance of incipient edema of the hemiplegic hand. This is associated with pain upon movement of the hand and the wrist, and there is usually pain of the shoulder. The full-blown clinical picture includes hyperpathia, changes in the color of the skin consisting of either pallor or cyanosis, and changes in temperature of the hand, which may be either hot or cold. Other symptoms are dyshidrosis manifested by sweating in the active phase and dryness in the late phase, subcutaneous nodules, atrophy of the skin and muscles with subcutaneous periarticular fibrosis, and contractures with limited range of motion. There is early radiographic evidence of osteoporosis.

The clinical course varies in severity from a mild self-limited form to a very severe intractable and unremitting form. Most cases respond to stellate ganglion blocks or systemic administration of corticosteroids; however, some cases show only partial recovery or no response at all, becoming a most difficult problem of management.

## MANAGEMENT METHODS

Sympathetic blocks are usually administered in series daily or every other day, but may be administered continuously for several hours or days. When administered early in the course of the syndrome, 10 to 12 blocks may be necessary, although on occasion we have administered as many as 15 to 17 blocks. I recommend that sympathetic blocks be performed on an inpatient basis and that environmental stimulation be confined to a minimum to enhance the effect of the block (see Chapter 7).

Steroids when administered should be given in sufficient doses to control the pain. The usually recommended dose is 30 mg of prednisone per day divided into three equal doses continued for two to three weeks and then tapered slowly.

Patients with mild to moderately severe cases respond well to one course of steroids, but those with more severe cases may suffer relapse as soon as the steroids are withdrawn, or the condition may recur shortly thereafter, necessitating additional courses of therapy.

In patients with intractable and unremitting cases of shoulder-hand syndrome in whom both sympathetic blocks and use of steroids have failed to arrest progression, sympathectomy must be considered and should be performed as soon as possible. In patients in whom sympathectomy is performed late in the course of this syndrome, the response may be either questionable or only partial. Following sympathectomy, patients may develop denervation hypersensitivity leading to more pain.

Other therapeutic measures have been used in the management of severe shoulder-hand syndrome. Systemic administration of intravenous procaine at doses of 4 mg per kg of body weight for 20 minutes has been used, the frequency of which depends on the patient's response to it. Regional sympathetic blocks produced by use of intravenous guanethidine have been advocated by British authors. The U.S. Food and Drug Administration has recently approved the intravenous use of guanethidine in the United States for experimental purposes. Reports indicate that most patients respond well with relief of symptoms to only one such block but occasionally may require more than one.

Oral sympathetic blocking agents have also been employed in unremitting cases, but they require close supervision and titration of dosage to avoid side effects such as hypotension. Propranolol has been advocated but guanethidine, which acts on sympathetic terminals, is the drug of choice.

The use of sedatives, tranquilizers, and antidepressants has been described but should be prescribed judiciously, as some drugs may have an adverse effect on pain in this condition. Use of phenobarbitol has been thought to predispose to shoulder-hand syndrome and we have found it to exacerbate pain in this syndrome. On the other hand, we have found that diazepam, a central nervous system depressant, greatly improves pain in shoulder-hand syndrome and that its effect is dose-related. We recommend that use of any drugs be avoided in shoulder-hand syndrome unless a clear-cut indication exists either for the shoulder-hand syndrome or an unrelated medical condition.

Anticonvulsants such as carbamazepine (Tegretol) and diphenylhydantoin (Dilantin) have been given in shoulder-hand syndrome with reportedly good results.

Application of heat or cold has been advocated, but they should be used only when tolerated by the patient. Intolerance to either heat or cold may exist in shoulder-hand syndrome and in such cases the offending modality should be avoided.

Massage has been given with beneficial results and can be applied if tolerated by the patient.

Behavior modification, including biofeedback (see Chapter 9), has been advocated for the control of pain as it has been in chronic pain in general.

It should be stressed that in the management of the patient with shoulder-hand syndrome, it is important to decrease sensory stimulation to the painful area. Handling of the involved extremity should be avoided and physical examination should be carried out with care to limit stimulation to a minimum. Often the patient exhibits delayed pain reaction following such stimulation, which may last for long periods of time.

Garments such as gloves and sleeves must be fitted in such a way as to produce the least possible stimulation. To-and-fro movement of garments over the painful area should be avoided for the same reason.

Splints and slings may also increase pain through just plain contact. Instead of using these, we recommend that the patient be allowed to hold the hand in the most comfortable position and that he be encouraged to perform active range of motion. Passive range of motion should be avoided because it requires manipulation of the extremity, and stretching is contraindicated. These techniques merely reinforce the abnormal reflexes, increasing pain and they result in greater limitation of motion, which they were intended to prevent.

On the other hand, the patient should be encouraged to use the extremity actively, but given the fact that active motion also may aggravate pain, exercise should be strictly graded to avoid exacerbation of pain. The exercise should be limited to tolerance; at times this may be minimal.

We believe that a regimen designed to limit sensory stimulation and to encourage active use of the painful extremity will ultimately result in lesser residual disability with better range of motion and function of the hand than if the patient were put through an aggressive program of physical and occupational therapy as suggested in the literature.

In our series of patients with stroke, we have had an incidence of shoulder-hand syndrome of 26.8 per cent. This high incidence may be partly due to a high index of suspicion and the early recognition of even mild forms that can remit spontaneously. In our series, all patients were treated and responded with complete remission to series of stellate ganglion blocks, our preferred method of treatment. Not a single patient went on to an unremitting intractable course, which may be attributed at least in part to early diagnosis and the early institution of therapeutic measures (see Chapter 2).

# Rehabilitation of the Hand in Children
by Phoebe Saturen, M.D.

Management of hand problems in the pediatric age group requires assessment of the child's developmental status so that evaluation of function and coordination can be contrasted with normal growth patterns, and so that age-appropriate activities can be selected in planning therapy. For example: at six to seven months, the hands are open, objects are transferred, and the child can hold a bottle and finger feed. At 10 to 11 months, a neat pincer grasp has developed, while dominance emerges in the second year. At 48 months a child can copy a cross and manipulate buttons (Table 14–3).

Initiation of therapy as early as possible is an important principle in working with children. For example, it was once believed that a child had to be mature enough to cooperate—even of school age—before a prosthesis could be prescribed. It is now clear that acceptance and utilization of upper extremity aids have the best hope of success when fitted during infancy so that the device is incorporated into the "body schema." The optimal time for prescription of an upper extremity prosthesis is when the child can sit with support and can bring the hands to midline to manipulate objects.

Treatment of a young child requires ingenuity on the part of the therapist. A play setting should be established in which the materials and activities offered accomplish the desired goals, if a youngster cannot cooperate in the practice of isolated movements. Since a child will neglect and deny a painful, weak, or sensorially impaired hand and rapidly shift to one-handed function, toys must be selected that foster bimanual manipulation, such as large lightweight blocks and wind-up toys.

Splints for children must be light, strong, and made of nontoxic materials with straps firmly attached. Above-elbow suspension may be necessary so that the child cannot utilize his flexible joints and chubby subcutaneous tissue to wiggle free. Sensory feedback is essential, and if parts of the hand cannot be left uncovered, part-time use of the splint during the day should be considered.

## CONGENITAL DEFORMITIES

Some anomalies of the hand should be carefully noted in the course of pediatric assessment, not because they impair function, but because of their diagnostic implications. The *transverse palmar* or *"simian" crease* and *clinodactyly* have increased prevalence in many malformation syndromes.

Although many hand abnormalities are isolated, a strong association exists between *abnormalities of the radial ray* and significant visceral anomalies. Hand pathology can vary in severity from total agenesis of the radius producing the radial club hand to mild proximal displacement of the thumb caused by first metacarpal hypoplasia. Radial club hand is seen with congenital aplastic anemia or renal abnormalities, while other radial deficiencies

**TABLE 14–3.** DEVELOPMENT OF MANIPULATIVE SKILLS IN CHILDREN

| | |
|---|---|
| Newborn | Hands in flexion, ulnar grasp obtainable |
| 3–4 months | Hands mostly open, midline play |
| 5–6 months | Voluntary reaching, palmar grasp |
| 6–7 months | Hands open, object transfer from hand to hand, finger feeds, holds bottle |
| 8–9 months | Index finger approach, lateral pinch |
| 10–11 months | Neat pincer grasp |
| 12–14 months | Voluntary release, uses spoon with spilling |
| 16–18 months | Emerging dominance |
| 24 months | Well-established dominance, builds 8-cube tower |
| 36 months | Copies circle, unbuttons garment |
| 48 months | Copies cross, can do buttons |
| 60 months | Sensory assessment possible |

such as absent thumb can be associated with congenital heart disease. Inheritance patterns and penetrance vary.

Partial hand deficiencies need individual solutions in which simple devices such as opposition posts are used, or deepening of the web space, so that the existing sensation of the remaining fingers is utilized.

When a thumb is missing or consists of a small dangling pedicle, pollicization of the index finger provides good function and adequate cosmesis.

*Camptodactyly*, congenital flexion contractures of the digits, may be familial or sporadic. Occasionally flexion deformities of the phalanges progress during childhood and may be mistaken for Dupuytren's contracture. Early onset, greater involvement of the fifth digit and of the proximal interphalangeal rather than the metacarpophalangeal joints, lack of nodules, and palmar fascial thickening are differential points. Early splinting can improve the deformity. By adolescence neither splinting nor surgery is helpful, although release of slips of the flexor digitorum sublimis tendon has been advocated in selected cases.

*Trigger thumb*, persistent flexion of the interphalangeal joint of the thumb, is a mild and isolated condition seen in infants and caused by tethering of the flexor pollicis longus tendon by a fibrous nodule at the level of the first metacarpophalangeal joint. During the first two years, the problem can be relieved by splinting the thumb in extension; with this treatment surgical correction later can be avoided.

*Arthrogryposis*, whether neurogenic or myogenic, can be associated with severe hand contractures along with generalized impairment of joint range. Usually the wrist is fixed in volar flexion and ulnar deviation and the fingers are in extension, with muscle weakness and hypoplasia complicating the picture. Whereas surgery has much to offer to improve alignment and stability of the lower extremities in this condition, efforts to improve position in the upper extremities may require a sacrifice of residual mobility.

Vigorous use of splinting with repeated modifications can do much to improve alignment of the hand during infancy. Splint adjustment or replacement may be necessary as often as weekly. Simple materials such as plaster of Paris molds secured by elastic bandages can be utilized. Because these deformities are notoriously prone to recurrence, night immobilization in the desired position should continue for years.

Improved hand position may not be useful to the arthrogrypotic child if there is rigid elbow extension. Capsuloplasty of the elbow with tendon transplant to provide a flexor motor can be offered. The triceps can be brought anteriorly, or if its sacrifice as an extensor is not desirable, the sterno-mastoid or pectoralis major muscle can be utilized, so that hand-to-mouth motion for feeding can be achieved. Usually only one arm is given flexor power and the other left in extension so that toilet activities can be performed.

## CEREBRAL PALSY

The term cerebral palsy applies to motor dysfunction caused by nonprogressive damage to the growing brain, and can result in a wide variety of clinical pictures and a broad spectrum of disability. In addition to delayed motor development and abnormal muscle tone, multiple handicaps are the rule. Rehabilitation planning must take into account the existence of intellectual deficit and involvement of vision, hearing, and peripheral sensation, the potential for development of head and trunk control and the prognosis for ambulation.

The key to maximizing functional hand use in cerebral palsy is proper positioning and stabilization of the head and body. An infant whose posture is dominated by tonic labyrinthine reflexes lies supine with the arms abducted and externally rotated, elbows flexed and hands positioned uselessly alongside his head. Prone positioning with the chest elevated over a small bolster can foster head control, protract the shoulders, and enable the hands to come to midline to facilitate the development of grasp.

Wheelchairs must be carefully prescribed and modified with a firm back and seat, lateral trunk supports, and selection of back-to-seat angle that minimizes extensor thrust. In the presence of severe spasticity the hips may need to be flexed past 90 degrees, and additional hip and thigh positioners may be added to encourage maintenance of hands and forearms in functional position. Elaborate commercial modular elements can be prescribed to achieve positioning, but easily lose adjustment. Homemade inserts of plywood with vinyl covered padding, custom fitted to the child, can be more effective.

In the neurodevelopmental approach to treatment, the therapist guides the child's active movements so that reaching and grasping occur without overflow of abnormal tone. Stereotyped and undesirable patterns such as excessive head and trunk extension or total flexor withdrawal of the extremity are prevented and the child experiences more "normal" movements. Although controversial, it is believed that therapy begun early and supplemented by a vigorous home program fosters optimal development and diminishes deformity.

In spastic cerebral palsy, the common forearm and hand deformities are limitations in elbow extension and supination, wrist extension, and radial deviation. The thumb is adducted or flexed into the palm. Night splinting can slow development of permanent contracture.

Surgery to improve hand function should be limited to carefully selected patients. A hand that has been ignored will not suddenly be utilized after an operation. Relative contraindications are severe mental retardation and in hemiplegic children severe cortical sensory deficit with impaired position sense and stereognosis. Although hand function can be improved, fine skilled opposition and rapid alternating movements will not be achieved by tendon release or transplantation, and the limited goals of surgery should be carefully explained.

Procedures commonly employed include release of tight forearm flexors, transfer of the flexor carpi ulnaris to the extensor digitorum communis to improve wrist extension, release of the thumb adduction-flexion contracture, and correction of swan neck deformities of the digits. Selection of muscles for transfer is done by electromyographic study in some centers. Splinting and use of procaine or phenol motor point block can be useful during preoperative evaluation. When the hand is tightly contracted and the palm macerated by the flexed fingers, flexor release and wrist fusion can be useful for both cosmesis and hygiene.

In athetosis, surgical procedures are unpredictable. Athetoid youngsters often learn tricks to stabilize their involuntary movements and produce function—for example, employing a tonic neck pattern to achieve elbow flexion by turning the head to the opposite side. Concentration on self-care skills and provision of adaptive equipment—non-slip tableware, built-up spoons and writing tools, and alternative devices such as modified typewriters—can be the keys to independence. These can be much more useful than hours of individual therapy with little hope of carryover.

## BIRTH INJURY TO THE BRACHIAL PLEXUS

Erb's palsy or injury to the upper trunk of the brachial plexus, comprising the anterior divisions of the fifth and sixth cervical roots, usually occurs after a difficult delivery of a large infant with shoulder dystocia, or by excessive traction on the neck in breach presentation. Although the shoulder and elbow are more affected than the hand, an extremity held in adduction and internal rotation at the shoulder with weak or absent biceps cannot be positioned for effective grasp. Scapular winging results from paralysis of the serratus anterior roots. Additional injuries such as fractured clavicle or humerus, diaphragmatic paralaysis, and involvement of the cervical cord itself should be ruled out. Inability to move the arm is usually noticed immediately after birth and can be observed by looking for asymmetry when eliciting the Moro reflex.

Initially there is hematoma around plexus elements, and manipulation of the arm should be avoided for the first few days. Positioning of the shoulder in abduction and external rotation by placing a soft roll of cloth in the axilla will avoid further traction on the injured structure. Pinning of the sleeve to the bed sheet is not appropriate, since more damage may ensue as the infant moves about. Rigid splinting of the shoulder is not recommended because it may foster permanent abduction contracture.

After seven to ten days, a program of regular range of motion performed at each diaper change should be initiated and taught to the family. External rotation and abduction at the shoulder and forearm supination and should be emphasized. If weakness of wrist extension persists, a cock-up wrist splint should be provided.

Electrical stimulation appears to retard muscle atrophy if treatment can be given several times a day. The use of the stimulator at home can be taught to reliable parents. Recovery is usually evident by six months of age and no further improvement is likely to occur after two years. Electromyography is useful prognostically, since return of voluntary potentials can precede clinical recovery by several weeks.

Late deformity of shoulder and elbow joint can occur with persistent elevation and rotation of the scapula caused by tight shoulder musculature. If there is fixed contracture or chronic posterior subluxation of the glenohumeral joint, capsuloplasty accompanied by muscle transfers, using the teres major and latissimus dorsi to enhance external rotation, can be performed. Derotation osteotomy of the humerus can provide improved forearm positioning.

In Klumpke's paralysis, there is injury to the lower trunk of the plexus with involvement of the C8 to T1 roots and often an associated Horner's syndrome. Sensory deficit is usually more severe, and splinting is essential to avoid the claw hand deformity resulting from intrinsic muscle weakness. Intensive stimulation to prevent neglect of the hand is needed even when motor involvement is not severe.

## JUVENILE RHEUMATOID ARTHRITIS

Although the mechanism of joint destruction in childhood arthritis is similar to the adult disease, the pattern of joint impairment differs. The proximal interphalangeal joints are affected early, producing "sausage fingers." With progression to the metacarpophalangeal joints, radial rather than ulnar deviation is a common deformity. In the pauciarticular type, large joints are generally involved, most often the knee, but wrist and elbow can be affected. In the polyarthritic type the cervical spine is involved. Although wasting and deconditioning are part of the arthritic process itself, the possibility of weakness due to cervical cord pathology should be borne in mind.

At times, children with JRA have a subacute inflammatory process and report little or no pain; they avoid discomfort by immobilizing the affected joints voluntarily. Thus a child may present with a fixed wrist or elbow contracture with advanced x-ray changes, having offered few complaints.

Adequate salicylate intake with prolonged treatment is the most effective therapy, although gold or steroid therapy may rarely be indicated, especially when systemic manifestations are severe.

The hands can be splinted at night. Splints should be constructed to avoid pressure over the radial and ulnar styloid processes and to prevent radial deviation. During the day regular activity and school attendance should be encouraged, although vigorous contact sports should be discouraged. In the absence of acute inflammation, heat can provide analgesia and should precede active range of motion that should be carried out at each joint daily.

# Occupational Therapy For The Rheumatoid Hand

by R. Chawla, O.T.R.

Rheumatoid arthritis is a chronic progressive systemic disease characterized by inflammation of the synovial membrane. Swelling, heat, redness, and pain are caused by the inflammatory process, thus leading to damage of joints, supporting soft tissue structures, and tendons. The course of rheumatoid arthritis is characterized by exacerbations and remissions, the process differing from patient to patient. The outcome is that most patients are left with varying degrees of deformities or disability or both. In this section I will discuss the occupational therapy management of the rheumatoid hand.

The chronic nature of rheumatoid arthritis requires that the patient be under supervision for extended periods of time in order to prevent or minimize deformity and maintain or improve function. An ongoing carefully planned occupational therapy program is therefore essential, starting in the early stages of involvement of the hand.

## EVALUATION

Standard manual muscle testing has limited value in evaluating muscle strength in rheumatoid arthritis because of pain or fear of pain. Deformities of the hand may also interfere with the proper interpretation of the test results. Therefore, evaluation of muscle strength may best be carried out by the testing of functional activities. However, when possible, objective means of measurements should be used. Grip strength can be measured with a Jamar dynamometer, if tolerated. When the grip is significantly weakened or painful, a sphygmomanometer may be used instead; this instrument is very sensitive and can accurately record even small changes in pressure. The cuff of the sphygmomanometer is held in the hand and adjusted to the appropriate size. Regardless of the method, for valid measurements the same instrument should always be used for repeated evaluations of the same patient. An average grip of 20 pounds is considered necessary for most activities of daily living.

Pinch strength can be measured by a standard pinch gauge, and both pulp-to-pulp and lateral pinch should be tested. Pinch strength is important for independent living because many activities require use of this motion, such as holding eating utensils, and buttoning. For most tasks an average pinch strength of five to seven pounds is necessary.

The measurement of range of motion by goniometry is important for the assessment of hand function, but when significant amounts of pain, swelling, and deformities already exist, functional interpretation of goniometic results is difficult.

Hand dexterity is tested by using objects of various size and shape. These are picked up and placed in a box within a certain time limit. This allows detection of fine motor involvement very early in the course of the disease.

Sensory evaluation ordinarily shows no deficit unless complications such as entrapment neuropathy or cervical spine involvement are present.

A detailed evaluation of activities of daily living should include self-care, communicative, and homemaking skills and job-related and other general day-to-day activities. Based on these results the patient may be given adaptive equipment to maintain or improve the level of independent function. Such an evaluation may also reveal the patient's own goals and degree of motivation, which should be taken into consideration in establishing rehabilitative goals.

## EXERCISE PROGRAM

The aim is to provide the patient with a well-balanced program of activities within the level of his tolerance interspersed with frequent rest periods. Pain limits the length and type of exercise program prescribed. The exercise program should consist of active range of motion just below pain for brief sessions several times a day. Activities that require full range of motion in a nondeforming direction are desirable, particularly those requiring reaching, picking up, and releasing light objects.

Flatt believes that resistive exercises should be avoided because they only contribute to the existing deforming forces, thereby increasing deformities because of the altered relationships between tendons, joints, and supporting structures.[1] Instead, he suggests that a carefully graduated program of exercises designed to protect the supporting structures be administered.

## JOINT PROTECTION

Joint protection cannot be emphasized enough, as this is one of the main goals of rehabilitative therapy. Furthermore, it should become an integral part of the patient's life style. This requires that the patient fully understand the principles and methods of joint protection in order to maintain a lifelong effort. This usually requires one-to-one instruction. A handout with descriptive illustrations may also be helpful.

The principles of joint protection include the following:[2]

1. Maintenance of muscle strength and joint range of motion. This is best achieved by a monitored program of activities of daily living and active exercises as just described, depending on individual deficits or needs or both.

2. Prevention of positions of the hand that tend to contribute to deformities by external or internal stress. An example of external stress is the rising from a bed or chair by supporting the body weight on the radial side of the hand; this would contribute to the development of ulnar deformities or aggravate existing ones. This should be avoided by exerting pressure on the "heel" of the palms of the hand instead and keeping the fingers straight. An example of internal stress is the effect of sustained muscular activity on joints such as the stress on the metacarpophalangeal joints when small objects are held that require strong grip. This stress can be reduced by using built-up feeding utensils, toothbrushes, razors, and so forth.

3. Utilization of the most stable joints and strongest muscle group for the task. For this, application of principles of body mechanics is essential. For example, instead of picking up a heavy pot with the fingers as is usually done, the patient should distribute the weight of the pot to the wrist and elbow by placing the palm of one hand under the pot while the other steadies it. If possible, the larger joints and muscle groups should be used as substitutes for smaller, more vulnerable joints and muscles, particularly in performing strenuous tasks.

4. Use of the joints of the hand in their most stable anatomical and functional position. When pain and limitation of joints in other parts of the body are present, the patient will resort to substitute motions, such as using his hands to pull himself up to rise from a chair, thus causing stress and strain on the hands, leading to joint instability. This could be prevented by the use of adaptive equipment that would raise toilet seats, or the use of cushions in chairs or wheelchairs.

5. Maintenance of correct patterns of movements and of good muscle balance. For example, finger flexion normally begins at the distal joints and finger extension begins at the metacarpophalangeal joints. This pattern should be preserved whenever possible so as to maintain a proper balance between intrinsic and extrinsic muscles and to reduce strain and fatigue.

6. Holding muscles or joints in the same position for prolonged periods of time is contraindicated and should be avoided, particularly if this causes pain. In performing activities that usually require sustained muscle action for long periods, as in writing, the patient should be instructed to take frequent breaks in the activity—every ten minutes or sooner if necessary—to prevent fatigue, joint wear, and ligament strain. If complete avoidance of a particular activity is desired, this also can be achieved by use of adaptive equipment. A book stand can be used while reading to substitute for continuous holding of the book.

7. Activities that prove to be beyond the power and endurance of the patient to complete should not be undertaken, or substitutes should be devised. An example is using a cart instead of carrying heavy or breakable items.

8. Application of energy conservation techniques, in which time and motion economy is observed, is an important principle in designing a therapeutic program for the patient. This can be done by rearranging equipment and tools either in the work place or in the home. In addition, extrinsic forces that put excessive stress on those joints

and periarticular structures that are most vulnerable should be reduced. For example, the patient should be instructed to slide objects instead of lifting them.

9. "Respect" for pain. It is well recognized that activities that produce pain must be either modified or omitted. In so doing, the patient must not confuse discomfort with pain. Extra caution is necessary when pain may not be felt by the patient either because of sensory deficit or administration of analgesic medication.

## SPLINTING FOR THE RHEUMATOID HAND

Splinting is always used in conjunction with a properly designed activity program. There are various materials available for fabrication of splints; however, the most commonly used by occupational therapists are low-temperature plastics such as Orthoplast, Aquaplast and Polyform. A splint pattern is cut from the material, which is then heated in water of 140 to 170°F temperature, then cooled to the patient's skin tolerance before the splint is shaped directly on the patient's hand. The advantages of using low-temperature thermoplastic materials are that adjustments and close contouring to conform to the anatomical part of the hand can be easily made and they are light in weight as well as washable. Splints should be modified or new splints made as often as necessary when changes in the hand warrant it.

### Indications for Splinting

1. Relief of pain.
2. Maintenance of good position, particularly during exacerbation of the disease process.
3. Prevention of limitation of joint range.
4. Stabilization of joints.

### Types of Splints

**Resting Hand Splint/Shell.** A resting hand splint (Fig. 14–10) is used at night but may also be used intermittently during the day to provide relief from pain and to maintain the wrist and fingers in a functional position.

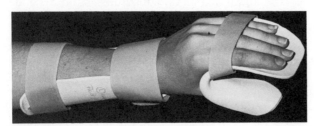

**Figure 14–10.** Resting hand splint/shell.

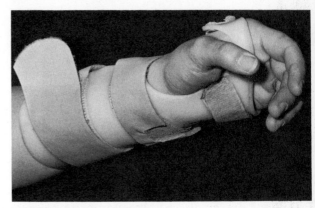

**Figure 14–11.** Wrist cock-up splint.

**Wrist Cock-Up Splint.** This splint (Fig. 14–11) is recommended for stability and relief of pain. It should be used for activities during the day that are stressful at the wrist. The splint can also be worn at night and may be used for relief of symptoms in carpal tunnel syndrome.

**Ulnar Deviation Splint.** It is designed (Fig. 14–12) to restrict full metacarpophalangeal flexion, thus preventing the development of subluxating torque forces that contribute to ulnar-directed deformities. At the same time it allows use of the fingers and thumb. Variations of this splint exist but the basic principle remains the same.

**Finger Splints.** The characteristic deformities of the fingers that are easily recognized in the rheumatoid hand are the swan neck and boutonniere deformities. Millender and Nalebuff have classified swan neck deformity[4] according to functional loss and the boutonniere according to severity.[5] Splinting is only effective during the very early phase of development of deformity.

The swan neck control splint (Fig. 14–13)[3] limits

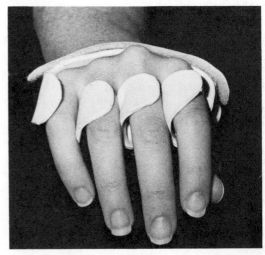

**Figure 14–12.** Ulnar deviation splint.

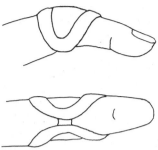

**Figure 14–13.** Swan neck control splint. The PIP joint is held in the desired amount of flexion to prevent hyperextension of this joint. (From Hollis, I. L.: Innovative Splinting Ideas. St. Louis, The C. V. Mosby Co., 1978.)

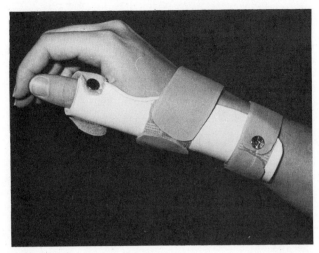

**Figure 14–15.** Thumb splint.

extension at the proximal interphalangeal joint but allows full flexion. Constant use of such splints may lead to tightening of volar structures and thereby prevent hyperextension.

The boutonniere control splint (Fig. 14–14)[3] holds the lateral bands above the axis of rotation and through prolonged use may lead to tightening of dorsal structures of the interphalangeal joints, thus stabilizing the joint.

**Thumb Splint.**   An unstable and painful thumb may interfere significantly with day-to-day activities. Though the carpometacarpal joint of the thumb is more frequently involved, the metacarpophalangeal joint may also be involved. Often the ulnar collateral ligament of the thumb may be weakened or destroyed. A splint designed to provide stability and good position to the carpometacarpal and metacapophalangeal joints, while the interphalangeal joint is left free to perform pinch activities, is recommended (Fig. 14–15).

When the interphalangeal joint is unstable, pinch-requiring activities are seriously hampered, particularly those involving small objects. A small ther-

moplastic splint on the dorsum of the joint can be applied to reduce stress and protect the joint, especially when early signs of involvement are present.

Postoperative splinting and occupational therapy treatment is an important aspect of the care of the rheumatoid hand, but it is beyond the scope of this chapter.

In conclusion, because of the systemic and progressive nature of rheumatoid arthritis, (see Chapter 13) application of the principles of joint protection, a monitored exercise program, and splinting techniques are important in the management of the rheumatoid hand so that the patient may lead a more productive life for a longer period of time and in greater comfort.

## REFERENCES

1. Flatt, A. E.: Care of the Rheumatoid Hand, 3rd edition. St. Louis, The C. V. Mosby Co., 1974.
2. Cordery, J. C.: Joint protection—a responsibility of the occupational therapist. Am. J. Occup. Ther. 19:285–293, 1965.
3. Hollis, I. L.: Innovative Splinting Ideas. In Hunter, J. M. et al. (eds.): Rehabilitation of the hand. St. Louis, The C. V. Mosby Co., 1978.
4. Nalebuff, E. A. and Millender, L. G.: Surgical treatment of the swan neck deformity in rheumatoid arthritis. Orthop. Clin. North Am. 6:733–752, 1975.
5. Nalebuff, E. A. and Millender, L. H.: Surgical treatment of the boutonniere deformity in rheumatoid arthritis. Orthop. Clin. North Am. 6:753–763, 1975.
6. McCann, V. H., Philips, C. A. and Quigley, T. R.: Preoperative and postoperative management—the role of the allied health professionals. Orthop. Clin. North Am. 6:1975.

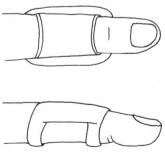

**Figure 14–14.** Boutonniere control splint. The PIP joint is held in extension thus stabilizing the joint. (From Hollis, I. L.: Innovative splinting ideas. St. Louis, The C. V. Mosby Co., 1978.)

# 15

# Shoes and the Foot

*by Lawrence Kaplan, M.D.*

Giannestras, in his text on foot pathology, re- marked that "one should be kind to feet, as there are twice as many as people." It has also been whimsically stated that since so many physicians have bad backs they prefer not to bend down to examine these lowly members.

Actually, proper shoe prescription is a relatively neglected medical art. Not infrequently the foot is relegated to the care of others. Part of the problem lies in the fact that there has been little basic re- search into proper correction of foot defects, and for that matter into shoe size standardization. It is difficult to believe, but it is nevertheless a fact, that there is no true national standard of sizes for shoes. There are certain gross measurements that are generally accepted, such as the fact that in the United States and England, length increases by one third of an inch per size and that width in- creases by one twelfth of an inch at the sole, the upper increasing only by one fourth of an inch. Furthermore, standards of size vary from manufac- turer to manufacturer and from one set of lasts to another. (The last is the device upon which the shoe is constructed, made of wood or metal.)

All of us have had the experience of finding that different pairs of shoes made even by the same manufacturer may or may not fit in spite of the listed size. Although foot coverings date back to the early history of man, their shape has varied for many reasons over the centuries. Originally, shoes probably were simply protection against rough, uneven ground. The first records of footwear go back three to four thousand years to the time of the Egyptians, who wore papyrus sandals made of grass, reeds, and hemp. Later, shoes were made with leather or hide held in place by thongs. The first woven stockings are known to have existed as early as 600 A.D.

Of interest is the fact that between the 11th and the 15th centuries shoes had an elongation of the toe tip reaching to absurd lengths from 6 inches for the lower classes to 18 inches for knights, 24 inches for barons and lengths so great that the tips were tied to the knees in the case of princes. These were called poulaines. The poulaine, however, was re- jected by Charles VIII of France because of his own swollen painful feet. The heel was in existence a little earlier than the 16th century. During the 17th century Catherine de Medici introduced the high heel at the French court as a compensation for her short stature. As with the poulaine, this exaggera- tion became so excessive that ladies of the court had to be physically supported in order to remain erect.

The first real attempt to establish shoe size was made by Edward II of England, who agreed that three average-size barleycorns equaled 1 inch; 39 barleycorns were determined to be the length of the longest foot, which was called size 13. Al- though the first differentiation of shoes between left and right actually dates back, as far as known, to the early 1800s (supposedly 1818), soldiers in the United States Union Army given separate right and left shoes subjected the shoes to derision as "crooked shoes."

The question of proper fit of shoes was so little understood as late as World War I that a study was done in 1914 by Dr. William Reno, a United States Army medical officer. He noted that of 2413 men examined, 2017 were wearing shoes that did not fit their feet; 1764 were wearing shoes that were either too narrow, too short, or both. He found that these men were suffering from corns, bun- ions, hammer toes, ingrown or deformed nails and many other similiar deformities.

All of us are familiar with the fact that even to the present day, to a large extent, style in shoes is considered more important than proper fit and comfort. It is a common experience on examining the foot to find that females, especially those who have worn high heels and pointed toes, suffer from numerous foot defects including tight heel cords, hammer toes, claw toes and bunions.

## NORMAL GAIT

In order to properly understand foot pathology and the principles of treatment by shoe corrections and other means, it is first necessary to understand how we walk in normal gait.

1. Heel strike: As the foot hits the ground at heel contact, the foot is in a position of varus, or turned in, with the sole facing the opposite foot, with only the lateral posterior portion of the heel in contact with the ground. This accounts for the greater wear of this portion of the heel in the normal well-shod foot. If the shoe is a flimsy slipper or sandal, it will tend to slide laterally on the foot and show wear instead on the mid-posterior aspect of the heel.

2. Foot flat: Shortly after the heel strikes the ground, the sole of the shoe of the same foot touches the ground. To arrive at this point in stance phase, the foot continues in its turned-in or varus pattern, with the greater weight being taken along the lateral border of the sole to the actual point where the foot is flat.

3. In mid-stance, the body weight is directly over the supporting extremity.

4. Push-off is divided into heel-off and toe-off. In heel-off, as the heel of the supporting extremity rises from the ground, the ball of the foot and the toes are still in contact with the ground. Beyond this point, however, there is a "roll-over" across the ball from lateral to medial with pressure being taken increasingly by the metatarsal and the phalanges of the medial toes. In toe-off, the push-off phase terminates when the entire foot rises from the ground and the extremity enters "swing phase," the point at which the foot is no longer on the ground. At this point of push-off the normal big toe must be in straight alignment with the rest of the foot, as per Meyer's line. Meyer stated that "the great toe must lie in such a position that its axis carried backward shall pass through the center of the heel." The longitudinal axis of the great toe carried backward passes through the center of the heel. Greater weight is borne by the medial aspect of the first toe.

The foot is a second-class lever. A second-class lever can be thought of as a wheelbarrow in which the power is supplied through the handle bars by the individual who holds and pushes the wheelbarrow. The weight being carried is in the center or container section of the wheelbarrow, and the fulcrum of the lever is the wheel of the wheelbarrow. In this sense the second-class leverage of the foot at the fulcrum is the first toe. The weight is the body located between the first toe and the power source, which is the calf muscles acting at the heel. The center of gravity of the foot is usually found just anterior to the ankle joint during mid-stance. However, when the first toe is in some degree of valgus (turned out toward the little toe) as it invariably is, not only among wearers of pointed shoes but also in older persons who have gone barefoot during their lives, the lever is twisted at its fulcrum and therefore is a disability, with inefficient movement in walking and running. Even in primitive populations, constant pressure against the medial aspect of the first toe during toe-off may account for the development of hallux valgus.

It has frequently been stated that shoes with pointed or cramped toe boxes are a major cause of hallux valgus. MacLennan, however, studied the prevalence of hallux valgus in an unshod neolithic New Guinea population.[10] He found that it was frequently severe, and increased with age, especially in women. Another study was done on the island of Tristan De Cunha, where it was found that in the unshod population over 60, there was a greater tendency to hallux valgus, in men as well as women. This tendency is probably due to the position of the foot during toe-off, with the increasing effect of pressure against the medial aspect of the first toe. In most instances in the small child the alignment of the first toe seems to follow the axis line.

Provided that one retains the concept of an anatomical metatarsal arch, with pressure being taken on the first and fifth toes and on the calcaneus, the three points of contact when the foot is on the ground, one half of the load is found to be at the hind foot and the other half is in the region of the forefoot. Of the aspect that bears weight in the region of the forefoot, one third is borne by the big toe and two thirds by the other toes. Other studies report 50 per cent of weight borne by the first toes in the forefoot and 50 per cent by the other four toes. However, during walking there is rapid movement from the calcaneus at heel strike along the lateral aspect of the foot across the metatarsals and phalanges to push-off on the big toe. On the other hand, during running with the heel off the ground, so-called toe-toe running as opposed to heel-toe running, weight is constantly borne by the metatarsals and the phalanges alone. One should not therefore think of the forces as static and unchanging. Even when one is standing still there is movement of the body; the foot must constantly adjust to the changing position. Unless the foot is healthy and shod in appropriate coverings, pain and disability can result.

## NOMENCLATURE OF THE FOOT AND THE SHOE

In order to understand the various disabilities and the means by which they are controlled, it is necessary to know some of the terminology used as well as to understand the types of shoe modifications that exist and the purpose for which they are used (Fig. 15–1).

The shoe consists of an upper part or the upper, the sole, the heel, and the lining present inside the shoe. The shoe itself consists of a posterior aspect in the region of the heel; the uppermost part of this area is called the *internal heel seat*, where the heel rests anatomically. Below this is the *base* of the heel, the section to which the heel is fastened. Finally, there is the heel proper, usually made out of leather or rubber. The anterior aspect of the heel is called the *breast* of the heel. The heel is also angled at the posterior surface to some degree and this is known as the *Pitch of the Heel*. The height of the heel is usually described as being measured by manufacturers in eighths of an inch, so that one refers to a three-eighths heel, seven-eighths heel, eight-eighths heel, and so forth. The sole also consists of an anterior aspect called the *ball* of the shoe, which is the widest part of the sole located at the metatarsal head. The *shank* is the area between the anterior aspect of the heel and the ball. In orthopedic shoes there is a piece of metal referred to as a *metal shank*, which is located in the area of the shank between the layers of the sole, which will be described. The tip of the outer sole anteriorly is spaced above the ground; this space is referred to as the *toe spring*, the space between the outer sole and the floor as measured at the tip. This allows the foot to rock through at push-off. The *sole* usually consists of at least two layers, the inner sole, seen on the inside of the shoe, and the outer sole.

In a well-built shoe as well as an orthopedic shoe the construction is commonly referred to as the *Goodyear welt construction*. This type of shoe has a space between the insole and the outersole called the filler.

The upper part of the shoe has an anterior portion called the *vamp*. Attached to the vamp is the *tongue* of the shoe, which is the strip of leather lying under the laces. The anterior end of the tongue is called the *throat*, being the point at which the tongue is attached to the vamp—that is, the base of the tongue. Quarters consist of the posterior aspect of the upper, sometimes separated from the anterior aspect by a stitched line referred to as *upper foxing*. It should be noted that in order to prevent contact and abrasions in the region of the lateral malleous, the lateral aspect is cut down lower than the medial.

The *lace stay* is the portion that contains the lace and that has eyelets. The eyelets are usually one-half inch apart from one another, and there are usually four eyelets on each side of the lace stay. Several types of lace stays are in use, which we have all seen but probably not noticed unless attention was directed to the differences. There is the so-called *Blucher* type, in which the lace stay can be pulled apart one side from the other as seen in Figure 15–2; the Blucher is part of the vamp. This allows for easy entry by separation of the two sides of the lace stay. There is the Bal,\* which is usually part of the quarters and is connected at its distal anterior aspect in a V shape. The Bal, which is also laced, is difficult to open fully in the region of the vamp. People with problem feet will find that a Blucher type of opening is easier to use than a Bal (Fig. 15–3).

The lining of the shoe should be perfectly

---

\*Shortening of the word Balmoral.

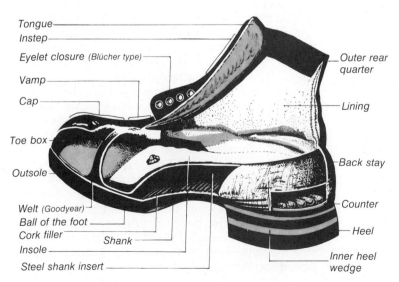

Tongue
Instep
Eyelet closure (Blücher type)
Vamp
Cap
Toe box
Outsole
Welt (Goodyear)
Ball of the foot
Cork filler
Shank
Insole
Steel shank insert

Outer rear quarter
Lining
Back stay
Counter
Heel
Inner heel wedge

**Figure 15–1.** Parts of a shoe.

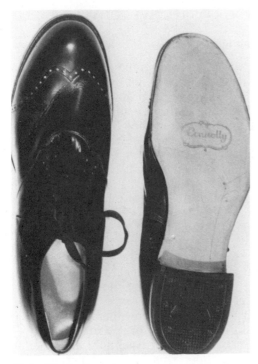

**Figure 15–2.** Blucher lace stay.

smooth in order to prevent contact pressure against the foot. The *toe box*, which is the very anterior part of the shoe, can be rigid and thus retain its shape and guard against injury to the toes or can be soft, without any stiff material. Furthermore, most good shoes have, in their posterior quarter, a *counter*, made usually from either a synthetic substance or ground leather, which is processed to become rigid and which is used to create a firm shape in the region of the heel. The counter usually extends to the heel breast, but special counters may extend either medially or laterally farther forward as well

as upward—over the malleoli, if necessary, for certain disabilities. The foot is also described as having certain areas such as the ball that are identical to the ball of the shoe, being that region at the level of the metatarsal heads. The waist of the foot is between the calcaneal area and the metatarsal heads or ball, as well as the instep, which is on the dorsum, somewhat anterior to the waist of the foot and basically in the region of the lace stay of the shoe.

## SHOE TYPES

The shoe with Goodyear welt construction is the most appropriate for adequate correction of foot disabilities, with the understanding that any shoe can be used, if necessary, to make sometimes fairly reasonable corrections when no other resource is permitted or available. This type of shoe serves to attach the upper and the lower through the welt, the upper being sewn to the welt and insole and the lower portion or sole also being sewn to the welt. The space in between, as mentioned earlier contains a filler material.

There is also the stitchdown type of shoe in which the upper is turned out and stitched down to the sole. The stitchdown and Goodyear welt shoes are the two most common types, and the Goodyear welt is more appropriate for corrective measures. The stitchdown consists of a lining cemented to the inner sole, a middle sole cemented to the insole, and an outer sole cemented to the middle sole. A small welt is added and stitched to all the layers.

Other styles of shoe include the strap and buckle closure, in which the shoe can be closed by a simple strap laced through a buckle. There is also a Velcro closure (Fig. 15–4) in which the Velcro passing through a wide buckle can be placed over the

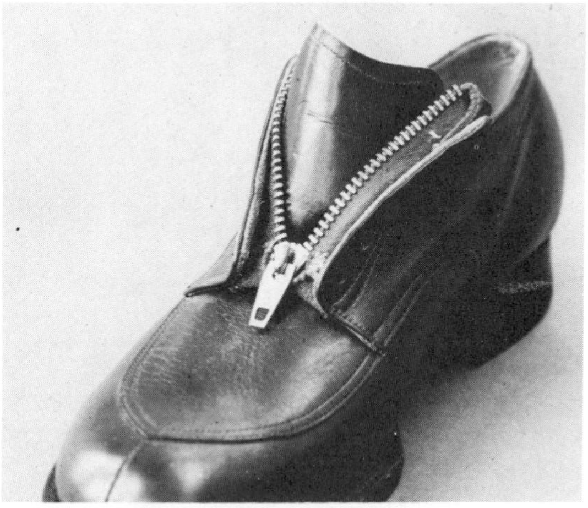

**Figure 15–3.** Zipper Bal lace stay.

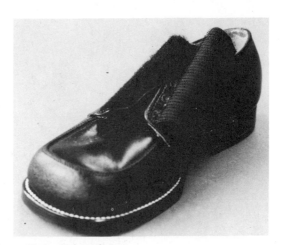

**Figure 15–4.** Velcro closure.

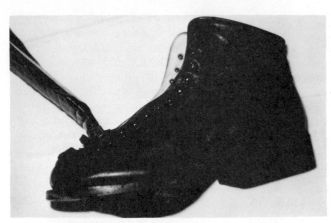

**Figure 15–5.** Surgical or convalescent shoe.

lace stay area and closed easily with one hand or simply by the palm of the hand pressing the Velcro sides together.

A shoe that is used to compensate for significant problems of putting on footwear is the so-called surgical or convalescent type, which is laced to the toe as is an athletic shoe. When great ease of entry is required, a shoe can be provided that has a posterior opening in the region of the back seam so that patients can insert the foot from the rear of the shoe, the closure being either lacing or Velcro (Figs. 15–6 and 15–7). This is an excellent shoe for someone who cannot bend the hip, the knee, or the back; the patient can simply place the shoe against a wall and slide the foot into it, closing from behind. This is also of value in someone who has no ankle motion and can therefore easily slide into the posterior aspect. There is also a common, easily purchased shoe with elastic material (goring). This is a type of low shoe in which the lace stay area simply stretches open for easy entry.

## FITTING CORRECTIVE FOOTWEAR

### PROPER FIT

For a proper prescription, the prescriber must determine whether or not the shoe is the appropriate size for the individual patient. Examination must be done with the patient in the standing position, and, if a laced shoe is used, it must be laced firmly, and any type of closure must be firmly closed.

In the case of the laced shoe the eyelets must be parallel and the two sides of the closure must be no closer than one fourth to one half of an inch to one another. The eyelets should be parallel to one another. If there is gapping at the top, the shoe is too tight across the instep. If there is gapping at the bottom, the shoe is too wide at the vamp. The length of the shoe should be one half to three fourths of an inch beyond the longest toe.

In rechecking to determine if a new shoe is required in a growing foot, there should be at least one fourth of an inch of spacing left between the longest toe, which is usually the first toe, and the tip of the shoe. This examination can be done in several ways. The patient, especially with a soft toe box, can push the big toe up against the toe box and this can be felt by the examiner and its distance from the toe tip determined. However, in the case of a rigid toe box in which the toes cannot be felt, the examiner measures at the ball of the foot and the ball of the shoe, which should be at the same point. This is referred to as the heel-to-ball length. The first metatarsophalangeal joint, which juts out farthest medially, can be palpated along the ball of the shoe just beyond the beginning of the turn in the shank of the shoe. Next, the exam-

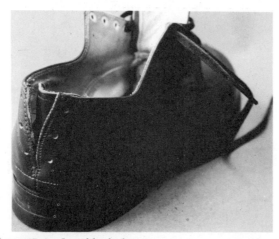

**Figure 15–6.** Laced-back shoe.

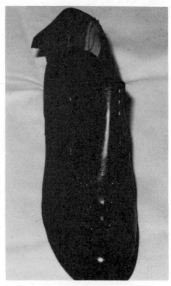

**Figure 15–7.** Velcro closure back stay.

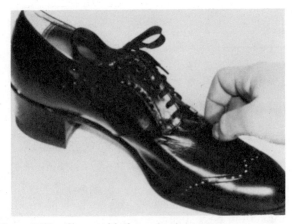

**Figure 15–8.** Shoe width determination.

iner should be able to gather, on pinching in the area of the vamp just distal to the lace stay, one-fourth inch of leather between the fingers.

In the erect position there should be no gapping at the sides of the shoe. If there is gapping, the shoe is probably too narrow. Furthermore, there should be no gapping at the back seam area; this should be a snug fit. When the patient walks there should be no piston action of the foot in the shoe in the area of the heel. A small amount is permissible if the shoe is new and stiff.

For a determination of whether or not the shoe has been worn properly, the greatest appearance of wear should be at the lateral aspect of the heel in the outer back corner. There should be a one-inch band of wear under the metatarsophalangeal joints across the sole of the shoe, and especially some wear under the first toe. In a child or an individual who runs, there may be greater wear under the toe tip in the region of the sole. This also occurs on riding a bicycle.

## PRESCRIPTION

Prescription is an art and not a science. The prescriber must take into account the individual and the particular pathology or failure will result. One other precaution that I practice is to have the patient bring the totally uncorrected shoe for my examination prior to having changes made. This prevents the dealer from having to throw out the already changed shoes and having to start anew. The prescriber should be warned, however, that some pedorthists, which is their title, object to what they feel is an encroachment upon their expertise. Nevertheless, I feel strongly that I would rather have the assurance that the shoe is the proper size before the dealer proceeds. This can prevent a lot of unhappiness and embarrassment on the part of the dealer. After the corrections have been made, I request the patient to wear the shoes

for one week and then to return for an examination of the shoe to make sure that the corrections are appropriate and the patient is comfortable, and that no minor changes are required.

### EXAMINATION OF THE FOOT

The patient should be stripped to underwear so that the entire alignment of the lower extremity can be evaluated. For example, patients with significant genu varum or genu valgum may, and commonly do, have malalignment of the feet because of the shape of the lower extremity and may therefore be in a forced situation of pes valgo planus or pes cavus. Further, if there is a knee disability with one lower extremity in valgus, not infrequently both feet will be totally different in their appearance, one being in valgus and the other in varus. This is important to be aware of in terms of the corrections given.

The patient is also observed walking (this is especially important in children), to see if there is eversion (toeing out) or inversion (toeing in). It is important to see the pattern of the movements and the corrections that might be needed during gait, especially in the presence of other types of disability such as results from trauma or poliomyelitis. The patient must be examined while supine. This is to determine the range of motion and malleability of the foot in the presence of callosities, corns, inappropriate positions of the toes such as hallux valgus, spreading of the foot, and so forth. With the patient in the erect position one can notice whether or not there are dropped metatarsals or whether the foot is spread out in the forward aspect (splaying), or has claw toes or hammer toes. On the table it is important to grasp the foot and to determine if the heel cord is contracted, if the foot is fixed in one position or another, such as in eversion or inversion, if there is loss of motor power and loss of active range of any of the ankle or foot directions, and if the foot is rigid or normally loose. Finally, it is important to determine if there is pain on manipulation of various parts of the foot, such as pain of the toes on manipulation in flexion and extension, tenderness of an area such as the metatarsophalangeal joints, pain over the ankle joint, medially or laterally, or pain on manipulation of the forefoot in relationship to the hindfoot. One also looks for tenderness over the sole in the anterior aspect of the calcaneus and over the plantar fascia of the heel or other parts of the sole. Careful examination is crucial and easily accomplished with practice.

Following the examination, a determination is made as to whether or not the foot disabilities should be corrected in alignment by the shoe or whether or not the disabilities simply should be accommodated for by elimination of foot movement

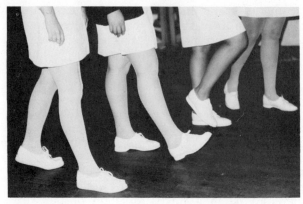

**Figure 15–9.** Walking in different phases of gait.

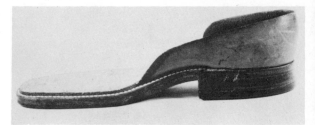

**Figure 15–11.** The long medial counter.

in the shoe and substitution for movement made through additions to the shoe. In the case of pain on movement or in the presence of rigid foot structure, it is necessary to accommodate. This implies making correction to the shoe, which will substitute for the rigid or painful movement. The preferable alternative is to correct the position of the foot with the shoe in order to return the patient to a more normal gait. This can be done only if the foot is malleable, and pain is not produced by the correction.

### REQUIREMENTS FOR SUCCESSFUL PRESCRIPTION

The first requirement is that the prescriber have *expertise in the dynamics of muscle movement*. This has already been discussed in terms of normal gait. (Figure 15–9 shows walking in different phases of gait.) The second is *knowledge of the pathomechanics of foot disabilities*.

The third is *a working knowledge of shoes and shoe modifications*. The prescriber should have a basic

understanding of how a shoe is constructed—the different materials that are used as well as modifications that have been developed to aid the disabled foot. The long medial counter shown in Figure 15–11 is used for extra support of the median longitudinal arch in pes planus and pes planovalgus, for example.

A *spirit of ingenuity and adaptability is essential* for the prescriber. For example, a well-dressed, appearance-conscious woman might ask, "How can I be seen in that kind of a shoe in public? I wouldn't wear it except for walking around the house—it's too ugly." In this situation a regular shoe can often be used, perhaps not as adequately but well enough, with external corrections (Fig. 15–12) or with insoles that are glued to the inside of the shoe and sometimes removable, sufficient correction or adaptation can be made so that the patient is quite comfortable. It is important to remember that "many roads lead to Rome." A wedge can be glued onto a dress shoe as an overlay on the sole or stitched to it, for the type of shoe that cannot be taken apart for sandwiching between the layers of the sole.

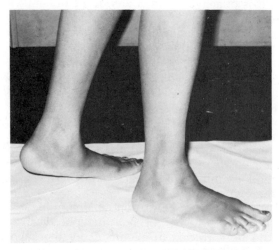

**Figure 15–10.** The planus foot showing the flattening arch and abnormal position of the foot.

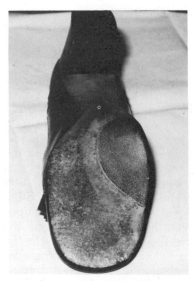

**Figure 15–12.** A glued shoe wedge overlay on an ordinary nonorthopedic shoe.

## ACHIEVING THE GOAL

It is important to have a clear idea of the treatment goal and to strive to meet this need.

RELIEF OF PAIN. Use is made of a dugout heel to accomplish this goal (Fig. 15–13). In the case of calcaneal discomfort, either due to calcaneal spur or to inflammation of the fascial tissue (calcaneal fasciitis), the region of the heel of the shoe can be dug out and the area filled with foam rubber, covered by a leather inner sole.

PROPHYLACTIC SUPPORT OF THE FOOT TO PREVENT PROGRESSIVE DEFORMITY (Fig. 15–9). The first staff member on the left wears a platform or wedge type of shoe. This type of shoe provides extra support under the shank in the other shoes as well. All this tends to help prevent descent of the medial longitudinal arch from either overweight or prolonged standing.

MECHANICAL SUBSTITUTION FOR LOSS OF MOVEMENT. In the case of a rigid ankle or foot, use of a SACH heel and a rocker bar from shank to toe tip can be used to substitute for lost ankle motion. The SACH heel (Fig. 15–14), whose name is an acronym for solid ankle cushion heel, is made of a rubber material that comes in three densities to allow for variable degrees of compression. This type of shoe heel is used in artificial limbs, when there is no ankle joint, to permit the heel to compress and to allow the patient to be able to reach foot flat without excessive motion. This same rubber material can be used as an insert into the heel of a shoe. It is referred to in this instance as a SACH heel and used to permit the patient to descend to the sole and then to rock through the sole through the extended "shank to toe tip rocker bar." This will substitute for a rigid foot or lost ankle motion. This same type of dual correction can be used to eliminate painful motion and to allow the sole of the shoe to do the work. The rocker bar itself, added to a sole, can be adapted in many ways in order to permit efficient lifting of the heel from the ground,

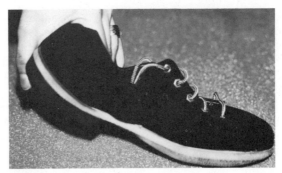

**Figure 15–14.** SACH heel with a long rocker bar.

followed by toeing off. It should be pointed out that there are several kinds of additions to the sole, such as the rocker bar and the metatarsal bar. The rocker bar may be very small and be found just posterior to the metatarsal heads, or it can be extended as shown in Figure 15–14. It is rigid so that it may be "fixed" upon certain lengths and apices. I frequently vary the position of the bar on the basis of the individual patient's need. If the foot is very sensitive, the apex can be "skived"—a shoe term meaning to cut down the height of the correction. Thus a patient with a feeling of being elevated too high on an involved foot or both feet can be given a skived apex that can be made higher at some future date when the patient is comfortable with this type of correction. Incidently, this is true of most corrections.

ELIMINATION OF MOVEMENT. Another method for eliminating motion is to use a semiflexible steel insert between the inner and outer sole or as part of a molded inner sole (Fig. 15–15). Such a steel insert is used for many foot conditions and for elimination of motion through the metatarsophalangeal joints, and so forth. Another purpose of this device is to accommodate a rigid deformity or a deformity that if corrected would produce only pain. This, in fact, is a prime principle: It is a mistake to attempt to correct what cannot be corrected or what would become painful when a correction is attempted.

PERIODIC RE-EXAMINATIONS. Periodic re-evaluations are an absolute necessity because, more than any other type of appliance, the shoe tends to wear and the distortion of weight bearing tends to

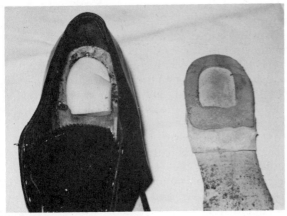

**Figure 15–13.** Dugout heel with covering inner sole.

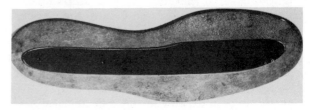

**Figure 15–15.** Semiflexible steel insert from calcaneus to toe as part of an inner sole.

produce changes in the correction, especially in the growing foot. Actual harm may be done when a growing foot is bound in a smaller shoe with all the corrections in the wrong places. This is particularly true when molded plates and arch supports are used.

There are several other precautions that must be taken on prescribing a corrective shoe and on re-evaluating the shoe after the patient has returned with the finished product.

AVOIDANCE OF SHOE WEIGHT OVERLOADING. It is important to consider the weight of the usual corrected orthopedic shoe as opposed to that of an ordinary shoe when treating people who are either markedly debilitated or who have weaknesses of the lower extremities, neurologic or otherwise. The weight of the shoe may be so great that the patient may be unable to lift the lower extremity from the floor appropriately; easy fatigability and an inability to walk may result. Poliomyelitis patients with paralysis or patients with peripheral neuropathy or significant paresis may find that the shoe is too heavy for their purposes, although it may very well solve the foot problem. In such an instance it is important to compromise and to provide a light shoe with corrections that do not act as a barrier to lifting the lower extremity.

Finally, it is important when evaluating the effect of the corrections to believe the patient. In most instances, even though the prescriber believes that the appropriate changes have been made, the patient who complains of pain or inability to walk properly will be in the right. It is crucial to listen carefully and to try to determine adjustments that can be made in the prescription to overcome the patient's discomfort.

There are two important physical laws in terms of correction that must be mentioned. The first is that *the pressure is inversely proportional to the square of the area*. This physical law is especially important in people with pain in the foot, such as in the metatarsophalangeal area, under the toes, in the region of the heel, or other locations. The concept is that the spread of weight throughout the entire foot by corrections considerably lessens the pressure at any tender point. For example, if the patient has a cavus foot (high arch), undue pressure is present in the region of the heel, as well as over the metatarsophalangeal joints. By filling in the longitudinal arch elevation with a scaphoid pad customized to match the arch height, the pressure will be extended along the midfoot as well as in the heel and the toe area. Furthermore, by using a SACH heel or digging out under the metatarsal heads and filling this area with foam rubber, the pressure gradient is softened as well.

This brings into play a second physical law, which is that *action is equal to reaction*. In other words, the harder the surface on contact, the harder the reactive effect against the foot. The softer the surface, the softer the reactive compression of the foot.

Correctional devices can be placed in one of three areas of the shoe:

1. As an insert on the inside of the shoe, called an inlay. These may be fixed or removable.

2. Sandwiched between the insole and the outsole. This can be done only on shoes such as the Goodyear welt, whose layers can be easily separated.

3. Modifications on the sole of the shoe, which are external, referred to as overlays or onlays.

Inlays commonly take up a size, especially if they are in the form of arch supports, either full length or three-quarter length. However, they do not easily erode unless made of soft materials. In some instances when there is no good counter material in the shoe, the insert may deteriorate and flatten out. Sandwiches in the shoe do not erode because they are not in contact either with the foot on the inside directly or with the ground on the outside. External sole corrections do tend to wear, but they do not reduce the size of the shoe, nor do they distort its inner surface.

## PATHOLOGICAL CONDITIONS

### PES PLANOVALGUS

Pes planovalgus, or flat foot, is an extremely common condition. In some instances the condition may be totally asymptomatic throughout a person's lifetime. In other cases it may cause considerable difficulty. The condition varies in degree from a minimal lowering of the longitudinal arch to complete collapse of the arch, the foot being flat on the ground with pronation of the hindfoot and abduction of the foot, which splays out laterally. One can classify the condition as first-, second-, third-, or fourth-degree pes planovalgus, depending on its severity. Anatomically the condition is characterized by a descent of the navicular and the cuneiform bones as well as a rotation of the talus downward and medially, in relationship to the calcaneus. In the more serious types of disability, the forefoot may be relatively internally rotated and abducted in relation to the mid and hind foot. Figures 15–16 and 15–17 show both anterior and posterior inversion of the ankle, flatness of the arch, and severe depression of the talus on the calcaneus, as well as loss of the longitudinal arch.

The objectives of corrections are to elevate the medial aspect of the calcaneus in order to reverse the rotational component of the talus to some degree and to support and raise the longitudinal arch in order to relieve stress on the foot and in some cases to derotate the forefoot into some degree of external rotation (pronation) relative to the hind-

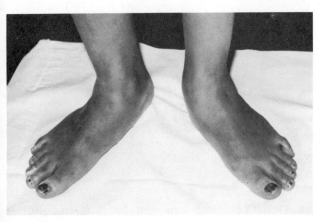

**Figure 15–16.** Pes planovalgus.

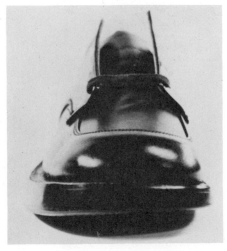

**Figure 15–18.** Orthopedic shoe with a lateral sole wedge.

foot. Figure 15–18 shows an orthopedic shoe that has a lateral sole wedge specifically designed to cause the relative external rotation of the forefoot.

A long medial counter (see Fig. 15–11) is sometimes necessary to support the longitudinal arch. This should extend beyond the breast of the heel to the first cuneiform or even beyond, in extreme cases, in order to provide greater support.

Scaphoid pads are placed under the medial longitudinal arch. They are usually made of a soft material such as rubber and usually covered with leather. Their height is determined by the severity of the planus deformity. A variation of the scaphoid pad is the "cookie" (Fig. 15–19). These are made of rigid leather for greater support. It has been my practice to use the softer scaphoid pad, which causes less initial discomfort and has a similar function.

Wedges made of leather can be placed as sandwiched material between the inner and outer sole, which is where they ordinarily belong. If necessary, because of the type of shoe the patient de-

mands, they can be glued as overlays under the sole. These wedges vary in thickness from one sixteenth of an inch to approximately one fourth of an inch, and the thickness will be determined by the severity of the problem. In a child one would start with one sixteenth and build up as necessary, usually to no more than one eighth. These wedges can be placed under the base of the heel medially to bring the foot into greater supination at the heel in order to counter the pronation that is present. These medial heel wedges are sometimes described as medial "roof" wedges, meaning that they are above the heel rather than on the inferior surface. Similarly, wedges can be placed under the lateral sole of the shoe in order to combat the relative internal rotation of the forefoot. If this is done, the steel shank must be removed in order to permit torsion of the shoe to take place. Steel wedges to supply a rigid shank are components of the manufacture of all orthopedic oxfords.

It should be mentioned that an orthopedic oxford, as usually described, has a medial long counter as part of its construction, as well as a straight inner border to the shoe and round toe

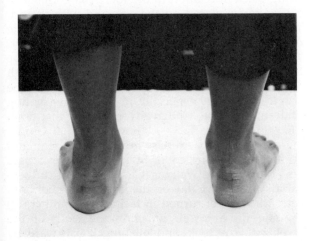

**Figure 15–17.** Pes planovalgus posteriorly with evident valgus heel.

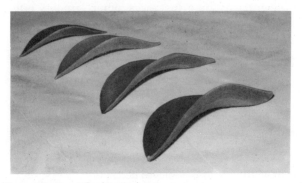

**Figure 15–19.** "Cookies" of various sizes.

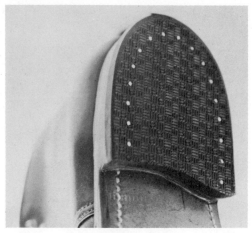

**Figure 15–20.** The Thomas heel.

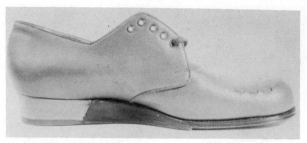

**Figure 15–22.** Medial shank.

box. This construction permits the first toe to remain in its normal position and prevents cramping of the toes. The wedge on a shoe usually extends to the midline of the sole, at which point it thins out to zero, a "feathering" of the wedge.

The aforementioned corrective devices will suffice for the average case, providing there are no complications such as dropped or painful metatarsals or plantar fasciitis. The prescription reads as follows:

Orthopedic oxford with long medial counter
medial heel wedge of $\frac{1}{16}$ or + thickness
and Thomas heel, with scaphoid pad

In more severe cases the entire anterior breast of the heel can be moved forward; the prescription would read, "Extended heel breast anteriorly." This will give even greater support to both the calcaneus and the longitudinal medial arch. Another means of increasing the correction is to extend the medial path of the heel all the way forward to feather out in the region of the ball of the foot throughout the shank, a medial shank filler (Fig. 15–22).

Ordinarily, for pes planovalgus, the combination of Thomas heel, long medial counter, medial heel wedge, and scaphoid pad in an orthopedic shoe is sufficient. In some instances when greater effect

must be obtained, one can order a straight-last shoe. An imaginary straight line drawn down the middle will divide this shoe into two equal halves, so that the normal medial curve of the forefoot aspect of the shoe has been removed. This allows for greater support of the forefoot in the shoe. Further, if the problem is even more severe and it is necessary to try to support the forefoot and hindfoot totally, one can prescribe a supinator last, or "turned-in" last, a corrective shoe whose front aspect is deviated medially to varying degrees on the basis of the last used on the posterior aspect of the shoe. With a line drawn through the middle of shoe, a greater part of the anterior aspect of the shoe would be located medial to the line than ordinarily. This can also help to correct the abducted forefoot and to support the longitudinal arch. In a supinator-last shoe, one can still add corrections; in fact, the shoe ordinarily is constructed with a Thomas heel, a long medial counter, and a medial heel wedge as well as the addition of a scaphoid pad to the prescription.

The child's foot must be evaluated every three months on an average, because this is the amount of time that it usually takes for growth to occur. Inserts such as arch supports are usually a poor idea in children, since even a small amount of growth will place every point on the internal device in the wrong place in relation to the foot. The corrections will be better placed on the sole and with the addition of a scaphoid pad, which can accommodate some degree of change in the size of the foot. When the shoe becomes too small, this will be shown by the fact that there is less than one-fourth to three-eighths inch from toe tip to tip of the toe box. In any case, especially in very active young children, the shoe will have worn out by that time.

EXERCISES FOR PLANUS FOOT IN THE CHILD. There is a place for exercise in the strengthening of the foot in a young child. Some of these exercises are: (1) practicing walking back and forth for several minutes every day on the lateral aspect of both feet with the feet turned in facing one another; (2) stepping on a towel, grasping the cloth of the towel with the toes, and pushing it backward by flexing the toes toward the rear of the foot, which

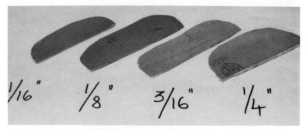

**Figure 15–21.** Wedges of various thicknesses.

also helps to strengthen the arch; (3) using resistive exercises for the muscles of the sole of the foot, with special emphasis on the peroneus longus, which supports the arch, and the tibialis posterior. These are done in a progressive resistive manner, starting with active exercises and building to maximum power for the muscle structures. It should be remembered, however, that with descent of the arch and malalignment of the bones, it is the ligamentous structures, which normally keep the foot in proper alignment, that have been weakened and stretched. These cannot be tightened. However, strengthening the aforementioned two muscles in particular helps in giving greater support to the arch. I have occasionally seen an improvement of the arch by several degrees through the use of this exercise. However, the child must be old enough, usually 8 to 10 years of age before cooperation can be expected for doing the exercises properly. This pertains to formal physical therapy, as well as a home exercise program, which should be prescribed.

## Pes Cavus

Pes cavus is as common a deformity as pes planovalgus. In pes cavus the medial longitudinal arch is curved higher than normal, forming a significantly high space between the walking surface or insole and the longitudinal arch. As a result of this situation the plantar fascia will tighten eventually in what is known as the windlass action (named for the windlass in a handle that is turned to bring a pail of water to the surface of a well). The fascia is inserted anteriorly over the superior surfaces of the proximal phalanges. Consequently, the proximal phalanges are pulled downward, putting the metatarsophalangeal joints into contact with the ground and destroying the transverse arch of the foot. As a result, the fat pads normally present under the metatarsophalangeal joints thin out, and these joints become compressed against

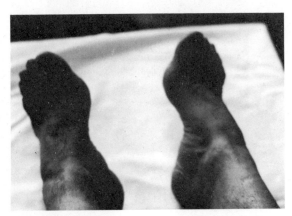

**Figure 15–23.** Pes cavus.

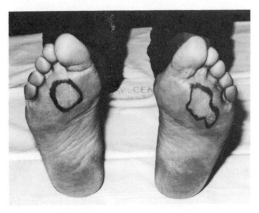

**Figure 15–24.** Callosities.

the bottom of the shoe. This results in what is called dropped metatarsals and, when pain occurs, metatarsalgia. Because of the undue compression in the plantar area, the foot may develop an inflammatory process (plantar fasciitis) in the region of calcaneal plantar tissue and a calcaneal spur, which can be quite painful at times. In this situation the foot is in supination or turned so that the sole tends to face inward to some degree. Simultaneously with the dropped metatarsals there is a tendency for the ligaments to weaken in the foot and to cause spreading of the forefoot so that the metatarsals are somewhat separated from one another more than is normal. This is referred to as a splayed foot.

As a result of the malalignment of the forefoot, calluses will form underneath the sole in the region of the metatarsophalangeal joints. These are seen in Figure 15–24, in which the area of the callosities has been circled.

Corrections for Pes Cavus and its Complications. There are several ways of dealing with the basic problem. The first treatment involves use of an orthopedic oxford with a long lateral counter rather than a medial counter to support the lateral aspect of the foot, which takes undue pressure because of the high arch and supinated position. If necessary, it is also possible to outflare the lateral aspect of the shoe by extending a wedged sole beyond the lateral borders. This may extend by one-fourth to as much as one-half inch in severe cases. The wedge height will be determined by the severity of the problem—from one-eighth to one-fourth inch. The arch itself is filled in with a scaphoid pad of sufficient height to contact the medial sole in the region of the elevated longitudinal arch. As mentioned earlier, it sometimes pays to start with a lower support and over a period of time elevate the scaphoid pad to full correction as the patient can tolerate this change. A reverse Thomas heel is prescribed, with the extension being on the lateral border of the shoe at least as far as the cuboid bone or beyond.

In less severe cases it may be sufficient to use an orthopedic oxford with a crepe sole, which softens the contact with the ground. The heel in this instance would be replaced with a SACH heel insert in order to permit the foot to come into contact with the ground more easily. This is helpful because pes cavus tends to be a rigid deformity that is not aided by correction as much as by accommodation to the deformity. A rocker bar can be added from shank to toe tip with an apex posterior to the metatarsal phalangeal joints. The insert of the shoe would contain a scaphoid elevation to fill in the cavus deformity.

Splayed foot, dropped metatarsals, and claw or hammer toes may be present, and metatarsalgia as determined by tenderness on palpation over the metatarsophalangeal joints, which are tender, particularly in the area of the second to fourth or fifth toes. To treat this, an inlay can be placed in the shoe and the scaphoid pad placed on top of this inlay. It will also be necessary to dig out the area of the inlay in the region of the metatarsophalangeal joints so that they are deeper than the rest of the support and the dugout area is filled, if possible, with foam rubber covered with leather. This adjustment also may be necessary under the toe tips, which may be pressing into the sole of the shoe and therefore require a dugout area as well. It is important in the presence of dropped metatarsals and claw and hammer toes to prescribe a high, wide, soft toe box with a straight inner border to permit the first toe to remain in normal position. A "deep shoe" is available that has extra room in the toe box and prevents development of corns and callosities over the upper surface of the toes, which in an ordinary shoe would be in contact with the toe box. Further, one would add a quadrilateral pad (or dancer pad, another name for this) to the shoe in order to take pressure off the metatarsal heads and to elevate them, if that is possible. If the toes are painful on manipulation, this correction may cause pain; therefore, it should be omitted and the rocker bar on the sole of the shoe will permit toe-off without pressure against the metatarsophalangeal joints lying in a dugout repository. In most instances, however, it is possible to use metatarsal pads. If there is undue pain at the calcaneal plantar surface, it is also possible to use a dugout heel as described earlier in the chapter. That, in combination with a SACH heel, is certain to relieve pain in the heel area. A rubber donut is sometimes used as a substitute for the dugout heel. However, in my experience this is totally inadequate.

In the presence of calcaneal fasciitis or a calcaneal spur, it is sometimes helpful to inject into the mid-calcaneal area in the case of fasciitis, or into the anterior border of the plantar surface of the cal-

caneus, a combination of 3 to 4 cc of lidocaine 1 per cent without epinephrine and 20 mg or 1 cc of dexamethasone. This can relieve to a significant degree the discomfort in this area.

If the patient with claw toe or hammer toe deformity is not helped by the deep shoe or high round wide soft toe box, it is possible, although somewhat less cosmetic, to balloon out the toe box of the shoe by cutting out the leather on the upper surface and sewing a large elevated patch into the cutout area to eliminate any conceivable pressure against the toes. In my experience with the deep shoe, however, I have not found this necessary.

## PES EQUINUS

This can be either an acquired or congenital deformity. It may occur as a result of weakness of the anterior tibial musculature in poliomyelitis, in multiple sclerosis with contracture of the forefoot and inability to dorsiflex, and in other similar diseases. The foot may be either in fixed deformity or flexible to some degree or on occasion it can be completely flexible. For the purpose of this discussion the rigid equinus deformity will be considered.

The object of the correction is to compensate for the equinus position and to hold the foot appropriately in the shoe while providing relatively simple entry into the shoe. Because of the equinus position, there is extensive pressure on the anterior aspect of the foot, with metatarsal compression on the plantar surface. As much as possible, if there is *any* flexibility in the position of the foot, this should be corrected.

In pes equinus of lesser severity, a high-topped

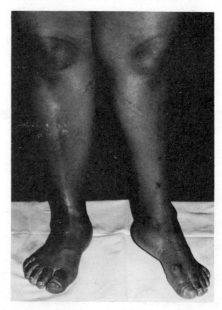

**Figure 15–25.** Pes cavus.

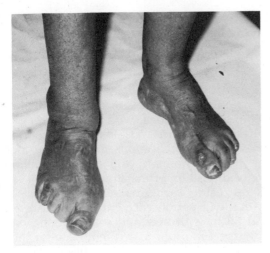

**Figure 15–26.** Equinus deformity in a poliomyelitis patient.

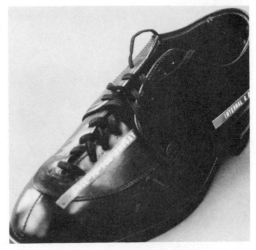

**Figure 15–28.** "Lace to toe throat" by slitting the vamp.

shoe is prescribed with either a convalescent or surgical lacing to allow for easy entry into the shoe. In some instances a regular shoe can be used with the addition of a "collar" that serves to keep the foot inside the shoe. The addition of elevations on the inside of the shoe is prescribed in order to compensate for the necessity of increased heel height. The shoe may also be revised to permit an extension of the lace stay through the vamp and the addition of eyelets to lace the shoe to the toe box. This is sometimes referred to as a lace-to-toe throat.

Figure 15–27 demonstrates a collar on a shoe, and Figure 15–28 shows the lace-to-toe throat. Another necessary modification is a medial longitudinal arch support to provide support to the medial aspect of the foot, which is under stress in the equinus position.

There are several ways in which the heel can be elevated to conform to the equinus position. Using the shoe with the collar, one can add as much as

three-fourths inch to the inside of the shoe as part of a full-length inlay placed in the region of the heel. If the required height is more than this, the inlay must be placed on the heel and inclined toward the sole of the shoe, using the formula shown in Table 15–1. (Naturally the elevation must conform to the configuration of the equinus deformity.)

If the patient also has disability in the forefoot because of pressure against the metatarsals and there is either metatarsalgia or dropped metatar-

**TABLE 15–1.** FORMULA FOR PLACEMENT OF INLAY IN TREATING PES EQUINUS

| Heel Height (Inches) | Ball | Toe |
|---|---|---|
| ½ | ½ | ¼ |
| ¾ | ½ | ¼ |
| 1 | ½ | ¼ |
| 1¼ | ¾ | ½ |
| 1½ | ¾ | ½ |
| 1¾ | 1 | ¾ |
| 2 | 1¼ | ¾ |
| 2¼ | 1½ | 1 |
| 2½ | 1¾ | 1 |
| 2¾ | 2 | 1 |
| 3 | 2¼ | 1¼ |
| 3¼ | 2½ | 1¼ |
| 3½ | 2¾ | 1¼ |
| 3¾ | 3 | 1½ |
| 4 | 3¼ | 1½ |
| 4¼ | 3½ | 1½ |
| 4½ | 3¾ | 1¾ |
| 4¾ | 4 | 1¾ |
| 5 | 4¼ | 1¾ |
| 5¼ | 4½ | 2 |
| 5½ | 4¾ | 2 |
| 5¾ | 5 | 2 |
| 6 | 5¼ | 2¼ |

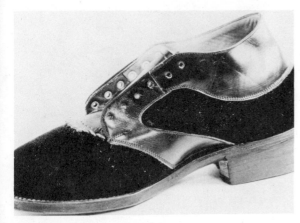

**Figure 15–27.** Shoe with a collar.

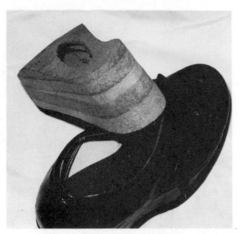

**Figure 15–29.** The sandwich between the inner and outer shoe.

sals, metatarsal pads or a rocker bar over the sole should be utilized, as discussed under pes cavus.

When the involved extremity is equal in length to the uninvolved one, it is also necessary to elevate the heel and sole of the normal extremity to permit the patient to swing through during gait with the equinus foot, since this will now be longer than the normal side. The normal side must be made equal in order to permit proper gait. Depending on the height of the elevations that are required, different substances may be used to make inlays for the lesser elevations that are placed inside the shoe. Cork or leather can be used, covered by an extra inlay of leather, if a full-length or three-fourths inch arch support is used. Overlays on the sole up to 1 inch or so can be made out of leather; beyond this, cork is preferable because with it extra weight for the shoe is avoided. In the higher degrees of elevation, it is crucial to use cork that has been hollowed out in order to make it light. This is placed between the inner and the outer sole, the outer sole being made of leather of one-fourth inch height. Figures 15–29 and 15–30 demonstrate the

hollowed-out cork elevation and the insertion between the inner and the outer sole.

### TALIPES EQUINOVARUS (EQUINOVARUS DEFORMITY)

As in equinus itself, it is important to make the same type of corrections, with the addition of corrections for the varus position of the foot. One either can add modifications to bring the foot, if flexible, into its normal position, or accommodate to the fixed position of the equinovarus.

Besides using the usual elevations and shoe types that will permit easy entry, it is also necessary to fill in with heel and sole wedging on the medial aspect in order to accommodate for the position of the foot and to place it flat on the floor. However, if the foot is flexible, the type of corrections should be used that will normalize the foot's position. This is done by adding lateral heel and sole wedging and outflares. A lateral long counter must also be used in order to protect the outer aspect of the foot, which will be taking increased pressure, as in pes cavus. Should there be excessive compression against the metatarsals, especially on the lateral aspect of the foot, insoles with dugout areas, filled with foam rubber in this area, must be utilized.

Figure 15–32 demonstrates the outflare of both the heel and the sole. The degree of flaring can vary, depending on the need, up to usually not more than one-half inch. If there is still undue pressure, especially with a high-topped shoe, the lateral counters can be made higher, up to and including the malleolus and sometimes almost to the top of the shoe. This gives added support to the lateral aspect of the ankle. If there is undue pressure caused by the high counter, it can be ballooned out to some degree to prevent pressure at

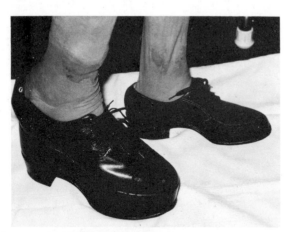

**Figure 15–30.** Hollowed-out cork elevation.

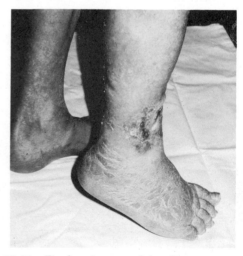

**Figure 15–31.** Fixed equinovarus deformity.

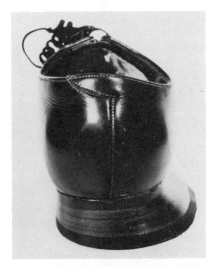

**Figure 15–32.** Shoe with outflare used for flexible varus deformity.

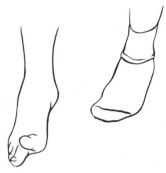

**Figure 15–33.** Stroke patient with hyperextension of the first toe during walking.

any particular point, much as one does with splinting or with prosthetic devices.

## SHORT LEG

In the case of a short lower extremity caused by a genetic or growth-related defect, such as fracture in a growing site prior to full growth or early poliomyelitis, it is necessary to add elevations to the shoe. The same principles apply as in the previous discussion of shoe elevations, with the same numerical formulas used for the elevations (see Table 15–1). However, it should be mentioned that for the one-half inch or less elevation that is required, except for certain instances in which the equinus position would be contraindicated, I do not add the sole elevation for cosmetic reasons. It is adequate to add to the one-half inch at the heel in several ways, one of them being by placing a heel cushion (hard rubber) as an inlay glued to the heel area. The other one-fourth inch can be obtained by either cutting the height of the opposite heel by that amount or elevating the heel on the involved side by a one-fourth inch addition.

## HEMIPLEGIA

In hemiplegia the foot problem is usually one of either flexible or fixed equinus deformity, not infrequently with some degree of varus. As may be seen on Figure 15–33, the first toe is in hyperextension and the foot is in varus. It is not uncommon for an examiner to miss the hyperextension of the toe, since the patient is usually examined with shod feet. The varus deformity, of course, can be seen shod or unshod. In the case of the hyperextended toe, which should be looked for, the shoe must have a high, deep, soft and wide toe box, in order to prevent pressure against the toe.

The patient may be given a short leg brace of metal; this must be attached to the shoe. An alternative is a Polypropylene brace, a widely used device that is inserted into the shoe. In any case the shoe must have the following characteristics: it must be an orthopedic shoe and in some cases a high shoe to prevent pumping of the foot in the shoe. It must have a rigid shank and a one-fourth inch leather sole. The lace stay must be of the Blucher type, preferably with some type of special closure such as Velcro, straps, or buckles to permit closing and opening of the shoe, especially if the patient also suffers from an upper extremity disability. The steel shank should be reinforced with a tongue in order to permit connection to the stirrup, which is the attachment of the sole for the brace, when necessary. Figure 15–34 shows a patient with hemiplegia with contracture of the ankle, fixed in plantar flexion. This is treated by an elevation at the heel, usually by the addition of a heel cushion glued as an inlay in the shoe, with or without the addition of a heel lift. If the foot is in varus and flexible, slight lateral heel wedge and sole wedges may be used to bring the foot into proper alignment during stance phase. If fixed, medial heel and sole wedges are used to accommodate to the contractures.

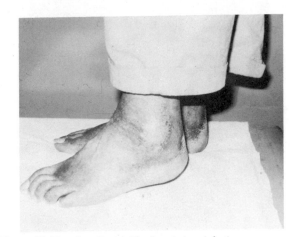

**Figure 15–34.** A patient with chronic hemiplegia.

## GASTROCNEMIUS-SOLEUS PARALYSIS

Occasionally, a patient will develop paralysis of these muscles. This was commonly seen in poliomyelitis. It may also be seen in peripheral neuropathy. As a result of weakness of the gastrocnemius muscle, the calcaneus tends to be pulled forward and the plantar fascia tends to contract and become stressed by this position. The peroneal muscles, in attempting to plantar flex the foot, increase the development of what becomes a cavus deformity with pes cavus. The patient ends up with toes in the claw and hammer position and with metatarsalgia and dropped metatarsals.

The treatment for this condition, which is usually a fixed deformity, is to accommodate as with the fixed deformity of pes cavus. The longitudinal arch area is filled with a scaphoid elevation, with a dugout area under the metatarsophalangeal joints and also under the toe tips in order to protect them preferably filled with foam rubber. The shoe should have a high, soft, wide, round toe box with a straight inner border. The shoe must also have a long lateral counter to protect the lateral aspect of the foot. In essence, the changes are similar to those described under pes cavus.

## CONDITIONS OF THE FOREFOOT

**Hallux Valgus (Bunion).** Hallux valgus is usually an acquired condition that results from a number of different situations, some of which have been mentioned earlier. It is much more common in females than in males and in the shod population, especially those who wear pointed or tight shoes with high heels. However, it is also seen as a result of certain congenital defects such as metatarsus varus or adductus, a condition in which the first toe is considerably separated from the second and consequently tends to be pushed toward the

second toe, creating a valgus deformity. It can be seen with a Morton's toe, a short first metatarsal, also a congenital defect. The degree of valgus tends to increase as the patient ages. Not uncommonly the first toe will ride over the second or force the second to ride over the third, causing overlapping. Consequently, an exostosis forms over the metatarsophalangeal joint on the medial aspect of the first toe, as well as an inflammatory process and chronic thickening of the connective tissue in the area superficial to the exostosis. The metatarsophalangeal joint is narrowed, with destruction of the joint space (Fig. 15–35).

Corrections for this disability are numerous. The basic objective is to allow for sufficient room in the area of the bunion in order to prevent further compression of the first toe and aggravation of the inflamed area, and to provide for proper gait as in the rule of the second-class lever. An orthopedic shoe with a so-called bunion last can be used. This is a shoe made on a last that, if bisected, would have a larger degree of widening in the region of the first metatarsophalangeal joint to allow for better spacing. This will correct moderate degrees of hallux valgus but will not be adequate for severe disability. The shoe must have a high, wide, soft, deep toe box with a straight inner border and the heel should be relatively low, not higher than 1½ inches and broad in type (1⅜ inches). The patient may also require a medial sole wedge of approximately one-eighth inch in order to shift the gravity forces toward the lateral aspect of the foot to some degree and away from the bunion. Next, in order to prevent pain, if the toe is very tender on manipulation, a Morton's toe extension (sesamoid platform) can be used. This device will immobilize, to some degree, the metatarsophalangeal joint and prevent pain. The shoe should also have a long medial counter for the longitudinal arch to also help in shifting the weight away from the first toe area. It is sometimes helpful to add a quadrilateral metatarsal pad in order to prevent the foot from slipping forward in the shoe.

I have not used the toe separator, a device placed between the first and the second toes, because I find that the majority of the patients do not feel comfortable with this correction. However, it can be used if found to be helpful. In the worst cases it is possible to remove the leather from the region of the bunion and to balloon out a patch of similar leather to give adequate room for the bunion (Fig. 15–36). The following figures show a typical hallux valgus deformity, as well as a shoe with a ballooned-out patch.

**Tailor's Bunion.** A not-uncommon deformity is the tailor's bunion. It takes its name from the traditional tendency of tailors to sit with legs crossed in the lotus position, with pressure being taken on the lateral aspects of the fifth toes. It is found in

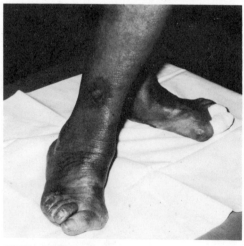

**Figure 15–35.** Hallux valgus.

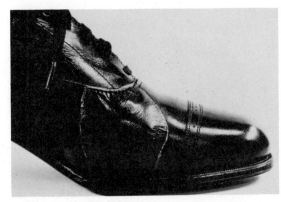

**Figure 15–36.** Balloon patch for hallux valgus.

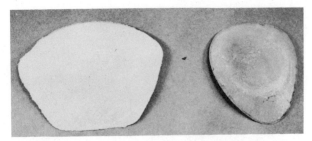

**Figure 15–37.** Triangular and quadralateral metatarsal pads.

several situations such as in a pes cavus deformity in which undue pressure is taken along the lateral aspect of the foot, in splayed feet with a spread forefoot such as in pes valgo planus as well as pes cavus, and is also seen in those who wear ill-fitting shoes. The condition is an exostosis of the lateral metatarsophalangeal joint with an inflammatory process similar to that seen in hallus valgus.

The treatment is usually relatively simple. The patient should have a wide, round, soft toe box with a lateral sole wedge of one-eighth inch thickness to move the center of gravity more toward the medial side of the foot. If other disabilities accompany the tailor's bunion, these too must be corrected. The objective of treatment is this condition is usually to accommodate rather than to correct the position of the toes, but frequently it is possible to support the flattened transverse arch, which is commonly flexible and pain-free. If there is marked tenderness of the metatarsophalangeal joints on palpation as well as significant pain in flexion extension of these joints passively, then accommodation rather than correction is made. The claw toe and the hammer toe differ.

**Claw Toes.** In this situation the metatarsophalangeal joint is extended, and the proximal and distal interphalangeal joints are in flexion. In hammer toes the metatarsophalangeal joint is extended, the proximal interphalangeal joint is flexed, and the distal interphalangeal joints are in extension with significant painful compression of these toes against the inner sole of the shoe. Because of the position of the toes there is a tendency to develop corns, especially over the proximal interphalangeal joints, as well as callosities under the metatarsophalangeal joints, especially in the area of the second to the fifth toes, and particularly the second, third and fourth toes.

Correction, when feasible, involves the placement of a metatarsal pad, either triangular or quadrilateral, to elevate the transverse arch. Several types of corrections may be added to the sole of

the shoe, including a metatarsal bar. This is a bar with abrupt edges, both anteriorly and posteriorly, just posterior to the metatarsophalangeal joints, used as an onlay on the sole of the shoe.

I believe that it is much more helpful to use the Denver bar. The Denver bar supports the entire metatarsal area, whereas the metatarsal bar supports only the distal aspect of the metatarsal. The bar consists of a leather extension on the sole. This is narrowed at the anterior aspect, posterior to the metatarsophalangeal joints, and widened to accommodate to the foot's flat position, passing backward along the metatarsal length. The anterior aspect can be slightly abrupt, or as I prefer feathered at its anterior end; that is, completely confluent with the sole.

In the presence of significant pain or rigid deformity, accommodation must be made. One would use an orthopedic oxford with a high, soft, wide, deep toe box, straight inner border, and with preferably a crepe sole of hard rubber, one-fourth inch thick. The placement between the inner and outer soles of a semiflexible steel shank from the calcaneus to the toe tip is necessary in order to allow for rigidity of the shoe, so that it does not flex at toe-off during the late aspect of stance phase. A SACH heel and a rocker bar are placed from shank to toe tip in order to allow the patient to pass through stance phase easily with significant toe spring. It is usually necessary to use an insert, either of leather with Neoprene material or Plastizote. This permits digging out of the insole under the metatarsopha-

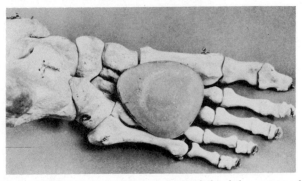

**Figure 15–38.** Metatarsal pad placement behind the metatarsal heads.

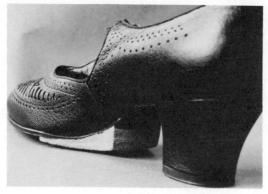

**Figure 15–39.** Denver bar.

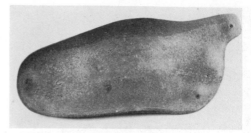

**Figure 15–41.** Arch support with Morton's toe extension.

langeal joints and the toe tips to allow for relief of pain in these areas during gait. This type of shoe is extremely comfortable and will eliminate the discomfort and disability. An occasional patient may require a balloon patch to be placed over the toe box to make extra room for the toes. However, with the deep shoe, this is rarely necessary.

It should be mentioned that, as an additional home treatment, the patient is advised to bathe the feet in warm water for about 20 minutes in the bath tub, sitting on a stool on the outside of the tub. Following this, the patient is instructed to use a no. 1 fine emery cloth, obtained in a hardware store, to gently brush away only the easily removable parts of the callus. This is done twice a week over a period of a few months, and with the corrections, the callus should disappear. Corn pads can be stuck to the corn areas to prevent contact with the top of the shoe and to allow healing.

**Hallux Rigidus.** In this condition there is either marked restriction caused by osteoarthritis or rheumatoid arthritis of the first metatarsophalangeal joint without the valgus deformity. To treat hallux rigidus, it is necessary to eliminate completely all motion at the metatarsophalangeal level in order to eliminate pain. The shoe must have a straight inner border and again, a wide, round, soft toe box. The shoe must be made rigid by placing a semiflexible steel shank straight through from the calcaneus to the toe tip and using a SACH heel and a rocker bar from shank to toe tip, usually skived because a large toe spring is usually not necessary.

There should also be a long medial counter and a scaphoid pad to prevent undue pressure on the first toe and to spread the variations of pressure throughout the foot.

Another method of handling this problem is to prescribe a full-length arch support with Morton's toe extension (Fig. 15–41). This is a soft leather extension under the first metatarsophalangeal joint that provides rigidity to the toe to some extent. This may help in milder cases but is ineffective in significant pathology. For these more difficult cases the earlier described adjustments to the shoe should be made.

**Morton's Toe.** In this condition the person is born with a short first metatarsal; this results in inappropriate toe-off and eventual disability in the area of the first and second toes. Since the first toe is inadequate for toe off, the second toe, which is longer, will be forced to take a greater amount of weight. This results frequently in a thickening of the second metatarsal shaft.

The treatment for this condition is the same as for hallux rigidus, either the use of a semiflexible steel insert (Fig. 15–42) through the sole, the rocker bar, and SACH heel, or the arch support with Morton's toe extension, depending on the severity of the disability.

**Morton's Neuroma.** Morton's neuroma is a common condition in which there is undue compression between the third and the fourth toes, with a neuroma of the digital nerves passing through the toe web, between the third and fourth anterior aspects of the metatarsal shafts. On palpation, this area will be very tender and the patient will complain of burning and tenderness on walking, felt in this region of the forefoot.

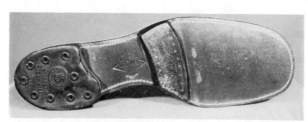

**Figure 15–40.** Rocker bar.

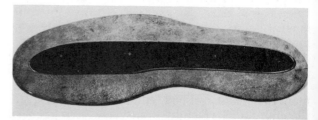

**Figure 15–42.** Semiflexible steel bar from heel to toe tip.

The mild neuroma will not uncommonly respond to injections of lidocaine and dexamethasone, plus a long-acting steroid of the triamcinolone type. I use 2 cc of lidocaine 1 per cent without epinephrine and ½ cc each of dexamethasone solution and ½ cc of triamcinolone suspension. This is injected into the toe web area of greatest tenderness between the third and the fourth toes. One may also use anti-inflammatory agents such as indomethacin or ibuprofen for a short period of time. Further, physical therapy is not uncommonly of help, with the prescription of whirlpool for 20 minutes, followed by dipping of the foot in paraffin for 15 minutes, followed by lidocaine 1 per cent without epinephrine, combined with hydrocortisone, iontophoresis, 5 to 15 milliamperes, for a period of 10 to 15 minutes.

The shoe corrections consist of simply the use of a lowered heel, usually of the solid ankle cushion heel type, and a rocker bar from shank to toe tip plus a scaphoid pad to distribute the pressure along the sole and make toe-off easy without much pressure over the neuroma. A quadrilateral metatarsal pad is placed as an inlay. Further, a lateral one-eighth inch sole wedge to move gravity toward the medial foot may help. If this does not bring relief within a reasonable amount of time, in my experience surgical excision is indicated.

## AMPUTATION OF THE FOREFOOT

In cases of amputation of the toes, a simple ordinary shoe, possibly with a rigid steel shank and a rocker bar, will allow for easy toe-off. Some patients can walk in an ordinary oxford with little problem. However, in amputations further posteriorly such as through the midtarsal area, it is necessary to use an appropriate filler. Shoes for patients with amputations at this level should include a semiflexible steel shank through the sole, as well as a rocker bar and preferably a SACH heel. The forefoot filler, made of foam rubber on an inlay inserted into the shoe, may also have a semiflexible

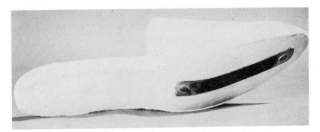

**Figure 15–44.** Semiflexible steel insert.

steel bar inserted onto the inlay itself. If the steel addition is added to the inlay, the long steel shank is unnecessary. The foam rubber filler must have a perfectly smooth posterior edge to prevent pressure against the stump. A leather liner on the stump end of the filler is helpful. It too should be absolutely smooth and wrinkle free.

## FRACTURES OF THE PHALANGES OR THE METATARSALS

Simple fractures of the phalanges require little support except during the first one or two weeks, when they may be quite painful. I have found it helpful to use a rigid shoe when the patient is capable of purchasing it for use such a short period of time. The shoe containing a semiflexible steel insert to the sole and a rocker bar from shank to toe tip will eliminate all motion. In my opinion, use of the technique of binding the fractured phalanx to the contiguous phalanx increases the pain by permitting the normal toe to tug on the fractured toe and to cause a greater problem than originally existed.

In the case of a metatarsal fracture, however, immobilization is of help. A full-length arch support incorporating a semiflexible steel bar and a rocker bar on the sole of the shoe, full length from shank to toe tip, will help considerably, diminishing the discomfort and allowing for healing.

## CONCLUSION

In conclusion, it should be pointed out that there are cases that are so complicated because of massive disability that only custom shoes or loose-fitting, simple coverings may be used. These cases include old severe poliomyelitis with distortion of the foot, peripheral vascular disease with partial amputations, and complete distortion, swelling, and malalignment of the foot from various severe ailments. Generally, however, with the understanding that the same goal can be accomplished in a number of different ways, almost all patients can be made comfortable. It is only necessary for the

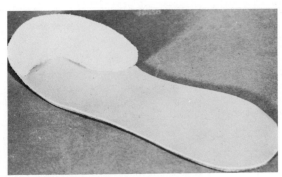

**Figure 15–43.** Foam rubber forefoot filler.

prescriber to be familiar with the underlying disability and the available methods for treatment and correction or accommodation to obtain proper results.

## REFERENCES

1. American Academy of Orthopedic Surgeons: Orthopedic Appliance Atlas, Vol. 1, 1952.
2. Hauser, E. D.: Diseases of the Foot. W. B. Saunders Co., Philadelphia, 1950.
3. Dickson and Diveley: Functional Disorders of the Foot. J. B. Lippincott Co., Philadelphia, 1953.
4. Bulletin of Prosthetics Research, Dept. of Medicine and Surgery, Veterans Administration, 10–2, Fall 1964.
5. Human Locomotion and Body Form, Morton, 1952.
6. Licht, S.: Orthotics. Physical medicine library. Vol. 9. 1966.
7. Kelikian, H.: Hallux Valgus, Allied Deformities of the Forefoot and Metatarsalgia. W. B. Saunders Co., Philadelphia, 1967.
8. Hauser, E. D.: Congenital Clubfoot, W. B. Saunders Co., Philadelphia, 1966.
9. Gamble, F. O. and Yale, I.: Clinical Foot Roentgenology. Williams and Wilkins, Baltimore, 1966.
10. MacLennan, R.: Prevalence of hallux valgus in a neolithic New Guinea population. Lancet 1:1398–1400, 1966.
11. Shoes for All People by Prescription, Reno, June 1914, The Medical Times.

# 16

# Rehabilitation in Fractures of the Limbs

*by James T. Demopoulos, M.D.*

In considering and planning the aftercare of an individual who has had primary management, conservative or surgical, of a fractured limb, one must differentiate between the patient with a simple fracture unassociated with major life style disruptions and the patient with a limb fracture that potentially can produce a near-total disability, including lifelong confinement to a dependent existence. For example, in an ankle fracture in a young, healthy individual, one would not anticipate functional complications, whereas a hip fracture in an elderly individual with pre-existing health problems could result in serious consequences. These could include inability to walk independently, cardiovascular and behavioral decompensation, decubitus ulcers, as well as specific limb deformities, weakness, and pain. However, it is important to recognize that this categorization of patients, young and aged, with simple and complicated fractures, does not address the multitude of patients classified between the two extremes. The point to be emphasized is that all patients with fractures require careful evaluation of their specific limb disabilities, anticipation of possible long-term sequelae and their recognition, and careful prescription and implementation of a formal treatment plan, be it the provision of a pair of crutches and ankle exercises or comprehensive management by a multidisciplinary team of health professionals. Further, successful functional outcome will ultimately depend on the referral of the patient for physical restoration and, if needed, rehabilitation. Rehabilitation is here defined as the process whereby the patient is returned to a maximum life style consistent with any residual permanent impairment.

It is the purpose of this chapter to provide the family physician and other interested health professionals with basic information on how to evaluate and restore to full function the patient who has sustained a limb fracture and received primary care for it.

## EVALUATION OF THE PATIENT

Evaluation of the patient with a limb fracture should conform to the basic principles used in evaluating all other instances of disease or trauma. Essentially, one must elicit a detailed history that includes the chronological events surrounding the injury, immediate post-traumatic care, significant previous medical and surgical history, review of other organ systems, description of the patient's prefracture functional level that includes locomotion ability, occupation, degree of socialization, and other life style factors, and finally, management of the patient up to the time of evaluation. A review of the pertinent radiographs and laboratory findings, together with communication with the surgeon, is vital; one must always be aware of possible contraindications and precautions.

Beyond the general examination, it is important to examine and record for later reference the exact status of the fractured limb: (1) Degree of active or passive motion of all the joints that can be safely moved, both proximal and distal to the fracture site. (2) Ability to contract the limb muscles and actively produce movement within the limitations imposed by the injury. Measurement of strength and endurance is often not possible or desirable because of pain, swelling, or feared disruption of the fracture alignment. (3) Sensory or motor disorders associated with peripheral nerve injuries. (4) Evidence of circulatory impairment of lymphatic, venous, or arterial origin, and findings suggesting superficial or deep thrombophlebitis. (5) Presence of reflex sympathetic changes producing pain, trophic changes, atrophy, and small joint motion limitations. (6) Atrophy secondary to the immobilization process. (7) Documentation of associated soft tissue injuries of the muscles, musculotendinous insertions, capsular and ligamentous tissues, as well as trauma to the skin and subcutaneous areas. (8) Pre-existing conditions affecting the injured limb such as osteoarthritis, other rheumatological entities, and neurovascular problems resulting from local or systemic diseases, or other causes.

## PRINCIPLES OF TREATMENT

In developing an aftercare program, there are a number of basic principles to be considered.

(1) The treatment plan must be individualized and directed to totally reversing, or maximally alleviating, all abnormalities of the fractured limb noted during the baseline examination.

(2) The status, or healing, of the fracture is always the major factor guiding treatment. Therapy needs to be applied with a full knowledge of all possible contraindications and precautions.

(3) All patients with a fracture require formal, professionally applied and directed treatment. One should never simply provide a patient with a few instructions to follow at home.

(4) A carefully constructed home program of exercises can and should supplement formal treatment. Again, printed instructions that are vague and apply to all patients should be avoided.

(5) Early referral maximizes the final outcome—before contractures, advanced atrophy, and other preventable complications develop. Physical restoration can begin even in early hospitalization of severely injured patients.

(6) Since each patient's response to a specific therapy format may vary, continuous assessment is necessary. For this reason, as well as others, active dialogue between the physician and the therapist often yields a more satisfactory outcome.

(7) The frequency and duration of physical or occupational therapy, or both, are highly relevant factors; treatment once or twice a week for 15 minutes or less can hardly be adequate to achieve the desired effect.

(8) Frequent re-examinations by the physician responsible for the restoration process permit interval adjustments of the treatment program. Comparisons with the previously noted baseline status of the fractured limb serve as a guide to improvement and signal onset of possible complications.

(9) Confronted with major complications and multiplying problems, the prescribing physician needs to consider consultation with a specialist in physical medicine and rehabilitation, either locally available or at a distance.

(10) Finally, as physical progress is achieved, attention must be given to the patient's pretrauma life style to ensure return to gainful employment, household duties, or education, and to leisure activities. Often other professionals are required to assist the patient to reach his normal functional level, or the most appropriate level.

## ELEMENTS OF THE TREATMENT PRESCRIPTION

A considerable array of therapeutic modalities and exercises are available, including those primarily provided by physical and occupational therapists. In order to reverse or improve the fractured limb's impairments and generally restore a patient to normal or near-normal functioning, one needs to choose from these modalities and organize their provision in a logical, effective manner.

Generally, initial application of some form of heat, particularly moist heat, induces general relaxation, reduces muscle spasm, improves tissue elasticity or elongation capabilities, alleviates pain and

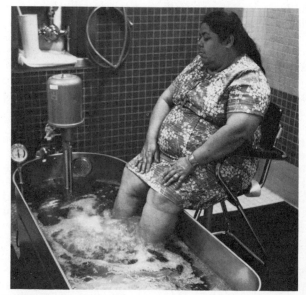

**Figure 16–1.** Whirlpool therapy following removal of an ankle plaster cast.

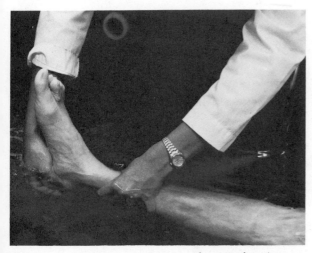

**Figure 16–2.** Underwater active-assisted range of motion exercises.

anxiety concerning therapeutic exercises, and often enhances the patient's motivation and participation in the overall treatment program. Heat as a treatment modality can be applied in many ways. *Hydrotherapy*, or the use of water in its liquid state, can include the use of a whirlpool or Hubbard tank, with the capability to vary water temperature and the direction and intensity of a swirling action. Various exercises can be performed while the limb is immersed in these water containers—ultrasound, can be applied underwater. Further, germicidal agents and other additives can be dissolved in the water.

A therapeutic pool is useful not only for heating but for the buoyancy effect of water, facilitating limb-unloading ambulation and exercise of weakened muscles.

Moist *hydrocollator packs* vary in size and shape and can be applied to all parts of the trunk or limbs. Heated in water to 150° F, wrapped in towels, and applied for approximately 20 minutes, these packs effectively provide superficial heating and other effects, notably muscle spasm relaxation.

*Paraffin units* are simply containers with heated liquid wax into which the limb is repeatedly immersed and then wrapped for 15 to 20 minutes. The wax coating prevents superficial heat loss and efficiently warms the limb segment as a prelude to exercise.

*Ultrasound* is a modality that emits mechanical energy as sound waves, deeply penetrating tissues and then being converted into heat. It is particularly useful for heating periarticular and articular surfaces and where adhesions limit joint motion.

*Shortwave* and *microwave diathermy*, as well as various lamps are other means of inducing deep and superficial heating of tissues.

Following the application of heat, if not contraindicated by systemic or local disease or injury, it is usual to prescribe one or more therapeutic exercises designed to increase joint motion, improve circulation by manual or mechanical means, strengthen muscles, improve coordination, mobilize limb segments by manipulation, free adhesions, and massage away muscle spasm. Further, individualized training sessions are used for improving ambulation and elevation activities and function in activities of daily living (dressing, feeding, and so forth).

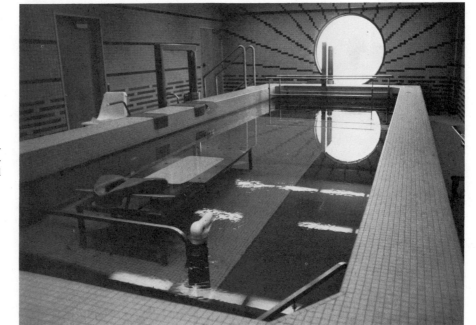

**Figure 16–3.** Therapeutic pool facilitates limb-unloading ambulation and exercises by weakened muscles.

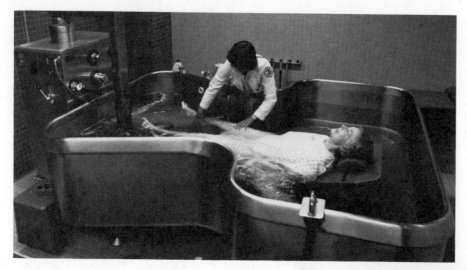

**Figure 16–4.** Passive range of motion exercises performed in a Hubbard tank.

**Figure 16–5.** Simultaneous knee and hip motion exercises in the Hubbard tank.

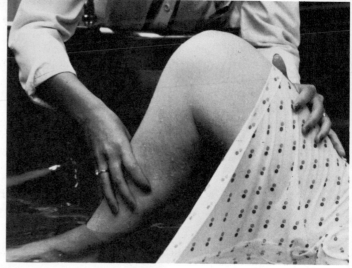

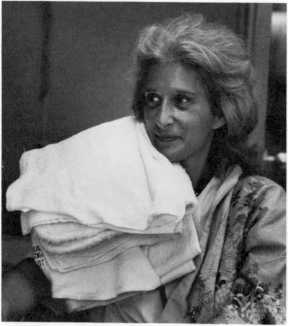

**Figure 16–6.** Hydrocollator packs applied to a shoulder.

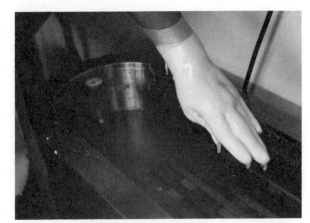

**Figure 16–7.** Paraffin immersions prior to exercising a fractured wrist.

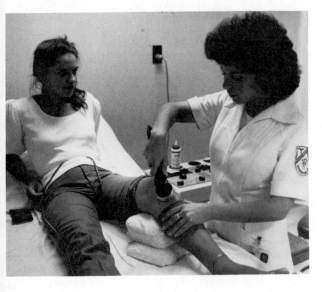

**Figure 16–8.** Ultrasound applied to the medial aspect of the knee.

**Figure 16–9.** Electromechanical equipment is used to efficiently regain motion and strength of the knee.

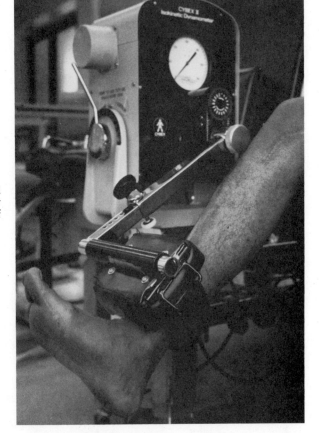

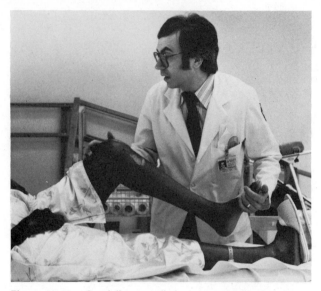

**Figure 16–10.** Carefully controlled exercises for hip fracture.

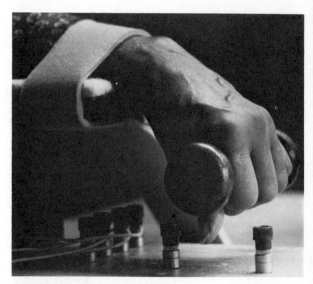

**Figure 16–12.** Progressive resisted exercises to redevelop wrist strength.

A description of passive, active, and active-assistive range of motion exercises as well as active and resistive strengthening exercises can be found in standard physical therapy texts, as can detailed descriptions of manipulation, massage, and other treatment modalities. Selection of the appropriate physical agents and exercise techniques is discussed when each different fracture site is considered.

In addition to prescribing the individual physical agents and exercises to be provided by physical and occupational therapists, one must prescribe splints, braces, assistive devices, other adaptive equipment, wheelchairs, special beds, and home equipment as needed. These items are mentioned as they apply to various fractures.

Finally, as one initially prescribes the physical restoration process, it is not too early to involve, as needed, trained rehabilitation nurses, social workers, vocational rehabilitation counselors, psychologists, and others.

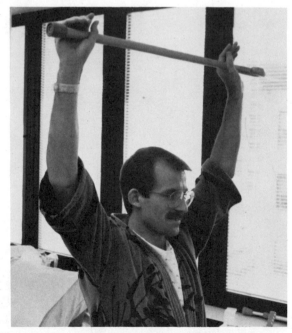

**Figure 16–11.** A cane is used to increase shoulder motion.

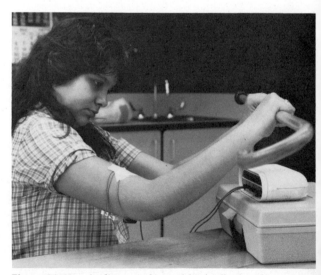

**Figure 16–13.** Auditory and visual biofeedback enhances motion of a fractured elbow.

## FRACTURES OF THE LOWER LIMBS

The major impairment resulting from fractures of the lower limbs involves ambulation. Essentially, the restorative process is directed to improving limb joint motion and strength and providing walking aids and braces if necessary to assist the patient to walk and to redevelop balance. The ability to ambulate is also dependent on normal or near-normal functioning of the other three noninjured limbs and the trunk. If there is evidence of dysfunction in these areas, exercises must also be prescribed for correction of any deficiencies.

Locomotion, particularly partial or non-weight-bearing on one limb, requires considerable expenditure of energy and careful concentration to avoid falling. A continuous assessment of the patient's cardiovascular status and ability to follow verbal orders is obviously essential. The therapist must monitor the patient's reaction to the ambulation training process and report abnormalities to the physician.

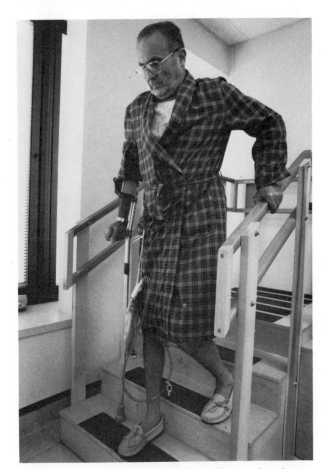

**Figure 16–15.** Stair climbing and descending with a forearm crutch.

## FRACTURES OF THE PELVIS

### AVULSION FRACTURES

This type of injury is usually seen in young individuals who strongly contract a muscle arising from the pelvis. Treatment includes:

(1) Bed rest and no weight bearing until pain is much alleviated.

(2) Application of moist heat at bedside to reduce muscle spasm around the injured site.

(3) Active range of motion exercises of the ankle-foot segments, active knee extension with support under the thigh, and as pain subsides, progressive active range of motion exercises of the hip joint.

(4) Ambulation with axillary crutches, first non-weight-bearing and then partial weight-bearing, depending on healing and reattachment of the avulsed fragment.

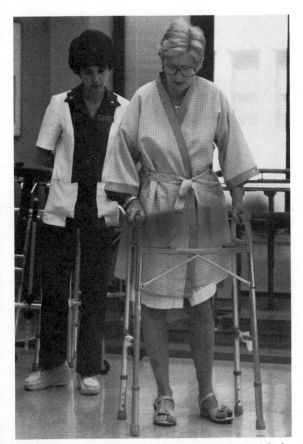

**Figure 16–14.** A walker is used to facilitate partial weight-bearing ambulation.

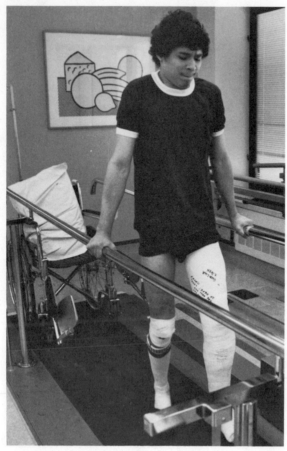

**Figure 16–16.** Parallel bars used to initiate nonweight-bearing ambulation.

(5) Subsequent range of motion exercises, active-assistive, to restore full motion.

(6) Progressive resistive exercises to regain full strength.

(7) Ambulation training proceeding to partial weight-bearing with one crutch, to one cane, to full weight-bearing.

### ISOLATED FRACTURES OF THE PELVIS

(1) Bed rest is prescribed until pain lessens considerably.

(2) During the bed rest phase, the patient is instructed to actively move the ankle-foot joints and upper limbs.

(3) With improvement, active exercises are performed, first internally and externally rotating the hip, then flexing the hip joint to 45 degrees by sliding the heel on the bed.

(4) Partial weight-bearing with a walker or axillary crutches is begun, depending on age, balance, and general strength.

(5) Progress is achieved to full weight-bearing, using appropriate walking aids for balance.

(6) Active and resistive exercises are done to regain normal motion and strength.

### DISPLACED FRACTURES

(1) Bed rest and traction are prescribed, depending on the fracture site and presence of associated dislocations.

(2) During traction, active ankle-foot exercises, upper limb active exercises, and deep breathing exercises are done.

(3) With bony healing and pelvic stability, active hip and knee exercises are added.

(4) Ambulation, partial weight-bearing, is begun with a walker or axillary crutches.

(5) If the patient is elderly, mobilization directed toward ambulation can begin by placing the patient on a tilt table, progressively increasing the angle and amount of weight-bearing. When the patient is able, progressive ambulation follows.

(6) Later, with complete fracture healing, exercises are increased to regain normal strength and motion of the involved lower limb.

## FRACTURES OF THE HIP

Fractures of the hip can be subcapital, intertrochanteric, or subtrochanteric and range from those with minimal roentgenographic findings to fractures with impaction, comminution, displacement, angulation, and severe malalignment. Primary treatment may include skeletal traction, pin fixation, open reduction, and fixation with an assortment of devices or replacement of one or more joint components.

The rehabilitative treatment plan must be carefully devised and phased in concert with the surgical care. Exercises and ambulation must be linked not only to the healing process but to the patient's general condition and response to treatment. Complications can include heart and lung disorders, decubitus ulcers, thrombophlebitis and embolic phenomena, other circulatory problems, and peripheral nerve dysfunction. A desirable final outcome clearly depends on a well-developed and monitored restorative program with professional diligence necessary at every phase of the long-term treatment plan. An elderly patient's ability to return to his pretrauma environment will be associated with success in ambulation and full or partial independence in self-care activities; all efforts must be made to achieve these goals.

Finally, it must be realized that the restorative processes to be described are broad outlines and are not intended to be effective in each variant of hip fractures. The point to be emphasized again is the need for individualized prescriptions, with constant re-evaluations and changes of treatment, daily if necessary.

## EARLY EXERCISES

Following definitive care for the fractured hip, early exercises are initiated at bedside, within a few days:

(1) Exercises to improve the patient's breathing capacity and ability to cough, i.e., chest physical therapy programs (see Chapter 22).

(2) Active and vigorous exercises of both feet to improve limb circulation and prevent ankle-foot contractures.

(3) Active exercises of the upper limbs: raising the arms to the side, front, and overhead, flexing and extending the elbows and wrists, and opening and closing the fingers.

(4) With stabilization of the pelvis, gentle and active exercise of the sound lower limb.

(5) "Quadriceps setting exercises" for the fractured hip limb.

(6) Positioning of the injured limb and avoidance of decubitus ulcers.

## MOBILIZATION PROCESS

(1) Patients are encouraged to gradually sit up in bed, assisted to dangle their legs, and continue deep breathing and active movement of their upper limbs.

(2) With assistance, the patient can stand at bedside without bearing weight on the affected side; if this is not feasible, the patient can be carefully lifted and placed in a wheelchair or appropriate bedside chair.

(3) If permitted by the status of the fracture, active exercises of the involved hip joint are added: abduction and supported hip-knee flexion and extension, sliding the heel on the bed, and gentle limited hip rotation.

(4) Assisted straight-leg raising is done, minimally at first.

(5) Knee extension and flexion can be added with the leg dangling over the side of the bed; slight manual resistance can be added.

(6) If necessary, early non-weight-bearing standing can be performed on a tilt table, increasing elevation angle and time to tolerance.

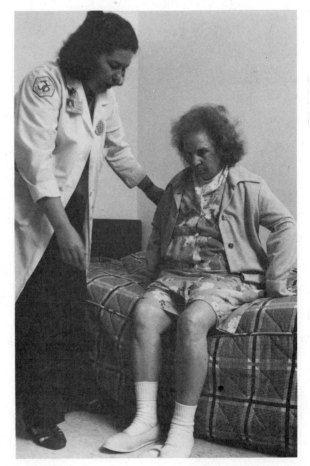

**Figure 16–17.** Learning to get out of bed following a hip fracture.

## AMBULATION

(1) Parallel bars are next utilized for standing and balancing; again, weight-bearing determinations are recommended by the attending surgeon.

(2) Depending on the patient's general status, short hopping maneuvers begin the ambulation process and strengthen the upper limb muscles.

(3) A walker is next employed, with maximal assistance and supervision, progressing to less-assisted ambulation. Independent use of a walker is usually the desired goal prior to discharge.

## ADDED EXERCISES

(1) Active range of motion exercises and manually resistive exercises are added for the involved limb, geared to each patient's status.

(2) Active exercises are continually encouraged for the other three sound limbs.

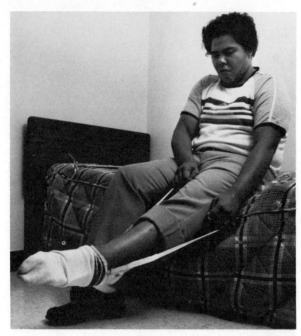

**Figure 16–18.** Assistive device for donning socks following hip fracture.

(3) Activities of daily living evaluations and training are added. Adaptive equipment for use at home could include a raised toilet seat, supports and bars in the bathroom, special bed needs, pulleys, weights, commodes, and other individualized devices.

### POSTDISCHARGE EXERCISES

(1) Continuation of formal exercises at home or at another less acute hospital setting should be provided for.

(2) The objectives are to achieve independent full weight-bearing ambulation, with a cane if needed for balance and support.

(3) Range of motion exercises and resistive exercises are upgraded in an effort to help the patient regain full motion and normal strength of the injured limb and the other limbs.

### ORTHOTIC DEVICES

If indicated, there are a number of lower limb orthoses (braces and splints) designed to support, unload, or realign the affected limb at the hip, knee, or ankle-foot areas, or at all joints. Shoe lifts are also used to equalize leg lengths.

### FRACTURES OF THE FEMORAL SHAFT

Fractures of the femur, distal to the hip joint, can occur at increasing distances distally, down to and including the knee joint, with disability including both the hip and knee joints. Since patients with this injury are usually younger and surgical fixation is more secure, the restorative process is less complex than that described for hip fractures in the elderly.

(1) Shaft fractures most often include soft tissue injury, with muscle spasms of the thigh groups, so moist heat is helpful before exercises are attempted.

(2) As soon as possible, depending on the fixation and stability of the fragments, active exercises are initiated to regain hip and knee motion in all planes—gradual progression is the guiding feature.

(3) General exercises for the three other limbs are encouraged as a preliminary to assisted, reduced weight-bearing ambulation.

(4) Ambulation usually begins with axillary crutches and partial weight-bearing. A tilt table, parallel bars, and a walker may be necessary in instances of more severe fractures and poor general condition of the patient.

(5) With healing, active-assistive range of motion exercises and manually resisted exercises are added for hip and knee.

(6) Ultimately, pulleys or weights or specially available equipment are used to regain normal strength of the involved lower limb.

(7) A four-point gait with crutches or canes follows, then a single cane, to discontinuation of walking aids.

### FRACTURES AT THE KNEE

The fracture can be of the patella, femoral or tibial condyles or combined, or associated with injuries of the supporting ligaments or capsular and musculotendinous tissues. The restorative process is based on the definitive care and involves restoration of knee function and ambulation.

(1) Moist heat is initially applied to the thigh region.

(2) Isometric quadriceps exercises are used during the early immobilization phase, together with active ankle-foot exercises.

(3) When indicated, gentle active knee flexion and extension exercises are begun, with gradual increases in the arc of motion, utilizing assistance by the therapist.

(4) Active-assistive range of motion exercises are used to regain normal motion; moist heat and

gravity can be used to supplement these exercises.

(5) Gentle manual resistive exercises are added in a prone position; this position can also be used for range of motion exercises.

(6) Ambulation with crutches is the usual starting point, with progressive increases to full weight-bearing and discontinuation of walking aids.

(7) Progressive resistive exercises, with weights, are used to restore normal strength.

(8) Knee orthoses are prescribed, if indicated.

## FRACTURES OF TIBIA AND FIBULA

Here again the fracture can involve the proximal shaft of the tibia and fibula, with a primary need to mobilize the knee, to midshaft fractures with both the knee and ankle joints requiring exercises, to distal tibial fractures that primarily involve the ankle. Definitive care is usually followed by application of a long plaster cylinder.

(1) Moist heat is applied to the thigh to produce muscle relaxation.

(2) Active exercises are initiated to help obtain full knee extension. Knee flexion active exercises are best done in a prone position.

(3) Active-assistive exercises are added to help the patient gain full knee motion.

(4) Active or active-assistive exercises or both are done to achieve full motion of the ankle and toes, including mobilization of the subtalar joints.

(5) Gentle massage of the distal leg can alleviate edema, as can carefully applied elastic bandages or a custom-fitted elastic stocking.

(6) Ambulation is begun with crutches, weight-bearing being increasingly permitted as the fracture heals.

(7) Assisted range of motion exercises and resistive strengthening exercises are added to regain motion and strength.

(8) In older patients, exercises are added for the hip and other limbs to avoid contractures and atrophy. Ambulation will require a walker in this group, with progression to other walking aids as healing progresses and more weight-bearing is allowed.

(9) Shoe lifts are added, if necessary.

(10) Exercises and ankle-foot orthoses may be indicated if there is associated peroneal nerve injury. Distal third fractures may interrupt posterior tibial nerve function, with weakness of the short toe flexors and intrinsic muscles of the foot.

(11) Patellar-tendon orthoses can unload the tibia.

## FRACTURES OF THE ANKLE

Fractures at this level can include the distal articulating aspect of the tibia, the lateral and medial malleoli, the supporting ligaments, and neurovascular structures, with pain, hemorrhaging, swelling, and motion limitations.

(1) Heat is applied in the form of hydrocollator packs or most often by using a whirlpool. The patient is instructed to perform underwater active ankle-foot exercises.

(2) Active and then active-assisted range of motion exercises are used to improve motion of the ankle and foot joints, including the subtalar joints and toes.

(3) If knee motion limitations and weakness are present, exercises are added to regain full motion and strength.

(4) Gentle, manual resistive exercises are later added to restore ankle-foot strength, followed in time by progressive resistive exercises for regaining normal strength.

(5) Ambulation is usually non-weight-bearing, crutch assisted, progressing in the course of time to partial and then to full weight-bearing with discontinuation of walking aids.

(6) Special shoes with internal or external modifications may be needed, together with a below-the-knee elastic stocking.

(7) Patellar-tendon orthoses can unload the ankle to expedite ambulation when non-weight-bearing ambulation is a problem.

## FRACTURES OF THE FOOT

This type of fracture can involve the talus (uncommon), the calcaneous (with or without comminution), the tarsal and metatarsal bones, or the phalanges. In most instances there is soft tissue injury, bleeding, pain, and swelling, with or without intra-articular damage.

1. Immersion in a whirlpool is used, together with active underwater exercises.

2. Gentle active, then active-assistive exercises are utilized to obtain full motion of the ankle and subtalar joints, as well as the toes.

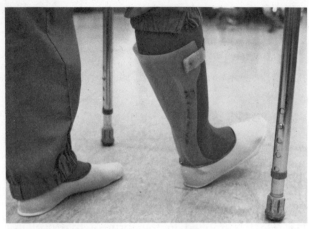

**Figure 16–19.** Plastic ankle-foot orthosis, or brace, to assist dorsiflexion following fracture-induced neuropathy.

3. Later, manual resistive exercises are added.

4. Ambulation is crutch-assisted non-weight-bearing or partial weight-bearing, progressing to normal gait patterns.

5. Shoes, with or without inner or outer modifications, are important for support and relief of pain, as are elastic stockings.

6. PTB orthoses can also unload more severe fractures.

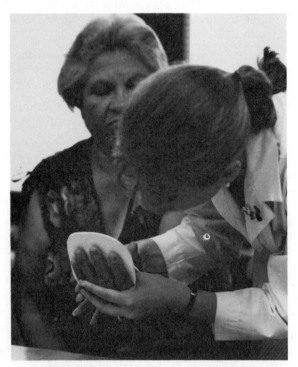

**Figure 16–20.** Initial measurements and fitting for an upper extremity splint.

# FRACTURES OF THE UPPER LIMB

The normal function of an individual's hand is dependent on full restoration of all impaired limb segments, regardless of the actual fracture site. Whereas one may accept less than full joint motion in the lower limb, particularly where ambulation and self-care are the major criteria for success, it is critical to strive for total restoration in fractures of the upper limb—vocational rehabilitation will greatly depend on the success of the restorative process, as will other life style elements.

# SHOULDER GIRDLE FRACTURES

Fractures, or fracture-dislocations that involve the sternum, clavicle, or scapula will interfere with glenohumeral motion because of protective immobilization secondary to pain or treatment. Following abatement of the acute process and healing, exercises are prescribed to produce normal function.

(1) Active and active-assistive exercises of the head and neck may be necessary to mobilize contracted adjacent joints.

(2) Deep breathing exercises, associated with motions of the clavicle and scapulae, can improve general motion of the proximal shoulder girdle areas.

(3) Active-assistive exercises are utilized to regain glenohumeral motion.

(4) Manual to progressive resistive exercises are added to obtain normal strength and endurance of the shoulder and arm muscles.

# FRACTURES OF THE SHOULDER

Fractures of this region include impacted fractures of the anatomical or surgical neck of the humerus, comminuted fractures of the humeral head with or without avulsion of the greater tuberosity, and associated shoulder dislocations. Neurovascular injuries are not common in impacted fractures but do appear in far greater frequency in combined dislocations and comminuted fractures of the head (brachial plexus or axillary nerve or both). Restoration is simpler in impacted fractures of this region; immobilization is also longer in the latter group so that therapy has to be more intensive and sustained to avoid permanent impairment.

### EXERCISES BY THERAPISTS

(1) Applications of moist heat to the shoulder area, with patient in supine position and shoulder abducted.

(2) The shoulder should be stabilized to prevent scapular motion, then active-assistive range of motion exercises are used to develop free glenohumeral motion. The arm is supported by the therapist, eliminating gravity and substitutions.

(3) Active range of motion of the elbow, wrist, and fingers; active-assistive exercises are used if there are deficits in these joints.

(4) With healing, active exercises of the shoulder are encouraged, against gravity. With assistance, full motion is attempted.

(5) With further healing, manual- and weight-resisted exercises are used for strength redevelopment.

### SUPPLEMENTAL OR HOME EXERCISES

(1) Functional and self-care activities are outlined and performed.

(2) Pendulum exercises, with the fractured limb fully extended at the elbow, are initiated early. Gravity is eliminated as the patient bends forward at the hip with the sound limb used for support—increasing rotary motions are used.

(3) Pulley exercises use an overhead pulley attached to a door to mobilize the injured shoulder with the sound upper limb.

(4) Wall-climbing exercises improve abduction while assisting the injured limb. Behind-the-back maneuvers assist redevelopment of abduction, internal rotation, and extension.

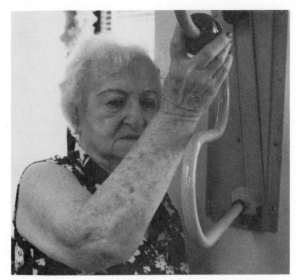

**Figure 16–21.** Wall-mounted device to improve shoulder motion.

(4) Wrist and fingers are exercised actively and vigorously.

(5) With healing and stability, resistive strengthening exercises, manual to weight-resisted, are ordered for the shoulder and elbow segments.

(6) Functional and self-care activities are a vital component of the program.

(7) In instances of radial nerve injury, additional techniques and exercises are employed, together with dynamic splinting.

## FRACTURES OF THE HUMERAL SHAFT

The fracture site can be at the proximal end of the humeral shaft, with shoulder dysfunction, distal or near the elbow with elbow motion impairments, or approximately midshaft with involvement of both shoulder and elbow. Fractures can be spiral or transverse with minor or major angulation and displacement—a therapy program must be carefully linked to the definitive care.

(1) Exercises to recover shoulder motion are similar to those described for fractures of the shoulder, including active and active-assisted exercises with stabilization of the scapula, first with gravity eliminated and then added.

(2) Pendulum exercises are useful, but pulley exercises can disrupt fixation.

(3) Active and active-assistive exercises are prescribed for elbow flexion and extension and forearm rotation.

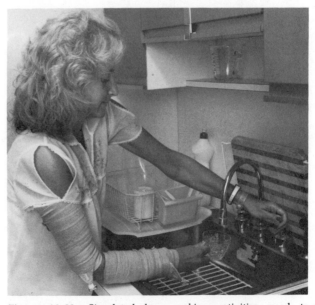

**Figure 16–22.** Simulated home-making activities used to strengthen the upper extremity.

## FRACTURES OF THE ELBOW

These fractures range from humeral supracondylar and intercondylar fractures, with or without extension into the elbow joint, usually with ligamental injuries, often with median and ulnar nerve injuries, less often with radial nerve lesions, to fractures that involve the olecranon or radial head. In all these injuries the problems are elbow motion and forearm rotation.

(1) Moist heat is applied to the elbow region, following removal of a cast, pins, traction, and so forth.

(2) With gravity eliminated and with the use of a powder board, active elbow flexion and extension are done, followed later by active-assisted range of motion exercises and repositioning to include antigravity exercises.

(3) Forearm rotation exercises are done.

(4) Wrist and finger exercises are added.

(5) Shoulder exercises come next.

(6) Functional and self-care activities need to be emphasized.

(7) Self-help devices and hand orthoses (splints) are fabricated when peripheral nerve injuries exist, together with specific restorative exercises.

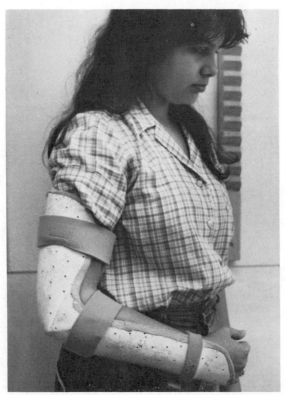

**Figure 16–23.**  Lightweight splint for a fractured elbow.

## FRACTURES OF THE RADIUS AND ULNA

In fractures of the forearm, one or both bones can be involved, proximally, midshaft, or distally; radioulnar articulations can be disrupted—peripheral nerve injuries are not common. The functional loss can involve elbow motion, forearm rotation, or wrist motion, or all three areas.

(1) Moist heat or whirlpool is initially prescribed.

(2) During immobilization, motion of the shoulder and fingers is maintained by active and active-assistive exercises.

(3) The elbow joint, and forearm rotation, are mobilized as previously described, including resistive exercises when appropriate.

(4) Massage is useful to reduce edema, particularly around the wrist and fingers.

(5) Active and then active-assistive range of motion exercises are used to improve wrist flexion and extension.

(6) Later, resistive exercises are added.

(7) Functional activities are provided to enhance restoration.

## WRIST FRACTURES

The most common wrist fracture occurs at the distal end of the radius; concomitant fractures of the ulna can be present, as can be injuries of supporting structures, blood vessels, and nerves with local painful trophic changes or shoulder-hand syndromes.

(1) Whirlpool therapy is used with active underwater exercises of the wrist and fingers.

(2) Active then active-assistive exercises are employed to restore wrist motion.

(3) Maintenance of normal motion of the fingers is vital during the immobilization phase.

(4) Elevation to minimize edema is also critical.

(5) Elbow motion and forearm rotation exercises are done.

(6) The patient performs funcitonal hand activities to enhance motion, coordination, agility, and strength.

(7) A detailed, well-understood home therapy program is devised to help in regaining motion and strength; this aspect of the program must be done hourly.

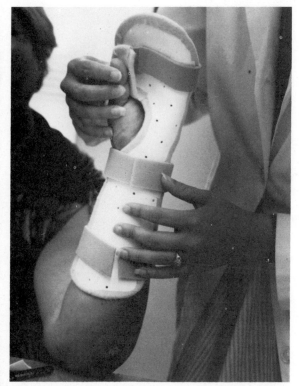

**Figure 16–24.** Completed hand orthosis, or splint, for wrist fracture.

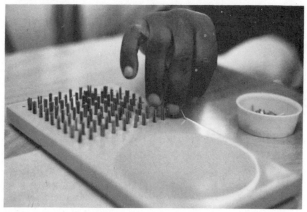

**Figure 16–25.** A pegboard used to redevelop fine hand function following fracture of two metacarpals.

## FRACTURES OF THE HAND

Fractures include those of the carpal and metacarpal bones and one or more phalanges. These can produce considerable impairment unless therapy is applied early and intensively. Therapy involves:

(1) Whirlpool with active exercises.

(2) Ultrasound, under water, to improve small joint motion when coupled with exercises.

(3) Paraffin immersions, another method for heating tissues.

(4) Careful joint-by-joint active, active-assistive, and passive range of motion exercises for the involved fingers.

(5) Manually resisted exercises for extrinsic and intrinsic muscles of the affected finger or fingers.

(6) Activities carefully constructed to enhance motion and total hand function.

(7) Use of individually designed hand orthoses for dynamic or static purposes.

(8) Provision to the patient of specially developed training devices to complement exercises at home.

(9) Frequent re-examinations, every few days, to evaluate the hand and alter the treatment.

(10) Continued intensive therapy until the therapist is convinced that there will be no further progress.

(11) Necessary corrective reconstructive surgery performed early, without delays of many months or a year.

# 17

# Peripheral Nerve Entrapment Syndromes

*by Aldo Perotto, M.D. and Edward F. Delagi, M.D.*

The term peripheral nerve entrapment syndromes includes those conditions in which nerve irritation or compression or both occurs when a peripheral nerve traverses an inelastic tunnel or a fibrous foramen, passes between hypertrophied muscle bellies, or is subjected to continuous or repetitive external trauma or pressure. The local anatomical changes produced in the nerve depend on the intensity and duration of the causative condition. When the intensity is low and the duration short, relatively minor pathological changes occur, mainly consisting of local segmental demyelineation and mild edema of the axons. The architecture of the nerve is well maintained. This results in slowing of conduction in the involved segment of the axons. If this is maintained beyond a critical time, neuropraxia will result; that is, the inability of a nerve impulse to cross the involved segment in spite of the anatomical continuity of the axons. Since Wallerian degeneration has not taken place, there is a prompt recovery when the offending condition is relieved. When the intensity of the cause is higher and the duration longer, the axon cylinders undergo Wallerian degeneration distal to the irritation or compression; however, the gross architecture of the nerve is maintained. This is referred to as axonotmesis. In such a lesion the removal of the cause results in slower recovery requiring the regrowth of axons from the point of compression to the muscle to be reinnervated.

In conditions of long duration and high intensity, the architecture of the nerve can be completely destroyed and fibrotic changes can take place. Called neurotmesis, this condition is found in long-standing cases of entrapment. Improvement cannot be expected in these cases even when the offending condition is corrected.

Most entrapped nerves have a combination of the first two levels of pathology, manifesting neuropraxia of some fibers and axonotmesis of others.

Axons that are compromised by a more proximal compression are vulnerable to more distal entrapment. When this occurs, it is referred to as a double crush syndrome. It is not unusual to have a combination of a C8 to T1 radiculopathy with a median nerve entrapment in the carpal tunnel. There is also some evidence that diabetic neuropathy favors the development of nerve entrapments.

In the upper extremity, the median, ulnar, and radial nerves are prone to entrapments that produce specific clinical syndromes. These are usually easy to differentiate.

## UPPER EXTREMITY SYNDROMES

Median nerve entrapment syndromes include pronator, supracondylar, anterior interosseus, and carpal tunnel.

### PRONATOR TERES SYNDROME

The pronator teres syndrome occurs when the median nerve is entrapped as it passes between the two heads of the pronator teres (Fig. 17–1B). The median nerve and the brachial artery descend together in the arm until they reach the level of the elbow joint. Here the nerve becomes more superficial and lies between the two heads of the pro-

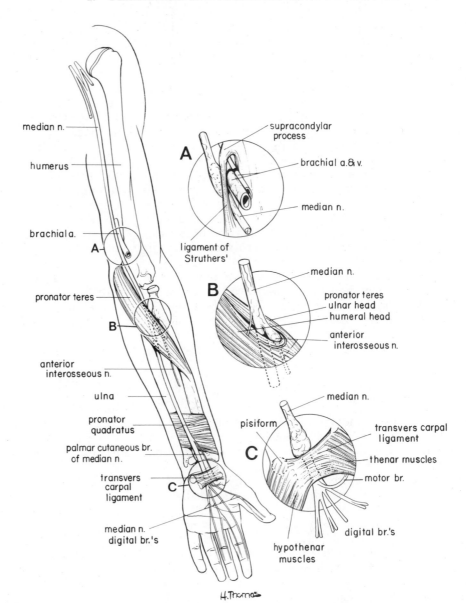

**Figure 17–1.** Common sites of median nerve entrapment. A, supracondylar; B, pronator teres; C, carpal tunnel.

nator, while the artery remains deep against the osseous structures, entering the forearm behind the pronator. Within the pronator teres muscle, it usually gives off branches to innervate this muscle and the anterior interosseous nerve. The most common causes of this syndrome are (1) narrowing of the space between the two heads of the pronator; (2) direct trauma of the volar upper third of the forearm with the development of local edema and subsequent scar formation; (3) repetitive motion of the limb with the forearm in pronation and the fingers in flexion (screwdriving); (4) an anatomical variation in which the nerve goes behind the pronator muscle rather than between its two heads; and (5) chronic external compression of the upper forearm.

When this condition is fully developed, its symptoms may be quite characteristic. Neverthe-

less, because of frequent anatomical variations and variability of the nerve involvement, accurate diagnosis may be difficult. Usually, the patient's initial complaint is one of discomfort or pain over the volar proximal third of the forearm, which is aggravated when the forearm is overpronated and the wrist is flexed. At the same time or soon after, paresthesia is noted in the radial 3½ digits.

The strength of the muscles in the forearm decreases, but the extent of muscle involvement and its severity vary greatly. The strength of the pronator teres muscle may or may not be affected, depending upon whether the innervation from the median nerve comes off at the level of the pronator muscle or above. Involvement of the muscles supplied by the anterior interosseous nerve may or may not be present; many times this nerve is totally spared. The muscle weakness most commonly seen involves the flexor capri radialis and the flexor digitorum superficialis in the forearm and thenar musculature and the median lumbricals in the hand.

Electrodiagnostic study is helpful in those cases in which the clinical evaluation leaves doubt. The nerve conduction velocity will demonstrate a slowing of conduction across the elbow, and the amplitude of the evoked response will be attenuated. Electromyography shows denervation activity in the flexor carpi radialis, palmaris longus, flexor digitorum superficialis, the thenar muscles, and the first and second lumbricals. As mentioned previously, the presence or absence of abnormal electrical findings in the pronator teres and/or muscles innervated by the anterior interosseous nerve is not diagnostic.

When the condition is mild and most of the signs and symptoms are experienced in the hand, carpal tunnel syndrome has to be ruled out. Unlike carpal tunnel syndrome, Phalen's sign is absent and the distal motor and sensory latency across the wrist is normal. Slowing of motor conduction across the elbow is present.

### SUPRACONDYLAR PROCESS SYNDROME

The supracondylar process syndrome (Fig. 17–1A) must be ruled out whenever a patient presents with pronator teres weakness. In about 1 per cent of limbs there is a bony process above the medial condyle that is frequently the origin of the ligament of Struthers, which runs to the medial epicondyle. The median nerve, accompanied by the brachial or ulnar artery, runs under this relatively inelastic band and may become entrapped here. The radial or the ulnar pulse or both may decrease or vanish when the arm is fully extended and supinated. Resting of the forearm and wrist is the treatment of choice in those conditions in which edema is thought to be responsible. Repeated local trauma or external pressure is to be avoided. In cases of anatomical variations or exuberant scar formation in the pronator teres muscles, surgical release is indicated.

### ANTERIOR INTEROSSEOUS NERVE SYNDROME

Anterior interosseous nerve syndrome (Fig. 17–1B) is a result of compromise of the anterior interosseous nerve at or near its site of origin from the median nerve. Entrapment may have several causes: thrombosis of the vessels that accompany the nerve, an accessory head of the flexor pollicis longus (Gantzer muscle), a tendinous origin of the deep head of the pronator muscle, an enlarged bicipital bursa, forearm fractures undergoing open reduction, and supracondylar fractures in children. The anterior interosseous nerve syndrome is characterized by pain or discomfort in the volar aspect of the proximal forearm area. This is followed by weakness or paralysis of the flexor pollicis longus, and flexor digitorum profundus slips to the index and middle finger and the pronator quadratus. As this nerve is purely motor (except for a few sensory fibers to the wrist joint), no sensory changes occur in the forearm or hand. Pain may be induced in the forearm by deep palpation over the pronator teres area or hyperpronation of the forearm. The patient will not be able to produce a terminal pinch between the thumb and the index or middle fingers because of inability to flex the distal phalanges. He will be able to pinch, opposing the pulp of his digits but will not be able to place them tip to tip. The patient will not be able to pick up a coin from a flat surface using his thumb and index finger. He cannot make an "O" between the thumb and the index or middle finger.

Manual muscle testing will demonstrate paresis or paralysis of the muscles involved. When the pronator quadratus is tested, it is very important to remember that the elbow must be fully flexed in order to eliminate the pronator teres. The electromyographic study shows denervation potentials in the flexor pollicis longus and flexor digitorum profundus slips to the index and middle finger and the pronator quadratus. All other median-innervated muscles in the forearm or hand will have a normal electrical output. Motor nerve conduction studies will be normal if the abductor pollicis brevis is used as the recording muscle. Motor conduction from the elbow to the pronator quadratus will be slowed and the amplitude of the evoked response decreased in proportion to the severity of the lesion.

In those cases caused by acute or chronic repetitive trauma, conservative treatment based principally on resting of the limb in supination is indicated. If this proves effective, modification of the responsible activity is indicated. If improvement is not obtained after six to eight weeks, or if the condition worsens, surgical exploration is indicated.

In all other cases, when mechanical compression is caused by thrombotic vessels, aberrant muscles, or a fibrotic deep head of the pronator teres, or when it follows fractures, surgical exploration should be carried out.

### CARPAL TUNNEL SYNDROME

Carpal tunnel syndrome (Fig. 17–1C) is produced by compression of the median nerve as it passes through the inelastic tunnel formed by the concavity in the two rows of carpal bones and the flexor retinaculum. It may be caused by hormonal dysfunction, as in the intermittent or "monthly" syndrome, pregnancy, or hypothyroidism. The cause may be inflammatory, as in tenosynovitis of the flexor tendons or ganglions and rheumatoid arthritis. Another cause is bony deformity secondary to fracture, acromegaly, or congenital stenosis.

The patient usually complains of paresthesias and pain involving the digits supplied by the median nerve. The skin over the thenar eminence and the palm is spared because sensation to these areas is supplied by the median volar cutaneous nerve. This nerve does not go through the carpal tunnel but enters the hand subcutaneously—under the skin of the volar aspect of the wrist. The paresthesias vary in type and intensity. Pain is referred to the hand but may radiate upward into the forearm. It may be present during the daytime but tends to be more intense at night, usually waking the patient one to two hours after he has fallen asleep. The patient will often state that shaking the hand relieves the symptoms. The patient frequently complains that the hand has become much more sensitive to cold. Differences in sweating between the ulnar and the radial sides of the hand are sometimes noted.

Another common complaint is accidental dropping of objects from the involved hand. Examination of the hand usually reveals some flattening (atrophy) of the thenar eminence muscles. There may be evidence of less moisture in the fingers served by the median nerve. The sensory examination shows decreased sensation of some or all of the fingers innervated by this nerve, but the skin of the palm and thenar eminence is spared. Manual muscle tests may show weakness in the abductor pollicis brevis, the opponens pollicis, and the first and second lumbricals.

When the volar aspect of the wrist is tapped, many patients report an electrical shock-like sensation radiating into the hand. The Phalen maneuver (hyperflexion of the wrist for one minute) will produce or increase the symptoms if they are already present. It has been demonstrated that acute flexion of the wrist produces compression of the median nerve between the long digital flexors and the retinaculum at its proximal edge.

The differential diagnosis should include all the other conditions involving the median nerve proximal to the wrist, the medial cord, the lower trunk, or the C8 to T1 nerve roots. The different pattern of sensory involvement in these conditions as well as weakness in muscle proximal to the wrist or ulnar-innervated intrinsic hand muscles will help in making the correct diagnosis. The clinical picture described leaves little doubt about the diagnosis. This means that the nerve is severely damaged and that the patient will most probably be left with some degree of nerve impairment. Fortunately, patients with such advanced pathology are seldom seen. Most of the patients seek help earlier, before the clinical findings are extensive enough to help make the diagnosis. In these cases, electromyography and nerve conduction studies are helpful. They not only give the data needed for a correct diagnosis but also provide an objective way of evaluating the course of the condition once the treatment has started.

At the early stage of the syndrome, when a mild demyelinating process is the dominant pathological picture, motor and sensory latencies across the carpal tunnel become of paramount importance. Values over 3.5 msec for sensory fibers and over 4.0 msec for motor fibers are indicative of entrapment, provided that the conduction velocity of the median nerve above the wrist is normal (more than 45 msec). When the values are close to the upper limits of normal, sensory conduction velocity across the carpal tunnel can be determined. This should exceed the distal velocity from the palm to the digit. In the early stages, the electromyogram will probably be normal or perhaps will show occasional denervation potential (fibrillation and/or positive sharp waves) in the abductor pollicis brevis or opponens pollicis.

When the condition is advanced, this test may not be needed for diagnostic purposes but is helpful in following the patient's course in an objective way. A decrease in the distal latency along with less fibrillation and more polyphasic potential are indicative of improvement.

The therapeutic approach in carpal tunnel syndrome depends on correcting the cause of the syndrome. When the condition arises because of hormonal disturbances, adjustment of the glandular dysfunction usually establishes normality. In cases in which the water retention from hormonal changes lasts for a known length of time (pregnancy) or is cyclic (menses), the approach should be different. In the latter, we are dealing with hormonal dysfunction resulting in water retention during the time that progesterone hormone production drops at the end of the second phase (progesterone phase) of the menstrual cycle. A few days of diuretics, starting at the time the patient usually becomes symptomatic, may prevent a recurrence of symptoms. In cases resulting from either cause, a resting splint at night may help in preventing the patient from flexing her wrist during sleep. Unless the symptoms are very severe, no further therapy is indicated.

In cases secondary to local nonseptic inflammatory processes, immobilization of the wrist and fingers in functional positions will control the edema. If the condition is not controlled in a few days and the symptoms of carpal tunnel syndrome persist, a local infiltration of the carpal tunnel region with a combination of local anaesthetics, 1 per cent lidocaine (1 cc) plus corticoid 40 mg/cc (1 cc), will decrease the local inflammatory changes in the tissues involved. A resting splint at night should be prescribed. In cases in which rheumatoid arthritis (acute) is responsible for the syndrome, complete immobilization of the wrist joint and fingers will prevent not only further compromise of the nerve but also irreparable damage to the wrist joint. This should be done simultaneously with the basic systemic treatment of the rheumatoid arthritis. If the symptoms are not controlled, surgical intervention is recommended. The aim of surgery is to decompress the carpal tunnel by incising the volar retinaculum.

In cases of bony deformity caused by fracture, acromegaly, or congenital stenosis, conservative measures do not usually control symptoms and early surgical intervention is indicated.

*Ulnar nerve entrapments* include cubital tunnel, flexor carpiulnaris, and Guyon tunnel syndromes.

### CUBITAL TUNNEL SYNDROME

This syndrome develops as a result of entrapment at the cubital tunnel, which is formed by the ulnar groove between the medial epicondyle of the humerus and the olecranon (Fig. 17–2B). This tunnel is covered by a loose aponeurosis that allows the nerve to move easily within the groove. The nerve normally stays within the groove from full extension to full flexion of the elbow. Cubital tunnel syndrome can be caused by ganglion formation, exuberant synovial tissue in arthritis, old fracture of the lateral humeral epicondyle (tardy palsy from excessive cubitus valgus), and dislocation of the ulnar nerve either permanently or intermittently when the elbow is flexed.

### FLEXOR CARPI ULNARIS ENTRAPMENT

Flexor carpi ulnaris entrapment takes place as the ulnar passes under the arcuate ligament between the two heads of the muscle (Fig. 17–2C). In both cubital tunnel and flexor carpi ulnaris entrapments the sensory involvement is localized over the ulnar aspect of the hand on both the palmar

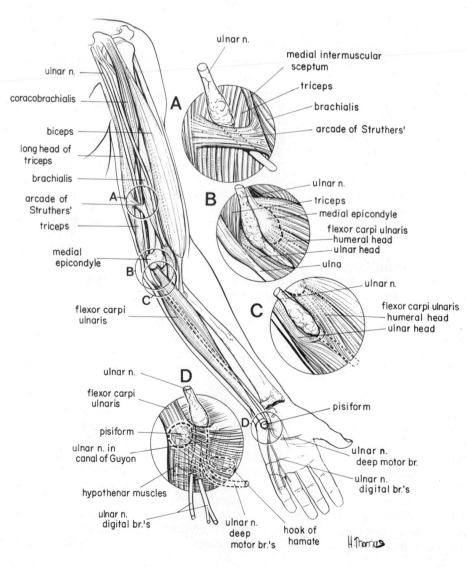

**Figure 17–2.** Common sites of ulnar nerve entrapment. A, arcade of Struther; B, cubital tunnel; C, flexor carpi ulnaris; D, Guyon's tunnel.

and dorsal aspects and may vary from slight dysesthesia to hypalgesia or complete anaesthesia or both. The motor weakness is manifested in the forearm by the flexor carpi ulnaris. This weakness results in radial deviation on wrist flexion and the flexor digitorum profundus producing weakness of flexion of the terminal phalanges of the fourth and fifth digits.

Mild clawing of the fourth and fifth fingers is present as a result of lumbrical weakness. Abduction and adduction of fingers is weakened because of interosseus muscle involvement. Adductor pollicis weakness causes the patient to substitute the flexor pollicis longus when he attempts to hold a piece of paper between the thumb and the proximal phalanx of the second digit (sign de Journal of Froment).

Tapping the nerve at the ulnar groove results in dysesthesia radiating into the fifth digit.

A segmental nerve conduction velocity study will show a significant slowing across the elbow segment as compared with the more proximal and distal segment. If the condition has been intense enough and present long enough, electromyography will show denervation of the flexor carpi ulnaris, the ulnar slips of the flexor digitorum profundus, and the ulnar-innervated intrinsic muscles of the hand. In addition, the ulnar sensory-evoked response will be of low amplitude or absent.

Splinting in extension at night is the treatment of choice when the cause is dislocation of the nerve caused by elbow flexion. During the day, protection of the nerve with a soft elbow pad will help to avoid further trauma. If this does not alleviate the symptoms, an anterior transposition of the nerve or a medial epicondylectomy should be considered. In patients with tardy palsy from cubitus valgus, one of these surgical procedures is indicated. For those patients with entrapment because of tight arcuate ligament, an incision of this ligament with resuturing of it underneath the nerve is indicated.

The arcade of Struthers (Fig. 17–2A), where the ulnar nerve passes through the intermuscular septum at the junction of the middle and lower third of the humerus, is rarely the site of primary entrapment. It is important because it can be the site of secondary entrapment if transposition of the ulnar is performed and it is not released at this point.

## ULNAR (GUYONS) TUNNEL SYNDROME

Ulnar (Guyons) tunnel syndrome occurs when the ulnar nerve is entrapped as it travels through the ulnar tunnel from the forearm into the hand (Fig. 17–2D). This tunnel is limited by the pisiform bone laterally and by the hamate bone medially. Its roof is the pisiform-hamate ligament. It is covered by a thickened aponeurosis originating from the flexor carpi ulnaris tendon. The nerve traverses the tunnel accompanied by the ulnar artery. It extends distally about 1½ cm from the distal skin crease of the volar aspect of the wrist joint. Usually the nerve divides within the tunnel into two branches, one superficial and one deep. The superficial, mostly sensory (except for few motor fibers for the palmaris brevis muscle) branch innervates the skin of the fifth digit and half of the fourth digit, as well as the skin of the ulnar side of the palm. The deep motor branch supplies all the interosseous muscles, the lumbricals for the fourth and fifth digits, the deep head of the flexor pollicis brevis, and the adductor pollicis.

Entrapment of the ulnar nerve at the wrist is usually caused by space-occupying lesions within the tunnel. Among these conditions, synovial thickening in rheumatoid arthritis and ganglions are the leading causes. It is also seen in patients in certain vocations in which they habitually press or bang with the hypothenar portion of the hand.

When the syndrome is complete, the symptoms and signs are characteristic. The patient may complain of pain over the palmar aspect of the ulnar side of the hand and the fifth digit and the ulnar aspect of the fourth digit. The dorsal aspect of the ulnar side of the hand as well as the dorsum of the proximal 1½ phalanges for the fourth and fifth digits will not be involved. This area is supplied by the dorsal cutaneous branch, which arises from the ulnar nerve about 10 to 15 cm proximal to the wrist joint and does not go through the tunnel.

Motor function shows the typical "preacher" or "benediction" hand. The fourth and fifth digits show mild hyperextension of the metacarpophalangeal joint, with slight flexion of the proximal and distal interphalangeal joints (intrinsic minus finger). The middle and index fingers will show a "pseudoclawing" (mild semiflexion of proximal and distal metacarpophalangeal joints), indicating the presence of lumbrical action.

The atrophy of the hypothenar and interosseous muscles, especially the first dorsal interosseous (guttering), may become quite obvious. Froment's sign will be positive because of the marked weakness or paralysis of the adductor pollicis.

Electrodiagnostic studies show a delay of the distal latency (latency across the wrist over 3.5 msec for the motor and sensory fibers). The electromyographic findings may vary according to the exact site of entrapment and its severity. When entrapment occurs at the proximal end of the tunnel, denervation potentials (fibrillation and positive sharp waves) will be found in both the hypothenar and the interosseous muscles. When the entrapment takes place at the distal end of the tunnel, the hypothenar musculature can be spared and only the interosseous muscles and the adductor pollicis will show denervation activity. In this particular instance, it will be helpful to obtain the distal latency from the abductor digiti minimi and the first dorsal interosseous. The former will show a normal latency while the latency in the latter will be prolonged (at least 1.5 msec difference).

This syndrome can be differentiated from cubital tunnel syndrome because in the latter muscles innervated by the ulnar nerve in the forearm will be involved and the sensory loss will include the dorsum of the hand. The distal ulnar latency will be normal, but the conduction velocity of the ulnar nerve across the elbow will be significantly decreased as compared with the velocity of segments proximal and distal to it.

In those patients in whom the condition is related to vocational or avocational activities, modifications to prevent recurring trauma to the pisiform-hamate region is indicated.

In all patients in whom the syndrome develops because of a space-occupying lesion, surgical exploration is indicated.

Radial nerve entrapments include the spiral groove syndrome and the posterior interosseous nerve syndrome.

### SPIRAL GROOVE SYNDROME

The spiral groove syndrome occurs as a result of either direct trauma or entrapment at the spiral groove of the humerus (Fig. 17–3A). As the radial nerve separates from the axillary nerve, it courses through the spiral groove between the medial and lateral heads of the triceps. Because of its close contact with the unyielding humerus, it is susceptible to compression at this point when external pressure is placed on the lateral and posterior surface in the middle third of the arm. This condition commonly occurs as a complication of humeral fracture or direct pressure on the nerve (bride groom palsy or Saturday night palsy).

When the condition is fully developed, the clinical picture includes drop wrist with the metacar-

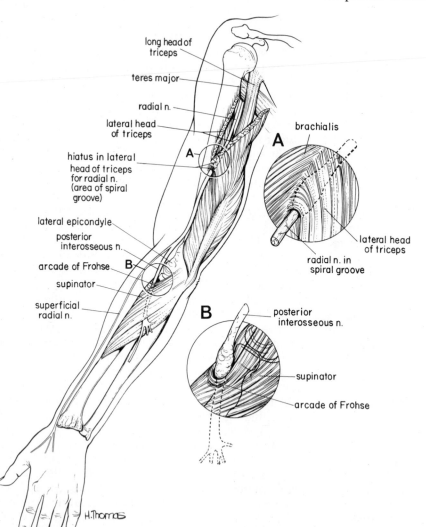

**Figure 17–3.** Common sites of radial nerve entrapment. A, spiral groove; B, arcade of Frohse.

pophalangeal joints flexed and the thumb adducted. There is an area of hypesthesia in the dorsal aspect of the forearm and hand down to the dorsal aspect of the second phalanx of the thumb, index, and middle fingers. An area of complete anesthesia the size of a dime is found in the dorsal aspect of the first web space. The triceps reflex is present. Muscle testing indicates that all muscles innervated by the radial nerve are paralyzed, except for the triceps. Therefore the patient is able to extend the elbow but is unable to dorsiflex the wrist, extend the metacarpophalangeal joints, abduct the thumb radially, and extend the interphalangeal joint of the thumb. With the metacarpophalangeal joints supported in extension, the patient can extend the proximal interphalangeal and distal interphalangeal joints of all fingers. There may be a weak extension of the distal phalanx of the thumb, but this motion is not carried out by the extensor pollicis longus but by extension action of the flexor pollicis brevis through the extensor mechanism of the distal phalanx of the thumb.

Elbow flexion is weakened when it is tested with the forearm in neutral position. This is because of lack of the brachioradialis strength. When the functions of the ulnar-innervated intrinsic muscles of the hand are evaluated, the patient's hand must be on a flat surface. If the test is done with the hand unsupported, one can erroneously diagnose an ulnar nerve lesion because of apparent weakness of the ulnar intrinsics.

The electrodiagnostic study will show slowing or lack of condition through the involved area but normal conduction distal to it, if the lesion is neuropraxic. If the lesion has progressed to axonotmesis, the electromyographic findings will be normal in the triceps but will reveal denervation potentials in the rest of the muscles innervated by the radial nerve, including the brachioradialis and the extensor carpi radialis longus. The compromise of these two muscles, together with the sensory impairment, are the two most important findings to make the differential diagnosis with the posterior interosseous nerve syndrome.

Treatment of this condition depends upon the cause; in case of tardy radial palsy secondary to fracture of the humeral shaft, an early surgical neurolysis is indicated. In cases of direct pressure (bridegroom palsy, Saturday night palsy), removal of the causal factor is usually all that is necessary.

## POSTERIOR INTEROSSEOUS NERVE ENTRAPMENT

The posterior interosseous nerve is frequently entrapped as it passes through the two heads of the supinator muscle. The radial nerve bifurcates just proximal to the elbow joint into two terminal branches: the superficial branch (mainly sensory) and the deep or posterior interosseous nerve (Fig. 17–3B). The latter enters the supinator muscle through an aponeurotic arch (arcade of Fröhse). Before entering the forearm, the radial nerve gives off two branches to the brachioradialis and the extensor carpi radialis longus. The extensor carpi radialis brevis innervation varies; sometimes it is directly from the radial nerve or the superficial division, but it is seldom from the posterior interosseous nerve. All other muscles in the dorsum of the forearm (supinator, extensor digitorum communis, extensor pollicis longus and brevis, and the abductor longus of the thumb) are innervated by the posterior interosseous nerve.

Most cases of spontaneous posterior interosseous nerve syndrome are found to be secondary to either thickening or narrowing of the arcade of Fröhse. Systemic diseases such as diabetes mellitus, periarteritis nodosa, leprosy, and heavy metal poisoning, are considered to be predisposing factors.

The complete syndrome presents a characteristic picture. The patient has discomfort or pain over the proximal and lateral aspect of the forearm (extensor-supinator area of the forearm) with no radiation or sensory changes in the limb. The patient can dorsiflex his wrist, but the hand will deviate radially. (The extensor carpi radialis muscles are not innervated by this nerve.) The fingers cannot be extended at the metacarpophlangeal joints, but the proximal and distal interphalangeal joints will be able to extend volitionally because these two joints are under the control of ulnar and median innervated muscles. The thumb cannot be extended at the metacarpophalangeal joint, but it will present a weak extension at the interphalangeal joint. This extension is not carried out through the extensor pollicis longus but by the short flexor of the thumb through the hood of the extensor mechanisms.

The sequence of involvement of the fingers may vary, and as the index and little finger have their own extensor muscle plus the head coming from the extensors communis, many times the middle and ring fingers are the first two that drop.

The electromyographic study shows that the muscles innervated by this nerve are undergoing a denervation process, the intensity of which will depend upon the severity of the entrapment. The supinator muscle may not show any evidence of denervation because the branches that supply it come off the nerve before they reach the arcade of Fröhse, and they may be spared. The nerve conduction study shows a slow velocity across the segment of the nerve that has to go through the supinator muscle as well as a low amplitude-evoked response if the entrapment is severe enough to have paralyzed a significant number of nerve fibers.

Nerve conduction velocities in the low 30's meter/sec and evoked responses under 1,000 μv are not unusual in well-established syndromes. The segment of the radial nerve from axilla to elbow shows normal conduction velocity. If the nerve was lacerated, no evoked response can be elicited.

In the differential diagnosis are considered lesions of the radial nerve proximal to elbow joint (crutch palsy, humeral shaft fractures). In these cases, the presence of sensory changes over the forearm's dorsal aspect and the radial aspect of the hand dorsum and the dorsum of the proximal one and one half phalanges of the thumb, index, and middle finger plus the inability of the patient to dorsiflex the wrist will suffice to locate the lesion as being proximal to the division of the radial nerve.

In cases of posterior interosseous nerve syndrome caused by thickening or narrowing of the arcade of Fröhse, immobilization of the wrist, fingers, and thumb in the position of function may be able to reduce the edema, diminishing the compression on the nerve. If after a six- to eight-week period there is no clinical evidence of improvement, surgical release of the nerve is indicated. Surgical exploration is also the rule in all traumatic cases. When systemic disease is responsible for the syndrome, full control of the basic disease may bring some improvement.

# LOWER EXTREMITY SYNDROMES

## PIRIFORMIS SYNDROME

Piriformis syndrome is the term used to describe entrapment of the sciatic nerve as it emerges from the pelvis through the greater sciatic foramen passing between the piriformis muscle above and the obturator internus below. The inferior gluteal nerve exits the plexus above the piriformis muscle and courses along the medial aspect of the sciatic nerve to reach the gluteus maximum muscle, which covers both nerves at this level (Fig. 17–4). The common causes of this syndrome are sustained piriformis muscle contraction and fibrotic changes in the muscle secondary to direct trauma, as in posterior dislocation of the hip joint.

When the syndrome is fully developed, the patient has motor and sensory changes involving the posterior aspect of the thigh and the entire leg and foot. Weakness can develop in the hamstrings group, gluteus maximus, ankle dorsi flexors and plantar flexors, and the intrinsic muscles of the foot. Pain and hypesthesia may be experienced mainly in the posterior aspect of the leg and in the sole of the foot. Because of the muscle weakness, the patient may present with a gluteus maximus lurch as well as difficulty in walking on toes or heels. Knee extension, hip abduction, and adduction are not involved.

The electromyographic study will help in arriving at the proper diagnosis. The hamstrings, ankle dorsi flexors, and plantar flexors and the intrinsic muscles of the foot demonstrate electrical abnormalities, as does the gluteus maximus muscle. The gluteus medius, tensa fascia lata and paraspinal muscles show normal electrical output. Nerve conduction studies usually show normal velocities with low amplitude-evoked responses in both motor and sensory fibers on stimulation distal to the entrapment. However, if nerve root stimulation of S1 is done with recording from the abductor hallucis or the extensor digitorum brevis, a significant delay in the proximal segment of either the tibial division or the peroneal division of the sciatic nerve can be demonstrated. When the process is in its early stage, treatment should consist of conservative measures such as local moist heat and/or local infiltration of the piriformis muscle with anesthetic agents, to release the muscle spasm. Rarely, surgical exposure of the sciatic foramen or excision of the piriformis muscle and neurolysis is necessary.

## MERALGIA PARESTHETICA

Meralgia paresthetica occurs when the lateral femoral cutaneous nerve is compressed as it passes under the inguinal ligament just medial to the anterior superior iliac spine into the thigh. The nerve arises from the posterior division of the anterior primary rami of the second and third lumbar nerve roots. It crosses the iliacus muscle under its fascia covering, crosses the deep circumflex iliac artery and passes through a fascial tunnel in the ligament's lateral attachment to the anterior superior iliac spine. As it exits from under the inguinal ligament, it lies under the fascia lata. The nerve becomes embedded in the fascia lata before it crosses the sartorius muscle. The nerve divides into an anterior division and a posterior division several centimeters after its exit from the inguinal ligament. The anterior division supplies sensation to the anterolateral and lateral aspects of the lower thigh, and the posterior division innervates the skin over the greater trochanter and the lateral aspect of the upper half of the thigh (Fig. 17–5).

The usual clinical presentation of this syndrome is complaint of discomfort in the lateral aspect of the thigh, variously described as pain, burning, numbness, formication, dysesthesia, and hyperpathia. The entrapment of the nerve is generally attributed to its anatomical arrangement, which makes it vulnerable to precipitating causes such as trauma, postural abnormalities, occupations requiring long periods of hip flexion, increased intra-abdominal pressure, obesity (particularly a sudden gain in weight), and wearing of a tight belt or truss.

It may be the first presenting symptom of a po-

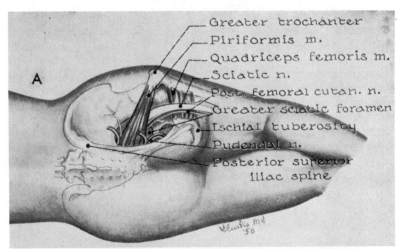

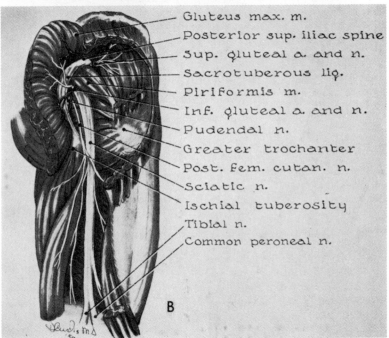

**Figure 17–4.** Site of piriformis syndrome. (From Moore, D. C.: Regional Block: A Handbook for Use in the Clinical Practice of Medicine and Surgery, 4th ed. Springfield, Charles C Thomas, 1971.)

lyneuropathy or a lesion of L2 or L3 or the lumbar plexus. An electrodiagnostic study designed to establish whether the condition is an isolated entrapment or a more diffuse or more proximal lesion is indicated. This should include conduction studies of these nerves: the lateral femoral cutaneous, the femoral, the peroneal, the tibial, and the sural bilaterally, and electromyography of the involved extremity including the iliopsoas and rectus femoris and the lumbar paraspinal muscles.

This condition usually responds to conservative measures, postural adjustments, and occupational modifications, and rarely requires surgical correction.

## POPLITEAL FOSSA ENTRAPMENT

Popliteal fossa entrapment is usually caused by compression by a Baker's cyst of the tibial nerve as it travels through the popliteal fossa. An effusion of the semimembranous bursa produces a popliteal tumor that, if sufficiently enlarged, may compress the tibial nerve. Depending upon the size, the common peroneal nerve and the sural nerve may also be involved. Other causes for this syndrome are proliferation of the synovial tissue in patients with rheumatoid arthritis and in cases of synoviomas of the knee joint. Aneurysm of the popliteal artery can also produce it (Fig. 17–6).

When the syndrome is fully developed, the patient has a tender tumor in the popliteal fossa. There is incomplete flexion of the knee joint and pain behind the knee or in the calf muscles when the foot is dorsiflexed. The gastrocnemius, the tibialis posterior, the flexor hallucis longus, the flexor digitorum communis, and the intrinsic muscles of the foot (with the exception of the extensor digitorum brevis) are weak or paralyzed. The entire plantar surface of the foot is hypesthetic or anesthetic. The patient is not able to flex his toes or to plantar-flex his foot and is unable to walk on his toes. If the common peroneal and the sural nerves are involved, the patient may also have weakness of the anterior and lateral compartment muscles of the leg with hypesthesia over the lateral aspect of the leg and the dorsal aspect of the foot and anesthesia over the lateral aspect of the foot and dorsal aspect of the first web space. In cases of complete paralysis of all three nerves, the patient shows complete paralysis from the knee down. The only area of the skin in which sensation is spared is the inner aspect of the leg supplied by the greater saphenous nerve, a branch of the femoral nerve.

The electrodiagnostic study will demonstrate slow conduction of the tibial nerve across the popliteal fossa. Similar findings could be present in the common peroneal nerve. The sural nerve–evoked response may not be obtainable. The electromyograph will demonstrate fibrillation potentials and positive sharp waves in all muscles innervated by the tibial nerve. If the process also involves the

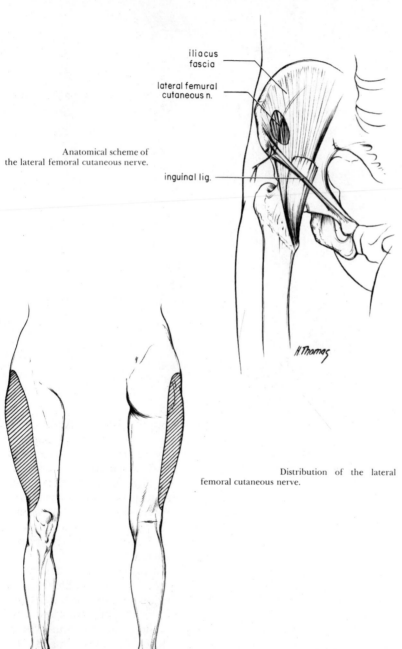

iliacus fascia

lateral femoral cutaneous n.

Anatomical scheme of the lateral femoral cutaneous nerve.

inguinal lig.

H. Thomas

**Figure 17–5.** Distribution of lateral femoral cutaneous nerve. (From Omer, G. E. and Spinner, M.: Management of Peripheral Nerve Problems. Philadelphia, W. B. Saunders Co., 1980.)

Distribution of the lateral femoral cutaneous nerve.

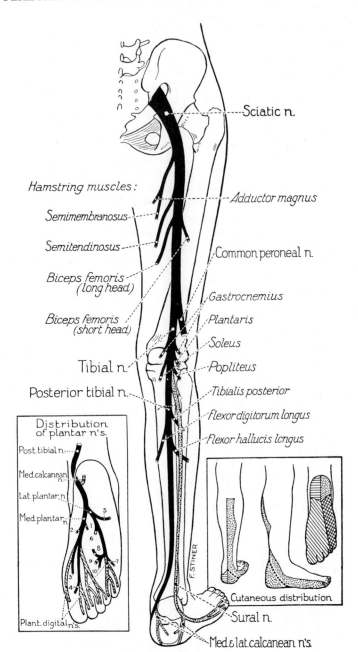

**Figure 17–6.** Course and distribution of the sciatic, tibial, posterior tibial, and plantar nerves. (From Haymaker, W., and Woodhall, B.: Peripheral Nerve Injuries, 2nd ed. W. B. Saunders Co., 1953.)

common peroneal nerve, the same findings will be present in the anterior and lateral compartment muscles. The hamstring muscles in the thigh will show normal electrical output. An arthogram of the knee joint will demonstrate if the cyst is or is not connected with the joint cavity.

The differential diagnosis includes lesions of the sciatic nerve at the thigh or higher. In these cases, the presence of symptoms above the knee and the absence of the "popliteal tumor" will help in making the diagnosis. In cases in which the cause is a popliteal artery aneurysm, the presence of the "pulsating" mass together with the presence of the arterial bruit help establish the diagnosis.

The treatment depends upon the cause. In cases of Baker's cyst, abundant synovial tissue, or synoviomas, removal of the "tumor" will not only help to determine the nature of the process but will relieve the compression. In cases of aneurysm, plastic reconstruction of the artery is the treatment of choice.

## COMMON PERONEAL NERVE SYNDROME

This occurs as a result of an injury or entrapment of the nerve at the point where it is superficial and therefore vulnerable. This point is located at the fibular head and neck, where the nerve winds around before dividing into two terminal branches, the superficial and the deep peroneal. The common peroneal nerve branches off the sciatic nerve at the proximal end of the popliteal fossa, where it is covered by the biceps femoris muscle. At this level it gives off the lateral sural cutaneous nerve, which joins the medial portion of the sural nerve coming from the tibial nerve. As the common peroneal nerve reaches the head of the fibula, it becomes firmly attached to it. The superficial division of the nerve innervates the peroneus longus and brevis and the skin of the distal half of the lateral aspect of the leg and dorsum of the foot. The deep portion of the nerve innervates the muscles in the anterior compartment (tibalis anterior, extensor digitorum communis, extensor hallucis longus, and peroneus tertius) and the skin of the first web space.

Among the most common causes producing this syndrome are excessive pressure from Ace bandages or poorly applied casts; excessive nerve pressure in bedridden patients who are allowed to remain for long periods of time with the leg in external rotation; this may produce excessive pressure upon the nerve. This syndrome has been described in normal individuals who habitually cross their legs, thereby producing excessive pressure upon the nerve. The superficial location of the nerve is the main reason for its vulnerability. Another reason is the firm attachment of the nerve to the fibula head, which does not allow the nerve to slide away from the excessive pressure. Other causes are fibula fractures at the neck, direct trauma to the nerve, severe acute genu varus, and acute inversion injuries of the ankle joint.

When the syndrome is fully developed, the symptomatology is typical. The foot of the patient appears in complete plantar flexion and slight inversion. There is hypesthesia in the lateral aspect of the leg and dorsum of the foot and complete anesthesia in the first web space. A complete manual muscle test reveals absence of muscle activity in all the muscles in the anterior and lateral compartment of the leg; the patient is unable to either dorsiflex or to evert the foot. Gait analysis shows that the patient brings the knee high in order to clear the floor during the swing phase, and the lateral border of the foot strikes the floor before the heel (steppage gait).

The electrodiagnosis shows a complete absence of nerve conduction after the fourth or fifth day after trauma, if the trauma was severe enough to produce axonotmesis of the nerve fibers. If the nerve fibers are neuropraxic, nerve conduction remains normal distal to the block, although there is no conduction across it. Electromyography shows no electrical activity either at rest or during voluntary effort within the two to three weeks following onset of the palsy. After this period of time, dener-

vation potentials appear (fibrillations and/or positive sharp waves) if axonotmesis has occurred. In cases in which the nerve lesion was incomplete, a combination is seen in which both deep and superficial branches are equally involved or in which the involvement of one is greater than the other. In each case, the symptoms and electrodiagnostic findings are commensurate with the extent of the lesion.

Three other conditions to be eliminated from the differential diagnosis are partial sciatic nerve injury at the thigh involving the peroneal division, lumbosacral plexus lesion, and L5 to S1 radiculopathy. In partial sciatic nerve injury, the short head of the biceps femoris muscle is compromised. This is best shown by demonstrating denervation potential electromyographically, since it is difficult clinically to uncover the loss of function of this portion of this rather large muscle. In lumbosacral plexus lesion, the sensory involvement is different and depends upon the extent of the lesion. The muscles weakened include some of those not innervated by the common peroneal nerve. Bladder function may also be altered. In L5 to S1 radiculopathy, the sensation of the sole of the foot is impaired, the Achilles tendon reflex is diminished, and the paraspinal muscles at the L5 to S1 level show denervation potentials (positive sharp waves and/or fibrillations).

Once the diagnosis is established, if excessive pressure was the cause of the problem, symptomatic treatment is indicated: removal of pressure and support of the foot drop in order to stabilize it. A plastic short leg brace with the ankle joint at 90 degrees will prevent the patient from suffering an inversion injury of the ankle. This condition is one in which prevention plays the most important role. Avoidance of pressure at the level of the fibula head and frequent changes in bed position in patients during the immediate postoperative period and in stuporous patients will save many individuals from developing this condition. The prognosis is usually good but it may take several months before recovery is complete.

## ANTERIOR COMPARTMENT SYNDROME

This occurs as a result of an increase in pressure within the anterior compartment of the leg. This osteofascial compartment contains the deep branch of the peroneal nerve, the anterior tibial artery and veins and the ankle dorsiflexors (tibialis anterior), toe extensors (extensor digitorum longus), the extensor of the big toe (extensor hallucis longus), and the inconstant peroneus tertius (Fig. 17–7). When the pressure rises within the compartment, which has a fixed volumetric capacity, the blood vessels are compressed and the blood supply to the muscle within the compartment is compromised. The

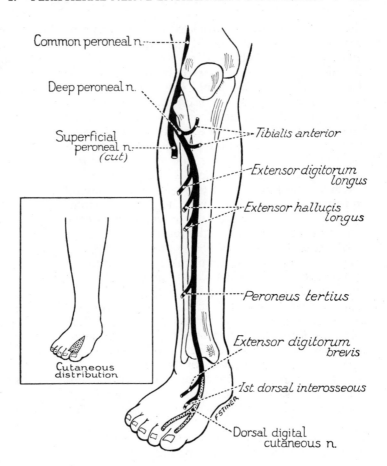

**Figure 17–7.** Course and distribution of the deep peroneal nerve. (From Haymaker, W., and Woodhall, B.: Peripheral Nerve Injuries, 2nd ed. W. B. Saunders Co., 1953.)

common causes of this syndrome are anterior tibial tendinitis caused by running long distances or a direct blow to the anterior aspect of the leg as in soccer or football or in an automobile accident. The overly tight application of a cast to the leg or swelling of the muscle because of a metabolic defect as in paroxysmal myoglobinuria may also produce increased compartmental pressure.

The most outstanding symptom is early, intense, and unremitting pain in the anterior aspect of the leg with signs of vascular depletion in the foot (coolness, paleness, and absence of dorsalis pedis pulse). The patient also complains of heaviness in the foot and of inability to dorsiflex the ankle, the toes, and the big toe. The patient retains his ability to evert and to plantar-flex the foot. There is hypesthesia or anesthesia in the dorsal aspect of the first web space.

The electrodiagnostic study shows no conduction along the deep peroneal nerve, but it will show normal conduction in the superficial peroneal nerve. Electromyogram of the involved muscles shows no electrical activity whatsoever during or immediately after the onset of the process. If the condition is severe and the ischemia to the anterior compartment muscles prolonged, the muscle becomes fibrotic. Electromyogram weeks later will

demonstrate no activity in these muscles, but the extensor digitorum brevis will have denervation potentials (positive sharp waves and/or fibrillations).

The differential diagnosis will have to be made mainly with an acute thromboembolic episode involving the anterior tibial artery. The lack of previous history of trauma and the history of conditions that may produce embolization will help in making the proper diagnosis.

Treatment for this condition is to decrease the intracompartment pressure as soon as possible before irreversible changes have occurred in the muscle and in the nerve. If the cause was direct trauma to the area, a generous fasciotomy is the treatment of choice. It should be kept in mind that elevation of the limb must be avoided; the ischemia and the pain will be increased with elevation because of a reduction in the lower extremity intra-arterial pressure. If a tight cast was the cause, removal of it may solve the problem; if not, fasciotomy is indicated.

### Tarsal Tunnel Syndrome

Tarsal tunnel syndrome occurs as the result of compression of the posterior tibial nerve or its branches as it passes under the flexor retinaculum behind the medial malleolus of the ankle joint.

This osteoligamentous tunnel is limited by the os talus medially and the medial malleolus of the tibia laterally. These two bones form a canal facing posteroinferiorly, which is covered by the flexor retinaculum of the ankle joint. The tendons of the flexor hallucis longus, the flexor digitorum longus, and the tibialis posticus accompany the neurovascular bundle containing the posterior tibial nerve through this tunnel. At the proximal end or within the tunnel the nerve divides into its three terminal branches: a cutaneous branch, the calcaneal nerve, which supplies the skin of the heel, and the lateral and medial plantar nerves. The lateral plantar nerve supplies the skin on the lateral aspect of the sole of the foot and half of the fourth and all of the fifth digit and innervates all the interossei, the second, third, and fourth lumbrical and the abductor minimi digiti. The medial plantar supplies the skin on the medial aspect of the sole of the foot and the first, second, and third digits and half of the fourth. In addition, it innervates the abductor hallucis, the flexor digitorum brevis, the flexor hallucis brevis and the first lumbrical (Fig. 17–8).

The most common causes of this syndrome are:

1. Tenosynovitis of the tendons within the tunnel caused by either local trauma or systemic disease (rheumatoid arthritis or other connective tissue disease).

2. Venous distention or engorgement within the tunnel from chronic venous insufficiency.

3. Distortion of the canal resulting from deformities of the ankle or foot, either developmental (pes planus, pes valgus) or traumatic (fracture of the medial malleolus or fractures or dislocations of the calcaneus or talus).

This syndrome usually presents with pain radiating into the foot and increasing on activity. Aggravation occurs on walking and on passive flexion and extension of the ankle joint. There is dysesthesia and decreased sensation in the sole of the foot medially or laterally or both. The skin of the heel is not affected when the calcaneal nerve runs superficial to the flexor retinaculum or the compression is distal to the tunnel. In cases in which the lateral plantar nerve is markedly involved, weakness and atrophy of the interosseus and lumbrical muscles results in the development of hammer toe deformity. Tapping behind the malleolus frequently causes an electric-like sensation to radiate into the foot.

Electrodiagnostically, the findings in this syndrome are normal motor conduction velocity in the tibial nerve from the popliteal fossa to the medial malleolus, and an increased distal motor latency either to the abductor hallucis (more than 6.5 msec) or to the abductor digiti quinti (more than 7.0 msec). If the latency to the abductor digiti quinti exceeds that of the abductor hallucis by more than 2.0 msec it indicates entrapment of the lateral plantar nerve.

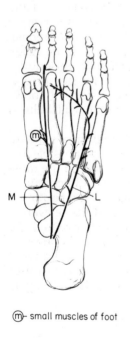

ⓜ- small muscles of foot

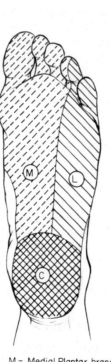

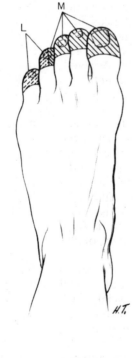

**Figure 17–8.** Cutaneous distribution of the posterior tibial nerve. (From Omer, G. E. and Spinner, M.: Management of Peripheral Nerve Problems. Philadelphia, W. B. Saunders Co., 1980.)

M – Medial Plantar branch
L – Lateral Plantar branch
C – Calcaneal branch

The common conditions that must be differentiated from this syndrome are peripheral neuropathy, posterior compartment syndrome, and S1 radiculitis. These can be easily excluded both clinically and electrodiagnostically. In peripheral neuropathy the sensory changes are usually "stocking" in distribution and not limited to the heel and sole of the foot. The extrinsic muscles of the foot may be involved.

In posterior compartment syndrome there is severe weakness of plantar flexion of the foot and edema in the back of the leg. In S1 radiculitis there is usually a history of low back pain with depression of the Achilles jerk, normal motor conduction, and distal latency in the tibial nerve; abnormal H-reflex and denervation potentials in the S1 innervated limb muscles and the S1 paraspinal muscles.

Conservative management includes correction of static deformities of the foot and ankle when possible and immobilization of the ankle joint. These simple measures favor the control of edema in the tunnel with a relative increase in space for the posterior tibial nerve. When the syndrome is caused by tenosynovitis of the tendons, the local infiltration with corticoids may reduce the inflammatory reaction and thereby reduce the pressure on the nerve. If these measures do not bring significant relief an exploration of the tarsal tunnel with opening of the flexor retinaculum is indicated.

## REFERENCES

Spinner, M.: Injuries to the Major Branches of Peripheral Nerves of the Forearm. Philadelphia, W.B. Saunders Co., 1972.

Omer, G. and Spinner, M.: Management of Peripheral Nerve Problems. Philadelphia, W.B. Saunders Co., 1980.

Haymaker, W. and Woodhall, B.: Peripheral Nerve Injuries: Principles of Diagnosis, 2nd ed. Philadelphia, W.B. Saunders Co., 1956.

Gray's Anatomy. New York, Bounty Books, 1977.

Lockhart, R. D. et al.: Anatomy of the Human Body. Philadelphia, J.B. Lippincott Co., 1965.

Aids to the Investigation of Peripheral Nerve Injuries. Medical Research Council—War Memorandum #7. London, Her Majesty's Stationery Office, 1943. (Reprinted 1967).

Nakano, K. K.: The entrapment neuropathies. Muscle Nerve 1:254–279, 1978.

Dell, P. C.: Compression of the ulnar nerve at the wrist secondary to a rheumatoid synovial cyst: case report and review of the literature. J. Hand Surg. 4:468–473, 1979.

Werner, C.: Lateral elbow pain and posterior interosseous nerve entrapment. Acta Orthopaed. Scand. (Supplement 174) 1–62, 1979.

Clark, C. B.: Cubital tunnel syndrome. JAMA, 24:801, 1979.

Macnicol, M. F.: The results of operation for ulnar neuritis. J. Bone Joint Surg., 61B:159–164, 1979.

Jones, R. E. and Gauntt, C.: Medial epicondylectomy for ulnar nerve compression syndrome at the elbow. Clin. Orthopaed. Related Res. 139:174–178, 1979.

Miller, R. G.: The cubital tunnel syndrome: diagnosis and precise localization. Ann. Neurol. 6:56–59, 1979.

Ring, H. et al.: Criteria for preclinical diagnosis of the cubital tunnel syndrome. Electromyogr. Clin. Neurophysiol. 19:425–34, 1979.

Odusote, K. and Eisen, A.: An electrophysiological quantitation of the cubital tunnel syndrome. J. Can. Sciences Neurolog. 6:403–10, 1979.

Kane, E. et al.: Observation of the course of the ulnar nerve in the arm. Ann. Chir. 27:487–496, 1973.

Lister, G. D. et al.: The radial tunnel syndrome. J. Hand Surg. 4:52–59, 1979.

Blakemore, J. R.: Posterior interosseous nerve paralysis caused by a lipoma. Coll. Surg. Edinb. 1979; 24:13–6, 1979.

Marquis, J. W.: Supracondyloid process of the humerus. Mayo Clin. Proc. 32:691–697, 1957.

Morris, H. H. and Peters B. H.: Pronator syndrome: clinical and electrophysiological features in seven cases. J. Neurol. Neurosurg. Psychiat. 39:461–64, 1976.

Rask, M. R.: Anterior interosseous nerve entrapment (Kiloh-Nevim Syndrome): report of seven cases. Clin. Orthopaed. Related Res. 142:176–81, 1979.

Nigst H. and Dick, W.: Syndromes of compression of the median nerve in the proximal forearm (pronator teres syndrome, anterior interosseous nerve syndrome). Arch. Orthop. Traumat. Surg. 93:303–312, 1979.

Stern, P. J. and Kutz, J. E.: An unusual variant of the anterior interosseous nerve syndrome: a case report and review of the literature. J. Hand Surg. 5:32–34, 1980.

Gelberman, R. H.: Carpal tunnel syndrome. J. Bone Joint Surg. 62A:1181–84, 1980.

Tanzer, R. C.: The carpal tunnel syndrome: a clinical and anatomical study. J. Bone Joint Surg. 41A:626–34, 1959.

Aminoff, M. J.: Involvement of peripheral vasomotor fibers in carpal tunnel syndrome. J. Neurol. Neurosurg. Psychiat. 42:649–655, 1979.

Kimura, J.: The carpal tunnel syndrome—localization of conduction abnormalities within the distal segment of the median nerve. Brain 102:619–635, 1979.

Harris, C. M.: et al.: The surgical treatment of the carpal tunnel syndrome correlated with preoperative nerve conduction studies. J. Bone Joint Surg. 61A:93–98, 1979.

McLaughlin, H. L.: Trauma. Philadelphia, W.B. Saunders Co., 1960.

Enright, T. et al.: Tarsal tunnel syndrome with ankylosing spondylitis. Rheumatism 22:77–79, 1979.

Bowrer, J. H. and Olin, F. H.: Complete replacement of the peroneus longus muscle: A. Ganglion with compression of the peroneal nerve. Clin. Orthop. Related Res. 140:172–174, 1979.

Menon, J. et al.: Tarsal tunnel syndrome secondary to neurilemoma of the medial plantar nerve. J. Bone Joint Surg. 62A:301–303, 1980.

Kopell, H. P. and Thompson, W. A. L.: Peripheral entrapment neuropathies. Huntington, N.Y., Robert E. Krieger Publishing Co., 1976.

# Section IV

# SYSTEMIC DISORDERS

# 18

# Cardiac Rehabilitation

*by Shanti S. Karwal, M.D.*

The total incidence and prevalence of coronary heart disease is not well known. We do know that over 3.9 million people in the United States have chronic coronary heart disease; 1.4 million people experience myocardial infarction annually. In addition, approximately 650,000 die of coronary heart disease each year. It has been estimated that about 160,000 cardiac deaths occur each year in individuals under 65 years of age.

Most studies indicate that the life style of an individual can predispose to coronary heart disease and increased mortality following myocardial infarction. Sedentary occupation has proved to be a major factor in the prevalence of coronary heart disease. There has been controversy in cardiac rehabilitation as to whether or not modification in the life style along with regular exercise can prevent or postpone the outcome of coronary heart disease. Nevertheless, early mobilization and resumption of daily activities after myocardial infarction is recommended. Patients with myocardial infarction are no longer confined to absolute bed rest as was the practice over a decade ago. The benefits of early rehabilitative measures have been recognized and these measures practiced increasingly by physicians. The complications associated with prolonged bed rest in the acute myocardial infarction patient, particularly physical deconditioning, vascular thrombosis, and pulmonary emboli, are reduced following early resumption of physical activities.

It has been observed and surveys indicate that about 85 per cent of patients under the age of 65 have returned to work within two to four months after an uncomplicated myocardial infarction. Over 75 per cent of patients resumed work at the same level of physical activity as before their myocardial infarction. About 15 per cent of myocardial infarction survivors under the age of 65 do not return to work each year. These are the patients who may have a special need for rehabilitation services, possibly because of increased impairment—physical, emotional, or educational. In addition, elderly patients or individuals with associated physical disabilities (neurological, muscular, skeletal, and so on, amputees and stroke victims) may require special training to enhance functions or to learn work simplification techniques to compensate for their disabilities. This can permit them to continue independent living and not to become cardiac cripples.

The purpose of this chapter is to review the contributing factors for coronary heart disease and the physiological effects of exercise and basic principles involved in cardiac rehabilitation. Emphasis is on the important role of rehabilitation medicine in managing patients with myocardial infarction. Cardiac rehabilitation is an important phase in the total management and demands an interdisciplinary team approach.

## DEFINITION OF TERMS

*Work* is defined as a product of force and the distance through which this force acts. Thus, lifting a 10-pound weight to a height of 5 feet will constitute 10 times 5 equals 50 foot-pounds of work. Pushing an object for a distance of 5 feet and applying 10 pounds of continuous pushing force constantly will also be 50 foot-pounds of work. Work has been classified as *concentric* when there is shortening of the working muscle, e.g., bending the elbows to lift an object. This is positive work. When there is lengthening of the working muscle, as in lowering an object, it is called *eccentric contraction* and is negative work.

Measuring the total mechanical work that involves muscle contraction and lengthening is difficult. Therefore, physical work or activity is measured by the amount of energy consumed during a particular activity. This can be calculated by the amount of oxygen and carbon dioxide exchanged.

A *calorie* is the unit of energy. One calorie is the amount of energy required to heat 1 kg of water 1° C (at 15° C). One liter of oxygen consumed is equivalent to about 5 calories.

*Power* is work performed per unit of time.

A *watt* is a measure of power. One watt is equal to 6 kilopound meters per min (6 kg meter/min).

The term *MET* expresses the amount of energy expenditure. It is a multiple of a basal metabolic unit independent of body weight: 2 METs represents an energy expenditure equal to twice the resting level (basal metabolic rate).

One MET equals 1.2 calories/min. The oxygen equivalent is about 3.5 to 4.0 ml oxygen/kg/min.

Physical efficiency is a ratio of the work done to the amount of energy used.

$$\text{Net efficiency} = \frac{\text{Work done} \times 100}{\text{Net energy used}}$$

Although the term *physical endurance* is used frequently, the definition remains ambiguous. To some students it means the duration of work performed. The best physiological index of total body endurance is the aerobic capacity of an individual—the highest level of oxygen consumption that an individual can achieve by dynamic exercises. This is called $Vo_{2max}$ (maximal oxygen consumption ml/kg/min).

$Vo_{2max}$ equals cardiac output times arteriovenous oxygen difference (A-$Vo_2$ difference), or heart rate times stroke volume tines A-$Vo_2$ difference. Cardiac output is the major determinant of $Vo_{2max}$ and indirectly of physical endurance.

*Cardiac output* is a product of heart rate times stroke volume. Either or both may vary with the physical activity. Stroke volume is the major determinant of maximal cardiac output. In a healthy young individual with heart rate of 75 beats/min and stroke volume of 75 ml/min, the cardiac output is 75 times 75 equals 4.1 liters/min.

$MVo_2$ (maximal myocardial $o_2$ consumption) equals heart rate times systolic blood pressure. It decreases with age and the presence of diseases of the myocardium and coronary arteries.

*Cardiac efficiency* is a ratio of $MVo_2/Vo_2$. High ratio is indicative of low cardiac efficiency.

Cardiac rehabilitation can be classified into five major categories: (1) preventive, diagnostic and therapeutic exercise in the coronary care unit, (2) endurance training programs designed to take place in a physical therapy gym or work physiology laboratory, (3) psychological and vocational counseling, (4) home exercise programs and (5) follow-up visits.

The concept of preventive cardiac rehabilitation has evolved because of the many preventable coronary risk factors that may lead to myocardial infarction, disability, and even death. These coronary risk factors can be classified as major and minor.

Major coronary risk factors include physical inactivity, cigarette smoking, hypertension, and hypercholesterolemia. The incidence of major coronary event, sudden death, and total mortality was found to be high when the three major risk factors—cigarette smoking, hypertension, and hypercholesterolemia—were present together. There are minor risk factors that contribute in the process of coronary heart disease. These include diabetes mellitus, obesity, hyperuremia, genetic predisposition, and Type A personality. Individuals with Type A personality are characterized by excessive striving for achievement, time urgency, and hostility. There may be many more factors yet to be discovered and studied, such as use of oral contraceptives.

It is important to emphasize the effects of physical inactivity and prolonged bed rest on the body. The rate of strength deterioration when a person is at complete bed rest is 3 per cent per day, and a decrease in activity causes a prompt fall in $Vo_{2 \text{ max}}$: A 20 to 25 per cent fall has been observed after 3 weeks of bed rest in young normal subjects. All this leads to limitation of work performance, decreased endurance, tachycardia during low level of work and even during rest, postural hypotension, easy fatigability and increased myocardial oxygen demand, increased blood viscosity, increased tendency to thromboembolic episodes and pulmonary emboli, negative protein and mineral balance, increased incidence of coronary heart disease, psychosocial and mental changes in the form of anxiety and depression, invalidism, and economic loss and suffering of the family.

Cardiac rehabilitation, including therapeutic exercise, improves the quality of life, enhances functional performance, improves the circulatory state and pulmonary ventilation, and maintains the physical, psychological, occupational, and recreational status of an individual.

Diagnosis for cardiac rehabilitation programs is the responsibility of the cardiologist; the diagnostic procedures include but are not limited to EKG, Holter monitoring, echocardiogram, radionuclide scans, coronary angiography, and stress testing. Those involved in physical therapy rehabilitation should have a basic understanding of the purpose and interpretation of findings of various tests.

The therapeutic exercise program in the coronary care unit is designed using a knowledge of work physiology. The program is designed for patients who have had myocardial infarction or coronary bypass surgery. Individuals with high coronary risk factors and atherosclerotic heart disease are treated in a different setting.

It is important that a careful evaluation be carried out before the patient begins the exercise program.

The patient population in a coronary care unit can be divided into four major categories.

1. *Uncomplicated completed acute myocardial infarction.* About 75 per cent of patients are in this category. They have small or moderate-sized infarcts and no evidence of continuous ischemia, left ventricular failure, cardiac shock, serious dysrhythmias, or conduction disturbances.

2. *Complicated myocardial infarction.* These are high-risk patients and have one or more of the previously mentioned complications.

3. *Uncomplicated high risk.* The condition of patients in this group may be uncomplicated initially, but they may have poor ventricular function and cardiac reserve or may have significant ischemia with a low level of activity.

4. *Acute myocardial infarction* (complicated or uncomplicated). These patients may also have neurological, muscular, or skeletal disorders such as stroke, amputations, arthritis, and fractures.

There may be a small group of patients with thyroid diseases, anemia, or chronic debilitating illnesses, and patients with cognitive disorders.

The physiatrist must be familiar with the nature

**TABLE 18–1.** NEW YORK HEART ASSOCIATION CLASSIFICATION SUSTAINED AND INTERMITTENT WORK LOADS

| FUNCTIONAL CLASSIFICATION | PHYSIOLOGIC SYMPTOMS | MAXIMAL CAL/MIN | | MAXIMAL METs |
| --- | --- | --- | --- | --- |
| | | Sustained | Intermittent | |
| I | Patients with cardiac disease but without resulting limitations of physical activity: ordinary physical activity does not cause undue fatigue, palpitation, dyspnea, or anginal pain | 5.0 | 6.5 | 6.5 |
| II | Patients with cardiac disease resulting in slight limitation of physical activity: they are comfortable at rest; ordinary physical activity results in fatigue, palpitation, dyspnea, or anginal pain | 2.5 | 4.0 | 4.5 |
| III | Patients with cardiac disease resulting in marked limitation of physical activity: they are comfortable at rest; less than ordinary physical activity causes fatigue, palpitation, dyspnea, or anginal pain | 2.0 | 2.7 | 3.0 |
| IV | Patients with cardiac disease resulting in inability to carry on any physical activity without discomfort; symptoms of cardiac insufficiency or of the anginal syndrome may be present even at rest; if any physical activity is undertaken, discomfort is increased | 1.5 | 2.0 | 1.5 |

of all existing problems before he can recommend patients for a program of therapeutic exercises in the coronary care unit. Physicians must be familiar with the energy expenditure or energy requirements for various activities. Subjecting patients with myocardial infarction to a high level of activity that increases the oxygen demand of the myocardium is dangerous.

The American Heart Association and the New York Heart Association have classified patients with cardiac disease into four functional classes according to the amount of work load tolerance, both sustained and intermittent (Table 18–1).

Work physiologists have classified normal daily activities according to MET required.

1. Minimal activities require less than 1.5 MET. Sitting in bed, semireclining, eating in bed and carrying on a conversation are a few examples of minimal activities requiring less than 1.5 MET of energy expenditure.

2. Light activities (1.5 to 2.5 MET): transfers from bed to chair, dressing and undressing, and washing hands and face in bed are light cardiac activities.

3. Moderate activities (2.5 to 3.5 MET): preparing meals, using a bedside commode, and walking at 2.0 to 2.5 mph are moderate cardiac activities.

4. Heavy activities (3.5 to 5 MET): bowel movement using a bed pan, bed making and sexual intercourse fall into the category of heavy cardiac activities.

5. Severe activities (5.0 to 7.0 MET): descending stairs and walking at 3.5 mph fall into the category of heavy cardiac activities.

6. Excessively severe activities (more than 7.0 MET): climbing stairs, fast bicycling, and jogging at 5 mph are excessively severe activities requiring over 7.0 METS.

MET requirements for some common activities are shown in Table 18–2.

Using this underlying principle and knowledge of energy requirements during various activities, patients are begun on rehabilitation programs in coronary care unit. Each patient requires individual assessment and care. The level of activities must be modified according to changes in the patient's clinical status during the course of illness. A rigid working protocol is not practical. The therapeutic exercise program in the coronary care unit is designed to deliver a low level of graded, dynamic, rhythmic, isotonic exercises—passive to active—with progression to activities of daily living and ambulation. Isometric exercises are avoided.

**TABLE 18–2.  MET REQUIREMENTS FOR COMMON ACTIVITIES**

| | |
|---|---|
| Passive ROM (range of motion) to arms (supine) | 1.2 |
| Active ROM to arms (supine) | 1.4 |
| Passive ROM to legs (supine) | 1.9 |
| Active ROM to legs (supine) | 2.0 |
| Active ROM to arms (sitting) | 2.0 |
| Straight leg raising (supine) | 2.5 |
| Straight leg raising (semisitting) | 2.9 |
| Transfer from bed to chair | 3.6 |
| Using bedside commode | 3.6 |
| Using bedpan | 4.7 |
| Doing pushups | 6.5 |
| Ambulation with braces, crutches | 8.0 |
| Sexual activity  a. Pre and postorgasm | 3.7 |
| b. During coitus | 5.0 for less than 30 sec |

There are many contraindications for the exercise program. Patients with crescendo angina or subendocardial infarction with persistent chest pain, are not candidates for starting therapy. Other contraindications are:

1. Cardiac shock

2. Ventricular arrythmias

3. Heart failure

4. Second- and third-degree heart block

5. Acute embolic episode (pulmonary or systemic)

6. Acute infections or sepsis

7. Thrombophlebitis

8. Acute myocarditis or pericarditis

9. Massive ventricular aneurysm

10. Severe stenosis of three major coronary arteries

11. Severe systemic or pulmonary hypertension

12. Severe ventricular outflow obstruction

13. Dissecting aortic aneurysm

14. TIA or acute stroke

There are relative contraindications and associated problems that require special consideration.

1. Uncontrolled supraventricular dysrhythmias

2. Moderate aortic stenosis

3. Uncontrolled metabolic diseases (thyrotoxicosis, diabetes)

4. Cardiomyopathy

5. Severe anemia

6. Acute fulminating arthritis

Patients with a fixed rate cardiac pacemaker, patients who are receiving such medications as digoxin, propranolol and quinidine, markedly obese individuals, and patients with psychoneurotic disturbances need special consideration.

During the course of therapeutic exercises in a coronary care unit it is essential to monitor the patient's clinical signs and symptoms, heart rate response, and changes in blood pressure. During the initial interview, the patient should be advised to inform his physician and therapist if he develops any of these symptoms:

1. Chest, shoulder, or jaw discomfort or chest pain

2. Palpitation

3. Severe dyspnea

4. Cyanosis

5. Excessive sweating, lightheadedness, dizziness, or fainting

6. Apprehension or confusion

7. Extreme fatigue, motor incoordination, or ataxia

8. Decrease in or failure to increase heart rate and/or systolic blood pressure during exercise

9. Heart rate above 115 beats/min during low level of exercise

10. Appearance of new murmurs or gallops

11. Detection of frequent ventricular premature beats, bigeminy, multiform or R on T phenomenon

12. PAT or atrial fibrillation

13. Second- or third-degree heart block

14. ST–T displacement from pre-exercise level

Leading questions may be asked during therapy sessions. The exercise program should be stopped, deferred, modified, or discontinued if the patient becomes symptomatic or if monitoring parameters become abnormal.

Every patient in a coronary care unit is under great psychological stress. Failure to detect the need for and provide early counseling and support may lead to permanent psychological dysfunction. One of the important factors that can modify the ultimate outcome in myocardial infarction patients is psychotherapy.

The psychological reactions that may appear include fear, anxiety, depression, and misconceptions. Psychotherapy must be included in the program of cardiac rehabilitation in the coronary care unit. The program should include education of the patient to allay fears of the environment and equipment in the coronary care unit. The purpose of the cardiac monitor and oxygen should be explained in positive terms. The patient should not have the impression that the equipment is there to keep him from dying. Misconceptions about heart attack, future employment, invalidity, and sex activity should be explored and dispelled. The patient should be helped to deal with fear, anxiety, and depression. This should be done with a team approach, and the active participation of a psychologist, trained nursing staff, and resident physician is essential.

Vocational counseling is important to help patients return to work or suitable placement so that after discharge from coronary care unit they do not become cardiac cripples.

A home program of endurance exercises to maintain physical and cardiac fitness is recommended. Instructions are given to patients at the time of discharge. Precautions, self-monitoring of pulse rate, and recognition of adverse symptoms are clearly explained. An endurance exercise program in the form of calisthenics, walking, and jogging to tolerance three times a week for 30 minutes is recommended. The upper limit of pulse rate (preferably heart rate) should be 80 per cent of maximum achieved heart rate during an exercise tolerance test. However, if the patient develops symptoms before the upper limit of heart rate is reached, the intensity of exercises should be modified after consultation with the physician in charge.

The purpose of cardiac rehabilitation is to let the patient live comfortably with an optimal level of functioning in life.

## SUGGESTED READING

1. Detry, J-M.: Exercise testing and training in coronary heart disease. H. E. Stenfert Kroese B. V./Leiden, 1973.
2. American Heart Association Cardiac Rehabilitation Committee: Guidelines for Cardiac Rehabilitation Centers, 2nd ed. 1982. Greater Los Angeles Affiliate.
3. Kottke, F. J., Stillwell, G. K. and Lehmann, J. F.: Krusen's Handbook of Physical Medicine and Rehabilitation, 3rd ed. Philadelphia, W. B. Saunders Co., 1982.

# 19

# Pulmonary Disorders

## Chronic Obstructive Pulmonary Disease

*by Horacio Pineda, M.D.*

Chronic obstructive pulmonary disease (COPD) refers to a group of diseases that generally includes emphysema, chronic bronchitis, and asthma. These diseases are characterized by persistent elevation of airway resistance. The condition in most patients suffering from either one or a combination of these diseases follows a chain of events that progressively leads to pulmonary insufficiency, pulmonary hypertension, and cor pulmonale. The airway obstruction and progressive lung destruction prominently observed contribute to altered mechanics of breathing. The resulting increase in the cost of breathing and ventilation-perfusion abnormalities ultimately results in hypoxemia and hypercapnia. The often protracted nature of these diseases exacts its toll in terms of personal suffering, disability, and financial drain on the patient, his family, and society as a whole.

Attempts at rehabilitating these patients are sorely lacking, particularly when one considers that untold millions worldwide suffer from or are disabled by these diseases. In the past few years alone, the United States Social Security Service spent between $750 and $900 million dollars in disability payments to these patients. Although some institutions around the country are striving to promote a comprehensive clinical and rehabilitative approach, the majority of these patients still receive little more than just symptomatic or emergency medical treatment. In spite of the great disability that results from these diseases and the potential for rehabilitation of a great number of these patients, the rehabilitation community as a whole has likewise paid little more than token at-

tention to these patients. It is therefore the purpose of this chapter to rekindle interest for these groups of disabled patients, as much as it is to present a bird's eye view of the problem and approach to therapy.

In clinical practice, these different obstructive airway diseases commonly occur in combination. It is, for example, rare to see emphysema in the pure form. Overlapping signs and symptoms of the different diseases in the same patient are therefore not uncommon. It is not within the scope of this chapter to present a complete clinical discussion of each of the diseases; rather, a brief clinical discussion on certain aspects pertinent to the rehabilitation practitioner will be presented. The reader is referred to standard medical textbooks to supplement the clinical material.

*Emphysema* is characterized by irreversible destruction of alveolar walls and the accompanying vascular bed, resulting in progressive dilatation of alveoli and terminal airways. The terminal and respiratory bronchioles lose their tissue support and become readily collapsible, resulting in incomplete evacuation of inspired air on exhalation. No single etiological factor has been found to explain all the pathological changes, but genetic predisposition (alpha$_1$-antitrypsin deficiency), autoimmune reaction, chronic inflammation, and air pollution, among many others, have been implicated. Men are affected more frequently than women. Typically, the patient is in the fourth or fifth decade of life when symptoms are first noticed. There is usually a smoking history. The patient presents with complaints of shortness of breath and easy fatigability.

331

Hyperinflation of the thorax and use of accessory neck muscles for respiration are prominent findings. These patients are seldom cyanotic unless their emphysema is far advanced. Some of them spontaneously do pursed-lip breathing. These two latter characteristics are responsible for the popular term "pink puffer" that is used to describe these patients. The cause of death in 75 to 85 per cent is secondary to cor pulmonale and right-sided heart failure.

*Asthma* is characterized by increased responsiveness of the tracheobronchial tree to various stimuli, resulting in bronchospasm that is at times accompanied by increased sputum production. There are two general clinical types, extrinsic and intrinsic asthma. Extrinsic, or allergic, asthma usually starts in childhood or early adulthood, presenting as episodic bronchospastic attacks that are generally allergic in nature. Two types of allergic reactions, types I and III, have been implicated. Type I allergic reaction is a reagin-mediated, immediate-onset reaction, while type III is the delayed reaction related to the Arthus phenomenon. Intrinsic, or infective, asthma on the other hand usually starts in adult life and is less episodic in nature, but rather produces manifestations of bronchial obstruction such as wheezing most of the time. Periodically, obstructive symptoms worsen, especially in the presence of upper respiratory infection. Both types of asthma prominently involve allergy-induced bronchospasm that responds favorably to bronchodilator drugs. Physical exercise and cold weather have also been observed to trigger wheezing in some patients. During severe bronchospastic episodes, cyanosis, hyperinflation of the chest, fatigue, and dehydration are commonly observed.

*Chronic bronchitis* is a disorder characterized by increased mucus secretion in the bronchi. These patients secrete a hundred milliliters or more of mucus a day for a minimum of three months in a year for two consecutive years. The character of the sputum varies from clear mucoid to yellowish or mucopurulent. The exact etiology is uncertain, but microscopic studies reveal hypertrophy of the mucus glands and goblet cells along the bronchial linings. These changes may be a response to respiratory irritants, mechanical trauma, or allergens. The typical chronic bronchitic usually is, again, a male urbanite who has a long history of smoking. The patient usually complains of a chronic productive cough that is usually worse in the morning. In contrast to the predominantly emphysematous patient, bronchitics develop cyanosis and signs of cor pulmonale earlier in the course of the disease. Thus they have been referred to as "blue bloaters." Again, symptoms are usually exacerbated by overlying infections of the respiratory tract.

*Bronchiectasis* is characterized by chronic, abnormal, irreversible dilatation of the bronchi. Three morphological types, cylindrical, varicose, and saccular, are usually found during bronchoscopic examination. Similarly, the exact etiology is unclear, but severe infections (pertussis), bronchial obstruction (endobronchial tumors, foreign bodies), and chronic inhalation of irritants have been implicated. The clinical manifestations vary depending on the severity of involvement and presence of complications such as long-standing infections. These patients present with chronic productive cough, easy fatigability, and loss of weight and appetite. The character of the sputum varies from dirty white to mucopurulent. Hemoptysis is occasionally present. In some patients, accompanying sinusitis and finger clubbing may be found.

## COMPREHENSIVE CARE FACTORS

For years, the therapeutic management of the patient with COPD has been mainly symptomatic outpatient treatment highlighted by repeated hospital admissions for treatment of exacerbation of symptoms or respiratory failure. Long-term management planning has been largely neglected, and the patient is commonly told to "take it easy and live with your disability." Hodgkin et al. published an excellent article on the subject and outlined not only the clinical manifestations of COPD but, more importantly, also suggested an approach to long-term management.[1] The general management of the COPD patient involves the harmonious interplay of the different therapeutic modalities, including general factors, medications, respiratory therapy, and physical therapy. Every physiatrist must have a working knowledge of these different modalities of treatment.

### GENERAL FACTORS

This extremely important but often neglected aspect of therapy many times spells the difference between the success or failure of any given therapeutic program. Most patients are not only in physical distress but are also often scared, confused, and misinformed, and feel neglected. It is not surprising to find that many patients fail to comply with immediate treatment modalities, much less follow through on a long-term basis. Therefore, it is important to start a treatment program by first educating the patient and his family about the disease, its treatment, and the many factors that influence its natural course.

The patient is advised to avoid smoking and inhaling airborne irritants. Patients are also advised to take precautions against respiratory infections and to seek immediate treatment if they occur. A high fluid intake together with a nutritionally balanced diet is encouraged. As much as possible, the patient should stay in an environment that is comfortable and moderate with respect to both humidity and temperature. Many times, patients will ask advice regarding relocation to a "better" environment. Any response concerning such questions necessitates careful consideration, because there is probably no "ideal" environment. A more prudent suggestion than the advice to relocate would be to have the patient try out the new place first. Among the things he should consider during this tryout period are weather conditions, air pollution, preponderance of airborne allergens, and availability of adequate medical, employment, social, and recreational facilities in the area. When appropriate, sexual counseling may be given. Many sexually active COPD patients often find the act of intercourse too strenuous. Shortness of breath or fear sometimes interferes with their enjoyment. For these patients, such measures as use of low-flow nasal oxygen, assuming the passive rather than active role, and using medications such as bronchodilators and cough suppressants prior to coitus may be of help. Finally, COPD patients should be encouraged to function and do as much for themselves as possible within the limits of their pulmonary reserve.

## MEDICATIONS

The pharmaceutical agents used in treatment of COPD are usually aimed at the many problems commonly encountered in these groups of diseases. These problems are increased airway resistance, tracheobronchial secretions, infection, allergic phenomena, and cor pulmonale.

The problem of increased airway resistance is common to all diseases that make up the group COPD. For many years, bronchodilator therapy has been the mainstay of treatment of these conditions. Bronchodilator preparations are numerous but the commonly used ones fall under two general types according to the mode of action. The first group is the adrenergic bronchodilators. This group of drugs acts on the different sympathetic receptors: alpha, beta$_1$, and beta$_2$. Since beta$_2$ receptors are largely responsible for pulmonary vascular and bronchial dilation, the more beta$_2$ specific a drug is, the more desirable it becomes. Unfortunately, most commercially available preparations also contain some factors that affect alpha$_1$ and beta$_1$, resulting in the undesirable side effects of increased heart rate and blood pressure. A comparison of the different sympathomimetic agents is shown in Table 19–1. These medications come in different preparations for oral, inhalation, or parenteral use.

The second group of bronchodilators is the theophylline derivatives (e.g., aminophylline, oxytriphylline). This group of drugs possesses a variety

TABLE 19–1. EFFECTS OF SYMPATHOMIMETIC AGENTS

| MEDICATION | PREDOMINANT EFFECTS | | |
|---|---|---|---|
| | Beta-2 | Beta-1 | Alpha |
| Isoetharine | * | | |
| Salbutamol | * | | |
| Isoproterenol | * | * | |
| Epinephrine | * | * | * |
| Ephedrine | * | * | * |

of systemic effects. These include bronchodilation caused by relaxation of the bronchial smooth muscles, central nervous system stimulation including the respiratory center, positive cardiac chronotropic and inotropic effects, increased diuresis from increased glomerular filtration and reduced tubular sodium reabsorption, and increased gastric secretion. The main indication for these drugs is for bronchodilation. Because of the many systemic effects that have been mentioned, they are also used as adjunctive therapy for such conditions as acute pulmonary edema, obesity-hypoventilation syndrome, and periodic respiration. These drugs should be used with caution in patients with intercurrent conditions such as peptic ulcer or cardiac arrhythmia.

A third class of drugs with bronchodilator effects is the anticholinergic agents (e.g., atropine, scopolamine). These agents produce some bronchodilation by inhibiting vagal parasympathetic nerve endings. They also reduce tracheobronchial secretions. Although they are popular as preanesthetic medication, they have little clinical value in the long-term treatment of COPD.

The problem of excessive tracheobronchial secretions is prominent in chronic bronchitis and bronchiectasis. This problem can be approached from many directions. First, an effort should be made to reduce sputum production by removing any known cause or aggravating factor. These factors usually include infection and allergy, which will be discussed in the following sections. Second, the remaining secretion within the tracheobronchial tree should be liquefied and rendered less viscous for easier expectoration. Improved hydration, expectorants, mucolytic agents, and detergents are frequently recommended in attaining this end. By far, improved hydration is still one of the most effective ways of liquefying sputum. Water can be taken orally, parenterally, or by humidifying inspired air. Expectorants work by facilitating water bonding with sputum (glyceryl guaiacolate), or by inducing proteolysis of sputum (potassium iodide). Mucolytic agents (N-acetyl L-cysteine) are effective in depolymerizing mucopolysaccharides. Introduced as aerosols, these agents are effective; however, they can be irritating to the bronchial mucosa. To prevent any resultant bronchospasm, they are therefore given with a bronchodilator. Detergents (Alevaire) are a drugs that decrease surface tension of secretions, thus reducing their tendency to adhere to the bronchial wall. Unfortunately, these drugs have a tendency to cause bronchial irritation and inflammation and should therefore be used with discretion. Enzymes such as dornase or streptokinase are seldom used in the routine treatment of the COPD patient but are sometimes used in the treatment of hematoma, hemothorax, empyema, and for clearing infected ulcers.

The problem of infection in these patients is especially important because many serious consequences may result. Respiratory infections are a common cause of exacerbation of symptoms among COPD patients. Infection causes inflammation and induces increased production of secretions; the accompanying fever tends to elevate metabolic rate. The combined result is increased difficulty of breathing sometimes leading to acute respiratory failure. For these reasons and because of the very little respiratory reserve that these patients have, antibiotic therapy is started at the earliest sign of infection. Oral tetracycline and ampicillin are usually given. In more serious infections, specific antibiotics are given, either singly or in combination, usually following the results of sputum culture and sensitivity studies. In some patients with chronic bronchitis and bronchiectasis, sputum culture may reveal chronic growth of microorganisms without any evidence of active infection. These patients do not usually require long-term antibiotic coverage, but they do require vigilant observation, especially for conditions that can reduce host resistance. As a preventive measure, COPD patients should receive annual innoculations against influenza and pneumonia.

Miscellaneous problems frequently encountered in this group of diseases include allergy and cor pulmonale. In some asthmatics and in bronchitic patients, an allergic component may be a prominent factor in their condition. For this reason medications with antiallergic properties are added to the regular therapeutic armamentarium. Adrenocorticosteroids are important drugs that possess a variety of actions utilized in controlling some manifestations of COPD. Steroids not only affect the immunologic response of the body, they also reduce the inflammatory response. Unfortunately, unwanted side effects such as increased gastric acidity, fluid retention, osteoporosis, and increased fat deposition frequently accompany any long-term use of these drugs. Their therapeutic value has been proven time and again in seemingly intractable situations. They have also been significantly valuable in controlling bronchospasm and acute respiratory failure when used in conjunction with bronchodilator therapy. To reduce unwanted side effects, these medications should be administered in the smallest effective dose for the shortest possible time. Most patients with COPD respond well to a 40- to 60-mg oral loading dose of prednisone given for a few days. This is then gradually tapered to the lowest possible maintenance dose, which is often as low as 5 to 10 mg per day. Whenever possible, these patients should be weaned off steroids completely or switched to inhalational preparations such as Vanceril. Prolonged use of steroids should be weighed carefully in patients suffering from diabetes mellitus, peptic ulcer, congestive heart failure, high blood pressure, and tuberculosis.

Of interest is a drug claimed to inhibit release of vasoactive mediators caused by antigen-antibody reaction. This drug is disodium chromoglycate. It is said to be effective in both the immediate and delayed types of allergic reactions. It is not a bronchodilator but is used for prophylaxis against acute bronchospastic attacks. It has no use in acute asthmatic attacks.

COPD patients who have signs and symptoms of cor pulmonale many times require the additional use of digitalis preparations and diuretics. Use of these drugs in COPD patients, however, requires careful monitoring of digitalis and electrolyte blood levels.

**Respiratory Therapy.** These modalities include aerosol therapy, oxygen therapy, and the use of the mechanical breathing devices. Combined with the other modalities of treatment, they are an important part of the total management in that they aid in maintaining ventilation and tissue oxygenation, as well as help in elimination of secretions.

Aerosol therapy is used to improve humidification, to facilitate elimination of tracheobronchial secretions, and for instillation of different medications into the respiratory tract. Aerosols are suspensions of very fine liquid or solid particles (0.005 $\mu$) in a gas medium. Using a variety of devices that range from freon-propelled hand nebulizers to compressors and positive-pressure breathing machines, medications such as bronchodilators, mucolytic agents, and steroid preparations may be instilled into the respiratory tract when mixed with the inspired air. More importantly, with this mode of therapy, water vapor may be aerosolized to prevent or correct humidity deficits, prevent crusting of secretions, and dilute mucus for easier expectoration.

Oxygen therapy is indicated when the blood level of oxygen is significantly low. Hypoxemia should not be confused with hypoventilation, since the former can occur at any level of ventilation, and the principle of therapy for each is not necessarily the same. Oxygen may be given on either a continuous or temporary basis. Temporary use of oxygen is indicated when patients who ordinarily maintain adequate oxygen levels develop an acute exacerbation. Supplementary oxygen may also be given to patients in order to improve their exercise tolerance during physical therapy or more strenuous daily activities. Similarly, temporary oxygen is prescribed following major surgery of a COPD patient. Continuous oxygen therapy, on the other hand, is indicated when patients with severely advanced disease are unable to maintain adequate oxygen levels in the blood at rest in spite of adequate drug therapy. It is difficult to set a certain arbitrary blood level of oxygen that would indicate necessity of continuous oxygen therapy because different patients react to hypoxemia in different ways. Although cell oxygenation is known to be critically curtailed when the $Pa_{O_2}$ drops below 30 mm Hg, the physician should not wait for this extreme situation before giving oxygen. Most patients present with distressful symptoms long before the $Pa_{O_2}$ reaches 50 mm Hg or lower.

When oxygen is being considered for a patient, it is still better to evaluate each case on an individual basis. Aside from improving tissue oxygenation, oxygen therapy is given to reduce pulmonary hypertension, reduce compensatory polycythemia, and improve the patient's overall physical and functional capacity. The smallest concentration given for the shortest possible time that will achieve adequate oxygenation is prescribed. It is known that prolonged administration of high concentrations of oxygen can result in toxicity characterized by thickening of alveolocapillary membrane, hyaline membrane formation, and focal atelectasis. Another danger that must be borne in mind is the possibility of oxygen-induced apnea caused by the removal of the anoxic drive to breathing in some patients. Bearing in mind these precautions, oxygen if indicated may be given by either nasal cannula, Venturi mask, or incorporated in the patient's intermittent positive-pressure breathing (IPPB) treatment.

Mechanical breathing devices are used mainly to assist, support, or assume control over the patient's ventilation. Assistive ventilation is indicated when the patient's own efforts are inadequate in maintaining acceptable blood gas levels. Controlled ventilation is indicated when the patient's condition is so severe that very little or no ventilatory efforts are evident. Unlike oxygen therapy, which is mainly designed to correct hypoxemia, mechanical ventilation is prescribed to correct reduced blood oxygen tension and carbon dioxide retention by improving effective ventilation. The beneficial effects of these devices in the treatment of acute respiratory failure are well established. Their long-term-use on COPD patients is, however, still of unproven value. Although they are not contraindicated for chronic use, prescriptions of such devices for this purpose should be carefully weighed and the patient's tolerance considered. Among the many mechanical breathing devices available, the most popularly used are the positive-pressure ven-

tilators. Intermittent positive-pressure breathing (IPPB) introduces air or an oxygen-enriched air mixture into the respiratory tract on a periodic basis. These machines can be set to operate cyclically by themselves at a predetermined rate and tidal volume or they may be triggered by the patient himself. IPPB machines may be pressure-cycled or volume-cycled. Pressure-cycled machines terminate the inspiratory phase after reaching a preset pressure. On the other hand, a preset volume determines inspiratory cutoff in volume-cycled ventilators. In both cases, expiration is usually passive. Despite the obvious benefits derived from these machines, their use requires judgment and caution. These machines, if misused, have the potential for causing harm. For example, improperly sterilized machines can spread infection throughout the respiratory tract. The higher the system pressure setting, the greater the risk of causing barotrauma (e.g., pneumothorax). There is also the danger of worsening hyperinflation in patients with expiratory obstruction and air trapping.

In some patients, hypoxemia persists, in spite of IPPB and ever-increasing inspired oxygen concentration. To maintain adequate oxygenation while at the same time the danger of oxygen toxicity is minimized, positive end-expiratory pressure (PEEP) is sometimes added to the set-up. This technique, which is commonly used in respiratory distress syndrome, many times enables adequate levels of oxygenation and ventilation to be given without need to resort to potentially toxic concentrations of inspired oxygen. PEEP is back pressure applied to the expiratory phase of breathing, which prevents the airway pressure from fully returning to atmospheric level. PEEP prevents the total collapse of alveoli at end expiration. This retards the tendency for atelectasis and at the same time improves the ventilation-perfusion relationship. However, PEEP produces an increase in functional residual capacity that is proportional to the amount of end-expiratory pressure imposed.

When these modalities are prescribed, consideration should be given the benefits that can be derived on one hand and the potential harm they can cause on the other.

## PHYSICAL THERAPY MODALITIES

Relaxation exercises, breathing exercises, postural drainage, and reconditioning exercises are the physical therapy modalities frequently prescribed for COPD patients. When used in combination with medications, respiratory therapy, and other general measures, they play an integral part in helping the patient with pulmonary disability to function to his maximal physical, mental, and vocational potential.

**Relaxation Exercises.** Patients with COPD readily experience shortness of breath. The severity of this shortness of breath varies but is usually increased by physical exertion, upper respiratory infection, or acute allergic episodes. In severe cases, this can be an exhausting and horrifying experience that the patient tries to avoid at all cost. Unfortunately, as the disease progresses, patients experience these feelings of suffocation at ever-increasing frequency. This sets in motion a chain of events that tends to aggravate rather than alleviate the problem. To avoid exercise-induced dyspnea the patient gradually reduces his physical activities, resulting in progressive physical deconditioning. Fear and anticipation of an attack of dyspnea leave the patient tense and anxious. This anxiety also contributes to increased muscle tension, inability to relax, assumption of a poor posture, and a tendency to panic in an impending bronchospastic attack. This anxiety sometimes results in the tendency of these patients to overmedicate themselves or resort to undue use of oxygen.

The objectives of relaxation exercises are to allay anxiety, reduce muscle tension, promote better posture, and gain better cooperation in performing the other therapy modalities. They also teach the patient to handle impending dyspneic attacks rationally. The classical relaxation technique includes placing the patient in a quiet, softly lit room in the most comfortable sitting or supine position. The exercise consists of a series of muscle contractions followed by a gradual, prolonged period of volitional relaxation. These exercises are first started on one muscle group and gradually other muscle groups are included. On a higher level, patient education and psychological counseling, if necessary, are incorporated. With a better understanding of his physical problem and his emotional reaction to it, the patient is more likely to succeed in cooperating and complying with the different modalities of therapy.

**Breathing Exercises.** The increased airway resistance encountered in COPD patients may be caused by bronchospasm, increased airway secretions, or, more importantly, small airway disease. In most cases, the increased airway resistance is manifested more on expiration than on inspiration. This impaired expiratory airflow and partial retention of inhaled air volume partially explains the hyperinflation frequently manifested by these patients. With hyperinflation, the diaphragm, which normally accounts for up to 65 per cent of inspiration, is kept at a depressed position, a mechanically disadvantageous state. To compensate, these individuals make use of their intercostal muscles and accessory neck muscles to augment the mechanically inefficient diaphragm during inspiration. Maintaining adequate ventilation in this manner is inefficient and the energy cost of the work of breathing is high. Consequently, these patients tend to breathe in a shallow rapid fashion, a pat-

tern of breathing that is itself inefficient. This breathing pattern, with a small tidal volume, results in wasted ventilation of the dead space.

The goals of breathing exercises are to improve alveolar ventilation, minimize air trapping and hyperinflation, and reduce the work of breathing as much as possible. To achieve these goals, the patient is taught to adopt a slower rate of breathing with a more normal tidal volume. Diaphragmatic breathing exercises are stressed in an effort to restore the diaphragm to function again as the main inspiratory muscle. This is done by placing the patient in supine or slightly head-down position and asking him to breath against abdominal weights (Fig. 19–1). The supine position tends to elevate the resting diaphragmatic position because of the weight of the abdominal viscera resting against it. The added abdominal weight provides resistive exercises to the diaphragm during inspiration. Several spirometer gadgets such as the Spirocare and the incentive spirometer may be used to regulate the size of the tidal volume.

Expiratory breathing exercises, on the other hand, are aimed at slowing the expiratory phase of breathing. This could slow down the expiratory flow rate, allowing more time for evacuation of air and at the same time minimizing terminal airway collapse. The addition of a proximal resistance to expiration (e.g., pursed lip expiration) is thought to increase intra-airway pressure, providing a splinting effect on the airways against early airway collapse. This explanation of the apparent benefits of pursed lip breathing is still debatable. Some think that pursed-lip breathing, a well-tolerated ex-

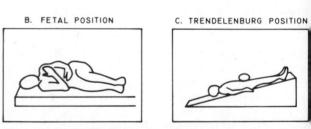

**Figure 19–1.** Diaphragmatic breathing exercises. (From Haas, A. et al.: Pulmonary Therapy and Rehabilitation: Principles and Practice. Baltimore, Williams and Wilkins, 1979.)

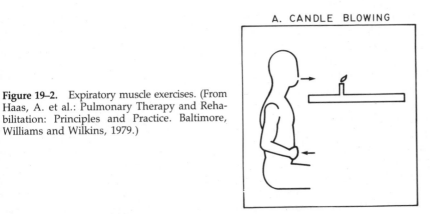
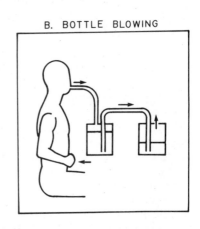

A. CANDLE BLOWING

B. BOTTLE BLOWING

**Figure 19-2.** Expiratory muscle exercises. (From Haas, A. et al.: Pulmonary Therapy and Rehabilitation: Principles and Practice. Baltimore, Williams and Wilkins, 1979.)

ercise sometimes adopted spontaneously by untrained patients, works mainly by slowing the expiratory flow rate. Whatever the real explanation is, expiratory exercises such as candle blowing and bottle blowing can be employed to achieve a controlled rate of expiration as well as the pursed-lip effect (Fig. 19–2).

**Postural Drainage.** The accumulation of secretions in the airways of COPD patients poses serious consequences if left untreated. Bronchial obstruction, atelectasis, pulmonary infection, and ventilation-perfusion abnormalities can result, as can spasmodic coughing resulting from local irritation.

Postural drainage, a set of noninvasive exercises used in conjunction with hydration, humidification, and medications, is designed to facilitate evacuation of secretions. This modality combines mechanical maneuvers (percussion and vibration),

gravity, and the coughing mechanism to expel acccmulated secretions. The patient is placed in different positions depending on the lung segment to be drained (Fig. 19–3) and vibration and percussion techniques are then applied. Any dislodged secretion is coughed up. The frequency of application of this modality depends on the amount of sputum to be drained. This frequency can range from one to four times a day. While these maneuvers are performed best by a trained therapist, the patient may perform self-percussion and drainage if no help is available.

Although recovery of sputum is greatly enhanced with these exercises, they should not be prescribed indiscriminately. Proper caution should be exercised in patients suffering from congestive heart failure, unstable cardiac arrhythmias, widespread malignancy, osteoporosis, and clotting defects. It is easy to see that complications such as

RIGHT UPPER LOBE

APICAL

RIGHT MIDDLE LOBE

MEDIAL

LATERAL

LEFT LOWER LOBE

SUPERIOR

POSTERIOR

RIGHT LOWER LOBE

ANTERIOR BASAL & MEDIAL BASAL

LEFT UPPER LOBE

INFERIOR

APICAL

TRACHEA

**Figure 19-3.** Postural drainage positions. (From Haas, A. et al.: Pulmonary Thearpy and Rehabilitation: Principles and Practice. Baltimore, Williams & Wilkins, 1979.)

exacerbation of heart failure, fractures, and bleeding manifestations may be produced in these patients. Finally, patients with loculated lung abscess should not be positioned with the abscess side up because of the danger of pus gravitating to the unaffected side. Percussion over an abscess must be avoided.

If the application of postural drainage fails in dislodging major mucus plugs, especially in the acutely ill patient, bronchoscopy and endotracheal suctioning should be considered.

**Reconditioning Exercises.** The basic purpose of these exercises is to achieve the maximal level of physical conditioning by employing gradually increasing levels of physical activities that are within the limits of cardiovascular and respiratory reserve. In COPD patients, this limit probably coincides with the patient's maximum aerobic capacity, which is related to his maximum oxygen consumption ($Vo_{2max}$). In reality, the patient's actual performance is often inordinately lower because other factors also come into play. These factors are mostly subjective and include dyspnea, motivation, or drive, as well as other psychological factors. Considering all these objective and subjective factors that can affect physical performance, aerobic exercise testing, in conjunction with the standard clinical evaluation, greatly enhances the accuracy of the overall assessment of these patients. In addition, an individually tailored exercise program geared to achieving maximum functional capacity can be prescribed with safety.

The exercises commonly employed include ambulation, stair climbing, treadmill, light calisthenics, stationary bicycle riding, and plain activities of daily living. The use of oxygen with these exercises is important, particularly in patients with significant hypoxemia. Arterial blood levels of oxygen of 55 mg Hg or lower (easily determined by microtechnique) generally require additional oxygen with exercise. The added oxygen in these cases helps to assure adequate tissue oxygenation during exercise, helps to delay or alleviate dyspnea and helps to increase endurance. Low-flow oxygen at 2 to 4 liters per minute is usually employed via a double-pronged nasal cannula. Progressively increasing loads of exercise are given until a plateau is reached. After this, a maintenance level of exercise is given for the patient to continue. Since $Vo_{2max}$ rates are sometimes observed to improve with reconditioning, some attempt must be made to try to wean the patient from oxygen if at all possible.

**Miscellaneous Exercises.** Biofeedback techniques have recently been reported to show significant promise in promoting general relaxation and bronchodilation and in altering the rate and depth of breathing. Biofeedback refers to the different techniques or instrumentation that provide immediate and continuous information on changes in bodily functions of which one is not usually aware. Electromyographic and electroencephalographic feedback have been employed in the treatment of COPD patients, but the practice is largely limited to specialized centers and is not yet widely used.

Of wider use and acceptance is a family of instruments designed to regulate and improve tidal volume, vital capacity, and inspiratory effort on a goal-oriented basis. Instruments such as the incentive spirometer and the Tri-Flo respiratory exerciser are examples of these and are designed to promote deep breathing. Prone immersion physical exercises (PIPE) have been reported to have significant value in reconditioning COPD patients. These exercises are done in a swimming pool with the patient swimming prone on a flotation board. The patient is asked to swim against a given weight placed on one end of the pool that is attached to the patient by means of a tether line and pulley system. This exercise is aimed at reconditioning the leg and arm musculature. Other reported benefits include reduction in functional residual capacity (FRC), reduction of cardiac stress, and promotion of better bronchial toilet by consequent breathing of warm, humid air. Again, actual clinical experience with this modality remains limited.

## CLINICAL APPROACH

The sight of a patient suffering from significant COPD at the office or clinic can be disturbing. The physiatrist sees not only an obviously disabled patient but also someone who appears to be in constant difficulty or outright distress. A way of approaching these patients without being overwhelmed is to organize thoughts on the interrelated problems at hand. The basic respiratory problem afflicting the patient should be identified. Knowing this allows a more rational approach to medical treatment and subsequent rehabilitative planning. A series of questions can aid in this.

*What is the clinical diagnosis?* In most cases, the answer to this is not difficult, since most patients referred to the physiatrist have been diagnosed beforehand by their primary-care physician. To update or confirm the diagnosis, a good history and physical examination coupled with the different diagnostic modalities of blood gases, pulmonary function testing, and radiographic studies can be reviewed or reordered. When evaluating these patients, one must bear in mind that a clinial diagnosis of either emphysema, asthma, chronic bronchitis or bronchiectasis in the pure form is rare. More commonly, a combination of two or more clinical conditions coexist.

*How severe is the disease and what is its rate of progression?* The answer to this question will allow more accurate immediate medical treatment as well as long-term rehabilitative and vocational planning. In spite of the myriad diagnostic modalities available, quantitating the severity of a particular disease process remains highly subjective and varies with each individual case. Rough estimates, however, are possible. A general guide, particularly in evaluating pulmonary function tests and blood gases, is to compare the patient's observed values with normal predicted standards. Values 65 to 80 per cent of normal predicted generally indicate mild impairment, 50 to 65 per cent indicate moderate impairment, and less than 50 per cent indicate severe impairment. The rate of progression of the disease may be evaluated by comparing past records with the present and doing follow-up studies at regular intervals.

*How does the disease affect the respiratory function in this particular patient?* Different diseases affect the respiratory system differently. While COPD manifests mainly as airway obstruction, some diseases affect lung volumes and the alveolar membranes readily; others affect the bronchial glands and smooth muscles. In any case, the specific approach to therapy depends greatly on the answer to this question. To further simplify the problem one can instead ask the question "Is ventilation adequate?" Knowledge of the ventilatory status is of prime importance, since effective gas exchange is the primary function of the respiratory system. Air flow and lung volume studies as well as minute ventilation and maximum breathing capacity contribute in assessing the status of the patient's ventilation. More importantly, the level of the blood gases usually sums up the adequacy or inadequacy of ventilation. $Pco_2$ in particular is directly related to the degree of hypoventilation. It is a better gauge than $Po_2$, since a low $Po_2$ may occur with either hypoventilation or hyperventilation. It may be worthwhile to point out that in emphysema, the $Pco_2$ may stay normal long after the $Po_2$ has deteriorated. However, in chronic bronchitis carbon dioxide retention and low oxygen tension may occur earlier in the course of the disease. Therapeutically, the presence of significant hypoventilation necessitates either one or a combination of breathing exercises or use of assistive mechanical breathing apparatus.

*What portion of the respiratory cycle is most affected?* It is important to know which phase of respiration is impaired in order to direct one's effort to the most appropriate mode of treatment. In general, COPD patients, particularly those with emphysema, suffer from airway obstruction primarily during expiration. Ordinarily, air flow is relatively unimpaired during inspiration. The seeming inspiratory difficulty that is manifested usually results from air trapping, which leaves the chest hyperinflated, limiting further inflow of fresh air. In addition, the hyperinflated state leaves the muscles of inspiration in a mechanically disadvantageous position. The treatment program should be aimed at alleviating the predominantly expiratory obstruction and consequent hyperinflation. This end can be approached in several ways: (1) use bronchodilator drugs to reverse any bronchospastic components; (2) reduce tracheobronchial secretions (which contribute to turbulence and increased airway resistance) by postural drainage, expectorants, mucolytic agents and hydration; and (3) use expiratory breathing exercises, which are designed to minimize the mechanical factors that promote early airway collapse. These exercises include pursed-lip breathing, bottle blowing, and candle blowing exercises.

*How is the problem of excessive tracheobronchial secretion approached?* Most patients with chronic bronchitis and bronchiectasis complain primarily of excessive secretions. This is caused by increased production rather than the inefficient elimination that might be found in a patient with neuromuscular disease. Drainage of secretions is important, since it not only causes an uncomfortable feeling of "congestion," but it may also predispose to complications such as atelectasis and infection. Clinical evaluation should include the character, amount, color, and even odor of the tracheobronchial secretions. During physical examination, the coughing mechanism should be evaluated, with particular attention paid to the status of the abdominal muscles and the expiratory chest muscles, the effort required during coughing, and the success at bringing up secretions.

Since the main objective is drainage of secretions, the treatment program should be directed at all the factors involved in the problem. These factors include the secretion itself, the cough mechanism, and the air passages.

Concerning tracheobronchial secretions, the goal is to reduce the amount as much as possible and liquefy whatever remains. These goals may be attained by reducing the factors that enhance mucus production such as irritants, inhaled allergens, and infectious agents. The patient is advised to stop smoking, avoid airborne pollutants and allergens, and avoid crowded places where he might be exposed to respiratory infection. Annual prophylactic immunizations against influenza and pneumonia are also recommended. Antibiotics are given at the earliest signs of upper respiratory infection. To facilitate expulsion of secretions, proper hydration and humidification are extremely important. In addition, the use of expectorants (glyceryl guaiacolate, potassium iodide), mucolytic agents (N-acetyl

L-cysteine) and detergents may help in liquefying and reducing the viscosity of secretions. The use of proteolytic enzymes to liquefy sputum is not popular in the routine treatment of COPD patients probably because of the irritation, odor, and potential allergic stigma associated with these drugs.

The cough mechanism and the ciliary action of the lining epithelium are the most important mechanisms in the clearance of secretions. To ensure optimal evacuation of secretions, both mechanisms should be in good working order. The sweeping motions of the ciliary projections of the lining epithelium propel mucus and small particulates toward the outside. Many factors can adversely affect its efficiency. Among these are inhaled pollutants, respiratory irritants, certain medications (such as general anesthetics and opiates), dehydration, poor humidification, and the presence of local infection. Fortunately, many of the measures used in dealing with tracheobronchial secretions (previous paragraph) may also be beneficial in enhancing mucociliary action.

Coughing not only eliminates excessive secretions but in addition prevents aspiration of foreign material into the tracheobronchial tree. This very basic bodily function is luckily both spontaneous, as with response to irritating stimuli, and voluntary. Its performance requires a series of well-timed steps. These include deep inspiration followed by glottic closure and expiratory muscle contraction resulting in a Valsalva maneuver. When sufficient intrathoracic pressure has been generated, a sudden glottic opening results in an explosive release. For a cough to be effective in expelling secretions, part of the inspired air must be more distal to the secretion so that during the explosive release phase of the cough, that bolus of air will help propel the secretion outward. Unfortunately, small airway disease is common among COPD patients. This renders the small terminal airways readily collapsible. During the expulsive phase of coughing some of these airways collapse, leading to air trapping and reduced efficiency of expelling the secretions. To gain the patient's utmost cooperation, a careful explanation of these events and maneuvers is important in helping him better understand the existing problems.

Some patients who have difficulty coughing, such as postoperative patients and those with stress incontinence, can sometimes benefit from "huffing" maneuvers. Huffing is similar to coughing in that a deep inspiration is first taken. Glottic closure and the Valsalva maneuver are similarly produced, but intrathoracic pressure is not allowed to build up as much as in a cough. Instead, a much lower intrathoracic pressure is released in stepwise fashion by alternately opening and closing the glottis. These coughing or huffing exercises are usually used with postural drainage and chest percussion and vibration techniques.

Finally, the airway should be maximally dilated to allow easier passage of secretions to be expelled. This can be accomplished by using bronchodilators prior to the drainage exercises.

*How does the pulmonary condition affect the patient's total physical and emotional well-being?* These aspects usually affect the patient's livelihood, interpersonal and family relationship, and, most of all, the patient's image of himself. For years, attempts have been made to quantify the disability that results from COPD. The problem is obviously difficult because so many factors, both objective and subjective, enter into the evaluation. Efforts range from the time-honored method of using pulmonary function tests (vital capacity, maximal voluntary ventilation, and $FEV_1$) to a combined consideration of pulmonary function, x-ray findings, and the degree of dyspnea. On the whole, no real satisfactory way has yet been devised that truly reflects the degree of disability that results from these diseases. Recently, more and more centers around the country are beginning to take a more positive point of view by assessing remaining functional ability rather than concentrating on disability. This viewpoint focuses more on what the patient can do rather than what he cannot.

This approach is accomplished by determining the patient's maximum oxygen consumption ($Vo_{2max}$) during a monitored exercise test. The patient is asked to do progressively increasing loads of exercise (by treadmill ambulation or bicycle ergometer) at the same time that the heart rate, EKG, blood pressure, and several ventilatory parameters are monitored. Aerobic monitors are able to measure oxygen consumption, carbon dioxide production, and minute ventilation at frequent regular intervals during the test. Derivation of MET* equivalent and respiratory quotient† are possible from these data. Subjective factors such as dyspnea, fatigue, dizziness, and chest pains are likewise noted. As in cardiac stress testing, the end point is determined by a preset target heart rate, electrocardiographic changes, ventilatory end points such as a plateau or decline in oxygen consumption and minute ventilation or progressively increasing respiratory quotient, and subjective complaints of fatigue, dyspnea, chest pain, or dizziness. The pulmonary exercise test shows the patient's maximum tolerable oxygen consumption, which may be expressed in METs. When the patient's maximum oxygen consumption is compared to existing data on the oxygen cost of different activities, a rough estimation can be made of the pa-

---

*3.5 to 4.0 ml of oxygen per kg body weight per minute.
†Volume ratio of $CO_2$ production and oxygen consumption.

tient's remaining functional capacity. The physical and vocational aspects of rehabilitation in this patient are greatly aided by such knowledge. In addition, follow-up testing at regular intervals may provide information on stability or progression and assessment of the effects of therapy and need for vocational retraining or household help. It is unfortunate that at this stage, this set-up is limited to a few specialized laboratories and is not yet in widespread clinical use.

## REFERENCES

Hodgkin, J. E., Balchum, O. J., Kass, I., Glaser, E., Miller, W. F., Haas, A., Shaw, B., Kimbel, P. and Petty, T.: Chronic obstructive airway diseases. Current concepts in diagnosis and comprehensive care. JAMA 232:1243–1260, 1975.

Haas, A., Pineda, H., Haas, F. and Axen, K.: Pulmonary Therapy and Rehabilitation: Principles and Practice. Baltimore, Williams & Wilkins, 1979.

Bates, D. V., P. T. Macklem and R. V. Christie: Respiratory Function in Disease, 2nd ed. Philadelphia, W. B. Saunders Co., 1971.

# Neuromuscular Disease with Respiratory Insufficiency

*by Augusta Alba, M.D.and Lou Ann Pilkington, Ph.D.*

Pulmonary disease is classified under two categories: restrictive and obstructive. Restrictive lung disease (RLD) is an abnormality of lung function defined by a decrease in lung volume. The primary malfunction of restrictive disease is a decrease in inspiration. There are extrapulmonary causes (kyphoscoliosis) and neuromuscular disease (NMD), and pulmonary causes with loss of lung tissue, air-containing alveoli, and/or lung compliance. Many of these disorders are interrelated. For example, in RLD secondary emphysema can develop from recurrent pneumonia.

The clinical course of neuromuscular disease, whatever its pathological origin, falls into two classifications: (1) respiratory muscle paresis or paralysis at the onset of illness and (2) progressive paresis or paralysis or both over a period of months or years. Thus, respiratory insufficiency can be sudden in onset or it can develop insidiously. Treatment requires repetitive testing of pulmonary function in order to provide artificial aid when needed and to check the efficacy of the respirator. The patient must have specialized nursing care and chest physical therapy. A single bout of pneumonia becomes a life-threatening "double jeopardy" to him.

The rehabilitation team must be included in the patient's regimen of care. The total care of the patient with neuromuscular disease and respiratory insufficiency is summarized in this section.

## DIAGNOSIS: NEUROMUSCULAR DISEASE WITH RESPIRATORY INSUFFICIENCY

The diagnosis of respiratory insufficiency is verified by clinical information demonstrating insuffi-ciency, by pulmonary function tests, and by arterial blood gas determinations.

I. Clinical data
   A. History. May include chest pains, fatigue, atelectasis, recurrent pneumonia, tracheostomy, need for artificial aid, hemiplegia, paraplegia, or quadriplegia secondary to neuromuscular disease.
   B. Admission evaluation. Fast respiratory rate (over 20 per min) with very shallow breaths; dyspnea, initially during exercise and later at rest; hyperventilation when it is still possible, poor breath sounds with rhonchi or rales; poor expansion of the upper and lower anterior or lateral rib cage and poor descent of the diaphragm with deep breathing; excessive use of accessory muscles of breathing: weak, non-productive cough, marked scoliosis or kyphoscoliosis, cyanosis, ventilation with respirator on admission, signs of right heart failure.
   C. Clinical evidence of hypercapnia. Peripheral vasodilation, bounding pulse, small pupils, engorged veins in the fundus, papilledema, confusion and drowsiness, depressed tendon reflexes, muscular twitching, extensor plantar responses, headache and coma. However, the presence of any one of these signs is very poorly correlated with the level of mixed venous $Pco_2$. Thus, it is important to obtain an arterial blood gas sample.

II. Pulmonary function tests
   Simple spirometry tests are performed at the bedside as soon as possible after admis-

sion. The rate (f), tidal volume ($V_T$), minute ventilation ($V_E$), vital capacity (VC), and end tidal carbon dioxide concentration ($ET_{CO_2}$ per cent) are the important measurements to be made. $ET_{CO_2}$ per cent should be converted to partial pressure, $PET_{CO_2}$ (torr). In the adult the rate is usually greater than 20 per min, $V_T$ less than 300 ml, $V_E$ is variable, and $PET_{CO_2}$ is generally over 45 to 50 torr. VC most often is less than 25 to 30 per cent predicted.

III. Arterial blood gas determinations

Arterial $Po_2$ generally is low, (less than 70 torr), percentage saturated hemoglobin may be above 90 per cent, and arterial $P_{CO_2}$ is low because of ventilation-perfusion unevenness and impairment (poor diffusion capacity).

IV. Other assessments of impairment include chest x-ray, sputum culture, echocardiogram, sophisticated pulmonary function tests, EKG (right heart hypertrophy), blood studies (polycythemia).

## TREATMENT AND THERAPY

### ARTIFICIAL VENTILATION

Goals are to keep the client's physiological environment as normal as possible during illness, recovery, and rehabilitation, and to enable the client to lead as active and comfortable a life as possible with his disability. Specific purposes of respirator therapy are to assist ventilation, to provide the sole means of ventilation, to improve alveolar aeration and chest expansion, and to promote bronchial drainage.

Criteria for respirator usage are that the machine provides adequate ventilation, is not confining to the body, is portable for use at the bedside or in a motorized wheelchair, and is acceptable to the patient.

## BASIC PRINCIPLES OF RESPIRATOR OPERATION

Artificial ventilation is best understood by placing it in the context of the vital capacity. The vital capacity can be defined as the combination of inspiratory capacity (full inflation) and expiratory reserve (forced expiration), both measured from the resting expiratory level. Inspiratory capacity can then be obtained by positive pressure acting on the airway (always artificial) or by negative pressure acting on the body.

Ventilation by positive pressure acting on the airway is either intermittent positive-pressure ventilation (IPPV) or glossopharyngeal breathing (GPB). IPPV is provided by the following types of respi-

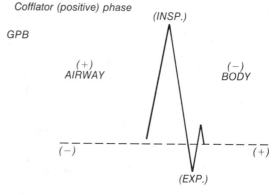

**Figure 19–4.** Respiratory assistive devices superimposed on a graphic representation of the vital capacity.

rators: volume respirator–console, pressure respirator–console, volume respirator–compact, pressure respirator–compact, and the Cofflator (positive phase) manual resuscitator or ventilator. It can also be provided by the following manual techniques: mouth to mouth breathing, mouth to mouth and nose (infant) breathing, and mouth to tracheostomy tube breathing.

Ventilation by negative pressure acting on the body is provided by these respirators: the iron lung or tank, the poncho, the cuirass or chestpiece, the rocking bed–head up, and phrenic nerve stimulation of the diaphragm. In the normal person it is provided by inspiratory muscles, intercostals, diaphragm, and accessory muscles of breathing of the head and neck.

The expiratory reserve volume can be obtained theoretically by negative pressure acting on the airway or by positive pressure acting on the body. In practice, negative pressure acting on the airway is utilized only for raising secretions. The machines used for this purpose are suction machines and the Cofflator (negative phase). Some patients can use a technique known as reversed glossopharyngeal breathing, in which they are able to develop a negative pressure in the hypopharynx that assists in raising secretions. The expiratory reserve volume can also be obtained by positive pressure acting on the body. It is provided by the following types of respirators: pressure respirator–compact, volume respirator–compact, both via the pneumobelt; and the rocking bed–head down. It is also provided by the old method of resuscitation in which force was applied to the lower rib cage. In normal persons it is provided by the expiratory muscles, including the abdominal and expiratory intercostal muscles.

## RESPIRATORY ASSISTIVE DEVICES

### INTERMITTENT POSITIVE PRESSURE VENTILATION (IPPV)

The ventilation mode most commonly used today is IPPV from a lightweight portable pump. The pump delivers filtered room air via oral or tracheal routes. It has a fixed pressure (15 to 50 cm $H_2O$) patterned to simulate normal breathing (40 per cent inspiration/60 per cent expiration). The rate and pressure are controlled. Newer models may be volume-controlled, may have the feature of assist and control, may have a variable I:E ratio, and may be set up with intermittent mandatory ventilation (IMV) assemblies. All units can be used with added oxygen. The machines can be run on AC or DC current, and can be mounted on either manual or motorized wheelchairs or used at bedside.

Mouth positive pressure is administered through a mouthpiece during the day. Some patients use the same mouthpiece in sleep by simply securing it near their person. Most use a Bennett mouthseal at night attached with either a plastic strap or with canvas straps and Velcro closure. Available masks are for the most part not comfortable enough for long-term use. It is the nurse's responsibility to watch for airway obstruction by noting expansions of the patient's chest, especially in sleep. The mouthpiece is held with teeth and lips and sits on the tongue. If the mouthpiece is not positioned properly, the tongue can obstruct air flow.

Tracheal positive pressure is used for patients with weak oropharyngeal muscles, with cycling disorders, with upper airway obstruction, or during sleep or coma. A closed system can be provided by cuffed tracheostomy tubes. However, in children, well-fitting tracheostomy tubes that are cuffless are used. Both children and adults who are not toxic or comatose and have strong oropharyngeal muscles can learn to close the lips, soft palate, and vocal cords during inspiration from the respirator. As a result they may need no cuff or may require only minimal inflation of a cuff. The need may vary in sleep as compared to the waking state.

In most cases a minimal leak technique is prescribed for ventilation, early in the course of respiratory rehabilitation. The cuff is inflated to the minimal occluding volume and then a small amount of air is withdrawn to create a partial leak. Machine settings are adjusted to compensate for the leak.

Potential damage to the trachea is avoided by this method.

Later, a tidal volume that may be two to three times the amount of air the patient needs for ventilation can be provided in order to improve vocal volume. The excess air is allowed to escape around the tracheostomy tube, which is cuffless or with a deflated cuff. The patient can use the air for sighing his lungs simply by consciously closing off the upper airway.

For adequate humidification cascade humidifiers (Bennett) are placed in the IPPV hose assembly at bedside, and cartridge inline humidifiers are used on respirators mounted on the wheelchair. The nurse must know how to troubleshoot the equipment, including how to recognize leaks, power or pump failure, and disconnections.

### GLOSSOPHARYNGEAL BREATHING; FROG BREATHING; GULPING

Glossopharyngeal breathing is a substitute method of breathing that decreases the patient's dependency on mechanical ventilation. Air is forced into the lungs by the muscles of the tongue, soft palate, fauces, pharynx, and larynx. The tongue moves posteriorly in a stroke-like action followed by a contracting action of the pharynx and closure of the lips and vocal cords between strokes. With each such stroke (gulp), air accumulates stepwise in the lungs. After approximately 20 strokes, the patient exhales. The volume of air he inspires per gulp can be from 30 to 90 ml; the tidal volume of one cycle can be from 500 to 2500 ml; the number of cycles per minute can be from 12 with the more shallow tidal volumes to 4 with the deeper. A minute ventilation of some 6 to 9 liters can be achieved. If the lungs are healthy, patients with essentially zero vital capacity from the usual respiratory muscles can maintain their arterial blood gas levels within normal limits for several hours without needing mechanical assistance.

Most patients must be taught to frog breathe. Some learn quickly; others take many months. Frog breathing not only allows the patient to stay off mechanical ventilators for longer periods of time but also inflates the lungs for effective coughing and increased compliance.

### IRON LUNG (TANK RESPIRATOR)

The iron lung or tank respirator is an airtight cylinder containing a stretcher-type mattress. On one end of the tank is a foam rubber or plastic collar that allows the patient's head to extend outside the tank. On the distal end or beneath the tank is a bellows of leather or rubber. The bellows acts to expand the area of the tank, thereby developing a negative pressure in the cylinder, to produce an inspiration. The patient in the tank is relatively inaccessible and must be carefully monitored. Nursing care can be administered through the portholes with the tank closed. It is easier to open the tank and have the patient use free time, mouth IPPV, or the dome adaptor, which on the later model Emerson tank provides cycled positive pressure to the nose and mouth. This form of ventilation requires the most organized and skilled nursing intervention. The patient's restriction and his sensory deprivation are given special consideration.

The iron lung is used by the neuromuscular disease patient without a tracheostomy with moderate to moderately severe respiratory infections in which he cannot handle the secretions. Severe infections with overwhelming sepsis and secretions are best handled in an intensive care setting with intubation and console volume ventilators. The patient usually recovers in one to two weeks with 24 hours a day of assisted ventilation in the iron lung, periods of mouth IPPV for deep breathing and coughing, chest physical therapy, and Trendelenberg positioning on every shift, in addition to the usual medical measures for treatment of the infection. The iron lung is also used for severe hypercapnia that has developed in the neuromuscular disease patient over a long period of time. The patient is ventilated continuously in the iron lung for one to two days until his end-expired carbon dioxide has dropped appreciably, and then other aids are tried. Careful attention to the airway is needed if the patient is comatose. The iron lung is preferred at night for sleeping by some patients.

### THE EMERSON PONCHO

The Emerson poncho has two components, a metal grid covering the chest and abdomen and a plastic poncho covering the grid and the whole body. The grid serves as a thoracic "tank," the poncho as the containing wall that, after all exposed edges have been rendered airtight, holds a vacuum. Negative pressure is obtained from the action of a chest respirator pump and exerts its effect on the thorax because of the space between the grid and the chest wall. The disadvantage is the difficulty in sealing the poncho and maintaining a good seal.

### THE CUIRASS (CHESTPIECE)

The cuirass is a shell or bubble that covers the patient's anterior and lateral chest wall and abdomen. The chest respirator pump provides the negative pressure for inspiration. The chestpiece is usually used at night during sleep; occasionally a patient also uses it throughout the day and even wears it in the wheelchair.

### THE ROCKING BED

The rocking bed is a hospital bed constructed with a motor system to rock the patient at a set rate and through a set arc, usually 30 degrees head up and 15 or 30 degrees head down. The patient can elect to raise the head of his bed into a semisitting position and still obtain good ventilation. The lungs are inflated as the head of the bed is raised because of the effects of gravity on the abdominal cavity contents and indirectly on the diaphragm. When the foot of the bed is raised, the reverse occurs and the patient exhales. Patients like to sleep on the rocking bed because it gives them a feeling of freedom and of movement.

A patient can be fed while he is using the rocking bed. Food is placed in the mouth while the bed is flat and the head of the bed has begun to rise. At first, small amounts are given slowly to avoid aspiration.

### ELECTROSTIMULATORS (DIAPHRAGMATIC PACEMAKER; PHRENIC NERVE PACEMAKER)

If an appreciable number of the anterior horn cells supplying the phrenic nerve are intact but cut off from the brain stem respiratory drive by high spinal cord injury, or not stimulated adequately by a defective respiratory drive, the phrenic nerve can be paced with an electrode placed over the nerve in the supraclavicular region of the neck.

A subcutaneous receiver is implanted with attachments to the electrode on the phrenic nerve. An external antenna is applied. A nine-volt battery-operated transmitter acts to stimulate the phrenic nerve via the antenna-receiver-conductor circuit. Usually a pacer for each phrenic nerve is inserted and they are used alternately or simultaneously. Any one pacer is usually used for periods of 12 hours. It is important for the nurse to handle this system as she would any electrical support system. All leads and connections must be checked and the battery supply tested. Care is used to avoid wetting the antenna during skin care. Vigorous scrubbing in the area of the implants that might twist or dislodge them is avoided. The patient who uses this form of ventilation enjoys increased mobility and privacy. Patients are taught not to readjust any pacer settings.

### PNEUMOBELT (ABDOMINAL EXSUFFLATION BELT)

A wide belt is designed like a corset with an inflatable rubber bladder inserted in the abdominal apron. The same portable respirators that provide cycled mouth IPPV can ventilate the bladder via a pneumobelt hose. Inflation of the bladder causes compression of the viscera; the diaphragm is forced upward causing expiration. Inspiration is either completely passive or assisted by the client's remaining inspiratory muscles. This ventilator is well accepted by patients because it leaves the face and mouth free and is easily concealed under clothing. The pneumobelt is essentially only effective with the patient in a sitting position of at least 45 degrees. A few elect to sit in bed during the night and use this aid for sleeping.

## THE COFFLATOR

The Cofflator is a portable cough machine that uses exsufflation with negative pressure to remove secretions from the respiratory tract. The client inhales from the machine during the positive pressure phase a volume of air large enough to expand his chest fully. At peak inspiration there is a sharp drop in pressure that causes the secretions to be swept toward the patient's mouth. The patient then has suctioning. Effective pulmonary toilet is achieved with two to three cough cycles given several times per day. The positive and negative pressures, volume, number of cycles, inspiratory and expiratory ratio, and time of each cycle are prescribed by the physician. The machine can be used with a tracheostomy adapter. If the patient has a tracheostomy tube that can be plugged, the treatment can be administered orally, and the patient then has suctioning via the tracheostomy tube.

## ALARM SYSTEMS

Alarm systems in respirator equipment are integral to the life support of this population. A variety of low or high pressure alarms and low volume alarms exist, as well as alarms for electrical failure. The nurse must recognize these signals, as well as the distress signals that the patient himself initiates by either using his tongue for clicking or using a patient-operated alarm.

## USE OF VENTILATORS IN RELATIONSHIP TO THE VITAL CAPACITY

If a patient's vital capacity is some 35 to 40 per cent of predicted, he should be introduced to the use of artificial aid. The tidal volume and minute ventilation as well as the $PET_{CO_2}$ should be obtained at variable settings of the respirator, and the optimal settings determined. If the patient's vital capacity is near 20 to 35 per cent, he should use aid for varying periods during each day determined not only by his blood gases but by his sense of well-being and absence of fatigue. Artificial aid throughout the night is highly recommended, especially if he is using accessory muscles to obtain much of the vital capacity. Patients with a vital capacity of 20 per cent or less are recommended to

use a respirator 24 hours a day. These figures are a rough guide; patients with intrinsic lung disease, emphysema, and/or kyphoscoliotic deformities of the thoracic cavity in addition to neuromuscular disease may need more aid sooner than someone without these added disabilities.

## GENERAL COMPLICATIONS

The patient in a respirator center is at high risk of contracting infection and atelectasis. The clearance mechanisms of ciliary transport and phagocytic activity are often abnormal, and the ability to cough or even breathe deeply is absent or very weak. Excessive mucus formation is often present; aspiration of pathogens from the nasopharynx into the tracheobronchial tree is often a source of pulmonary infection. Preventive treatment includes suctioning, voluntary deep breathing exercises when possible or deep breathing exercises with intermittent positive pressure breathing, postural drainage, chest physical therapy, and assisted coughing. Frequent change of position must be utilized.

Tracheal injury, localized trachiectasis, and stenosis can be caused by intubation.

## RESPIRATORY DISABILITY AS RELATED TO DISEASE

The degree of ventilatory impairment of the patient with spinal cord injury is related to the level of the cord lesion and, of course, the degree of involvement. Patients with high cervical lesions can show complete loss of vital capacity; those with low cervical lesions may retain 30 to 60 per cent of predicted vital capacity, whereas those with thoracic and lumbar lesions show only a minimal 10 to 20 per cent loss of vital capacity.

If patients with lesions above $C_4$ survive the initial injury, life-long tracheostomy and maintenance on respiratory equipment are necessary.

Injuries from $C_4$ to the high thoracic segments of the cord may also produce severe respiratory embarrassment during the acute stage and intensive measures as described must be taken to prevent complications.

Even in patients with no signs of respiratory distress on admission, problems may develop several days later. Increased neurological damage and depression of the medullary respiratory center can occur. Pneumothorax, fatigue to the point of exhaustion, and aspiration of food or gastric contents resulting from inability to cough may further compromise respiration.

In the patient with progressive neuromusucular diseases such as amyotrophic lateral sclerosis, multiple sclerosis, or syringomyelia and syringobulbia, restrictive pulmonary insufficiency becomes progressively worse over several months or several years, and bulbar involvement occurs. In the early course of the disease, the patient has a compromised ventilatory system but requires no artificial aid; however, in the final course of the disease respiratory distress may become so severe as to require a mechanical ventilator 24 hours a day.

With bulbar involvement the patient experiences dysphagia, dysarthria, and difficulty chewing. Weakness of the laryngeal muscles and soft palate and muscles of the pharynx can result in partial closure of the airway and upper airway obstruction, and a tracheostomy may be required.

In the patient whose respiratory condition has become stable, such as the patient with poliomyelitis, symptoms of alveolar hypoventilation can still occur. This happens from the normal aging process, from incomplete recovery after a severe respiratory infection with residual lung pathology, from inadequate ventilation with an artificial respirator, or from all three causes.

Many of the patients experience symptoms of alveolar hypoventilation immediately upon awakening. This is of interest because studies of respiration during sleep have shown that hypoventilation with increased alveolar $PET_{CO_2}$ occurs in the normal individual when asleep. Fishman has stressed the fact that while nocturnal hypoventilation poses no clinical problems in normal subjects, it may seriously derange the blood gases and control of ventilation in patients who already have compromised pulmonary function.*

Scoliosis or kyphoscoliosis may occur because of progressive deformity of the spine and bony structure of the thorax. Severe narrowing of the thoracic cavity can occur in the anteroposterior diameter. Scoliosis further limits expansion of the chest wall and further decreases vital capacity. If the deformity is serious enough, there is added danger of upper airway involvement; if a tracheostomy tube has been inserted, it may even become difficult to maintain in correct placement.

Chronic alveolar hypoventilation can precipitate cor pulmonale. Hypoventilation disturbs the $\dot{V}/\dot{Q}$ ratio and results in abnormal gas tensions. It is well documented that cor pulmonale and pulmonary hypertension occur only in those patients in whom the gas tensions of arterial blood are abnormal.

*Fishman, A.P.: Pulmonary Diseases and Disorders. Inadequate ventilatory drive, New York, McGraw-Hill, pp. 429–430, 1980.

# Nursing Management of Patients With Respiratory Insufficiency

by Alice Mertz Nolan, R.N., M.A.

Nursing management of the severely handicapped respiratory patient is both a challenge and responsibility. The challenge stems from the integration of a wide range of disciplines. Responsibility for clinical expertise and thoughtful nursing care underlies this complex practice.

The nurse views the total patient, and deals with existential issues such as change in body image, peer interaction, intellectual growth, sexuality, and family adjustment in light of respiratory insufficiency. Inasmuch as direct nursing care is delivered around the clock, continuity in total care is allowed for. Communication and support are essential in this process.

A coordinated nursing care plan is the sine qua non for rehabilitation.

The nurse helps the patient distinguish priorities and manage daily personal care. As individual needs are identified, patients' abilities are utilized in planning for realistic goals. A balance is achieved between overprotection and permissiveness.

The respiratory rehabilitation nurse in a respiratory care center is knowledgeable in each of the following areas. She:

1. Understands the mechanics of normal blood flow and diffusion.

2. Receives training in identification of restrictive and obstructive respiratory diseases.

3. Understands the physiological basis for pulmonary function testing and identifies factors governing prescription of pulmonary function tests and more frequent usage of capnograph levels rather than invasive arterial blood gas studies.

4. Is able to explain to patients and families the need for annual testing based on changes in lung function.

5. Monitors patient respiratory status, understanding limitations of the patient's vital capacity.

6. Can perform a physical assessment of heart, chest and lungs.

On the ward, specialized training includes management of patients with chronic respiratory insufficiency. This includes those with relatively normal lung tissue with ventilation impaired by neuromuscular disease. Distinction is made between upper and lower motor neuron disease and respiratory system diseases (central cycling problems) in planning nursing care. Specifically polio, amyotrophic lateral sclerosis, muscular dystrophy, and multiple sclerosis are emphasized.

Patients with abnormal lung tissue are reviewed to show differences in the nursing approach to several conditions. This includes cases of airway obstruction such as bronchitis, emphysema, asthma.

The implications of cerebral trauma and drug intoxication are reviewed in relation to respiratory drive and prescription of medications.

The nurse understands the cough mechanism and its impairment by neuromuscular disease and spinal cord injury. She utilizes specialized equipment as prescribed, such as the Cofflator, vaporizers, and cascade humidifiers to encourage coughing and pulmonary toilet. Changes in patient temperature and in the color, amount, and consistency of secretions are documented. She understands the use of mechanical respirators, ventilation patterns, and principles involved in use of equipment.

The nurse is responsible for ensuring proper rates and pressures as prescribed by the physician while monitoring the patient's tolerance of treatment methods. This includes checking on tubing for proper connection, patency, and leaks. She maintains a safe environment for patients and staff by ensuring proper grounding of electrical equipment, including checks on integrity of wires and plugs. She utilizes sanitary techniques in maintenance of the patient's immediate environment. This includes cleansing of equipment and proper disposal of secretions. It is also her responsibility to discourage superinfection of patients by nosocomial agents and iatrogenic routes.

## MEDICAL REGIMEN

The nurse in managing the prescribed medical and nursing regimen becomes aware of the range of behaviors that are usual for each patient. The subtle nuances of each patient's attitudes in routine activities are the best indicators of total wellbeing. Slight changes in outlook, mentation, and energy levels are noticeable long before manifestations of respiratory failure come to light. Cyanosis is not a reliable sign in a population in whom many compensatory mechanisms have been brought into play. Hypercapnia is often reflected in general mood and energy levels.

Similarly, the nurse is the first to notice changes in muscle tone, strength, and functional activities. She is responsible for supervising range of motion exercises and passive stretching motions as tolerated to retard functional impairment.

Vigilance is needed to keep the patient active and involved. Since skeletal contractures and paralysis make positioning and transfers difficult, Hoyer lifts are utilized for most transfers from bed to chair.

## NURSING MANAGEMENT

Basic nursing procedures take on new implications for the immobilized respiratory population. In turning and positioning the patient, the nurse must consider his special respiratory needs and equipment. Air, foam, and water mattresses are utilized for skin protection. Special foam mattresses can be cut for accommodation to pressure-sensitive body areas for use with rocking beds. Pillows are used for support in muscle imbalance and weakness, thus preventing compensatory muscle habitus.

**Skin Care.** While providing skin care, the nurse teaches to patients position techniques and prevention of decubitus ulcers.

**Bracing.** Nursing management of bracing includes the proper positioning and application of splints, braces, and Orthoplast jackets. Bracing in the scoliotic patient allows for improved pulmonary function and chest expansion.

**Chest Physical Therapy.** Principles of chest physical therapy are utilized in turning and positioning patients. Postural drainage is routinely performed to limit the potential for respiratory infections. Cupping and clapping are performed on an ad lib basis during personal care activities. Once secretions are mobilized, the nurse will suction the patient or help with assistive coughing. Cofflator therapy is also used. Thoughtful practice schedules chest pulmonary toilet before or in between meals.

**Activities of Daily Living (ADL).** Nursing utilizes and protects the communication and assistive devices prescribed when giving care to patients. By generalization of activities, nurses support efforts in independence training.

**Nutrition.** Special encouragement is given to maintaining proper nutritional balance while allowing for the patient's respiratory limitations and need for variety. Solid food is available to those with reliable gag and swallow reflexes. Gastrostomy tube feedings are given when muscle loss has affected the patient's swallowing mechanism. When the patient with a tracheosotomy is fed, a number of precautions must be taken. Feedings can be given with the cuff inflated or deflated as discussed later. Generally the patient is fed while sitting in the wheelchair or in a semi-Fowler's position (while in bed). When possible the patient remains seated for 25 to 45 minutes after the meal. This assists gravity in the movement of food and prevents regurgitation and aspiration.

As a rule, cuffs are inflated to minimize aspiration risks. In some cases an exact tracheostomy tube fitting is achieved. For these patients (cuffless or with deflated cuffs), aspiration risks are minimal. Cuffless tracheostomy tubes provide the advantage of easy swallowing because the inflated cuff does not bulge into the esophagus.

In some instances a patient is tested to evaluate aspiration dangers. This procedure involves swallowing colored gelatin or a methylene blue cocktail (5 cc:30 cc $H_2O$) with the tracheostomy cuff deflated. The trachea is then suctioned. If the colored gelatin or dye is present in the aspirate, the tracheostomy tube cuff is reinflated during feedings. This process indicates competence of the glottis during feedings.

The same test may be performed with the cuff inflated. This determines if aspiration is occurring around the cuff or through a tracheoesophageal fistula.

**GI Function.** Immobilization and ventilation lead to changes in gastrointestinal function. Diet is modified to include fruit juices, fluids, and high fiber when tolerated, to compensate for changes in gastrointestinal mobility. Feedings are encouraged to prevent gastric ulceration and bleeding. Hypercarbia and hypersecretion of acid combined with stress and drug therapy (antibiotics, steroids) without proper management often lead to ulceration.

Fecal impaction reduces vital capacity. Nursing management of bowel routines is mandatory for spinal cord–injured patients.

**Fluid Management.** Nurses also develop a sense for monitoring their patient's fluid balance. Relative overhydration can occur with positive pressure ventilation. Factors include the increased production of antidiuretic hormone, reduced serum oncotic pressure, elevation of mean airway and intrathoracic pressures, reduced lymphatic flow, subclinical cardiac failure, and hydration from ventilator humidification and nebulization systems. Swelling of extremities and moist breathing not relieved by expectoration and suctioning should be brought to the attention of the physician.

## TRACHEOSTOMIES

A variety of tracheostomy tubes are used. These are prescribed by the physician after consideration of many factors.

### TYPES

**Jackson Silver (Pilling tube)** consists of three parts: obturator, inner cannula, and outer cannula. This tracheostomy tube, with swivel adapter, includes a screw-on adapter to the inner cannula that connects with the ventilator tubing.

**Plastic (Silastic) tracheostomy tubes** are used for the majority of patients requiring inner cannulas. High volume low pressure cuffs are used most frequently, but cuffless tracheostomy tubes are also used. Both cuffed and cuffless tracheostomy tubes are used if an individual is able to breathe through his mouth with or without mouth IPPV.

Cannula size and cuff pressure are prescribed by the physician to achieve a snug fit without producing complications. Sizing aims to prevent tracheal stenosis. Cuff pressure is low to prevent impairment of mucosal circulation and necrosis. Proper fitting prevents hemorrhage, tracheal scarring, obstruction, and stomal infections.

The following devices are used when patients gain improvement in their respiratory status.

**Fenestrated Tracheostomy Tubes.** These tubes have a "window" or opening in the superior-posterior wall of the cannula. As the patient breathes, air moves both around and through the tube from the upper airway. The nurse verifies patency of the fenestration and observes for respiratory distress. This tube can be plugged to test the success of upper airway ventilation.

**Tracheal Button.** The tracheal button (Kistner button) is used to maintain an open stoma for emergency management or pulmonary toilet. It has a flared flange in the anterior aspect of the trachea, preventing closure of the tracheostomy. (A tracheostomy tube can be reinserted when necessary.) The button allows the patient to assume a normal breathing pattern and to talk. It is changed weekly, but stoma care is given every day. The patient has the security of an accessible airway with the freedom of decannulation. A disadvantage is that the button can easily dislodge; if the patient does not have a surgically permanent tracheostomy, the tracheostomy can shrink in size or close before the extrusion of the button is discovered.

It is a nursing responsibility to check the type and size of the tracheostomy tube before insertion. Cuffed tubes are tested for the integrity of their balloons. Symmetry of inflation and position are determined before insertion.

Traditional methods are used for routine cleansing of tracheostomies: they are cleaned with hydrogen peroxide and normal saline in between tracheostomy tube changes. (Sterile technique is utilized.) Stomal dressings are changed whenever they are soiled.

### SUCTIONING THE PERMANENT TRACHEOSTOMY

Noisy moist respirations accompanied by increasing pulse and respirations indicate the need for aspiration of secretions. Assisted respiration should be quiet at the end of this process. Good nursing judgment is imperative in deciding whether suctioning is necessary. The following guidelines are used.

1. Minimal negative pressure is used (100 to 150 cm water in adults).

2. Suctioning is brief to avoid hypoxemia, cardiac arrhythmias, and trauma to the mucous membranes.

3. A sterile rubber catheter half the diameter of the tracheostomy tube (inner cannula) is inserted and rotated.

4. Suction is applied only during withdrawal of the catheter.

5. If secretions are thick, 2 to 5 ml of sterile normal saline can be instilled to loosen secretions. This is suctioned immediately after instillation.

6. Common sense is used during this procedure. Gross contamination is avoided by meticulous handwashing with Betadine (povidone-iodine) scrub solution before suctioning. A sterile catheter is used for each suctioning period. The modified surgically clean technique is used for the chronic tracheostomy patient. After eight weeks the tracheostomy site becomes colonized by bacteria; therefore, clean technique is permissible. Disposable sterile catheters with sterile solutions are used without gloves. In contrast, for recent tracheostomies, strict sterile technique is observed.

After suctioning, several hyperinflations with a manual resuscitator act to mobilize secretions and re-expand atelectatic areas. Suctioning is repeated if needed.

### COMPLICATIONS

**Infection.** Monitoring tracheal secretions is an important part of infection control. Suspicious secretions are collected and cultured. The nurse watches for the following changes in the patient: elevation in temperature or WBC count, pain, or malaise. In this instance, changing the ventilator (and oxygen) tubing is important intervention. Nebulizers are changed and filled with sterile solution. Special efforts are taken to avoid contamination. Antibiotic therapy is managed as prescribed by the physician.

**Bleeding.** Bleeding is rare in the patient with chronic tracheostomy. It may be caused by trauma from improper suctioning or cannula insertion. More often it involves external tension on the tracheostomy tube from the ventilator tubing. When the client turns his head or extends beyond the limits of his tubing, trauma can occur. The physician will evaluate the cause of large amounts of blood.

## DOCUMENTATION

Nursing documentation for the respiratory patient includes graphing of mechanical assistance. This includes type and period of time for each form of assistance and free time. General condition and tolerance are also noted.

## NURSING APPROACH

Nursing approach in a respiratory rehabilitation center allows patients to have freedom of choice in activities and recreation, taking into account ventilatory support and time off the ventilator. All patients are showered regularly using manual ventilation if necessary. Patients are dressed and assisted out of bed each day, so they can participate in a program of activities. Regardless of prognosis, patients are kept active for as long as possible and encouraged to maximize their abilities regardless of medical limitations.

Care is also provided to children with neurological diseases and respiratory insufficiency in a manner similar to that in adults. The minimum admission age to a long-term rehabilitation respiratory center is 3. These children become a particular challenge in management as they grow and mature.

# The Role of the Physical Therapist in the Care of Patients with Neuromuscular Disease and Respiratory Insufficiency

*by Linda Snyder, R.P.T., M.A.*

As in all rehabilitation efforts the emphasis in physical therapy is placed not only on rehabilitation but also on prevention. Physical therapy techniques used in rehabilitation of persons with neuromuscular disabilities include improving strength and endurance of remaining musculature to produce an effective breathing pattern, maintaining or increasing chest expansion or both, and teaching the use of aids to maintain or increase breathing reserve. In other words, whatever muscle power or rib cage expansion the patient has is maximized to the fullest to maintain respiratory homeostasis and thereby allow the patient to lead a more active life.

Breathing exercises include relaxation exercises, diaphragmatic breathing exercises, mobility exercises (passive range of motion and manual stretching of arms and trunk), chest expansion exercises (with incentive spirometers), coughing techniques, positioning, and frog breathing.

Physical therapy techniques used to prevent further problems include bronchial drainage and deep breathing and coughing exercises with manual assistance to clear mucus. All the methods cited that improve chest expansion improve both the patient's ability to breathe on his own and make it easier for a respirator to be effective.

In the area of education the patient is taught to breathe synchronously with the respirator. He is made aware of signs and symptoms of respiratory infection such as increased production of mucus, change in color and consistency of mucus, and feelings of congestion in the lungs and a decrease in inspiratory volume with the spirometer. He is trained to be alert to the need for increased ventilation and for aggressive measures to combat infection when these signs and symptoms occur. Family and aides are trained to assist the patient in these techniques and to re-enforce the patient's use of them.

# The Role of the Occupational Therapist in the Care of Patients With Restrictive Pulmonary Disease

*by Elaine Bennethum, M.S., O.T.R., R.P.T., Joyce Sabari, M.A., O.T.R., Doris Schanzer, O.T.R. and Judith Wasserman, O.T.R.*

Occupational therapy is geared toward enabling individuals with restrictive pulmonary disease to achieve their maximum potential for independent performance of life skills and activities to enrich the quality of their lives. Occupational therapists focus treatment on the neuromuscular residuals of the primary diagnosis. They apply their expertise with adaptive equipment, in combination with knowledge of body mechanics, in designing devices to ensure adequate positioning of respiratory equipment and lead to productive and meaningful use of residual physical and intellectual capacities.

## POSITIONING OF RESPIRATORY EQUIPMENT IN BED

To stabilize the respiratory hose in a consistently accessible position in bed, a "gooseneck,"* (a flexible metal rod used for microphones and desk lamps), is attached to the headboard or siderail with "hoseclamps."† The respirator hose is placed into a "broom clip" or "tool holder."‡ fastened to

---

*Available from electronic supply distributors.
†Available from automotive supply distributors.
‡Available in hardware stores.

the end of the gooseneck. This gooseneck apparatus can be easily adjusted or repositioned and decreases the danger of accidental removal of the hose from the trachea. It also ensures that hosing will be available to the quadriplegic patient who uses the respirator aid orally and is unable to manually realign the hose to his mouth.

A small foam cushion with a Velcro strap can be placed on the patient's chest, with the respirator hose placed on top inside the Velcro strap to provide consistency of positioning between the hose and the tracheostomy tube. This prevents pull on the trachea and irritation of the hose to the patient's skin.

For individuals who use intermittent positive-pressure breathing devices during sleeping hours and are unable to manually readjust their hosing, the plastic lipguard can be attached to a custom-fitted figure-of-eight strap fastened with Velcro around the head and the back of the neck. This stabilization could save the life of a patient who may not awaken if his mouthpiece drops while he is asleep. Pneumobelt liners, fabricated from mattress pads, are used to improve comfort and prevent skin breakdown.

## PATIENTS IN WHEELCHAIRS AND POSITIONING OF RESPIRATORY EQUIPMENT

Selection of and training in the use of an appropriate motorized wheelchair system for independent mobility is a major priority with the quadriplegic patient. The inclusion of equipment for mechanical respiratory assistance poses an additional challenge in meeting this goal. The occupational therapist collaborates with the physician and other team members in selection and prescription of a mobility system. The occupational therapist trains the patient in the operation of the wheelchair and familiarizes him with all aspects of its care and maintenance so that he will be able to give clear instructions to anyone assisting him.

The respirator is mounted on the back of the wheelchair, away from the battery, to protect it from leaks of battery fluids. Batteries are placed on an appropriate-sized supporting tray on the wheelchair. It is frequently convenient to mount the battery charger on the chair so that it is always available. The respirator hose can be positioned in a gooseneck apparatus on the wheelchair push handle.

It is recommended that the patient who uses a motorized wheelchair also possess a manual wheelchair. Although the motorized unit offers independent mobility, it does not substitute for the reliability and portability of a manual wheelchair. A respirator user's manual wheelchair needs to be equipped with a 12-volt battery, a charger, a battery tray, and a hanging rack for the respirator unit.

## FUNCTIONAL ACTIVITY

The occupational therapy treatment program for these patients is geared toward eliciting maximal functional potential from remaining head, neck, and limb musculature. When potential remains in upper extremity musculature, every attempt is made to improve strength and to translate this into functional activity with adaptive equipment. Individuals who have motor innervation in head and neck musculature only are trained in the use of mouthsticks, headsticks and/or electronic environmental control systems. This can enable them to turn pages, use a telephone, type, operate computers, calculators, and tape recorders, and participate in adapted crafts and leisure activities.

Environmental control systems use electrical wiring to attach various electrical appliances to a panel of switches that is accessible to the disabled individual. The patient can control lights, radio, television, page-turning, door locks, intercom systems, and so on. Although a reliable environmental control system can be a valuable tool, it cannot take the place of a mouthstick or headstick or eliminate the need for a personal attendant.

Additional considerations regarding psychological adjustment arise with those who must depend on respiratory assistance. Even after their conditions are medically stable, their self-image of a "sick patient" can impede progress in resuming a productive life. The respirator-dependent patient often feels extremely vulnerable, and may be fearful of any new activity because of its possible effects on the operation of his respiratory equipment. The feelings of independence and productivity resulting from successful completion of tasks can help to allay these fears. Individuals who have had opportunity for independent mobility, exploration, and mastery of tasks and life skills with the guidance of the occupational therapist find it easier to resume satisfying lives in the community after discharge.

# The Role of the Speech-Language Pathologist in the Care of Patients with Respiratory Insufficiency

*by Carol Manly, M.A., C.C.C.*

The patient with neuromuscular disease who requires pulmonary care and treatment may also show symptoms of an accompanying speech or swallowing impairment or both. The expertise of the speech-language pathologist can be utilized in diagnosing and rehabilitating this patient. The speech symptomatology seen in pulmonary care patients can be separated into two major categories: functional and organic speech disorders.

## FUNCTIONAL SPEECH DISORDERS: APHONIA AND INCOORDINATION

Functional speech disorders have no underlying neurological basis and are caused by mechanical interruptions to the speech system. An open or cuffed tracheostomy causing functional aphonia is an example of a functional speech disorder. When there is not an adequate amount of air flow to the vocal folds, an individual cannot produce voice. Usually the condition is temporary, but the patient requires a mode of communication in the interim even if mouthing movements of the articulators is good.

One mode of communication may be writing, but another efficient mode of communication is the use of an electrolarynx, which vibrates the vocal mechanism. The electrolarynx is a mechanical means of producing voice in the patient with intact articulatory ability. The electrolarynx and writing will not help the quadriplegic patient. In these cases, nonelectronic and electronic communication systems must be considered. These systems are discussed later.

Another functional speech disorder is incoordination of the inspiratory air cycle with speech production. This disorder occurs when a patient is placed on a respirator for the first time. A short period of treatment in which the patient is taught to become aware of the respirator cycle and inspiratory air flow for speech purposes is usually ameliorative.

## ORGANIC SPEECH DISORDERS

### DYSARTHRIA

Organic speech disorders are most prevalent among pulmonary care patients; the primary disorder seen is dysarthria. Dysarthria is a collective term used to describe various types of speech disorders resulting from neurological damage that causes disturbances in muscular control over the speech mechanism. Dysarthria is not a language disorder and is differentiated from aphasia. The dysarthric individual comprehends language, is able to read and spell, but shows a breakdown in the motor output system for speech. In the pulmonary care patient, the breakdown is primarily caused by weakness or spasticity or both. Historically, dysarthria was thought to be solely an impairment of articulation, but now the literature delineates the parameters of speech that are affected by dysarthria: respiration, phonation, resonance, prosody, and articulation.

### Classification of Dysarthria Types

The patient with neuromuscular disease who requires pulmonary care may exhibit a certain type of dysarthria that is directly related to the specific type of neurological deficit. For example, the patient who suffers a brain stem stroke will exhibit a flaccid dysarthria characterized by hypernasality, nasal emission, imprecise consonants, and breathy voice. Another type of dysarthria is spastic dysarthria, which is characterized by imprecise consonants, monopitch, monoloudness, and reduced stress. Phonatory changes include harsh voice and strained-strangled voice, in which the voice seems to be squeezed through the glottis. A patient with amyotrophic lateral sclerosis (ALS) will exhibit symptoms of a mixed flaccid and spastic dysarthria because the disease shows both bulbar and pseudobulbar characteristics.

### DYSPHAGIA

Dysphagia which is a swallowing impairment may accompany the dysarthric impairment. The symptoms of the dysphagic impairment are identical to the dysarthric symptomatology. Dysphagic symptoms in the pulmonary care patient are classified as bulbar impairments or pseudobulbar impairments or both.

### GENERAL TREATMENT PROCEDURES: DYSARTHRIA AND DYSPHAGIA

Once an in-depth differential diagnostic speech examination is performed to diagnose the speech dysfunction appropriately in the patient with neuromuscular disease and respiratory insufficiency, a differential treatment program is developed. General treatment procedures are employed differentially according to the type of dysarthria that has been diagnosed, as well as the specific parameter or parameters of speech that are affected. The dysphagic treatment program is an aspect of the total speech and voice treatment program.

A rehabilitative medical protocol is utilized at Goldwater Memorial Hospital for dysphagia diagnosis. Special tests and diagnostic equipment outlined in the protocol are indirect laryngeal examination, nasopharyngoscopy, cinefluorography, blue dye test, and a complete speech test battery of the oral-peripheral and laryngeal structure and function. Results of the testing determine candidacy for the dysphagia treatment program. The dysphagia treatment program is usually a precursor to the speech treatment program, and many of the treatment techniques are applicable both to swallowing and speech function.

There are general treatment guidelines that are assistive during feeding for either type of dysphagic impairment:

1. The patient should be sitting in an upright position at a 90-degree angle.

2. Use food such as apple sauce that is easily manipulated on the patient's tongue.

3. Avoid liquid because it is the most difficult substance to swallow.

4. Instruct the patient to tilt the head forward (chin down) in preparation for swallowing (Fig. 19–5).

Conceptually, a speech and dysphagia treatment program involves use of specific neuromuscular facilitation techniques and within that framework re-

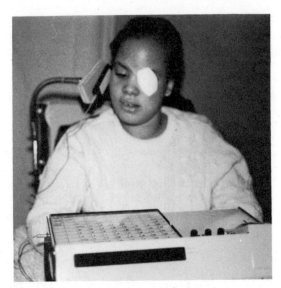

**Figure 19–6.** Patient with electronic device.

training normal synergistic movement pattern for both speech and swallowing. The speech-language pathologist works in a team with the occupational and the physical therapists in developing trunk stability and normal postural tone. Postural tone and trunk stability are the foundations for a successful program.

The emphasis of the treatment program for the patient with the primary symptom of flaccidity is to increase and strengthen muscle movement. Neuromuscular facilitation is used to activate and strengthen oral, pharyngeal, and laryngeal muscle groups to reinstate normal movement pattern for speech and swallowing function. A specific symptom of flaccidity can be an organic aphonia in which there is inadequate vocal fold closure. The speech-language pathologist initiates intrinsic laryngeal exercises to increase vocal fold movements that, in turn, increase the patient's ability to produce voice and to swallow. A biofeedback device, VISIPITCH, is also used to improve voice production. The device provides the patient with a visual display and at the same time gives the clinician objective information concerning the patient's performance.

A discussion of treatment procedures and techniques would be incomplete without a description of the anarthric patient and augmentative communication systems.

## ANARTHRIA: AUGMENTATIVE COMMUNICATION SYSTEMS

Anarthria is the most severe form of dysarthria and is the total loss of speech. Language is not affected and the patient maintains adequate cognitive and linguistic skills. The anarthric or nonspeaking pulmonary care patient may also have

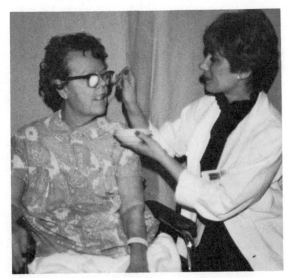

**Figure 19–5.** Therapist and patient in assistive feeding.

quadriplegia or paresis and may not be able to communicate through writing. The anarthric condition may be temporary until speech returns through treatment. It may also be a permanent condition, as is seen in progressive diseases.

An augmentative means of communication supplements whatever means of communication the nonspeaking patient uses—for example, eye movements and head nods. Augmentative communication systems are both nonelectronic and electronic.

Some of the nonelectronic devices involve special ways of pointing to letters to spell messages. For example, a quadriplegic patient may have good head movement and may be able to spell by using a light beam worn on the forehead. This enables him to shine the light on each desired letter.

Electronic devices involving microprocessors can also be provided to the nonspeaking patient. For example, a patient may require a device that can be programmed to store and print out frequently used sentences and phrases so that each message does not have to be spelled out letter by letter. Other electronic devices can print out messages as well as produce synthesized speech.

Every nonspeaking patient should be provided with a nonelectronic communication system and, if needed, a more sophisticated electronic system.

# Psychological Aspects of Respiratory Treatment: Management of Respiratory-Related Anxiety

by Christopher MacDonald, M.S.

The interruption of respiration, even for short durations, can produce painfully agitated states of physiological arousal, probably reflexive in origin because the response can be observed in earliest infancy as well as in later life. If the person is conscious, the arousal is experienced subjectively as terror. When this experience comes to be associated with a chronic condition of respiratory insufficiency, the patient becomes exceedingly vulnerable to heightened levels and acute onsets of anxiety. Behaviorally, this anxiety is transformed into fearful concerns about the adequacy of the life-supporting respiratory equipment. These patients may become overly cautious and self-protective, refusing to be weaned from equipment that is no longer needed or refusing to experiment with other kinds of respiratory assistance. The treatment of such patients requires special psychological considerations.

## THE PSYCHOLOGICAL MILIEU

One of the chief concerns in the management of anxiety in a long-term respiratory facility should be the creation of a healthy psychological milieu. To minimize the disruptive effects of anxiety, the patients must be able to perceive the ward as a safe, stable environment with a competent, caring staff and adequately maintained equipment. Under-

standably, the patients' relationship with the physician is of paramount importance to their emotional adjustment. They need to be assured of the physician's medical skill and of the physician's empathetic concern for their emotional needs as well.

Patients regularly develop powerful transference reactions to the physician, who comes to symbolize the "good or bad mother or father figure," and the loss or absence of a particularly trusted one can cause general unrest on the ward.

It is also impossible to overestimate the importance of the nursing staff to the patient's psychological well-being. Nurses have the closest and most prolonged contact, and it is the nurse who is ultimately entrusted with the patient's sense of safety and security. The nurse represents the caring, nurturing, protective maternal function and as such embodies the most elemental, original, and powerful of psychological figures.

Considering the importance of the patients' physical priorities and the intensity of their attachments to the staff, it is not easy to establish the type of relaxed, nonauthoritarian atmosphere that is conducive to psychological growth. It is advisable, therefore, to give the patients as much autonomy as possible in their medical care, treatment decisions, and future discharge planning. Ward councils run by patients, which are allowed to exercise an influence on the management of the ward, contribute to the psychological stability of the patients by giving them a sense of control over their own environment. Social and recreational activities as well as opportunities to develop intellectual and aesthetic interests are provided. Therapeutic home visits should also be encouraged to help acclimate the patients to life outside the hospital during the difficult transition to independent living.

## ROLE OF THE PSYCHOLOGIST

### EVALUATION

The psychologist attempts to evaluate the patient on admission and periodically during the course of treatment. Psychological data are shared with the staff to help in the construction and modification of the overall therapy program. Cognitive functioning, memory and learning capacity, self-awareness, and general achievement motivation are important determinants, hence predictors, of a patient's success in achieving a treatment goal.

It must be remembered, however, that in respiratory rehabilitation the overriding criterion for admission is the existence of a treatable respiratory insufficiency. Therefore, we cannot always be selective from a psychological point of view. When patients exhibit serious psychological deficits, the psychologist's evaluation helps in setting realistic expectations and reasonable limits to the treatment so as to best utilize the resources of the staff. For example, when a serious learning and memory deficit intersects with vocal paralysis, as may occur in anoxic brain damage, it becomes impractical for the speech pathologist to attempt to train the patient on an alternate communication device, and the psychologist's evaluation may help to accelerate the decision process.

### CONSULTATION

The consultative role of the psychologist is quite varied. Often the special in-depth testing skill of the psychologist is required to clarify problems in vocational planning, ability to use special equipment, or readiness for discharge. Basically the psychologist's consultative role is an adjunctive one to the other members of the rehabilitation team. Nurses often express concern with a change in the patient's affective or behavioral status and want to know how to understand and cope with it. Physical and occupational therapists are often confronted with the patient's anxiety or depression over the slowness of motor return and may report a decline in the patient's motivation. Physicians occasionally report that a patient is refusing medication or other necessary treatment. The busy pace of an active treatment center simply does not allow for the development of deep empathic relationships between patients and most of the members of the staff. Changes in the patient's behavior may therefore be experienced by a staff member as abrupt, inconsistent, capricious, and unpredictable.

In order to understand it, a standard or stereotyped explanation may be invoked. As an example, a patient may be said to be refusing treatment because he is "entering the denial phase." Another approach is to seek causal explanations for the behavior change in the circumstances that immediately preceded it. The frequent failure to find satisfactory explanations in these approaches may result in a somewhat intolerant or otherwise negative view of the patient. Because the psychologist's interest and training lead him to focus on the patient's underlying dispositions and motives, he is often in a better position to make sense out of the behavior, to explain its logic and its continuity, thus helping to remove some of the staff's doubts.

### PSYCHOTHERAPY

The primary role of the psychologist is as a psychotherapist, employing the traditional techniques of individual or group psychotherapy. Treatment may be supportive, that is, helping a patient to cope with some immediate problem or emotional reaction. It may be insight-oriented, that is, helping the patient to become more aware of the unconscious motivational influences on his behavior. Occasionally treatment may involve intensive "crisis intervention" to rescue a patient from a serious suicidal path or an incipient psychotic episode. Therapeutic techniques for the cognitive behavioral control of pain are being used with greater frequency by psychologists with respiratory patients. Electronic biofeedback technology, combined with psychological theories of learning, is a new form of psychophysiological therapy designed to increase the patient's control over autonomic functioning, muscle training, and pain management.

# The Role of Social Service in Treatment of the Respiratory Insufficient Patient

by Gail M. Herring, M.S.W., A.C.S.W.

## PREADMISSION SCREENING

The role of the social worker in treatment of the patient with respiratory insufficiency begins with the preadmission screening process. After the patient has been medically approved for admission, the social worker will attempt to gather patient and family history and evaluate planning goals from a psychosocial and financial point of view. The primary goal is for the patient to return to community living, either living independently or with others. While discharge planning depends on physical rehabilitation, without adequate psychosocial functioning and financial resources, discharge planning can be extremely complex. After the preliminary assessment, the social worker makes a recommendation to the medical team whether this applicant has the necessary tools (combination of emotional support, self-directedness, and financial support) for community living.

## HISTORY

The psychosocial history is the social worker's tool for assessment and planning. The patient can be viewed in a familial, cultural, ethnic, religious, and socioeconomic framework. Family and social relationship—the ability to relate—will be of particular importance to all treatment modalities. The patient's support systems and pre-existing coping mechanisms are very important for motivation and adjustment, and for discharge planning. The pre-existing life style of the patient plays a significant role in these areas. The action-oriented young adult, in particular, has more difficulty adjusting to disability with respiratory insufficiency and therefore needs consistent emotional support as well as assistance to develop coping mechanisms and begin to deal with the environment. For action-oriented persons and artistic and sports professionals, this is a change in physical, and therefore mental, status. It can take years of support and psychological help before the new role is adequately integrated.

Another factor that will determine areas of intervention and concern for the social worker is the age of onset. Young adults and adolescents have more difficulty in adjusting to disability. Psychosexual development will be of particular concern for the child and the adolescent, as self-image is of greater significance when body image and functioning are seriously impaired before self-identification takes place. Self-esteem, self-image, social skills, and coping mechanisms are significant to all age groups, and treatment planning needs to address these issues appropriately.

## REALITY TESTING

The social worker as well as all team members must provide a realistic base for the patient and family in treatment and planning. The patient or family who insist that the patient will "walk out of the hospital" is encouraged to discuss the patient's current physical functioning to facilitate realistic discharge planning. The social worker uses a variety of tools to help with adjustment, such as meetings with rehabilitation professionals and constant support and reality testing.

## DISCHARGE PLANNING

The discharge of the patient with respiratory insufficiency depends on many factors, not the least being available services in the community. The social worker will need to explore options with the patient and follow through in obtaining home attendant services, finances, Medicaid, wheelchair-accessible housing, appropriate furniture, and medical supplies. Of even greater importance is the social worker's assistance to develop and enhance patients' independence, support system, and coping mechanisms. This is extremely complex because of the amount of services needed for these severely disabled patients, and the Medicaid laws, especially outside New York City, cover the costs of fewer services than the patient requires. The social worker needs to be very creative and persistent in efforts to discover new financial resources and appropriately use already existing ones. This usually means a considerable amount of advocacy to make Medicaid officials, politicians, and social service and public health agencies aware of the lack of funds and services and engage them in helping to obtain these services for the respirator-dependent patient. The social worker then needs to impart this information to the patient so that he has a clear understanding of what to expect upon discharge.

The discharge process begins at admission and is re-evaluated throughout treatment. In order for the discharge to be successful, the social worker must be an active advocate and provide significant clarification and information throughout the process.

While the medical treatment team is preparing patient and family for the physical and medical aspects of life in the community, the social worker must prepare all concerned for the psychological, social, and economic contingencies of community living. The social worker may have to be creative in developing alternatives to traditional discharge plans, such as planning for group living or shared homes. The special needs of this patient can be met outside institutional life with proper planning.

# Discharge Planning and Home Care

*by Carmel A. Tuths, R.N., M.A.*

The time arises when the patient with neuromuscular disease and subsequent respiratory insufficiency no longer requires intensive rehabilitation services. The goal of care for these patients is return to the community with supportive care and services. This is a viable cost-effective alternative to long-term institutionalization that maximizes the patient's psychological well-being.

There are many unique considerations for the respiratory-impaired neuromuscular patient who is returning to the community. The public health nurse facilitates this process through coordinating a discharge planning program that is an integral part of the rehabilitation program. Multidisciplinary team intervention, education of the patient and family, and coordination of community services are essentials of discharge planning. The commitment and enthusiasm of professionals to mainstream patients provides the support and encouragement in this endeavour.

Community discharge plans are implemented when several patient criteria have been met: stable medical condition, plateau in rehabilitation therapy, available community care providers, active medical insurance, and commitment of the patient to meet self-care needs with supportive services. The goals of the preliminary phase of the discharge planning process focus on education, coordination, and communication to anticipate and prepare all aspects of care required for community living. The patient and family are interviewed by the public health nurse to develop a suitable discharge plan. Areas of assessment include functional capabilities, required surgical supplies, appropriate medical and rehabilitation follow-up, and required adaptive and respiratory equipment.

A home evaluation is completed early in the discharge process by the public health nurse and occupational therapist with the patient to determine accessibility and safety of the environment. Recommendations for architectural adjustments and adaptive equipment are made by the occupational therapist at this time. This activity helps to allay the anxiety and concerns that patients have in returning home. All equipment necessary for home maintenance is coordinated by the public health nurse; this includes respirators, activities of daily living devices, adaptive equipment, and surgical supplies. Patients are instructed in procedures for obtaining supplies and repairs in the community. They receive medical, nursing, and rehabilitation follow-up through their local community health facility after discharge. Complete multidisciplinary summaries with care plans are forwarded to the appropriate agencies. The type of follow-up care chosen depends upon the patient's medical and functional status and can include home care agency, outpatient department, or private physician.

Prior to discharge, the public health nurse instructs the patient, family, and home attendant on special diet, medication regimen, appropriate activity levels, adaptive equipment, and medical emergency plans. Psychological preparation and emotional support is rendered by the rehabilitation team to relieve the stress that the patient with a severe respiratory impairment experiences in returning to the community.

Coordination of information from the institutional providers to community providers is a paramount factor in the success of the actual discharge. The public health nurse assures her availability at the time of discharge to intervene expediently for any unanticipated problems and provide further follow-up when required. A home visit will be made when necessary to evaluate the adequacy of services. Open channels of communication and availability provide continuity of care in the discharge process.

The respiratory-impaired patient receives long-term supervision at home by community nursing, social service, and rehabilitation specialists. Home care respiratory vendor agencies provide ongoing equipment repair and maintenance while Visiting Nurse Service provides supportive care, health teaching, and supervision of home attendant care. Respiratory re-evaluations are done at the respiratory care center on a yearly basis or as necessary, and the information is forwarded to the community agencies that need it.

Psychological and emotional adjustment of the patient occurs as he becomes reintegrated into the community. Re-establishing relationships with family and friends, relating to other primary care providers, and resuming meaningful activities are indicators of a healthy community adaptation.

Patients with respiratory insufficiency secondary to neuromuscular disease are enjoying life in the community despite sometimes severe impairments. They face challenging problems that include financial, social, and health care accessibility. However, they benefit with greater emotional and psychological well-being outside of institutional care. These patients have shown that they can live and thrive with reasonable safety with proper preparation and coordination of professional and support services.

# 20

# Rehabilitation and the Chronic Renal Disease Patient

by Diana D. Cardenas, M.D., Nancy G. Kutner, Ph.D. and
J. Robin deAndrade, M.D.

ACKNOWLEDGEMENT
We are grateful to John D. Bower, M.D., Professor of Medicine,
University of Mississippi Medical Center, for his critical and
helpful review of this chapter.

The patient with chronic renal failure, or end-stage renal disease (ESRD), faces many of the problems common to patients with other chronic disabling diseases, yet few efforts have been made to provide ESRD patients with comprehensive rehabilitation. In the United States alone, approximately 57,000 persons were receiving maintenance dialysis therapy in 1981. The vast majority of patients are on hemodialysis; the remainder are on some form of peritoneal dialysis. There are also approximately 15,000 living renal transplant recipients in the United States. For those who have a successful transplant, the quality of life is preferable over life on dialysis; in one patient's words, "When I was on dialysis I was breathing—now I am living." Most chronic renal failure patients are not transplant recipients, however. We need to maximize the quality of life of dialysis patients and not be satisfied with just keeping them alive.

The distribution of primary diseases leading to chronic renal failure varies in different areas of the United States and between the United States and European countries. Table 20–1 approximates the etiology of chronic renal failure in the United States.

Both dialysis and transplant patients experience social, psychological, and financial stresses in addition to medical complications. Self-image and self-respect are impaired not only by physical

**TABLE 1.** USUAL DISEASES RESULTING IN KIDNEY FAILURE

| | PERCENTAGE |
|---|---|
| Glomerulonephritis | 38 |
| Interstitial disorders | 15 |
| Primary hypertensive disease | 12 |
| Polycystic kidney disease | 8 |
| Diabetic nephropathy | 7 |
| Collagen and vascular disorders | 3 |
| All other hereditary disorders | 2 |
| Miscellaneous causes | 5 |
| Unknown cause | 10 |

*From Klahr, S.: Overview of the pathophysiology of chronic renal disease and uremia. In End-Stage Renal Disease: Pathophysiology, Dialysis, and Transplantation. National Center for Health Care Technology Monograph Series, U.S. Dept. of Health and Human Services, 1981.

changes but also by loss of job, changes in roles performed within the family unit, changes in relationships with friends, and dependency on medical personnel.

Chronic renal failure patients commonly experience one or more of the following symptoms in addition to the complications of their underlying disease:[2]

1. Fatigue and insomnia

2. Symptoms of peripheral neuropathy, e.g., "restless" legs, paresthesias, sensory or motor loss or both

3. Muscle atrophy

4. Skeletal problems including bone pain, fractures, osteonecrosis, or other forms of renal osteodystrophy

5. Itching (pruritus)

6. Gastrointestinal disturbances, especially nausea and vomiting, constipation, diarrhea

7. Decreased mental acuity, apathy, irritability

8. Depression

9. Sexual dysfunction

## FATIGUE

With adequate dialysis therapy, which restores a more normal fluid and electrolyte balance and raises the patient's hematocrit, organic sources of fatigue are reduced, but many patients continue to complain of fatigue. We have found that patients who complain of severe fatigue are significantly less likely to be employed or to be students than are patients who categorize their fatigue as "moderate" or "mild." Anemia in dialysis patients is a chronic condition that may be a cause of continuing fatigue among dialysis patients. Other possible contributors include undernutrition, acidosis, and the level of parathyroid hormone. In our research, cardiovascular disease does not seem to be correlated with high fatigue levels among dialysis patients. We have found, however, that the modality of treatment may be important; hemodialysis patients more often complain of severe fatigue than do patients on peritoneal dialysis. Similarly, hemodialysis patients often require time to "recover" or feel good again following their treatment, especially with larger fluid removal, while peritoneal dialysis patients do not experience this.

Although the etiology of fatigue in dialysis patients is undoubtedly complex, we suggest that depression is the etiology of fatigue in a subset of patients. In the general population, fatigue that is worse in the morning and tends to improve during the day is commonly due to emotional problems, a phenomenon frequently seen in patients on dialysis. In a study of 137 dialysis patients, we found that those patients reporting significant fatigue upon arising also evidenced significant levels of depression even when questions related to fatigue were deleted from the psychological test.[1]

Deconditioning enhances fatigue, and there is growing interest in examining the potential benefits of aerobic exercise for dialysis patients. In research to date, measurements of oxygen consumption before and after exercise training have shown improvement in $VO_2$ max. The data also suggest better control of hypertension, possible improvement in hemoglobin levels and other laboratory studies, and a reduction in depression and anxiety.[4] Patients participating in this research are exercised under supervision after undergoing a symptom-limited graded exercise treadmill test following the Bruce protocol.

Stationary bicycling at home is the focus of exercise studies underway in Michigan and Wisconsin, with phone contacts, home visits, and office visits used for follow-up. Patients generally exercise on nondialysis days. Bicycling and walking on a treadmill can be easily supervised when patients can come to a gym or physical therapy department. Swimming is another alternative. In addition to stationary bicycling and rapid walking, jogging on an indoor track has been used under physician supervision in Washington University's exercise research program. However, it is generally believed that jogging may be contraindicated for many renal patients because of potential bone problems.

A regular program of walking, e.g., at a temperature-controlled shopping mall, can be prescribed for many patients who are not able to participate in a more strenuous exercise program. Patients might be instructed to walk half a block a day for the first week, a block a day for the next week, and gradually build up until they are walking eight to ten blocks at a steady rate every day.

One must remember that chronic renal failure patients have a tendency to develop hyperkalemia because the major route of excretion of potassium is via the kidney. If a patient does not comply with diet prescriptions and eats foods high in potassium such as bananas, nuts, and citrus fruits, he is at greater risk of sudden death from cardiac arrhythmia. Obviously, emergency equipment should be available if the patient is exercising strenuously. Patients on continuous ambulatory peritoneal dialysis (CAPD) should be monitored for possible exercise-related complications with catheter exit and intra-abdominal fluid. Exercise programs for both hemodialysis and CAPD patients should be graded, with patients progressing to higher levels of activity as they become stronger and more independent. Muscle atrophy and patient motivation are important factors determining the patient's initial level of exercise.

Exercise may significantly reduce feelings of fatigue in some patients, and psychological intervention may be helpful for other patients. Overexertion and inadequate rest should be avoided by all patients. The occupational therapist can teach the patient energy-saving techniques such as proper posture and breathing, organizing a daily schedule, and establishing a regulated work pace and a balance between activity and rest. It may be helpful to have patients keep a diary of their activities so that the occupational therapist or other personnel can help individualize daily tasks and goals. Counseling in work simplification and energy saving enables patients to gain independence in self-care, homemaking, vocational, and avocational activities.

## PERIPHERAL NEUROPATHY

Uremic polyneuropathy, a common concomitant of end-stage renal disease, has been well described in the literature. It has been reported that about 65 per cent of the patients who go on dialysis therapy have clinical evidence of uremic neuropathy.[14] Clinically, the neuropathy in its milder form affects predominantly the lower limbs with symmetrical numbness, paresthesias of the feet, and "restless" legs. More severe forms affect the upper extremities as well, with loss of sensation and strength distally. We have observed decreased grip strength, i.e., values below the tenth percentile for their age, in 70 per cent of a sample of dialysis patients. Peripheral neuropathy is probably a significant contributing factor, although factors such as disuse atrophy or fear of injuring the vascular access may also be involved. The patients we have studied demonstrate normal pinch strength, suggesting that activities such as feeding, dressing, or personal hygiene are not likely to present problems, while activities requiring a forceful grip are likely to be difficult for many patients.

If foot drop develops, light-weight shoes and plastic ankle-foot orthoses can be prescribed, but care must be used with the patient who has insensitive feet or significant pedal edema. A light-weight metal "piano wire" brace can also be used. Generally, the patient with marked paresis in the lower extremities will have weakness in the upper extremities and thus be unable to utilize more extensive bracing such as knee-ankle-foot orthoses. Mild strengthening exercises, range of motion exercises, and training in activities of daily living can benefit the patient with peripheral neuropathy, but one must be aware that the patient's work capacity is generally decreased. As mentioned, general conditioning exercises should not be overlooked.

Often the patient with severe polyneuropathy has diabetes mellitus or some other systemic disease as the underlying cause of renal failure. In cases in which the patient is nonambulatory, CAPD or overnight peritoneal dialysis (continuous cycling peritoneal dialysis [CCPD]) can permit the patient's participation in an inpatient rehabilitation program without the disruption of scheduling dialysis hours or transporting the patient to a dialysis unit. CAPD or CCPD exchanges can be performed by rehabilitation nurses once they are taught the technique in cases in which grip, sensory loss, or visual loss prevent the patient from performing the exchanges independently. The times for CAPD exchanges can coincide with meals and bedtime and thus not interfere with a full day's rehabilitation program. Not all patients are candidates for CAPD or CCPD but, when possible, such modalities obviously provide greater opportunities for comprehensive rehabilitation in the severely disabled patient as well as for travel and employment in the mildly disabled patient.

## MUSCLE ATROPHY

Disuse atrophy may not be apparent because of edema in chronic renal failure patients. Contractures, especially in the hips, knees, and ankles, may develop. Range of motion exercises are beneficial in such cases, and splinting may be necessary.

As noted, dialysis patients are likely to have significantly weaker grip strength than normal persons, suggesting the potential benefit of exercise that is specifically designed to improve viable upper extremity muscles. One easily instituted exercise is repeated squeezing of a rubber ball, which can even be done while the patient is undergoing dialysis.

## SKELETAL PROBLEMS

The skeletal problems of major significance are renal osteodystropy, osteonecrosis, skeletal pain and fractures.

### RENAL OSTEODYSTROPHY

This is an established entity and is a combination of osteomalacia (or rickets in growing children), hyperparathyroidism, and osteoporosis.

The osteomalacia is due to the nonavailability to osteoid of calcium and phosphate, because of the profound alteration of calcium and phosphorus balance and changes in pH. Furthermore, calcium absorption from the gut may be diminished because vitamin D is not converted to its active form by the kidney.

Because of the tendency to a lower serum calcium and a high phosphate level, parathormone is secreted, and this eventually results in secondary hyperparathyroidism.

Osteoporosis occurs because of lowered protein availability caused by anorexia and loss in the urine. Other factors may also operate.

As a result of these biochemical changes in the milieu interieur, the following clinical problems may be found: bone pain, pathological fractures, bony deformities, secondary osteoarthrosis, slipped upper capital femoral epiphysis, soft tissue calcification, and fatigue.

Slipping of the upper femoral capital epiphysis has been reported in children. Following satisfactory dialysis, the incidence of slipping of the epiphysis was markedly reduced. This is a problem that is amenable to satisfactory treatment, and hence it should be kept in mind and the appropriate x-rays taken to identify this condition.[9]

Erken[3] found that among 42 patients on maintenance hemodialysis, secondary hyperparathyroidism was present in 34 per cent; osteomalacia in 56 per cent; osteosclerosis in 12 per cent; osteopenia in 61 per cent; and extraosseosis calcification in 40 per cent.

The severity of these manifestations is a function of time and available dietary calcium. It takes years to develop these problems and generally a decade for them to produce significant disability. Homeostasis mandates a certain level of serum calcium; this demand may be satisfied by leaching this element out of the bone, hence the clinical skeletal problems. Dietary calcium can satisfy the needs of homeostasis. However, dietary restrictions may interfere with an adequate supply. Furthermore, excessive ingestion of calcium, or even a reasonably normal amount, may result in the deposition of this substance in unwanted locations such as the kidney parenchyma, the blood vessels, and in other soft tissues, and the production of urinary calculi.

Optimal management of renal failure by dialysis or transplantation significantly minimizes, but does not eliminate, renal osteodystrophy. Hence, early control before the syndrome is clinically apparent goes a long way to prevent these skeletal manifestations.

## OSTEONECROSIS

Osteonecrosis seems to be related to the use of steroids for immunosuppression in transplantation. The dosages of corticosteroids used for renal transplantation are generally higher than are used for the majority of other clinical conditions.[9]

The incidence of osteonecrosis varies. Erken noted that after renal transplantation, 60 of 100 patients showed evidence of osteonecrosis. The femoral head was involved in nine occasions, and femoral condyle in ten. These are the two more common sites for this condition. Radiological surveys of the skeleton will increase the harvest of lesions in different parts of the body in post-transplant cases. Osteonecrosis in the head of the femur, where for the most part it is symptomatic, ranges from 7.5 to 15 per cent.

The natural history of osteonecrosis in different parts of the body indicates that only a few are symptomatic. Symptoms commonly occur when the condition affects the femoral head and the femoral condyles. In probably about half of the instances after a period ranging for months to years of increasing severity, the condition stabilizes. In some cases, less pain is noted.

For the most part, definitive treatment means a surgical operation. Non-weight-bearing probably does not significantly alter the course of the disease or diminish symptoms. In these patients, the irksome manner required to maintain a non-weight-bearing posture probably imposes too great a burden, considering the myriad other problems that are present. If the condition is bilateral, this form of treatment becomes virtually impossible.

In the case of the hip, surgical management includes strut bone grafting, curettage and bone grafting, subtrochanteric osteotomy, transtrochanteric rotational osteotomy,[11] and total hip replacement. Of these, the rotational osteotomy is a most promising approach. It shifts weight-bearing from an abnormal, collapsed portion to one with a better contour and with better weight-bearing characteristics.

The results of the total replacement are gratifying, and are almost as good as when done for conditions other than avascular necrosis secondary to renal transplantation. This condition is amenable to treatment with the conventional total arthroplasty, as well as double shell surface replacement and an articulated Bateman type of implant.

In deAndrade's series of 20 hips in 16 patients, treated by total hip replacement in adults, the results were as follows: excellent, seven hips in five patients; good, nine hips in seven patients; fair, two hips in two patients; poor, two hips in two patients. One hip in the excellent category sustained the technical problem of fracture of the shaft of the femur during surgery. This problem was treated with a long-stem prosthesis and with cerclage wiring. Both patients whose hips were rated as poor complained of pain for no apparent reason. Loosening is a possibility in these. All patients had had steroids. Thus, replacement surgery produces results that are acceptable and gratifying, although not quite as good as those in patients without end-stage renal disability.

## SKELETAL PAIN

Pain of skeletal origin is for the most part managed symptomatically with rest and exercise, splints and appliances, counterirritation, counseling, and orthopedic measures.

Rest should never be prolonged for fear of aggravating osteoporosis. It should be guided by the need for symptomatic relief. Most patients with skeletal problems can benefit from an exercise maintenance program. It should be similar to that used in the management of arthritis. The purposes of such a program are to keep neuromusculoskeletal functioning at the optimal level and to prevent or to minimize the effects of secondary osteoarthroses. (Swezey[12] presents examples of such routines in his book.) Exercises tailored to specific needs are almost always needed. Splints are of particular value for resting specific parts because they provide rest without courting generalized osteoporosis.

Appliances include walking aids such as canes, crutches, and walkers. On rare occasions, a wheelchair may also be needed. Another aid is a three-wheeler motorized cart for mobility for distances longer than 50 feet.

Shoes may need to be modified. The most useful alteration is provision for a heat-molded Plastizote insole. This will require shoes a size larger. The modifications used in the management of rheumatoid arthritis may also be required, such as lightweight space shoes with soft uppers and metatarsal bars or rocker soles.

As in the case of other types of pain, counterirritation is a simple, safe, and useful form of management. These techniques should be utilized to the fullest extent. Simple forms of heat and cold are most appropriate. Other therapeutic entities include ultrasound, especially for localized pain, transcutaneous electrical nerve stimulation (TENS), and acupuncture. The fact that anesthetic areas may be present because of peripheral neuropathy must be kept in mind. Counseling includes information about the disease and its symptoms, body mechanics, contingency management, operant conditioning, relaxation training, and self-hypnosis.

Narcotics and analgesics may be used in the case of pain secondary to end-stage renal disease. Because of the changes in metabolism produced by this disease, the selection and methods of use of these drugs are different from those in patients without renal disease. This subject is beyond the scope of our consideration here.

Orthopedic measures include the management of deformities, fractures, and secondary osteoarthrosis. As a rule local injections of steroid should not be given. Management resembles that of rheumatoid arthritis, especially in respect of the need to avoid long periods of immobilization, and the pos-sibility of the need for multiple surgical procedures. Total joint replacement is a useful procedure in selected cases, and the results are comparable to those obtained in the absence of renal disease. Renal disease appears not to compromise the use of polymethylmethacrylate cement, which is customarily utilized in these procedures.

## FRACTURES

Fractures that occur in the weakened bone associated with end-stage renal disease, as a general rule, heal in a manner similar to that in bones of patients without renal disease. This is to say, non-union or delayed union are not special problems, and these fractures take no longer to heal. Other problems, however, must be kept in mind in their management. Immobilization for long periods should be avoided because it may aggravate osteoporosis. Furthermore, the presence of other bone and joint problems such as secondary osteoarthroses may influence the selection of methods of management, with a greater bias toward internal fixation and early mobilization.

## ITCHING

High amounts of urea deposited in the skin when the patient's blood urea nitrogen is elevated often produces itching. Increased calcium concentration in the skin as a consequence of secondary hyperparathyroidism also contributes to intense itching. Removal of the parathyroid glands brings relief for some patients from this symptom, but this is not uniformly true. Itching is also relieved by good control of the serum phosphorus level through diet and aluminum compounds.

## GASTROINTESTINAL DISTURBANCES

Nausea and vomiting are frequent gastrointestinal complaints of patients with chronic renal insufficiency. It has been speculated that ammonia produced from the breakdown of urea, rather than urea itself, is a source of these symptoms. With proper diet, especially limitation of total protein intake but sufficient high biological value protein, production of ammonia decreases and nausea and vomiting tend to subside. Nausea and vomiting may also be related to the hemodialysis procedure, necessitating alteration in the size of or technique of operating the artificial kidney. Too rapid removal of fluid can also produce nausea and vomiting.

Constipation is another frequent complaint of dialysis patients because of their need for aluminum compounds that function also as phosphate binders.

Other gastrointestinal complaints may include diarrhea, flatus, hiccoughs, or gastrointestinal bleeding.

## DECREASED MENTAL ACUITY, APATHY, IRRITABILITY

One of the first signs of uremia is decreased power of concentration. The patient feels apathetic and has difficulty keeping his attention on what he is doing. Symptoms can proceed to pronounced lassitude and confusion. Treatment of the renal failure with either dialysis or transplantation reduces the symptoms, although dialysis patients' concentration span tends to be relatively short, and some report having periods of disorientation. Some investigators recommend the serial use of cognitive testing to monitor the adequacy of dialysis.[10,13] Such data may also assist in the selection of vocational goals and appropriate counseling.[2]

## DEPRESSION

It is common for patients who have lost kidney function and face dependence on dialysis therapy for the remainder of their lives to experience a stage of depression in the course of adjusting to their illness. Denial, anger, depression, and bargaining stages are likely to precede acceptance of the chronic illness. Some patients may be unable to move beyond deep-seated depression, perhaps making conscious or unconscious suicide attempts, necessitating psychological counseling or psychiatric treatment or both. Even for relatively well-adjusted patients, there may be recurrent bouts of depression accompanying events such as painful medical complications, job problems, or sexual and marital difficulties. The renal failure patient's most important resources for dealing with these episodes of depression are a sense of purpose and meaningful activity in his life and the availability of significant others who provide social and emotional support.

Employment and a sense of being self-sufficient can be very important buffers against depression in the dialysis patient's life. We have found that both men and women who are employed have lower depression scores than patients who are unemployed.[8] It may be beneficial for patients who could take an early retirement to continue working on a part-time basis because of the reassurance that their skills and knowledge are still valued and they as individuals are still "needed." Even if the job provides little intrinsic reward itself, the employed patient may value the fact that he is still able to support himself. Regardless of the prestige level of the job, employed patients have peer and co-worker associations that are potentially supportive. These opportunities for self-esteem and social support are lost when patients accept disability benefits and avoid employment.

Patients can also gain a sense of purpose and meaningful activity in a number of ways other than employment. Both men and women can gain satisfaction from caring for children and from taking responsibility for various homemaking activities. The goal of seeing a young child or grandchild grow up may be the most important thing in a patient's life, giving him a reason for living. Some patients value the challenge of volunteer or community service activities, which may involve them in numerous organizations or political groups.

Activity—whether employment, family-centered, or community involvement—should be encouraged by the rehabilitation team that deals with chronic renal failure patients. The patient's family must also be encouraged to expect the patient to do as much as possible for himself. This may conflict with the family's initial desire to take care of and protect the sick member, but it encourages acceptance of responsibility and independence on the patient's part and avoids potential build-up of resentment on the part of family members who, perhaps unconsciously, may begin to perceive the chronically ill person as a burden.

Availability of social and emotional support from others is a very important resource for the chronic renal failure patient who has a tendency to become depressed. If family or friends cannot provide this support, dialysis staff or rehabilitation personnel or both can be a "second family." Two categories of patients are particularly likely to need this outside support. One category includes young, unmarried adults who want to remain independent of their parents and whose ties with peers are limited by their inability to share activities such as strenuous sports or social drinking. Widowed older patients are another category whose depression is as much a function of loneliness as it is of their chronic renal failure.[7] Both of these groups often depend heavily for support on their associations with other patients at the dialysis clinic and their associations with professional staff.

Finally, a regular exercise program will be beneficial in helping patients improve their physical strength and self-concept and experience less depression.

## SEXUAL DYSFUNCTION

Sexual dysfunction in chronic renal failure patients can be caused by physical, pharmacological, and/or psychological factors. A marked reduction in sexual interest and the impaired ability to perform sexually are common among dialysis patients. A large majority of the patients we have studied have reported decreased satisfaction with their sexual life compared to their satisfaction with their sexual life before the onset of dialysis. Treatment of sexual dysfunction is aimed at the cause or causes and requires a willing patient and partner and trained professional counselors. It is important for the professional to understand the couple's past relationship and to discuss openly with both partners the range and acceptance of each other's sexual expressions (see Chapter 28).

## CONCLUSION

In order to successfully rehabilitate the chronic renal disease patient, several conditions are desirable:

(1) The patient's medical and emotional condition should be reasonably stable.

(2) It is important to evaluate the patient's stage of adjustment to his illness. A patient who is still in the denial stage probably does not follow his diet and fluid restrictions and may even miss dialysis treatments. Rehabilitation of the chronic renal disease patient requires that the patient accept and comply with treatment prescriptions.

(3) The patient should be motivated sufficiently to make efforts to reach specific rehabilitation goals. Many patients receive Social Security or other disability benefits and fear that if they were to become employed they would lose this income. This partially accounts for the unemployment that characterizes an estimated 40 per cent or more of the dialysis population.[5]

(4) The patient should have the opportunity to learn and a willingness to change habits and apply new skills. There is growing consensus that assigning patients whenever possible to treatment modalities that maximize their involvement in their own care—especially home hemodialysis, CAPD, CCPD, or self-care within a dialysis facility—fosters patients' independence and self-confidence.

Rehabilitation personnel who have been extensively involved with chronic renal failure patients in the past have been the social worker and the nutritionist. The physiatrist has been largely underutilized, as have the physical therapist, occupational therapist, rehabilitation nurse, psychologist, and vocational counselor (except in states with very active vocational rehabilitation programs).

Team evaluations of the needs of chronic renal failure patients, when utilized, have proven very helpful, making possible the development of a program geared to the status and needs of the particular patient. As nephrologists and their patients become more aware of the benefits of rehabilitation (for example, the benefits of regular physical conditioning), greater utilization of the (rehabilitation) system can be expected.

## REFERENCES

1. Cardenas, D. D. and Kutner, N. G.: The problem of fatigue in dialysis patients. Nephron 30:336–340, 1982.
2. Chyatte, S. B.: Rehabilitation medicine in chronic renal failure. In Chyatte, S. B. (ed.): Rehabilitation in Chronic Renal Failure. Baltimore, Williams & Wilkins, 1979, pp. 28–45.
3. Erken, E. H. W.: Skeletal changes before and after renal transplantation. J. Bone Joint Surg. (Br) 60-B: 285; 1978.
4. Goldberg, A. P., Hagberg, J., Delmez, J. A., Carney, R. M., McKevitt, P. M., Ehsani, A. A., and Harter, H. R.: The metabolic and psychological effects of exercise training in hemodialysis patients. Am. J. Clin. Nutri. 33:1620–1628, 1980.
5. Gutman, R. A., Stead, W. W. and Robinson, R. R.: Physical activity and employment status of patients on maintenance dialysis. N. Engl. J. Med. 304:309–313, 1981.
6. Klahr, S.: Overview of the pathophysiology of chronic renal disease and uremia. In End-Stage Renal Disease: Pathophysiology, Dialysis, and Transplantation. National Center for Health Care Technology Monograph Series, U.S. Dept. of Health and Human Services, 1981, pp. 1–22.
7. Kutner, N. G. and Cardenas, D. D.: Rehabilitation status of chronic renal disease patients undergoing dialysis: variations by age category. Arch. Phys. Med. Rehabil. 62:626–631, 1981.
8. Kutner, N. G. and Gray, H. L.: Women and chronic renal failure: some neglected issues. J. Soc. Social Wel. 8:320–333, 1981.
9. MacGeown, M. G.: Immunosuppression for kidney transplantation. Lancet I:310, 1973.
10. Ryan, J. J., Souheaver, G. T. and DeWolfe, A. S.: Intellectual deficit in chronic renal failure: a comparison with neurological and medical-psychiatric patients. J. Nerv. Ment. Dis. 168:763–767, 1980.
11. Sugioka, Y.: Transtrochanteric anterior rotational osteotomy of the femoral head in the treatment of osteonecrosis affecting the hip—a new osteotomy. Clin. Orthop. 130:191, 1978.
12. Swezey, R. L.: Arthritis: Rational therapy and rehabilitation. Philadelphia, W. B. Saunders Co., 1978.
13. Teschan, P. E., Ginn, H. E., Bourne, J. R., Ward, J. W., Hamel, B., Nunnally, J. C., Musso, M. and Vaughn, W. K.: Quantitative indices of clinical uremia. Kid. Int. 15:676–697, 1979.
14. Thomas, P. K., Hollinrake, K., Lascelles, R. G., O'Sullivan, D. J., Baillod, R. A., Moorhead, J. F. and Mackenzie, J. C.: The polyneuropathy of chronic renal failure. Brain 94:761–780, 1971.

# 21

# Sports Medicine

*by Vojin N. Smodlaka, M.D., Sc.D.*

Physical education, sports, and dance are movements that have become part of our way of life. Millions of Americans are involved in all kinds of exercises, training, and competitions. These are people of both sexes and all ages. They start exercising and competing as children and continue late in life. These exercises may be of light, moderate, or high intensity, of short or long duration, and may reach an extent that can lead to acute fatigue or exhaustion. Table 21–1 illustrates the amount of training undertaken by members of some national athletic teams.

Performance in different sports may reach high levels and speeds in some sports such as skiing and cycling can be dangerous. A fall at high speeds may cause multiple injuries.

During competitive athletic effort the body reacts according to certain patterns. When work is of submaximal level the physiological parameters are in a steady state, but when the athlete performs on a maximal or near maximal level, the body's maxima reactions take place. At the end of such maxima efforts physiological values have been registere such as a heart rate of 220 per min, blood pressure of 250 mm Hg, respiration rate of 50 per min, axi lary body temperature of 40.3° C after a 10,000 meter run, weight loss of 6 kg in cyclists; hematu ria with albumin and casts after a marathon run o a soccer game.

When such efforts are made too often in a perio of months, without adequate rest in between, th athlete may fall into a state of "overtraining," syndrome often seen when athletes or their coache are overambitious. In rare cases, when trainin and competition are in excess, the athlete may b permanently damaged—he may be "burned out, a poorly understood syndrome. To explain suc athletic efforts, the following statement was mad "The art of record-breaking is the ability to tak more out of yourself than you have. You punis yourself more and more and rest between spells Athletes call such training or competition PAT pr grams: pain, agony, torture!

Effects of these maximal efforts, extreme speed maximal body reactions and accompanying traun have been investigated. Little by little, investig tion research, and experiments have provided a swers and explanations. A body of knowledge h accumulated that forms the basis of sports medicir

## WHAT IS SPORTS MEDICINE?

Sports medicine is a new specialty in Medicir The first important attempt to form and define t

**TABLE 21–1.** ESTIMATED AMOUNTS OF TRAINING

| | |
|---|---|
| Runners, joggers | 25 km/day |
| | 150 km/week |
| | 3,000,000 steps/yr |
| Swimmers | 6 hrs/day |
| Gymnasts | 3–4 hr/day |
| Weightlifters | 20,000–30,000 kg/day |
| Javelin throwers | 6,000 times/season |
| | 50,000 during career |
| Divers | 150,000–200,000 dives |
| | during career |
| Soccer players | 70–80 games/yr |

From Franke, K.: Traumatologie des Sportes. VEB Verlag Volk und Gesundheit. Berlin, 1980.

area of sports medicine was made in Dresden, Germany, at the 1911 World Hygienic Exposition, with the creation of a special department of physical exercise (Smodlaka).

We may define from the view point of a scientist or that of a clinical practitioner. The scientist is interested in studying the positive and negative effects of physical exercise and competition on all human bodies—both sexes, all ages, normal persons and patients with diseases or disabilities. The practitioner of sports medicine is interested in utilizing the positive effects of exercise and competition and in preventing or curing the negative ones.

All kinds of scientists are involved in sports medicine research, including biologists, anatomists, physiologists, biochemists, biomechanics, clinicians of the various medical and surgical specialities, psychologists, engineers, architects, economists, sociologists, and many others. All are contributing to the theoretical and practical knowledge of the field. The practitioners include physicians, health professionals, physical educators, coaches, trainers, masseurs, referees, and all others involved in the field of physical education, sports, recreation, and dance. Gradually, physicians and trainers started to devote part time, and later full time, to sports medicine, working as team and club physicians and trainers.

In many countries sports medicine has become a recognized medical specialty with a three- to five-year residency training program and a specialty board. These specialists work in medical schools as professors, researchers, teachers, and residency program directors. This is the case in Europe, where the system of socialized medicine has made it possible.

In the United States sports physicians are self-made and self-educated. They participate in courses and symposia organized around the country. They become competent in this field and usually work part-time as sports physicians.

National societies of sports medicine were first organized in central Europe before World War I. The American College of Sports Medicine was formed in 1954 and is today the largest such organization in the world, with almost 12,000 members. The International Federation of Sports Medicine (FIMS) was formed in 1928 during the Winter Olympic games in St. Moritz, Switzerland. Many national organizations publish journals of sports medicine; today there are about 20 such publications in different languages.

Physiatrists as specialists in physical medicine and rehabilitation are competent to prescribe therapeutic physical exercises to patients who need them. They know the effects and values of exercise and are competent in prescribing and supervising exercise and training of nonathletes and athletes. They also prescribe physical therapy for patients with all kinds of diseases and injuries as well as treating highly trained athletes.

Some physiatrists are not only involved in sports medicine but also in sports and competition for disabled persons such as the blind, deaf, and paraplegics and serve as team physicians for these groups.

Sports medicine may be divided in two main parts: biological and medical aspects and traumatological and rehabilitative aspects.

## BIOLOGICAL AND MEDICAL ASPECTS OF SPORTS MEDICINE

Since earliest times, teachers who accumulated empirical knowledge and experience observed that a gradual increase in physical exercise develops the strength, endurance, skill, and speed of their students. The law of gradual increase of intensity and duration of training was discovered. Well known is the story of the ancient Greek Olympic athlete, Milon of Crotona, who started to lift a calf every day from its birth to increase his strength and was eventually able to carry a four-year-old bull!

Lamark, a modern scientist, developed the biological principle that the "function develops the organ." Darwin defined the principle of adaptation of the organism. Pflüger, a physiologist, stated that "Weak stimuli stimulate the vital processes, the average enhance them, the strong inhibit them, and the too-strong destroy them." Schultz-Arnod's law is laconic: "Use maintains, effort develops, and exhaustion damages." Roux said on one occasion: "Too strong or too long a function weakens the organs."

These principles still guide physical educators, trainers, and sports physicians when prescribing physical exercise and training. Finally, Hippocrates recommended over two thousand years ago the following rule for daily living: Work, food, drink, sleep, sex, all in moderation. But what is moderate for a highly trained person will be excessive for a feeble elderly man! Applying these recommendations in the process of training, we may enhance physical condition, increase working capacity and fitness, and improve performance. The human body is able to adapt to a prescribed single effort instantly. If the effort is near maximal or maximal, the body will use all its physiological reserves to the point of exhaustion. However, if the body is exposed to a gradual training program over several months or years, it will adapt gradually two ways: morphologically and functionally. If the body is immobilized with bed rest, a general atrophy and loss of functional capacity will occur. For this reason it is said that immobilization is the enemy of the athlete.

## MORPHOLOGICAL ADAPTATION

The cardiovascular system was the main target of investigation of many sports physicians. A large amount of information on its functions has been accumulated through the years. The concept of the "athletic heart" was introduced as early as 1899, when it was discovered by simple digital percussion that well-trained endurance athletes have a larger heart. This has been confirmed by modern investigators using all kinds of diagnostic methods.

It was well documented that wild animals forced to lead an active life for survival have a larger heart in relation to body weight than domestic animals. Grober calculated that for 1000 gm of body weight the domestic rabbit has 2.40 gm of heart, the wild rabbit has 7.75 gm, the domestic goose has 6.98 gm, and the wild goose has 11.02 gm. A domestic horse has a heart of 3.5 kg, a racehorse a heart of 7 kg.

Reindell et al. published a similar list of relative heart rate in different animals to show the relationship between activity and size of the heart (Table 21–2).

The same process of adaptation of the heart occurs in athletes who live an active life. They develop a large heart, heavier by weight and larger by volume. Reindell et al. published the comparison in Table 21–3.

Friederich and Medved reported the average anthropometric values of the Yugoslav national waterpolo team: height of 185 cm, weight of 91 kg, age 25, 12 years of training and a heart volume of $1263 \pm 29$ cc.

The heart is very adaptable to instant and ongoing exertion and changes its volume accordingly. Reindell et al. measured the volume of the heart during Valsalva phenomenon in six normal persons and found that the volume declined from 755 cc to 457 cc, which is 39 per cent. In six athletes the heart declined from 1082 cc to 553 cc, or 49 per cent.

**TABLE 21–2** HEART SIZE RELATED TO BODY WEIGHT IN KG

| Animal | Body Weight | Relative Heart Weight |
|--------|-------------|------------------------|
| Pig | 49.7 | 4.52 |
| Calf | 280.0 | 5.35 |
| Human | 58.0 | 5.88 |
| Sheep | 20.6 | 6.17 |
| Horse | 493.0 | 6.77 |
| Hare | 3.70 | 7.70 |
| Doe | 20.6 | 11.55 |

$$\text{Index} = \frac{\text{Heart Weight} \times 1000}{\text{Body Weight}}$$

From Reindell et al.: Herz., Kreisslaupkrankheiten und Sport. Munchen, Johann Ambrosius Barth, 1960.

**TABLE 21–3.** COMPARISON OF HEART SIZES AND VOLUMES

| Heart Weight | | Heart Volume | |
|--------------|---|--------------|---|
| 300–350 gm 6 cases | 790 cc | Average persons | (67) |
| 350–400 gm 9 cases | 782 cc | Sprinters | (86) |
| 400–450 gm 14 cases | 876 cc | Middle distance runners | (66) |
| 450–500 gm 2 cases | 923 cc | Long distance runners | (66) |
| 500–550 gm 3 cases | 1104 cc | Professional cyclists | (18) |

From Reindell et al.: Herz., Kreisslaupkrankheiten und Sport. Munchen, Johann Ambrosius Barth, 1960.

During a training period the heart volume changed, depending on the activities, as shown in Table 21–4.

The heart of a pregnant woman increases in size and weight, with the greatest increase at the end of pregnancy. It returns to almost normal after pregnancy. This adaptability of the heart and other organs is a characteristic of living beings and is well developed in highly trained athletes.

Capillarization of trained muscles is a morphological way of adaptation. Petrén et al. showed that the number of capillaries increased in the muscles of trained animals. Smodlaka et al. demonstrated that the spleen is larger in well-trained athletes and that it became smaller at the end of an extreme effort. Training also increases the size of the muscles and bones. It may be concluded that some training methods increase the morphological values of the trained person.

Functional adaptation to exercise occurs during training. It has been well established that endurance athletes have a very slow heart rate at rest; it may decline to values of 40, 35, and 32 per min, especially in professional cyclists. This condition is called athletic bradycardia.

The slowing-down of the heart rate occurs during normal athletic training, and also affects patients in the course of rehabilitation. This is a universal phenomenon not well explained.

I demonstrated in 1960 that the heart rate decreased in a group of cardiac patients who were rehabilitated after heart surgery using endurance interval training.

Blood pressure is lower in trained athletes. It also declines in average persons and patients at the end of an exercise and rehabilitation training program. Mellerowicz drew a curve expressing this difference of systolic blood pressure in the average population and athletes.

A training program increases the heart's maximal stroke volume. It is especially high in endurance athletes. The maximal cardiac output in-

**TABLE 21–4.** GERMAN MASTER ON 800 M

| DATE | TRAINING CONDITION | HEART VOLUME IN CM | O₂ PULSE 200 WATTS | HEART RATE |
|------|--------------------|--------------------|--------------------|------------|
| 5– 1–56 | Training | 975 | 18.8 | 138 |
| 9– 5–56 | After injury | 860 | 17.2 | 153 |
| 9–21–56 | Training | 935 | 18.4 | 140 |
| 3– 2–57 | Training | 1080 | 20.9 | 115 |
| 4–18–57 | Sickness | 950 | 19.3 | 150 |
| 5–11–57 | Training | 1000 | 20.2 | 145 |
| 6–22–57 | Training | 985 | 21.0 | 134 |
| 10–26–57 | 14 days influenza | 1015 | 19.2 | 143 |
| 3–22–58 | Training | 975 | 18.8 | 138 |
| 3–22–58 | Training | 1000 | 20.6 | 134 |
| 5–10–58 | Training | 1040 | 21.6 | 128 |
| 7–25–58 | Training | 915 | 19.7 | 142 |
| 12–20–58 | Little training | 870 | 18.0 | 157 |
| 12–12–59 | Moderate training | — | 19.4 | 143 |

From Reindell et al.: Herz., Kreisslaufkrankheiten und Sport. Munchen, Johann Ambrosius Barth, 1960.

creases with training. Many other organs and systems react to training programs with increased morphological values on exertion and decreased physiological values at rest. Explanations of these adaptation processes and phenomena may be found in textbooks of sports medicine and work and sports physiology (Astrand and Rodahl, De Vries, Hettinger, and Mellorowicz-Smodlaka).

Observing development of morphological and functional qualities of the body during a lifetime, we see that they develop from the moment of birth until they reach their maximal value. After that time these values start to decline as a result of three factors: aging, inactivity, and pathological conditions. This increase and decline may be expressed with a curve that is more or less parabolic. We call this the biological curve of height, vital capacity, strength, endurance and cardiac output. All of these morphological and functional qualities may be developed during the growth period of life. Physical education of youth in schools is based on this fact. During the middle- and old-age period, physical exercise will eliminate the decline due to inactivity, because "what we do not use, we lose." We cannot stop the aging process, but we can cure or control many diseases, and we can prescribe exercise and training programs for elderly persons.

Adaptation to an acute intensive effort occurs

**TABLE 21–5.** PHYSIOLOGICAL VALUES OF AN AVERAGE MAN AND A WELL-TRAINED ENDURANCE ATHLETE

| PARAMETER | AVERAGE | MINIMAL | MAXIMAL |
|-----------|---------|---------|---------|
| Heart rate | 70–75 | 28 | 270 |
| Respiration rate | 16 | | 46 |
| Blood pressure | 125/70 | 90/60 | 270/90 |
| Heart weight | 300 gr | | 550 gr |
| Heart volume | 300 cc | | 1700 cc |
| Heart index | 11.3 | | 15.48 |
| Heart stroke | 65 cc | 44 cc | 300 cc |
| Cardiac output | 5 L | 1.8 L | 40 L |
| Heart work | 14.000 mg/24 h | 7.500 mg/24 h | |
| Circulation time | 15″ | 43″ | 8″ |
| Oxygen pulse | 5 | | 25 |
| Vital capacity | 4500 cc | | 8000 cc |
| Tidal volume | 350 cc | | 50% of V.C. |
| MVR | 4–5 L | 3 L | 170 L |
| O₂ Consumption | 300 cc | | 6000 cc |
| CO₂ Production | 400 cc | | |
| Resp. equivalent | 0.85 | | 1.5 |
| Ventil. equivalent | 2.5 | 1.7 | |
| O₂ Debt | | | 22.8 L |
| Aerobic capacity | 45 cc O₂/kg/w/min | | 90 cc O₂/kg/w/mi |
| Loss of weight | 2.5 kg | | 6 kg |
| Body temperature | 36.6° C | | 40.3° C |

immediately. The body uses its reserves. In our daily life, we usually use only a fraction of any organ's capacity. At rest we breathe with a tidal volume of around 500 cc, but with exercise the tidal volume increases.

The human may live with a fraction of the capacity of most organs, as the following list shows:

1. With one half of a lung
2. With one third of a kidney
3. With one sixty-fourth of a liver
4. With one half the normal volume of blood
5. Without a stomach
6. Without a cerebral-frontal lobe
7. Without a spleen, gallbladder, genital organs, eyes, ears, extremities, and part of the intestine.

Athletes develop large organ reserves as a result of training and effort: weightlifters develop their muscles, swimmers their lungs, and cyclists their cardiovascular system. These reserves make the difference between the athletic performance of champions and average individuals.

The adaptation process of the human body to athletic training may be demonstrated in Table 21–5.

## MEDICAL SUPERVISION OF SPORTS

Physicians and sports practitioners such as physical educators, coaches, instructors, trainers, referees, and officials have to maintain a constant control and supervision of participants in physical education, sports, recreation, and dance. This supervision may be divided in two main areas. The first is control of the health and status of training of participants, and treatment and rehabilitation after disease or injury. The second is supervision of all facilities such as gymnasiums, pools, athletic fields, and trails, and all equipment and uniforms to ascertain that they are constructed and maintained to follow public safety regulations. This control and supervision is a basic part of sports medicine.

Many sports organizations provide mandatory periodical medical examinations, especially before competition, to ensure that only healthy and fit individuals take part in extreme competitive efforts. It is absolutely necessary to eliminate from competition athletes with disease and injuries to prevent aggravation and worsening of the pathology.

Sudden cardiovascular deaths are not rare in sports. Hornof et al., Reindell et al., Oberlander, Letounov et al., Toker, and Wolffe have reported such cases. Brković and Ivankovic, supervising thousands of athletes in the Institute of Sports Medicine in Belgrade, reported cases of rheumatic endocarditis and carditis and found many athletes with focal infections of many organs and systems. These were all sources of potential complications.

I have personally witnessed six deaths on the field involving several sports during my long career as a sports physician. It was a painful experience and tragic event for the family and community. I became very aware of the danger involved in sports.

At the end of many types of competitions it is important to perform check-ups. The organizers of marathon runs and similar endurance competitions have a large staff of practitioners who take care of exhausted competitors. The best way for a physician to obtain clinical experience in this area is to become a volunteer member of such a staff.

Evaluating the physical condition and training of an athlete is a special task that requires stress testing in a well-equipped human performance laboratory. These time-consuming, expensive tests are reserved for highly trained candidates in the process of Olympic preparation. These tests help team physicians and coaches evaluate the level of training and prescribe further training.

## SPORTS TRAUMATOLOGY

All human activities are dangerous, as are physical education, sports, recreation, and dance. Some exercises are more dangerous, some less. We have to study athletic injuries, their etiology, biomechanics, prevention, and treatment, and the athlete's rehabilitation, to be able as physiatrists to help athlete patients. Analyzing sports injuries, we see that these are really common injuries that may occur in regular daily life, at home, on the job, or in traffic. Some of these common injuries occur more often in one sport or another. Very few injuries are typical of only one particular sport, as are tennis elbow, javelin elbow, wrestler's ear, and boxer's nose.

Breitner published a monograph titled "Sportschäden und Sportverleztungen" differentiating sports injuries and "sport damages." The concept was accepted and sport damages are called "overuse injuries" or "stress injuries" today. They are the result of multiple minimal injuries accumulated in a long period of athletic training and competition.

Stress injuries usually affect the legs and pelvis and less often the upper extremities: overuse injuries are treated conservatively with rest and physical therapy modalities. The most important principle is prevention and early diagnosis to prevent stress fracture if a bone is affected.

Sports injuries may be wounds, contusions, concussions, muscle or ligament injuries, luxations, fractures, and others.

### LOCATIONS OF SPORTS INJURIES

Many years ago Wachsmuth et al. and Petitpierre published statistics concerning the relation-

**Table 21–6.** RELATIONSHIP OF INJURY TO BODY AREA

| BODY AREA | WACHSMUTH AND WOLK ALL SPORTS | PETITPIERRE WINTER SPORTS |
|-----------|----------------|----------------|
| Head | 6.1% | 3% |
| Body | 10.9% | 7% |
| Arms | 23% | 23% |
| Legs | 59.9% | 67% |

From Wachsmuth, W. and Wolk, H.: Über Sportunpälle und Sportschadën. Leipzig, Georg Thiene, 1935; and Petitpierre, M.: bie wintersportverletzungen. Stuttgart, Publisher Enke, 1939.

ship of injury to body parts (Table 21–6). All other statistics to date, though collected in different environments, are basically similar to these.

In some sports some parts of the body are more affected than in other sports. For example, injuries of the arms occur more often in goalkeepers than in other soccer players. The right side of the body is more affected than the left side, and males are more often injured than females.

Injuries may be divided according to their severity, and Wachsmuth reported his findings in Table 21–7. It is estimated that 90 to 95 per cent of all injuries require conservative treatment, and only few need surgical care. The physiatrist is best qualified to treat sports injuries using conservative modalities, including physical therapy and rehabilitation.

The difference between treating average patients as opposed to highly trained athletes is in the final goal. Athletes expect to be able to return to their extreme efforts and competition after complete rehabilitation. Athletes are very concerned about their health, physical and athletic condition, and performance ability. They will do everything to build and maintain their athletic prowess and work toward rehabilitation after injury. Athletes are highly motivated patients. The athlete demands that the diagnosis be accurate, the decision prompt and unequivocal, and the treatment definitive (Quingly). When sports participants are injured, they ask immediately, "When I will be able to exercise again?"

## CAUSES OF INJURIES

The causes of injury have been divided into five categories:

1. Inexperience of beginners
2. Poor or inadequate equipment
3. Poor field and weather conditions
4. Fatigue and lack of fitness
5. Foul play and incompetent referees, coaches, instructors and officials.

The beginner does not have the theoretical or practical knowledge, technique, or skill of his sport. He is inexperienced and does not know how to protect himself or how to escape an injury, a fall, or a collision. He has to be taught by a good teacher—coach, instructor, trainer, parent, or referee.

Equipment is designed to protect a sports participant from injury. It should be of good material and quality, well fitted and maintained, and properly used. Coaches, trainers, parents, referees, and physicians should check the equipment and its application prior to training and competition. Field and weather conditions are of great importance in many sports. Fields, trails, and gymnasiums have to be well built, safe, clean, and well maintained.

Weather is an important factor, in outdoor sports especially in the mountains, both in summer and winter. Cold weather, snow, ice, freezing temperatures, and wind have an effect in cold climates, as has hot, humid weather in hot climates. Cold may cause frostbite of the nose, ears, fingers, toes, breasts, and penis. Hot weather provokes dehydration and heat stroke. Rain and fog are also important weather factors.

Fatigue at the end of a training session or competition and at the end of the season provokes general weakness, slows the reflexes and all reactions, and diminishes coordination and skills. The fatigued sports participant is prone to falls, being unable to avoid collisions and loss of balance on slippery ground. It is well known that skiers at the end of a full day of skiing can injure themselves due to exhaustion. Good physical condition is important in preventing injuries caused by fatigue.

Good teachers, coaches, trainers, instructors, referees, parents, and physicians, teach sports participants the dangers of sports, fair play, the rules of the games, and prohibit foul play. A strictly officiated competition and game reduces injuries.

## TREATMENT OF SPORTS INJURIES

Treatment of sports injuries starts immediately on the field with first aid and continues until the sports participant is able to return to the sport and compete again. The team physician provides treatment and follow-up care. The injured athlete is immediately restricted in movements and is partially or totally immobilized.

The acute injury provokes a local inflammatory reaction of the injured tissues expressed in five

**TABLE 21–7.** SEVERITY OF INJURY AND DAYS LOST

|  |  | No. SICK DAYS |
|---|---|---|
| Insignificant | 11.5% | |
| Light | 63.5% | 10–15 sick days |
| Moderate | 22% | 15–30 sick days |
| Severe | 3% | over 30 sick days |

From Wachsmuth, W. and Wolk, H.: Über Sportunfälle und Sportschadën. Leipzig, Georg Thiene, 1935.

clinical symptoms and signs: pain, loss of function, swelling, redness, and warmth. Loss of function is a natural defense mechanism that immobilizes the injured part. This defense reaction may be explained in several ways.

The first is *voluntary immobilization:* the pain of the injured area forces the athlete to keep the injured part immobilized. He knows that every movement will provoke pain. The second is *Payr's defense reflex:* pain provokes this mechanism. Pain stimuli reach the posterior horn cells, inhibit the anterior horn cells of the pain level that innervates the muscles of the injured segment, and provoke paresis or paralysis of these muscles. The injured person cannot move the injured part. This forcible natural reflex and involuntary immobilization lasts a relatively long time and subsides slowly. This fact has to be taken into consideration during rehabilitation. The third is *development of edema.* Edema occurs because of extravasation of blood, lymph, or synovial fluid in or around the muscles, tendons, joints, or other tissues. Edema, especially when extensive, makes the entire area stiff and hard, with tension caused by high pressure in the tissues, and takes a long time to be resorbed and eliminated. Athletes, especially professionals, cannot afford to be immobilized for long periods; therefore it is important to prevent extravasation and edema by immediate, energetic, and proper first aid.

A fourth reason for immobilization is *disturbance in the vasomotor neurovegetative trophic functions of the injured area.* Following Leriche's theory, this disturbance is caused by a reflex provoked by pain, which specially affects the sympathetic system and disturbs the trophic functions, prolonging the reparative process of the injured tissues so that edema and immobilization last longer. Leriche recommended immediate elimination of pain and cutting the reflex by injecting lidocaine to provoke a pharmacological local sympathectomy—a sympathetic block. This method is accepted by many physicians. It consists of injecting 0.5 to 1 per cent of 1 to 10 cc of Xylocaine in selected cases (see Chapter 7).

It is important to emphasize that injecting lidocaine on the athletic field to eliminate pain and sending the athlete back to compete immediately is a dangerous policy. The local anesthesia eliminates pain and limping but impairs the natural coordination of players and exposes them to a new injury. Some physicians may be tempted to give lidocaine under pressure from the player, coach, officials, or fans. This policy must be considered as malpractice.

Fifth is *therapeutic immobilization* using slings, splints, bandagings, casts, crutches, wheelchairs or bed rest, when indicated. The basic rule of therapeutic immobilization is to make it as localized and as short as possible.

In conclusion, first aid should consist of the prevention of extravasation with edema, elimination of pain to reduce Payr's defense reflex and Leriche's sympathetic reflex, and to enhance healing and rehabilitation.

First aid consists of several steps:

1. Immobilization of injured part
2. Elevation of the part
3. Compression
4. Application of cold
5. Elimination of pain.

Immobilization as first aid helps eliminate the pain and decreases local circulation, extravasation, and edema. However, immobilization provokes atrophy very fast, especially in highly trained athletes and professionals.

Deitrick et al. studied the effect of immobilization in bed on human metabolism of calcium, phosphorus, sulfur, and nitogen. They found a negative balance soon after the beginning of absolute bed rest, which was corrected after resumption of regular activity. They did not investigate how long it took to replace the lost minerals.

Saltin et al. studied the effects of bed rest on three college students and two athletes. They were stress tested before and after three weeks of bed rest, and following 55 to 60 days of intensive rehabilitation. These investigators found a significant reduction of the subjects fitness, maximal oxygen intake, and heart volume, and increase of heart rate. It took them 50 to 60 days to regain the same values and reach previous fitness. Other investigators also reported negative effects from complete bed rest.

Kottke has emphasized that immobilization combined with hematoma, lymphedema, and effusion in or around the joints, tendons, or capsules stimulates the formation of fibrotic fibers, adhesions, and contractions. Histological evidence of fibrosis may be documented on the fourth day of injury.

Clinical experience teaches us that strong muscles protect the joints and prevent injuries. It is axiomatic that the muscle is the strongest ligament and prevents distortion of the joint.

Each sport develops strength and endurance of the muscles to the level necessary for the usual motions involved in performing that sport. If we want to increase the strength of muscles and their flexibility to respond to unusual demands, we have to expose these muscles to a "special conditioning training" before an injury occurs, and especially after in the process of rehabilitation.

Bender et al. have shown how important it is to build up strength. They exercised two groups of 150 cadets. The first went on a regular conditioning training program, the other a special program to build the strength of the quadriceps muscles. The second group sustained fewer injuries during the year. The cadets who sustained new injuries had

58 days of duty loss and 14 days of hospitalization without surgery. Cadets with reinjuries had 72 days of duty loss, 131 days of hospitalization, and 4 surgical interventions.

When to stop immobilization and start mobilization and therapeutic exercises is quite a difficult decision. George Perkins in his Robert Jones Lecture in London, 1952, stated: "It is difficult to say when the inflammation has ceased and repair has begun. It is difficult clinically to determine when to change from one treatment to the other." This is a matter of personal clinical experience because we do not have reliable clinical research to guide us.

Sorensen experimented with two groups of patients after menisectomy. The first group started weight bearing the fourth day and the other the tenth day using a cane. He did not find any difference in the occurrence of complications such as hydrarthrosis. Erikson et al. studied the effect of a "movable cast" recommended by Burr et al. after anterior crutiate ligament surgical repair. The patients with a movable cast started athletic training earlier (1.5 as opposed to 3.75 months) and they also had less muscle atrophy (circumference of the thigh 0.5 cm as opposed to 3 cm). These patients were trained with isometric exercises of the legs but without any specific general reconditioning program and suffered a marked reduction of endurance. Erikson et al. recommend general endurance training.

The present treatment of choice is to begin early rehabilitation with gradual mobilization, combining exercises for strength and endurance. The injured part may stay immobilized, but the rest of the body should be exercised to prevent deconditioning.

Until the early 1920s athletes were rehabilitated in the hospital to reach some independence in daily activities. After discharge they were left to decide when to return to athletic training and competition. At that time physicians did not assume the responsibility of rehabilitating the athlete for competition. This was left to the coach and trainer. Today, the team physician follows the athlete from the moment of injury to the moment of returning to competition.

I became involved in sports medicine in 1934, and in 1937 used a well-developed system of manual progressive resistive exercises in the rehabilitation of athletes. Since that time, the only difference in my prescription for the rehabilitation of athletes is the amount and intensity of reconditioning exercises, imposed by the contemporary level of physical conditioning of Olympic athletes and professionals.

Rehabilitation of athletes is a team effort of the athlete, physician, trainer, and coach. Facilities and sufficient time must be available for the athlete to reach a high level of physical conditioning and fitness.

Elevation is a therapeutic modality, used as first aid to help prevent extravasation and development of edema and later to promote resorption of this edema. Use of gravity is a simple, cheap, and practical measure, and a good home remedy. Edema in the lower extremities forms faster because of gravity, and remains longer. However, it is often not easy for a young person to accept bed rest with elevation of the leg or of the lower part of the bed.

## APPLICATION OF COMPRESSION

I remember my grandmother using a large knife to apply compression to the foreheads of my younger sisters when they hit the corner of a table, to prevent the formation of a lump. She combined the pressure with the cold blade. This method of compression is universally accepted as first aid, to prevent extravasation and formation of edema.

The injured part may be compressed with the fingers, the hand, a piece of ice, or an elastic bandage, and compression should last 20 to 30 minutes. The compression may be continued with elastic bandages with padding around the uneven joints. Mechanical alternating compression is done with Jobst boots, used with 50 to 100 mm Hg pressure, in cycles of 60 seconds on and 15 seconds off, for 20 minutes. Compression may be applied for several days to treat sustained edema of the joints and the area outside the joints. Compression may be combined with other physical therapy modalities (cold or heat).

## USE OF COLD AND CRYOTHERAPY

Application of cold is a universally accepted therapeutic modality, used as first aid and as therapy for the first several days after injury. Cold suppresses pain, extravasation with edema, and local inflammation with heat and redness, and constricts the vessels. Trainers always keep an ice bag with crushed ice handy, to apply immediately on an injured part on the field and in the locker room. Some use ethyl chloride, spraying the injured part for one to two minutes.

Cold therapy may be applied with different methods—placing the injured part under running water, submerging it in a bucket of cold or icy water, using cold compresses, performing ice massage (cryotherapy) or whirlpool. This therapy lasts for 24 to 72 hours.

Cold is used to calm the strong inflammatory reactions in severe bursitis, tendinitis, synovitis, and similar inflammations.

## USE OF DRUGS

Pain is a natural warning symptom, a defense, which forces the subject to protect the injured part by immobilization voluntarily or involuntarily.

Some other reflex mechanisms occur as was described. Pain provokes immobilization and immobilization provokes atrophy, especially when it lasts too long. For these reasons pain should be suppressed and eliminated.

Analgesics and anti-inflammatory drugs are recommended by many sports physicians. The list of recommended drugs is a long one. Each physician has to accumulate personal clinical experience in using these drugs in combination with physical therapy modalities.

Lidocaine injections in combination with corticosteroids are in use. Some sports physicians are very cautious with cortisone and recommend only one or two injections, afraid of complications such as rupture of the tendons. We have seen a couple of ruptures after several injections of cortisone.

Use of analgesics in carefully selected cases is recommended in order to start early mobilization, passive and active range of motion, and active progressive exercises, in spite of pain. The tablets are given half an hour prior to treatment.

## MOBILIZATION

Mobility of the affected part of the body starts as soon as possible. Movement of the rest of the body starts the second or third day, when the injury is stabilized. Therapeutic exercises are the most valuable modality in the process of reconditioning and rehabilitation. To achieve mobility, all kinds of therapeutic physical exercises are in use.

Therapeutic exercises should be prescribed as digitalis is—carefully. This is a slogan to remind the physician to study "the pharmacology of physical exercise," which is not well understood, for the simple reason that medicine did not take exercise seriously.

There was a period in the history of use of digitalis when people discovered empirically that a tea brewed from the digitalis leaf had a positive effect on cardiac patients. They did not know what was in the leaf. Little by little medical science and pharmacological research extracted and purified the pharmacological contents of the digitalis leaf and developed the pharmacology of digitalis.

Today therapeutic exercise is in this early period of its history that digitalis was years ago. We know that exercise has positive effects, but we do not know the single, daily, maximal, toxic, or lethal dosage of physical exercise. Therefore we do not prescribe them as exactly as we do drugs.

Physical exercise adequately prescribed develops the strength, endurance, speed, or skill of the body and its parts. Isometric exercises predominantly develop strength, and isotonic exercises develop endurance, the two main qualities of athletes.

When prescribing exercises we have to define the intensity and duration of each isometric or isotonic exercise. To do so, we use as a base line the maximal capacity of isometric or isotonic performance and prescribe 100 per cent of maximum, or 90, 80, 50, and so on. We should prescribe the duration of each of these exercises, of each work load, resistance, and power.

The question that arises immediately is the appropriate duration for each exercise. How long can a person maintain the isometric or isotonic performance with maximal effort of so-called 100 per cent, how long with 90, 80, 70 per cent, and so on?

The thousand-year-old empirical experience of weightlifters teaches that they can maintain a maximal weight over their heads for three to four seconds. The rules of competition require that the weightlifter keep the weight up for three seconds. Less than maximal weight they are able to support longer.

Mondgil and Karpovich studied the duration of maximal isometric contraction of the elbow under three different angles with and without support of the elbow on the table and established that student volunteers were able to maintain their maximal contractures for 3.8 to 4.3 seconds.

The maximal isometric contraction may be prescribed with a maximal duration of four seconds or with a shorter duration of three or two or one second.

DeLorme recommended a maximum of 10 repetitions to recondition the strength and started the first 10 exercises with full range of motion and 20 per cent of maximum. Each movement up lasted usually one second, the return to basic position one second, followed by a short rest of one second. Then he gave a one-minute rest to have time to increase the weight by 10 to 30 per cent increments of maximum. The patient then performed the next 10 repetitions and so on, finally reaching the level of 100 per cent—the maximum. The duration of each movement lasted one second, which for the last repetition is 25 per cent of the maximal duration of four seconds. He did not recommend a duration of four seconds for the maximal weight.

The question is: Should we prescribe maximal isometric contraction with maximal duration? To answer this question, we will use the empirical experience of weightlifters. When they train, these athletes do not use maximal weight and maximal duration. They train with 75 to 85 per cent of their maximum. Only when competing do they push to the maximum to break their personal records. My recommendation is to start with a very low isometric effort of short duration of one to two seconds and increase gradually to 75 to 85 per cent of the maximum effort and duration.

To find the maximum strength of the affected site, nonaffected site should be tested, assuming that they were equal before injury.

What is the maximal capacity and duration of isotonic efforts? Jokl et al. studied the world records in running and calculated the relationship between

**TABLE 21–8.** RELATIONSHIP BETWEEN RUNNING EFFORT AND EXERTION

| DISTANCE METERS | RECORD TIME | % MAX VELOCITY |
|---|---|---|
| 100 | 9.95 | 100.00 |
| 200 | 19.80 | 100.51 |
| 400 | 43.86 | 90.74 |
| 800 | 1.43.50 | 76.91 |
| 1,500 | 3.32.20 | 70.33 |
| 3,000 | 7.35.20 | 65.58 |
| 5,000 | 13.13.00 | 62.74 |
| 10,000 | 27.30.80 | 60.27 |
| 42,000 | 2.08.34 | 54.17 |

From Jokl et al.: Running and swimming records. Br. J. Sport Med. 10: No. 4, 1976.

effort of running and duration (Table 21–8). They took the effort of a 100-meter run as the maximal possible dynamic isotonic human effort and calculated the effort when athletes ran 400 m, 800, 1500, etc. They found that the longer the distance the less was the effort. The marathon runner ran with 54 per cent of the maximal capacity needed for running 100 m.

Zeljaskov calculated the speed of Bulgarian runners (Table 21–9). The longer the distance the slower the speed and consequently the effort.

It is clear that in prescribing running as reconditioning therapeutic exercise, the distance, the speed, and duration have to be specified. Again, the runner should start with low speed and increase gradually to no more than 75 to 85 per cent of maximum capacity. It would be very helpful in the process of reconditioning to know what was the runner's best running time for different distances prior to injury to establish the speed of reconditioning running. In our eagerness to help the patient, we are inclined to start with high specifications and increase them too fast. Reconditioning and adaptation take time.

To prescribe physical exercises, some authors use and recommend physiological parameters, such as maximal heart rate, maximal oxygen consumption, maximal blood pressure, or a percentage of these. To do so for each individual, the max-

imal parameter should be established with a stress test or estimated using different recommended formulas or tables. To stress test a person takes time, proper equipment, and experience acquired in a human performance laboratory.

In daily practice the heart rate is the most commonly used parameter. The following formula is used to estimate the maximum heart rate:

$$HR\ max = 220 - age$$

When prescribing therapeutic exercises such as running, swimming, and cycling, the target heart rate has to be defined. This is the target that the person must try to maintain when exercising.

We recommend starting with 50 per cent of maximum heart rate and increasing gradually to 75 to 80 per cent of maximum heart rate. Only highly trained distance runners may maintain a high heart rate. For example, a 25-year-old long distance runner is able to run 5000 m maintaining a very high rate, near 180 per min. This is close to the maximum heart rate estimated with the recommended formula.

## MUSCLE GROUPS

We differentiate three main groups of muscles: flexors, pronators, and adductors, and their antagonists—extensors, supinators, and abductors. The arm uses the first group of muscles when performing work. The other group, the antagonists, are used to stretch and extend the arms and put the arms in a position to act again.

The first group is stronger than the second one. When immobilized, the second group loses strength relatively faster than the first one because of lower muscle reserve. For this reason we have to rehabilitate the second group with special care.

The extensors of the hand and foot are generally very weak. After immobilization they become weaker and unable to keep the wrist and ankle under control and prevent distortion.

Strong extensors prevent injuries of the wrist in boxers, and the ankles in different participants in sports.

Extensors, abductors, and supinators are at the same time antigravity muscles, fighting gravity all the time and keeping a good erect position and posture. These muscles are sensitive and atrophy easily. They have to be specially rehabilitated. Extension exercises—"antigravity exercises"—have to be part of daily conditioning training of an average man, especially when aging starts.

In the phylogenetic development of the human race, some muscles have changed their function because of erect position and have become extensors instead of flexors and vice versa. These muscles are very sensitive to injury and immobilization and atrophy easily and quickly. For these reasons these muscles need special attention for prevention

**TABLE 21–9.** RELATIONSHIP BETWEEN DISTANCE AND TIME

| DISTANCE | SPEED M/SEC | TIME |
|---|---|---|
| 100 m | 8.92 | 11.2 |
| 200 m | 8.47 | 23.6 |
| 400 m | 7.72 | 51.8 |
| 800 m | 6.89 | 1.56.1 |
| 1,500 m | 6.29 | 3.58.3 |
| 5,000 m | 5.15 | 16.10.1 |
| 10,000 m | 5.05 | 33.13.6 |

From Zeljaskov, C.: Teorija i Metodika na Sportnata Trenirovka. Sofija, 1981.

of atrophy, and early and prolonged rehabilitation. The deltoideus, vastus medialis, rectus femoris, and extensors of the hand and foot are especially sensitive.

Because of the modern concept of fitness, which has been accepted as a new way of life to enhance wellness, millions of people are exposed to possible injury and millions of such injuries occur. Up to 95 per cent are treated conservatively. The physiatrist is especially well equipped to treat these injuries.

# REFERENCES

Astrand, P. O. and Rodahl, K.: Textbook of Work Physiology, 2nd ed., New York, McGraw-Hill Book Co., 1977.

Bass, A.: Treatment of muscle, tendon and minor joint injuries in sports. Proc. Roy. Soc. Med. 62:925–928, 1969.

Bass, A.: Rehabilitation after soft tissue trauma. Proc. Roy. Soc. Med. 59:653–656, 1966.

Bender et al.: multiple angle testing method for the evaluation of muscle strength. J. Bone Joint Surg. 45A:135–149, 1963.

Boyne et al.: Oral antiinflammatory enzyme therapy in injuries in professional footballers. Practitioner 198:1186, 543–546, 1967.

Breitner, B.: Sportschäden und Sportverletzungen. Neue deutsche Chirurgie, Bd. 58. Stutgart, Ferdinand Enke, 1937.

Brković, I. and Ivankovic, D.: Zarisna zapaljenja srcanog misica u sportista. Sportska Praksa 1–2, pp. 31–34, 1974.

Brković, I. and Ivankovic, D.: Oligosimptomni oblici reumatickog endomiocarditis-a u sportista. Sportska Praksa 11–12, pp. 4–7, 1972.

Burr et al.: Funktionelle Behandlung nach Bandnaht und Plastik am Kneegelenk. Langenbecks Arch. Klin. Chir. 122: 1971.

Deaver, G. G.: Arch. Phys. Ther. X-ray, Radium. pp. 415–418, July 1931.

Deitrick et al.: A study of the effect of immobilization upon various metabolic and physiologic functions of normal men. Am. J. Med. 4, 3:1948.

DeLorme, T. L.: Restoration of muscle power by heavy resistance exercises. J. Bone Joint Surg. 27:645–647, 1945.

De Vries, H.: Physiology of Exercise. Dubuque, Iowa, Wm. C. Brown Co. Publishers, 1966.

Dreisiljer, J.: Gefahren der lokalen Cortisosteroid Injektionen an der Achillessehne. 24 Sportärztekongress Würzburg, 1971.

Erikson et al.: An attempt to shorten the convalescence period in athletes for major knee injuries. Proceedings of the XX World Cong. Sport Med., Melbourne, 1974.

Fitch et al.: Indomethacin in soft tissue injuries. Proceedings of the XX World Cong. Sport Med., Melbourne, 1974.

Franke, K.: Traumatologie des Sportes. VEB Verlag Volk und Gesundheit, Berlin, 1980.

Friederick et al.: Das grösste registrierte absolute Herzvolumen eines gesunden Leistungssportlers. Med. Sport Hf. 2, III, 1965, pp. 43.

Glick, J. M.: Therapeutic agents in musculoskeletal injuries. J. Sports Med. 3:136–138, 1975.

Hansen, S. E.: Eine medizinische Sportstudie. Skidlauf und Skidwetlauf in Mitteilungen aus der Medizinischen Klinik zu Upsala, Bd. II. Jena, G. Fischer Verlag, 1899.

Hettinger, T.: Isometrisches Muskeltraining. Stuttgart, Georg Thieme, 1972.

Hollmann, W., and Hettinger, T.: Sportmedizin-Arbeits-und Trainingsgrundlagen. Stuttgart, F. K. Schattauer Verlag, 1976.

Hornof et al.: Les accidents mortels dans le football. Proceedings of the XVI Int. Cong. de Medic. del Deporte, Santiago, Chile, 1962.

Huskinson et al.: Indomethacin for soft tissue injuries. A double-blind study of football players. Rheumat. Rehab. 12:159–160, 1977.

Jokl et al.: Running and swimming records. Br. J. Sport Med. 10: No. 4, 1976.

Karpovich, P.: Physiology of Muscular Activity. Philadelphia, W. B. Saunders Co., 1966.

Keul, J.: Limiting factors of physical performance. Stuttgart, Georg Thieme, 1973.

Kottke, F., Stillwell, G. K., and Lehmann, J. F.: Krusen's Handbook of Physical Medicine and Rehabilitation. W. B. Saunders Co., 1982.

Krahl, H.: Is local corticosteroid therapy indicated in the tendopathies? Med. Klin. 65:29–30, 1970.

Kretzler, H. H.: Tendons and cortisone. Proceedings AMA ed. Aspect Sports 16:31–33, 1974.

Leriche, R.: A propos du traitement par infiltration novocainique de l'epicondilique des joueurs du tennis, des maladies post-traumatiques de même ordre, de soi-disant apophysites de croissance, de certains fracteurs, sans deplacement et des sequelles osteoarticulaires. Pres. Med. 5:99, 1936.

Letounov, S. P. et al.: L'influence de la pratique durable de football a la sante au developpement physique et aux resources functionnelles de l'organisme. Proceedings of the XIV Cong. Int. de Medic. del Deporte, Santiago, Chile, 1962, pp. 57–76.

Mellerowicz, H.: Ergometry: Basics of Medical Exercise Testing. Smodlaka, V. and Rice, A. L., tr. Munchen, Urban and Schwarzenberg, 1981, p. 154.

Mondgil and Karpovich: Research Quarterly, 40:536–539, 1969.

Muckle, D.: A comparative study of flurbiprofen and aspirin in soft tissue trauma. Br. J. Sports Med. 10:11–13, 1976.

Oberlander, W.: Primare operative Versorgung einer traumatischen Ruptur der Aorta abdominalis. Zbl. Chir. 89:376–380, 1964.

Ochsenhirt, N.C. et al.: Arch. PM and R.V.4, 1953.

Payr, E.: Zur Meniscusfrage, Vor-und Nachbehandlung des Gelenkes, Sportunfull, Berufsschaden Folge. Z. Chir. 16:976–980, 1936.

Perkins, G.: Rest and movement. J. Bone Joint Surg. 35:521–539, 1953.

Petrén, T. et al. Arbeitsphysiologie 9:376, 1936.

Petitpierre, M.: Die Wintersportverletzungen. Stuttgart, Publisher Enke, 1939.

Quingly, T. B.: Contribution of Sports Medicine. AMA Proceedings of the 7th Nation Conference on the Medical Aspects of Sports, 9–11, 1965.

Reindell et al.: Herz, Kreisslaufkrankheiten und Sport. Munchen, Johann Ambrosium Barth, 1960, p. 43.

Saltin, B. et al.: Response to exercise after bed rest and after training. Circulation 38:5 Suppl. 8, 1–78, 1968.

Smodlaka, V.: Sports medicine in the world. J.A.M.A. 205:762–763, 1968.

Smodlaka, V.: Interval training in heart disease. J. Sports Med. Phys. Fitness 3:93–99, 1963.

Smodlaka, V.: Uvod u sportskomedicinski rad (Introduction in sportmedicine practice). Belgrade, Sportska knjiga Publisher, 1961.

Smodlaka, V. N.: The cause of sports injuries (0 uzrocima povredjivanja u sportu). Fiskult. 3–4, 1949.

Smodlaka, V.: La rate sportive. Proceedings VII Int. Congress Sports Medicine, Prague, 1938.

Smodlaka, V., et al.: Exhaustive exercise: effects on size of spleen. Arch. Phys. Med. Rehabil. 54:421–423, 1973.

Sorensen, K.: Effusion in the knee following meniscus operation. V. Ugeskr. Laeg. 131:2142–2144:1969.

Toker, Y.: Herzinfarkt bein einem 24-jahrigen auf dem Fussballplatz. Med. Welt, Stuttgart 15:757–760, 1965.

Unverferth et al.: The effect of local steroid injections on tendons. J. Sport Med. 1:31–37, 1973.

Wachsmuth, W. and Wolk, H.: Über Sportunfälle und Sportschäden. Leipzig, Georg Thieme, 1935.

Wolffe, J. B.: Football in relation to the young with special reference to the cardiovascular system. Proceedings of the XIV Cong. Int. de Medic. del Deporte, Santiago, Chile, 1962, pp. 77–82.

Zeljaskov, C.: Teorija i Metodika na Sportnata Trenirovka. Sofija, 1981.

# Section V

# SPINAL CORD

# 22

# Spinal Cord Injury

## *Introduction*
*by John F. Ditunno, Jr., M.D.*

The incidence of spinal cord injury in the United States is 7,000 to 10,000 and the estimated prevalence is 200,000 patients.

As a result of improved care, as documented by the National Spinal Cord Injury Model Systems Program, morbidity and mortality has been decreased, hospital stays and readmissions are decreased, and presumably patients will live longer and function better.

Although spinal cord injury centers provide lifelong follow-up care, they must rely on practitioners in the local community to provide certain elements of primary care within the community's resources. It is because of this ongoing responsibility that we recognize the need to assist individuals with spinal cord injuries and their local medical practitioners with a systematic approach to the problems most commonly encountered. This concern is well described in Dr. John Young's editorial on Follow-up care in the Spinal Cord Injury Digest in which he underscores the need for a "lifeline" between the patient/client, community resources, and the center.

This section chapter is an orientation and guide for the family physician and the physiatrist (rehabilitation physician) to aid in the evaluation and management of problems that occur in follow-up care of individuals with spinal cord injury.

In order to understand the evolution of the problems that occur following discharge from a spinal cord injury (SCI) center, it is essential that the local practitioner be aware of the phases of acute, rehabilitation, and follow-up care that such a center provides.

The Spinal Cord Injury Table of Contents (p. 380) serves as a reference in using the article. The problems encountered in follow-up care begin the discussion. Next, a description of the problems that occur during the phases of care from admission to discharge are outlined under the categories of (1) Medical-Nursing, (2) Functional, and (3) Psychological, Social, and Vocational. Finally, a summary of problems is listed in the context of differential diagnosis, therapeutic intervention, and considerations for referral and triage with the regional spinal cord injury center.

The authors include physiatrists (rehabilitation physicians), nurses, physical therapists, occupational therapists, social workers, and psychological and vocational counselors, all of whom work primarily with spinal cord–injured patients. In the planning, preparation, and development of the chapter, members of the Department of Family Medicine of Jefferson Medical College assisted us and reviewed the manuscript for emphasis and relevancy.

It should be understood that the presentation cannot address every problem or the many nuances of individual circumstances as they relate to the patient, family, or community, and is based on a conceptualized model that must be modified according to the individual circumstances.

The temporal relationships of the problems are portrayed graphically in Table 22–2. The acute medical problems such as atelectasis, deep vein thrombosis, and pulmonary emboli have a high incidence and morbidity early but may become of little or no significance after discharge, whereas the

**TABLE 22–1.** SPINAL CORD INJURY TABLE OF CONTENTS

psychological, social, and vocational problems, although present in the acute phase, become the major factors after discharge.

The functional problems will not be great if the patient remains reasonably healthy and is effectively coping.

Whatever the cause of spinal cord injury, the period between the accident and the patient's arrival in the hospital emergency department is critical, since an estimated 25 per cent of the fatal complications of cervical spine injuries may occur during this time. Even though most fatal complications occur from the force of impact, proper management by the rescue team is vital to protect survivors and decrease mortality.

**TABLE 22–2.** TEMPORAL RELATIONSHIP

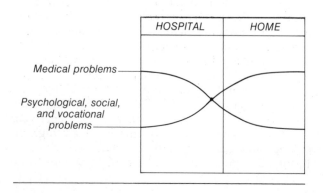

## OVERVIEW

Spinal injury is a worldwide problem and one of increasing importance. Approximately 70 per cent of all cases of spinal cord injury impairment are caused by trauma and 30 per cent by disease (cancer, neurological disease, and congenital anomalies). While paraplegics tend to have a higher percentage of complete lesions (60 per cent) than do quadriplegics (50 per cent), there are an equal number of quadriplegics and paraplegics. Spinal cord injury occurs predominantly in males (80 per cent). Spinal cord injury occurs most frequently in the younger age groups, 60 per cent in the 15 to 29 age group and 80 percent under 40 years of age. In the older age group, falls are most often responsible for the injury, while in the 0 to 14 age group penetrating wounds are the most common etiology. Vehicular mishaps account for 50 per cent of all spinal cord injuries.

## FIRST AID MEASURES AT THE SCENE OF THE ACCIDENT

Adequate and appropriate first aid measures are needed to reduce further neurological sequelae and to lower mortality. The first priority is the life support system, with assessment and maintenance of the basics—airway, ventilation, circulation. If cardiopulmonary resuscitation is needed, the neck must not be extended, but a "jaw thrust" or "chin lift" technique can be used to open the airway with the neck in a neutral position.

The emergency care of the spinal cord–injured person can be divided into four primary stages: (1) identification, (2) immobilization, (3) extrication, and (4) evaluation. Identification is that period in which recognition of possible spinal cord injury is made. It is best to assume that there is spinal cord injury in the patient with head injury, sensorimotor loss, pain in neck or back, or an impaired level of consciousness. In some instances, motor weakness may be subtle, with manifestations such as inability to make a fist with an extended wrist or slight difficulty in moving the toes. After the identification of possible spinal cord injury is made, a careful but rapid evaluation should be made to determine the need for treatment of a potentially lethal situation such as hemorrhage, shock, or cardiac arrhythmia.

Emergency treatment of the patient with spinal cord injury is aimed at supporting vital functions and preventing further spinal cord damage through immobilization prior to transportation of the patient. The patient should be protected from active and passive motion of the spine during these initial phases. Immobilization, therefore, is critical during emergency treatment. A sandbag placed on either side of the head can properly assist in this maneuver. Once the cardiopulmonary status has been stabilized, the patient should be immoblized in a Philadelphia collar. A short spinal board should be used prior to extrication to be replaced by an orthopedic stretcher or a long spinal board. Immobilization of the spine prior to extrication must be kept in mind at all times, particularly in those situations such as an automobile collision or when the patient has been injured in water. Although the extrication must be rapid, it should be done with the greatest of care. If the patient is in the sitting position, he should be cautioned not to move during the procedure. After the extrication, 5 per cent glucose and water should be given intravenously with an infusion rate not to exceed 30 minidrops per minute; the IV site also serves to keep a vein open for future medication administration. Oxygen via a mask at a flow rate of 6 to 8 liters per minute should be initiated to be followed by the insertion of a nasogastric tube and indwelling Foley catheter. A bolus of 50 cc of sodium bicarbonate should be given to be followed by 100 mg of Solu-medrol or its equivalent. After these measures, the patient should be transported to the spinal cord injury center. If, in the opinion of the emergency care team, the patient cannot survive transport to the spinal cord center because of the distance involved and the instability of vital signs or life-threatening injuries, the patient must be taken to the nearest acute care hospital for emergency care. The spinal cord center should be noti-

fied, however, regarding the injury and the plans so that the patient can be transferred as early as possible.

## MANAGEMENT IN THE ACUTE CARE HOSPITAL

All treatment personnel should have access to an adequate history of the accident. This will help in diagnosis and future management. A complete neurological examination should be done and recorded with careful observation of respiratory movements.

Experienced and knowledgeable personnel must assume the management and care of these patients in order to prevent further neurological injury. The airway, ventilation, circulation, and vital signs should continue to be assessed and maintained. A bag-valve mask, nasotracheal intubation, or an esophageal airway may need to be used to maintain the airway. Oxygen should be administered and, if necessary, assisted ventilation. Careful pulmonary toilet with assisted coughing should be carried out to prevent early infection or aspiration. A careful examination should be done to rule out other major associated injuries such as fractures, ruptured viscus, or head injury. A central venous pressure and indwelling Foley catheter can assist in making judgments about fluid replacements.

Long bone fractures should be splinted; open fractures have second priority to abdominal, chest, or head injuries.

The patient must be turned; log-rolling is used with a minimum of two people to turn and a third person to immobilize and support the patient's neck and head in neutral alignment. The neck should not be moved unless the airway is blocked. Sandbags around the head will help maintain the neutral position and immobilize the neck.

When a patient is in cervical traction, a rough guide is that 5 pounds should be used for each level of cervical injury.

Depending on the level of neurological injury and associated injuries, the patient will probably be immobilized either in cervical traction or placed on a Stryker turning frame, Roto-Rest, or regular hospital bed. All patients in cervical traction must be turned every two hours. In the Stryker turning frame, the patient is turned prone to supine every two hours. In the Roto-Rest bed, the patient is rotated to 145 degrees every 4 to 5 minutes automatically, obviating the need for manual turning. In a regular hospital bed, the patient is turned manually, side to back to side every two hours, with the head, shoulder, and pelvis moving simultaneously to maintain proper alignment. The skin requires careful attention during the immobilization techniques. Back care, including massages of the bony prominences, should be done as the patient is turned off that side. Utilization of foam padding and elevation of the heels and elbows will help prevent abrasions and pressure ulcerations. In addition to the bony prominences of the posterior body, the patient's knees, ankles, and thighs are particularly prone to breakdown. This can be avoided by the use of pillows between the lower extremities during the sidelying position. Although the plastic halo jacket is lined with sheepskin or synthetic material, breakdown can occur, especially in those who are insensate. Careful attention should be given to all these areas as outlined so that any possible breakdown may be noticed early and treated adequately.

Joint mobility, particularly at the shoulders, is limited by the application of cervical immobilization devices; therefore, these patients should receive passive range of motion exercises every two hours. These individuals should be provided with elbow pads to prevent abrasion from contact between elbows and the plastic and metal buckles over the halo device. The patient should never be supported or lifted by grasping of the anterior metal bars but rather by support from the back. The outriggers of the metal device frequently present a problem, especially in those patients who lack elbow extension. In this situation, the arms will fall on the outriggers during some activities, causing mild to moderate degree of injury. The use of thick foam rubber attached to these metal bars will help minimize this problem.

Difficulty in chewing often occurs in patients in this apparatus and the use of chewing gum between meals may help to facilitate chewing while adjustments are being made to the halo.The pin sites in the skull require local care similar to that suggested for the Gardner-Wells tongs, namely cleansing these areas with one half strength peroxide and normal saline followed by the application of Betadine ointment with sterile cotton swab during each nursing shift.

The orthopedic surgeon should indicate the status of stabilization and mobility on the patient's chart on admission and for each intervention including the placement of the halo, the immediate postoperative period, and on transfer to another facility.

Traumatic spinal cord–injured patients are particularly vulnerable to the threat of spinal cord edema, hematoma, and hemorrhage during the stage that follows injury. Because of these complications, the life and function of the patient may be seriously threatened. Medical-surgical intervention may minimize these risks if progression of symptoms is noted early before irreversible damage has occurred. Therefore, it is necessary to monitor and record the neurological examination at frequent regular intervals during the acute phase of hospital care. All patients admitted with the diagnosis of spinal cord injury should be placed on a "neurowatch" routine to determine the level of function and stability of signs. All data should be recorded on a flow sheet, which should be kept at the patient's bedside. The daily monitoring must include the neurological assessment, immobilization status, bowel and bladder function, lung status, extremity evaluation with particular emphasis on deep vein thrombosis screening, and skin checking.

To provide maximal coordination of acute phase management of the spinal cord–injured patient and family, the appropriate physician should speak to the family regarding the future considerations for surgery. A family meeting should be held within the first week in order to discuss the neurological impairment, associated injuries, decision for the future surgical intervention, functional prognosis, various facilities of care, and projection of length of stay.

# Immobilization and Stabilization Evaluations (Surgical Considerations)

by William E. Staas, Jr., M.D. and Jay D. Roberts, M.D.

Surgical management may involve three factors: general surgical problems, neurosurgical interventions, orthopedic considerations.

Since these patients may have sustained multiple injuries, surgical intervention may be necessary if abdominal or chest injuries have occurred. If such is the case, the team should quickly determine the stability of the spine prior to surgery, especially in those patients who have incomplete lesions. The orthopedic members of the team, therefore, are critically involved in decision-making relevant to definitive management of the unstable spine.

For the cervical spine, maximum immobilization is obtained with halo-skeletal fixation. However, this is rarely indicated today because adequate fixation can be obtained with a halo jacket. (Fig.

22–1A). This consists of a metal tiara fixed in four opposed positions by pins inserted into the skull. The tiara is attached to a frame by rods that are in continuity with a molded plastic body jacket. The stability of the system is attained through placement of the supporting rods into the mounting brackets attached to the body jacket. This device permits early mobilization of the patient in contrast to the traditional skeletal immobilizers, which require the use of a bed or frame and a prolonged period of total immobilization. Complications are related to the pins themselves; they include slippage, cellulitis with occasional severe infection, and occasionally osteomyelitis of the skull. In rare instances, the skull may be pierced by pins. This usually occurs if frequent tightening of the pins is required.

In the past, ulceration under the jacket was a problem, especially in the presence of loss of sensation over the thorax. More recently, lining the jacket with lamb's wool or synthetic materials has lessened this problem considerably. Nonetheless, periodic inspection of the skin should be done to treat the problem if it does occur. In individuals with marked pulmonary impairment related to the level of neurological injury, the jacket may further add restriction to ventilation. Finally, in the event of cardiopulmonary arrest, the anterior portion of the jacket must be disengaged, necessarily requiring a delay in the resuscitative efforts. It is important, therefore, to keep the tightening devices attached to the patient's jacket to deal rapidly with the problem of cardiopulmonary arrest.

The halo device should remain attached until such a time as there is x-ray evidence of bony stabilization or fusion or both. This will require fre-

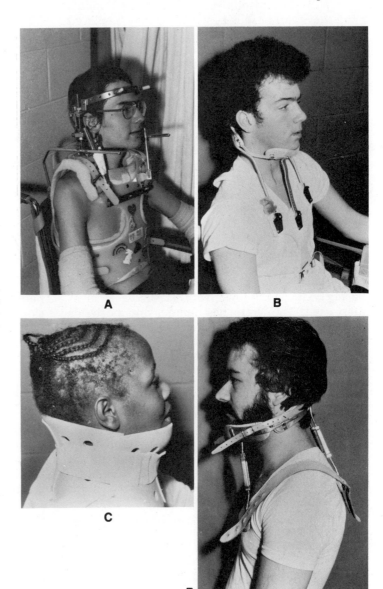

**Figure 22–1.** Cervical immobilization and stabilization devices. *A,* Halo jacket; note tightening devices taped to right upright. *B,* SOMI (sternal occipital mandibular immobilizer). *C,* Four-poster collar. *D,* Plastizote Philadelphia collar.

quent x-rays and evaluation by the orthopedic surgeon.

For a lesser degree of immobilization of the cervical spine, the SOMI (sternal occipital mandibular immobilizer) (Fig. 22–1B) or the four-poster collar (Fig. 22–1C) may be considered. For the patient who requires still lesser degrees of immobilization, the molded Plastizote Philadelphia collar (Fig. 22–1D) may be used. Although this is more comfortable than the SOMI or four-poster collar because of its compressibility, it provides lesser degrees of immobilization. The main problem with this device is skin irritation caused by friction, which occurs under the chin. The use of materials that will decrease shearing, such as a silk scarf, will help avoid this problem. When the halo device is removed, patients should be placed in the Philadelphia collar for a prescribed time, depending upon individual needs. Likewise, those patients using the SOMI or four-poster collar may be placed in a Philadelphia collar before immobilization is discontinued completely.

Once a decision has been made to discontinue all devices, the patient should be weaned slowly. It is best to start with one hour out of an immobilizer per day, gradually increasing this time to the patient's pain tolerance. As the weaning process proceeds, cervical isometric exercises can be initiated to strengthen weakened muscles. The weaning process should take no longer than two weeks, at which point the patient would be free of the device and without pain. Muscular discomfort while in the device, particularly in the halo, is very common and responds to reassurance and mild analgesia. The same is true of the discomfort experienced during the weaning process from the immobilizing device.

For the thoracic and lumbar spines, a molded plastic body jacket lined with Plastizote is most often used. The jacket has anterior and posterior shell components that are attached by Velcro closures on either side. In the patient with a high thoracic injury, a SOMI device is attached to the jacket to provide further stabilization of the spine. Most patients can tolerate the jacket well, although it will require frequent minor revisions during the initial stages because of pressure points and mild discomfort. The anterior-inferior portion of the jacket can be cut away to permit suprapubic tapping or performance of the Credé maneuver for patients who are involved in bladder retraining programs. The jacket is usually worn until that time when the spine is deemed stable by the orthopedic surgeon.

As with the cervical devices, a gradual weaning process is necessary to minimize patient discomfort. While the body jacket is worn during the initial phases, the skin should be examined frequently for breakdown. During the day or evening, while self-care is going on and prior to the appli-

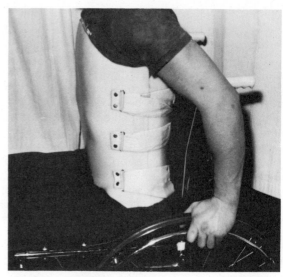

**Figure 22–2.** Thoracic/Lumbar immobilization and stabilization device. Molded plastic body jacket.

cation of the jacket, the patient can be log-rolled from side to side for cleansing of the skin and inspection for ulceration. Depending on the individual circumstances and the status of the spine, the jacket may be removed while the patient is in bed or sleeping. Again, log-rolling is used for removal. The neurosurgical members of the team are involved not only in the decision on immobilization but also in the decisions for possible surgical intervention. The clinical presentation, the type of fracture, the degree of instability, and the findings on the myelogram or computerized axial tomographic (CAT) scan will dictate possible surgical intervention. Myelography is indicated, especially in incomplete lesions, since disc or bony fragment compression may be responsible for part of the neurological picture. Although surgical decompression is still controversial in such situations, operation for removal of pressure is believed by many to be indicated.

A treatment protocol should be developed for the acutely injured spinal cord patient that would include high-dose steroids and osmotic diuretics to minimize cord edema and possibly to limit the degree of further neurological damage. Because of the initial trauma that occurs, as well as the use of steroids, immediate treatment should also include the use of antacids in addition to $H_2$ histamine antagonists to minimize the development of stress ulceration, which is so common in these patients. The use of prophylactic heparin to lessen the risk of pulmonary embolism in these patients at extremely high risk is also open to question because of the danger of further bleeding locally, in the cord, or elsewhere. Although it has been believed by many that low doses of heparin are not effective as a prophylaxis of thromboembolism in this group of patients, most centers will initiate a program of 5000 units every 12 hours as the patient's condition is stabilized.

Orthopedic surgical considerations include evaluating the instability of the spine, prescribing the appropriate immobilizing device, and making the decision for or against use of stabilizing procedures. Some patients will also need attention to other fracture sites. Long bone fractures of the up-per and lower extremities are not uncommon in such patients and will require operative fixation or splinting or both. This will further impair the functional level of the patient, particularly if this extremity has motor and sensory capabilities intact. An opinion from the orthopedic surgeon is expected in the initial rehabilitation process to determine the time at which these bones are healed enough to support weight.

## Fractures

*by William E. Staas, Jr., M.D.*

Long bone fractures in spinal cord–injured patients may occur at the time of spinal injury or later. Those occurring in the subacute or chronic phase are either caused pathologically or by trauma.

Acute fractures occurring at the time of spinal injury most often result from high-energy forces, thus the location of fracture as well as the pathomechanics are no different from that in other patients. The management may require internal fixation; many orthopedic surgeons think this can be done safely and with good results. Some of the earlier thinking regarding avoidance of operative procedures and internal fixation has changed as more experience has been gained. It is still accepted, however, that when open techniques are contraindicated, a Hoffman device or use of pillow splints and avoidance of a plaster cast, especially in the totally insensate patient, offer the safest alternatives with fewer complications.

Pathological fractures occur most commonly in the distal femur and proximal tibia (Fig. 22–3) and often are associated with minor trauma such as turning in bed, transfer activities, and therapeutic range of motion exercises. Operative management is usually not recommended. Well-padded splints or pillow splints will usually suffice. This is in contradistinction to the principles discussed for acute phase fractures. It is well known that in spinal cord–injured patients with long bone fractures healing of these fractures occurs quite readily, with exuberant callus formation. Every effort must be made to maintain adequate alignment during the

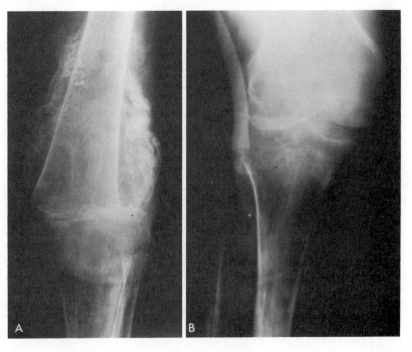

Figure 22–3. Pathologic fractures at the most common sites. *A*, distal femur; *B*, proximal tibia.

healing process, at the same time that the patient is kept as functional as possible. Cast or plaster immobilization has been a problem, especially in patients with severe or total sensory loss, because of skin breakdown.

In the spinal cord–injured patient who sustains a traumatic fracture in the chronic phase, these injuries are most often due to high-energy forces as is true in the acute phase. Internal fixation may be appropriate, but whenever possible, nonoperative management should be considered, including the use of well-padded splints and pillow splints. Again it is important to individualize treatment, to maximize patient independence during management of fractures, and to minimize the risk of skin breakdown.

For the patient who is ambulatory or has potential to be ambulatory, union at the fracture site is imperative. For the nonambulatory patient, this is less critical and nonunion may be acceptable.

# Respiratory System Management

by Stanley R. Jacobs, M.D. and Jay D Roberts, M.D.

## THE ACUTE STAGE

In the early phase, the major life-threatening complications that occur in cervical and high thoracic spinal cord–injured patients are hypoventilation, atelectasis, pneumonia (bacterial aspiration), pulmonary emboli, pulmonary edema, and pulmonary arrest. Respiratory death is the leading cause of mortality in acute spinal cord injury.

Pathophysiological changes with C5 to T1 quadriplegic patients include ventilatory, cough, and sigh alterations. Loss of the intercostal muscles leaves only the diaphragm and sternocleidomastoid muscles intact. Vital capacity averages between 1000 and 1500 cc initially and increases to 2000 to 2500 cc after two months. Blood gases show an average partial arterial oxygen pressure ($PaO_2$) of 70 to 80 mm Hg acutely but as the vital capacity increases to 2000 cc, the $PaO_2$ will approach normal values. With a vital capacity of 1000 cc or greater, there is usually no need for assisted ventilation, but when the vital capacity drops to 600 to 700 cc or below, a ventilator is mandatory. The diaphragm, which contributes 40 to 60 per cent of the tidal volume, does most of the ventilatory work. The accessory muscles of breathing—the sternocleidomastoids—should be strenthened and are believed to be able to contribute to the increased vital capacity.

Immediate studies should include a chest x-ray, arterial blood gases, pulmonary function studies such as a vital capacity by portable respirometer, complete blood count, and 12-lead EKG with continuous EKG monitoring.

When there is airway obstruction, the major responsibility is to maintain or achieve an adequate airway without moving the neck so that further spinal cord damage will be avoided. Adequate ventilation is assured if the partial arterial carbon dioxide pressure ($PaCO_2$) is 40 mm Hg or less. At no time should adequate oxygenation be compromised to avoid assisted ventilation; a $PaO_2$ of 60 mm Hg is the minimal acceptable value. In addition, many centers suggest fractional inspired oxygen concentration ($FIO_2$) supplementation to give added protection to the spinal cord.

The vital capacity of 1500 cc is needed for an effective cough. Loss of the active expiratory muscles (abdominals and internal intercostals) makes assisted coughing mandatory. Expiratory flow rates less than 40 cm $H_2O$ indicate poor cough capability. The best way to ensure bronchial cleansing is to assist coughing and maintain chest wall range of motion. In the acute phase the chest wall and diaphragm will not fibrose and develop fixed contractures; however, this can occur and gradually become a serious impediment to adequate ventilation. Therefore, chest range of motion exercises and assisted coughing should be started frequently within a week of injury by inflating the chest either by a deep breath, intermittent positive pressure breathing (IPPB) machine or Ambu bag, and then expelling the air by thoracic abdominal pressure. A nasogastric tube may have to be inserted to prevent gastric dilitation because such distention can easily block diaphragm muscle descent. Without adequate diaphragm excursion and rate of descent, ventilation may be inadequate and so-called *meteorism* can be a cause of apnea and sudden death in these patients and is preventable.

The normal person deep breathes six to eight times per hour, but sigh depth and frequency diminish greatly in quadriplegia. The sigh optimally spreads surfactant and stimulates its production.

*Text continues on page 392.*

**Figure 22–4.** Assisted cough technique to assure bronchial cleansing, demonstrated here by inflating chest with Ambu bag and then expelling air by thoracic pressure. (From Shapiro, and Harrison: Clinical Application of Respiratory Care. Chicago, Yearbook Medical Publication, Inc., 1979.

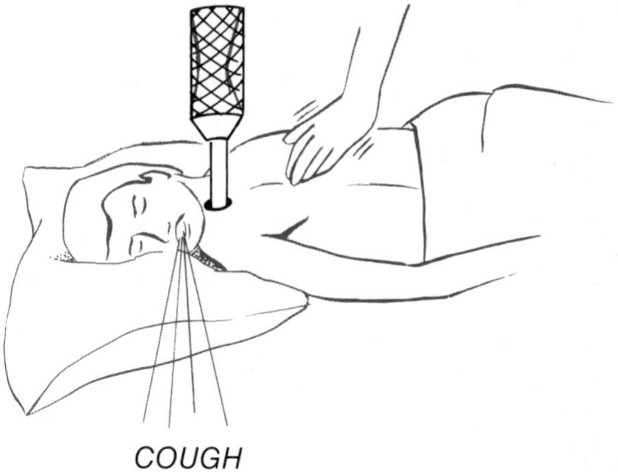

COUGH

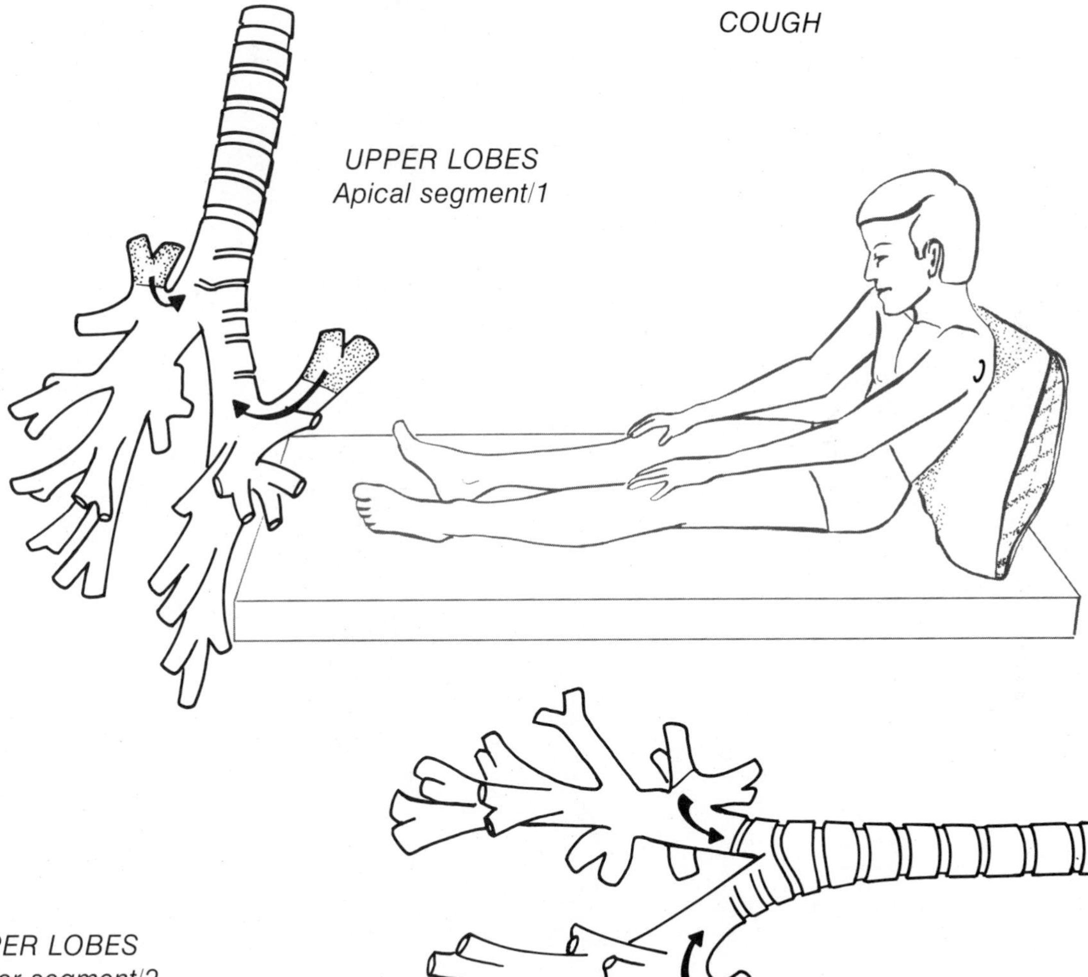

UPPER LOBES
Apical segment/1

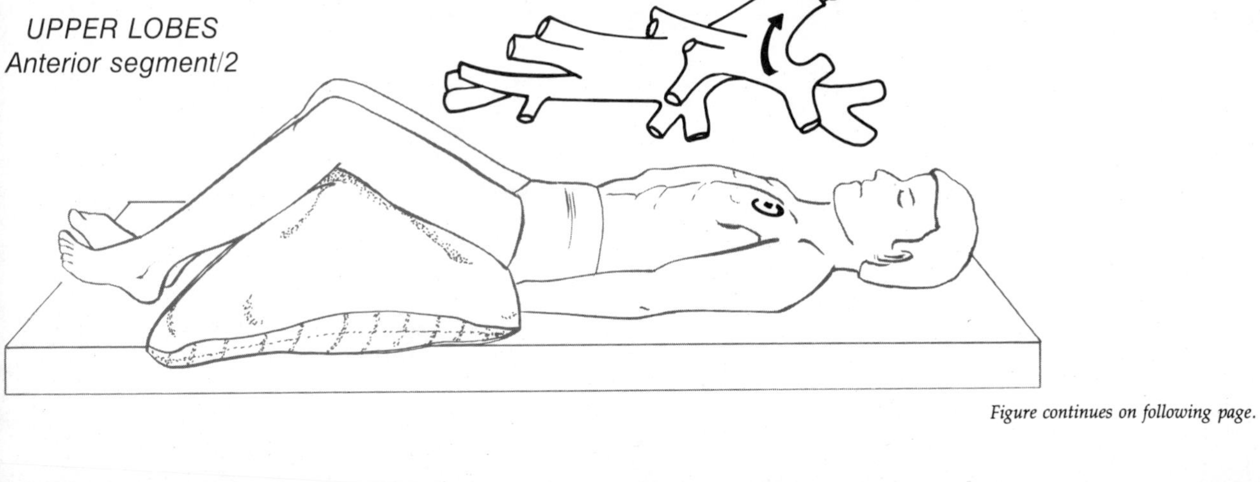

UPPER LOBES
Anterior segment/2

*Figure continues on following page.*

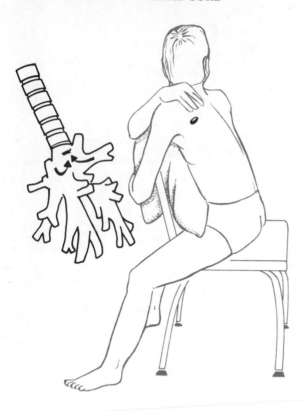

**Figure 22–4** *Continued.*

**UPPER LOBES**
*Posterior segment/3*

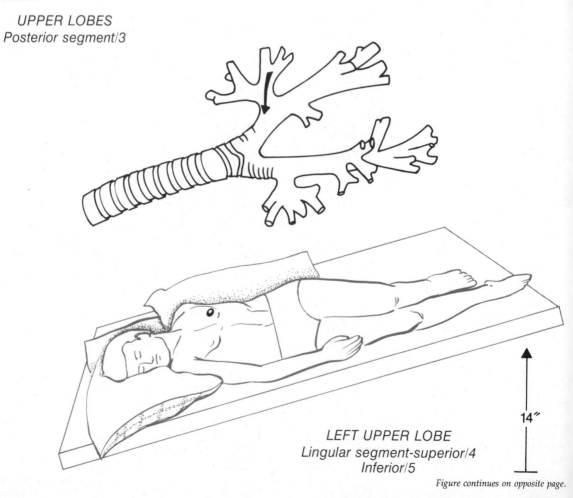

14″

**LEFT UPPER LOBE**
*Lingular segment-superior/4*
*Inferior/5*

*Figure continues on opposite page.*

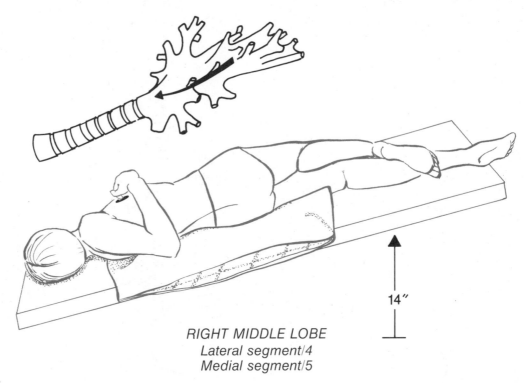

RIGHT MIDDLE LOBE
*Lateral segment/4*
*Medial segment/5*

**Figure 22–4** *Continued.*

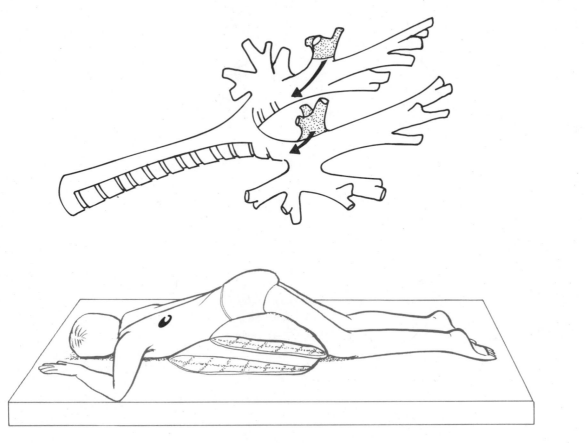

LOWER LOBES
*Superior segment/6*

*Figure continues on following page.*

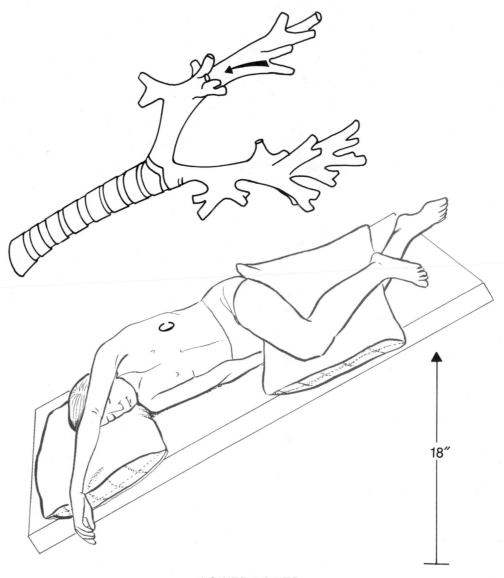

*LOWER LOBES*
*Anterior basal segment/8*
**Figure 22–4** *Continued.*

*Figure continues on opposite page.*

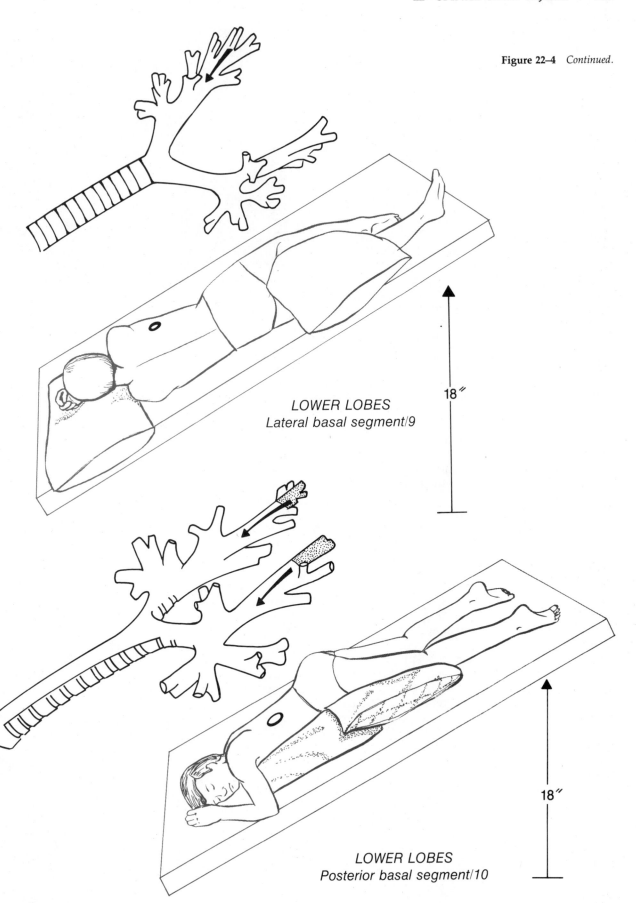

Figure 22–4 *Continued.*

*LOWER LOBES*
*Lateral basal segment/9*

18″

*LOWER LOBES*
*Posterior basal segment/10*

18″

Without adequate surfactant, alveolar tension remains equal and small alveoli collapse into the larger alveoli, causing progressive atelectasis and hypoxemia. Utilizing IPPB for these patients restores the sigh function and prevents hyposurfactant atelectasis. Any continuous ventilator used must have automatic sigh control.

When the diaphragm work-up reveals unilateral loss of diaphragm function and the patient is positioned on the side, the weak diaphragm should be uppermost, with the strong diaphragm closest to the bed surface. When the patient is sidelying, the hydrostatic recoil effect of the abdominal viscera is strongest on the lower diaphragm. This maximizes remaining force and excursion. The amount of air the diaphragm can move is directly dependent on the amount of passive dome effect caused by abdominal recoil. In the normal person, this recoil is passively maximized by abdominal wall tone as well as the hydrostatic recoil of the intra-abdominal viscera. The patient with high spinal cord injury in the acute phase loses recoil of the abdominal wall. If the strong diaphragm is placed uppermost when the patient is sidelying, the only force left to return the diaphragm to a maximally domed preinspiratory position is lost. The amount of inhalation is directly proportional to the amount of air exhaled, and this exhalation depends entirely on the passive recoil of the compressed abdominal viscera.

If the patient with high spinal cord injury whose ventilation is marginally satisfactory is placed in a sitting position without careful study, acute hypoventilation and respiratory failure may result. These patients usually have isolated weakened diaphragmatic breathing. Sitting them erect causes the abdominal contents to drop away from the diaphragm. The diaphragm assumes an end-expiratory (preinspiratory) flattened position instead of the usual normally domed preinspiratory position. Therefore, the total inspiratory excursion is significantly decreased. With a 60-degree head-up elevation, the vital capacity drops approximately 30 per cent compared to the supine vital capacity. This drop can be enough to trigger respiratory failure.

If the prone position is used, the effect on tidal volume, respiratory rate, vital capacity, and blood gases should be carefully monitored. Many patients cannot tolerate the prone position because abdominal content descent is blocked and inspiratory capacity is greatly compromised. This may precipitate sudden cardiac or respiratory arrest or both.

The recommended therapy is application of an abdominal binder or sometimes a corset without stays. This corset or binder prevents decrease in abdominal visceral hydrostatic pressure. Proper elevation of the diaphragm, inspiratory reserve, and vital capacity are maintained.

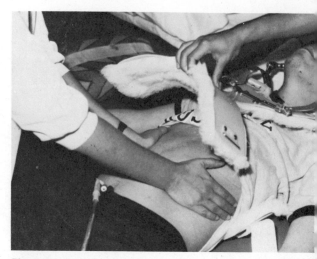

**Figure 22–5.** With halo jacket; side straps are loosened and jacket front is lifted to allow access to thoracic abdominal area for assisted cough technique.

Before oral intake is allowed, the patient's ability to swallow should be evaluated. The neck should be stabilized prior to eating in the event that an oral or pharyngeal phase swallowing defect exists; aspirated food could provoke severe coughing and uncontrolled neck motion. Swallowing can be tested with small amounts of dextrose and water and if it is satisfactory, liquids may be started. The patient may then progress to pureed, soft, and regular food. If there is a swallowing problem, it is helpful to evaluate vocal cord motion, provided that neck motion can be controlled safely. The supine position should be avoided for two hours after meals, and large meals should be avoided initially.

It is recommended that fluid intake be less than 1500 cc the first 24 hours because excessive fluid can easily result in pulmonary edema from loss of sympathetic tone and increased vessel permeability. A low blood pressure does not require volume replacement unless true shock or preshock exists. Central venous pressure, pulmonary wedge pressure together with blood gases, pH, and urinary output are more reliable indicators.

## WEANING THE SPINAL CORD–INJURED PATIENT FROM THE VENTILATOR

Intermittent mandatory ventilation is not helpful in weaning the severely compromised patient. The traditional method of starting a patient with a few minutes off the ventilator two or three times a day and gradually increasing time off acts as a safe, graded exercise; emotional support and monitoring of symptoms, vital signs, and arterial blood gases should be provided.

## THE CHRONIC STAGE

If a patient is to be transferred after the acute phase of injury to a center, the status of secretions and the effect of transport on respiratory function as it relates to time, method, and personnel must be carefully evaluated. If the patient has marginal respiratory function or is on a ventilator, special arrangements for staff and equipment should be made in advance.

Approximately only one in ten quadriplegic patients who are placed on a ventilator will remain on it, and most will increase their initial vital capacities dramatically by about one liter. Once the respiratory system has stabilized, it is hoped that the patient will still have normal lungs. Pathophysiologically, only the ventilatory system is weakened. Even with quiet breathing, the ventilatory energy needed to breathe is greater in these patients than normal. However, without the added stress of pneumonia and hypersecretion, the elevated energy cost of breathing lowers endurance reserve but by itself, is rarely the cause of ventilator dependence.

### SPECIAL PROBLEMS

**Unilateral Diaphragmatic Paralysis.** Diagnosis is determined by double-exposed full inspiration/ expiration plain film and vital capacity. It may require up to 18 months for a lower motor neuron–injured phrenic nerve to regenerate, but most injuries begin to improve in three to five months. Electrodiagnosis may be of value. Essential features in the treatment are use of incentive spirometry, evaluation of the effects of sitting up on vital capacity, and use of a custom-made corset or pneumobelt.

**Elderly Patients.** These patients may have prior respiratory system disease such as chronic obstructive pulmonary disease or asthma and a careful history is important. Certain changes in the respiratory system occur with aging, and, despite normal vital capacities, the normal values for $PaO_2$ in the elderly are less than in younger patients. For example, in the 60-year-old person, the lower normal limit $PaO_2$ is 80 mm Hg and in the 80-year-old, 60 mm Hg. This change may be caused by pulmonary shunting. When quadriplegia is superimposed on the aging lung, the patient may need greater than usual amounts of oxygen support. To be effective, this support may have to be by face mask. Despite reasonable vital capacity, these patients may need ventilator support. Because of the loss of oxygen absorption reserves and the increased ventilatory demand that this creates, they might require this for several months. In addition, they are more susceptible to atelectasis, cardiac arrhythmias, and ischemia in the acute phase. The usual methods of postural drainage, percussion, clapping, suctioning, and assisted cough are effective. Sometimes bronchoscopic lavage is necessary. Should atelectasis develop, close monitoring with x-rays and blood gases is essential.

**High Quadriplegia, C1 to C3.** These patients obviously require assisted ventilation indefinitely. The high quadriplegic patient does not experience dyspnea or labored breathing; therefore, ventilatory failure without fail-safe alarms can cause quiet death. While it is not the purpose of this chapter to discuss the management of the permanently ventilator-dependent quadriplegic patient, several suggestions to improve the patient's environment appear appropriate. A simply battery operated horn or bell attached to a low-pressure signaling device can supplement the usual alarm system to permit the patient to signal nurses for usual needs. In addition, an electrolarynx may be used to facilitate communication with staff and family.

# Cardiovascular Problems

*by Frank Naso, M.D. and William E. Staas, Jr., M.D.*

There are a number of phenomena that occur with relative frequency in the spinal cord–injured patient that can be grouped as cardiovascular problems. In some instances these phenomena are only minor; when treatment is necessary, it is effective and without major sequelae. Such is the case with orthostatic hypotension, which is prominent in quadriplegia but is easily treated. On the other hand, there are instances of life-threatening complications that require interventions which are unusual in rehabilitation medicine. Such is the case with reflex bradycardia and cardiac arrest. Each of the common areas is reviewed and an accepted protocol of treatment is outlined.

## ORTHOSTATIC HYPOTENSION

Orthostatic hypotension is characterized by a precipitous drop in systolic and diastolic blood pressure along with an elevation in heart rate. It has been demonstrated that a significant change in pulse and blood pressure can occur in high spinal cord–injured patients. Among the activities associated with this phenomenon are postural changes, such as changing from the recumbent to the sitting position, transfer activities, eating, and drinking. In the neurologically intact individual, similar activities are more commonly associated with a rise in blood pressure and heart rate. The cause for postural hypotension seems to be related to the pooling of blood in dependent extremities and the absence of reflex vasoconstriction in those with lesions above the sympathetic outflow (T5 to T8). Although tachycardia occurs (vagolytic response via carotoid body), it cannot maintain an adequate blood pressure. Patients complains of dizziness, lightheadedness or a feeling of faintness. On occasion, they may suddenly lose consciousness without preceding complaints. Immediate treatment includes placing the patient in the recumbent position with the head down and legs elevated. If the syndrome occurs while the patient is sitting in a wheelchair, tilting the wheelchair backward will relieve the symptoms.

Once the problem is recognized, preventive measures should be instituted. Among those that have been found to be helpful are the following: use of thigh-length elastic stockings and abdominal binder, very gradual change in body position from supine to sitting prior to the major position change, rest periods between changes from supine to sitting, and elevation of leg rests when in the wheelchair. Occasionally, ephedrine sulfate in doses of 25 to 30 mg once to four times daily with sodium chloride and fluid supplementation may be necessary.

Generally, the use of elastic stockings along with abdominal binders and gradual change in body position will be adequate to prevent this problem. Some patients with protracted cases will require supplemental medication. If ephedrine, salt and fluid-loading are inadequate, fluorinated steroids may be needed. Gradually as the patient spends more time in the sitting position, orthostatic hypotension tends to resolve as a clinical problem. Generally, this is in a time frame of several months. When the situation resolves, the treatment measures may be gradually withdrawn. Indeed, the low blood pressure may be replaced by episodic hypertension and the syndrome of autonomic hyperreflexia as spasticity appears.

## AUTONOMIC HYPERREFLEXIA

The syndrome of autonomic hyperreflexia, first described in 1917 by Head and Riddoch, is characterized by a sudden onset of hypertension, bradycardia, sweating, piloerection, flushing, dilated pupils, nasal stuffiness, blurred vision, and headache in high spinal cord–injured patients. It usually occurs with lesions at or above the T6 level and characteristically appears within several months after injury as the phase of spinal shock subsides. The incidence has been reported as high as 85 per cent in quadriplegic patients. Although it may be present for many years, it classically subsides within three years of injury but may reappear at any time, following a symptom-free interval. Numerous stimuli have been associated with the syndrome. Distention of the bladder or rectum is a not uncommon cause. It is not unusual to see the problem with fecal impaction or with rectal stimulation that occurs with evacuation. Bladder calculus, decubitus ulcers, and ingrown toenails are also causes. In a small number of patients, no known etiology can be found. Hypertension is clearly a major danger because seizures and even death as a result of cerebral hemorrhage may ensue, especially in the elderly patient.

The pathophysiology of autonomic hyperreflexia is complex and involves afferent impulses initiated by the noxious stimuli. These impulses then enter the posterior horn of the spinal cord where segmental reflexes may be initiated. Impulses also ascend the spinal cord, synapsing with neurons of the intermediolateral column in the thoracic spinal cord initiating vasoconstriction, which is particularly intense in the splanchnic bed. The thoracolumbar sympathetic trunks are activated; this results in sweating, vasoconstriction, and piloerection. Above the level of injury, and in some cases below it, hyperhidrosis is observed. As a result of vasoconstriction, severe hypertension is produced with headache and typical flushing above the level of injury along with pallor below the level of spinal injury.

In the neurologically intact human, inhibitory impulses from higher centers in the brain stem counteract vasoconstrictor reflexes. In the high spinal cord–injured patient, however, the descending inhibitory impulses are ineffective because of the spinal cord injury so that the spinal reflexes are left unchecked. Bradycardia is seen in approximately 40 to 50 per cent of patients during the acute episode, is initiated by baroreceptors in the carotid sinus, and is aortic arch–mediated through the medullary vasomotor center. This is a compensatory mechanism that is ineffectual in reducing blood pressure during acute episodes. Other cardiac findings include premature ventricular contractions, bigeminal pulses, elevation of the T wave, and the appearance of U waves on the electrocardiogram.

In view of the severity of the problem, it is imperative that the syndrome be recognized and managed properly and promptly. Any spinal cord–

injured patient with a level of injury above T6 who complains of headache or sweating should have the pulse and blood pressure recorded. If hypertension is present, with or without bradycardia, appropriate measures should be taken to eliminate the noxious stimuli. In most cases, this entails establishing free bladder drainage or evacuation of the bowel. For the patient with an indwelling Foley catheter, it may mean changing the catheter and later evaluating for bladder calculi. For the patient on intermittent catheterization, prompt evacuation of the bladder and re-evaluation of the frequency of catheterizations are required. In the presence of fecal impaction, the bowel should be decompressed digitally if necessary, or by rectal wash. Occasionally, a high colonic enema is necessary.

Pharmocological agents including amyl nitrite, guanethidine and mecamylamine are occasionally indicated. Amyl nitrite pearls may be inhaled for rapid reduction in blood pressure. Its effect, however, is short term. Mecamylamine in divided doses of 2.5 to 12.5 mg per day offers effective control by producing ganglionic blockade and is said to be relatively free of side effects in the doses indicated. Guanethidine is a peripheral sympatholytic agent that has a longer duration of action than mecamylamine and is effective in 2.5 to 15 mg doses per day. However, because of its longer duration of action, a single daily dose is effective in controlling the problem. Rarely, with an acute life-threatening episode, one must use more drastic means to produce an effective reduction of blood pressure. In this situation, intravenous agents or occasionally, spinal anesthesia may be necessary.

In the patient who experiences the dysreflexia syndrome, with minor stimulation such as occurs with rectal manipulation or colonic irrigation, it may be well to consider using the appropriate drug prior to instrumentation. This is particularly true for the procedures of cystoscopy and cystometrogram, which are frequent causes for dysreflexia. If hypertension does occur with the instrumentation, management should include immediate cessation of the instrumentation and decompression of the bladder or bowel. If this is inadequate, pharmacological agents might be used.

## REFLEX BRADYCARDIA AND CARDIAC ARREST

Reflex bradycardia with and without cardiac arrest has been observed and reported in high cervical spinal cord injuries. This is primarily a problem occurring in the first six weeks following injury during the phase of spinal shock. Classically, it occurs during tracheal stimulation and is more likely to occur in the presence of hypoxia. It is believed to be caused by a vasovagal reflex that normally is counteracted by sympathetic response. In the spinal cord–injured patient, however, sympathetic outflow is impaired as a result of the injury. Treatment for the acute episode includes administration of oxygen and atropine. Adequate oxygenation may prevent recurrent episodes, but, if this is not the case, maintenance atropine may be necessary. If these agents are not effective, rarely, insertion of a cardiac pacemaker may be necessary. This is particularly true in elderly individuals who have cardiac disease and who cannot tolerate the lower cardiac output related to the bradycardia. If cardiac arrest occurs, the emergency team must be called to assist in cardiopulmonary resuscitation. This CPR, however, must be initiated by the treatment team. Those involved in resuscitation should keep in mind the unique problems of dealing with this situation in the cervical spinal cord–injured patient. Such problems as dealing with the neck-immobilizing device and the surgical stability of the spine must be considered with insertion of the endotracheal tube. Esophageal airways are available for effective ventilation in situations involving instability of the spine.

## THROMBOEMBOLISM

Thromboembolic phenomena are common in spinal cord–injured patients, and it is quite likely that phlebitis is present in well over half the cases. The chief cause of death in acute spinal cord injury is either pulmonary infarction or pulmonary infection. Although most patients survive the pulmonary embolism, the rehabilitation process is temporarily interrupted. Pulmonary ventilation is further impaired with recurrent embolism, producing dangerous hypoxia, especially in the high quadriplegic. Ventilatory assistance, including tracheostomy, is sometimes indicated in this situation. Close clinical observation is in order in these patients, but since many cases of phlebitis escape detection, the physician must retain a high index of suspicion because physical findings may be absent in many cases. Some centers routinely perform screening procedures of the lower extremities in patients with complete lesions. Doppler ultrasound, and impedance plethysmography can identify significant clot in the deep venous system of the thigh in over 90 per cent of cases; however, it is ineffective in the calf. On the other hand, the $I_{125}$ fibrinogen scan can identify clot in the calf in over 80 per cent of patients. When there is doubt, a venogram may be used for definitive diagnosis.

Prophylactic heparin in doses of 5000 units every 12 hours subcutaneously may be of help in decreasing the incidence of thromboembolism. This should be done as early as possible if no contraindication exists. It is generally believed, however, that this is not as effective in prophylaxis as it is with other high-risk patients. Multiple trauma patients may well be hypercoagulable when the prophylaxis is intiated too late in the process to be effective. Using herapin in prophylactic doses along with platelet-inhibiting agents may be more effective. The problem of pulmonary embolism continues in spite of aggressive prophylaxis and screening procedures. In this situation, the quadriplegic may not present with typical signs and symptoms. The absence of sensation below the level of the lesion frequently will eliminate the presence of pleuritic chest discomfort. However, some patients will complain of shoulder pain, which may be confused with musculoskeletal or radicular discomfort. Therefore, in the presence of the abrupt onset of shoulder pain, one should suspect the possibility of pulmonary embolism. Arterial blood gases are frequently not helpful, especially in those patients who already have ventilatory impairment and low arterial oxygen. A sudden change in vital signs with tachycardia and fever along with tachypnea may be the only signs. Indeed, if the fever persists in the absence of clinical or laboratory signs of infection, a diligent search for thromboembolism should be made. The ventilation perfusion scan is frequently helpful in diagnosing pulmonary embolism, but more diagnostic is a pulmonary arteriogram.

If phlebitis or pulmonary embolism is identified, full courses of continuous intravenous heparin, averaging 1000 units per hour, is the safest method of treatment. Partial thromboplastin time (PTT), monitored daily, will help in adjustments of infusion dosage. Optimal dosage will prolong the PTT twice normal. Treatment should continue for 7 to 10 days to be replaced by Warfarin until the patient no longer is immobilized. In the presence of pulmonary embolism, treatment should continue for 6 to 12 months. It should be kept in mind that these patients are at high risk for thromboembolism each time they are immobilized. It is not uncommon to see the problem cropping up after a surgical procedure such as a flap rotation for decubitus ulcers. Continued clinical and laboratory evaluation is important at this stage as well.

# The Neurogenic Bladder: Physiologic Mechanisms and Clinical Problems of Bladder Control

by William E. Staas, Jr., M.D. and Janet G. LaMantia, R.N., M.A.

Impairments in normal bladder function are common in patients with neurological disease. Most physicians have experienced the frustration of attempting to evaluate and manage such patients without achieving the desired goals. A referral to the urologist should be preceded by a thorough work-up and basic understanding of the problems and a plan for treatment. We will review the physiology of urination, the mechanisms and physiology of urinary continence, outline a classification of neurogenic bladders, and discuss bladder management. In addition, common problems associated with the neurogenic bladder are discussed.

## PHYSIOLOGY OF URINATION

In the neurologically intact adult, micturition is a coordinated act under reflex and voluntary control. Retention and expulsion of forces are balanced at all times and can be inhibited or facilitated by higher brain centers. In the infant bladder, emptying occurs solely as a spinal reflex. As the child develops it begins to perceive detrusor activity and associates this with desire to void. Between 18 and 30 months of age, the child learns inhibition contraction of pelvic floor muscles with reflex inhibition of the detrusor when the desire to void is experienced. Between 30 and 48 months of age, the child learns to urinate on command with associated volitional detrusor facilitation.

The events that occur during the two types of urination (desire and command) have been documented by electromyographic, cystometric, and radiological studies. On desire, the detrusor muscle is contracting in association with opening of the vesicle neck–internal sphincter. Then the pelvic floor relaxes and the bladder base lowers, followed by relaxation of the external sphincter. There is disagreement over the sequence of events during micturition on command. Langworthy reports initiation by facilitation of the detrusor, which contracts followed by relaxation of the pelvic floor and lowering of the bladder base. This is followed by relaxation of the vesicle neck and finally the external sphincter. Muellner suggests that voluntary urination is initiated by the diaphragm or abdominal muscles or both, with increase in intra-abdominal pressure. This is followed by relaxation of the pelvic floor muscles and descent of the vesicle neck with reflex contraction of the detrusor. Opening of the internal and external sphincters then follows in sequence.

Inhibition or interruption of urination begins at the external sphincter and is followed by elevation of the bladder base and closure of the vesicle neck–internal sphincter in association with relaxation of the detrusor. The contractions of the external sphincter occlude the urethral segment distal to the prostatic urethra. However, in the male the vesicle neck remains open and thus urine remains in the prostatic urethra at the termination of urination.

## MECHANISMS AND PHYSIOLOGY OF URINARY CONTINENCE

Bladder emptying and continence are dependent upon reciprocal balance of the forces of expulsion and retention. Continence is primarily dependent upon physical force and spinal reflexes, both of which can be facilitated or inhibited by the higher brain centers.

Continence depends on an intraurethral pressure that exceeds intravesical pressure. Pressures can be calculated by using Laplace's formula, $P = T_r$. P is pressure, T is wall tension, and $r$ refers to radius for a cylinder. The radius of the closed urethra is small. Therefore, even low wall tension will result in a high intraurethral pressure. Bladder pressure that rises slowly with increasing volume is thus opposed by a high intraurethral pressure. Grieve has reported the resting bladder pressure in normal individuals to be 10 to 20 mm Hg, whereas intraurethral pressures are 20 to 45 mm Hg. Other contributing factors include elastic, smooth, and striated mucle fibers of the urethra, as well as tissue tone, which tends to decrease with age.

## INCONTINENCE

Specific characteristics of the voiding pattern may aid in diagnosis. Precipitate voiding is typical of an incomplete upper motor neuron lesion. This may be found with brain or spinal cord disease and has been termed the *uninhibited neurogenic bladder*. Stress incontinence is associated with lower motor neuron lesions. Laughing, coughing, sneezing, lifting, and stair climbing are examples of precipitating stress. The problem may be neurogenic or muscular; the former is related to lower motor neu-

ron dysfunction of the detrusor and pelvic floor muscles, whereas the latter is associated with damage or relaxation of the pelvic floor muscles. This has been called the *autonomous bladder*. Overflow incontinence may occur in upper motor neuron or lower motor neuron lesions in association with acute urinary retention. Reflex incontinence is seen in patients with upper motor neuron lesions. This has been termed the *reflex* or *automatic bladder*. Dribbling occurs in patients with decreased or absent resistance to urine flow, such as may occur in spina bifida with spastic detrusor muscle and flaccid pelvic floor muscles.

## REFLEXES

Bladder function is controlled by three reflex centers: (1) ganglia within the detrusor muscle that maintain bladder tone as the volume of urine increases; (2) the spinal center located in the sacral spinal cord (S2 to S4); and (3) the supraspinal centers in the hypothalmus, limbic system, and midbrain, which facilitate and inhibit the spinal reflex center.

Voluntary and reflex voiding are under the control of the parasympathetic and the somatic systems. The sympathetic nervous system is not critical. Preganglionic parasympathetic fibers originate from the second, third, and fourth segments of the sacral spinal cord in the anterior and lateral horns. They exit with the ventral roots and become the pelvic nerves, synapsing with postganglionic fibers within the bladder wall. The somatic fibers also arise from the second, third, and fourth sacral segments in the anterior horns and exit in the ventral roots, subsequently becoming the pudendal nerve fibers to the striated muscles of the pelvic floor and external sphincter. Sensory input from both systems enters the dorsal roots and subsequently posterior horns in the same sacral segments as the efferents.

If the influence of higher centers in the brain is interrupted as occurs in spinal cord injury, the spinal center then is the only neuro-resource for reflex voiding. If the spinal center is injured, reflex voiding may be impossible. Six reflexes have been described in association with the sacral spinal center: (1) there is a gradual increase in bladder wall tension as urine volume increases. When threshold is reached, intramuscular sensory fibers are stimulated, sending impulses through the pelvic nerve to the sacral parasympathetic center. Motor impulses return in the same nerve and produce detrusor contraction. (2) As the result of detrusor contraction, proprioceptive fibers send impulses via the spinal nerve to the spinal center. They synapse and cause inhibition of somatic motor fibers of the external sphincter. Thus the pudendal nerve is inhibited and the pelvic floor relaxes. (3) Contraction of the pelvic floor and external sphincter initiates proprioceptive impulses, which traverse the pudendal nerve and subsequently inhibit the pelvic nerve. The detrusor muscle then relaxes. (4) Fibers within the bladder mucosa sensitive to chemical, thermal, and mechanical stimulation facilitate detrusor contraction via the pelvic nerve. (5) These same impulses from the bladder mucosa facilitate pelvic floor contraction via the pelvic nerve–pudendal nerve arc. (6) The passage of urine within the urethra inhibits the internal sphincter, as well as the external sphincter, resulting in relaxation. This is mediated via the pudendal nerve–pudendal nerve arc.

## CLASSIFICATION OF NEUROGENIC BLADDERS

The term neurogenic bladder does not connote a specific diagnosis or a single etiology. Rather it embraces the entire field of neurological urology. The patient's history, physical findings, and laboratory results permit establishment of the diagnosis and classification of the urological disturbance. Of importance are the neurological pathways involved, the extent of the lesion, and the voiding disturbance. Numerous classifications have been suggested, ranging from the most complex to the simplistic. In our opinion, the system proposed by Bors is the most physiologic and functional. It is summarized as follows:

  I.  Sensorimotor neuron lesion
      A.  Upper motor neuron lesions (above the conus—spinal reflex center)
          1.  Complete
          2.  Incomplete
      B.  Lower motor neuron lesions (below the conus)
          1.  Complete
          2.  Incomplete
      C.  Mixed lesions
          1.  Complete
          2.  Incomplete
 II.  Sensory neuron lesions
          1.  Complete
          2.  Incomplete
III.  Motor neuron lesions

The degree of bladder function or dysfunction can be estimated by determining the percentage of residual urine as it relates to total bladder capacity. Bors has found that residuals up to 20 per cent in patients with upper neuron lesions, and up to 10 per cent in those with lower motor neuron lesions, is compatible with satisfactory bladder function.

In contrast with the neurologically impaired, the normal bladder has intact sensation for temperature and distention. Saddle sensation and motor function are normal. Intravesicle pressure remains below 20 cm of water until the urge to void occurs between 350 and 500 cc. At that point, pressure rises to 60 to 80 cc of water. Uninhibited bladder contractions are absent during bladder filling. Vesicle capacity is 350 to 600 cc with no residual urine.

## BLADDER MANAGEMENT

Early urological management in the acute stage immediately after spinal cord injury involves continuous bladder drainage with a Foley catheter. In the 72 hours immediately after spinal injury the patient is in a catabolic state with accompanying diuresis. Intermittent catheterization is difficult at this stage because of the high bladder volumes within acceptable range. Once the patient's condition is medically stable, and he is no longer in need of intravenous therapy and can be fluid restricted, bladder training can begin.

Bladder retraining consists of a combination of modalities that include an intermittent catheterization program (ICP), fluid restriction, reflex stimulation of bladder, Credé maneuvers, and pharmacological intervention. Not all of these modalities are necessary in each patient. Bladder training can begin prior to specific diagnostic testing; however, the need for complete urodynamics is important in achieving a balanced bladder. The nature of vesicourethral function and the involvement of the autonomic and somatic nervous systems is very complex, and diagnosis of bladder type on symptoms or single urodynamic test can be misleading.

In early stages of bladder training, laboratory evaluations should be done weekly: urinalysis, culture, SMA 6-12, free fatty acids. Every other week blood urea nitrogen and creatinine levels should be tested, especially when nephrotoxic drugs are being used. As the bladder becomes balanced, cultures will only need to be done monthly and during the first year after discharge at three-month intervals.

The aim of bladder retraining is based on a functional approach to urinary drainage:

  I.  Unrestricted flow of urine from kidneys
      A.  Bladder and urethra catheter free
      B.  Relief of urethral obstruction
 II.  Abacterial state
      A.  Sterile intermittent catheterization
      B.  Frequent emptying of bladder at spaced intervals
III.  Bladder continence
      A.  Complete emptying of bladder at each voiding by developing enough force of expulsion for a long enough period of time.

Although it may be desirable to keep a catheter out of the bladder to decrease the risk of infection, urinary retention requires that a catheter be used. Intermittent catheterization is a bladder training technique developed to keep the catheter out of the bladder for a greater part of the time, and to eventually achieve the catheter-free state.

Continuing with the functional approach, the next step is relief of urethral obstruction. This needs specific diagnostic evaluation and may be treated by pharmacological or surgical intervention or both. In upper motor neuron lesions urodynamics may show that the external urethral sphincter displays high resistance, especially in early stages of spinal injury. There is also the possibility of obstruction of the posterior urethra, secondary to pressure in the upright sitting position. Occurrence of high residual urine is common in upper motor neuron injuries because of the incoordinated activity of the external sphincter and the bladder wall.

The abacterial state is maintained by strict adherence to a sterile intermittent catheterization program and frequently spaced intervals of bladder emptying (see later discussion).

The third part of the functional approach to bladder retraining is maintaining bladder continence, in which the bladder will empty completely, maintaining a force of contraction that is sufficient to expel urine and for a time long enough to empty the bladder. Again, urodynamics is very important in assessing detrusor dysynergia or hypotonicity. This can be done through pharmacological and reflex stimulation or manual Credé technique.

Specific urodynamic testing when correlated with the physical examination will lead to diagnosis of the specific dysfunction. It enables the physician to correctly intercede with a plan based on physiological data. Tests of the lower urinary tract that should be included in the complete urodynamic work-up are:

1. Electromyography—to evaluate striated external sphincter function by assessing the innervation and integrity of the reflex pathway during rest and voluntary sphincter contraction and reflex detrusor contraction.
2. Urethral pressure—to evaluate bladder neck and urethral smooth muscle function. The intraurethral pressure along the length of the urethra is measured.
3. Cystometry—to evalute detrusor function in terms of sensation, pressure volume responses, reflex detrusor contractions, and voluntary ability to suppress detrusor contraction.
4. Uroflowmetry—to evaluate function of urethra and bladder by giving normal or abnormal flow rate reading; is not specifically diagnostic.

The repeated use of urodynamics during the bladder retraining program will give the practitioner information about which stimuli need to be strengthened or which need to be inhibited to encourage proper voiding and bladder emptying.

The intermittent catheterization program can be started when urodynamic testing is started or completed. There are a number of situations in which ICP is contraindicated, and a better method is to use an indwelling catheter or a suprapubic cystostomy. In the early phase of injury, in the postoperative period, or when major illness intervenes, it will be impossible to restrict fluid intake, especially if intravenous fluids are necessary. Temporarily using an indwelling catheter is clearly a more reasonable alternative until fluids can be restricted. ICP is also contraindicated when major anatomical abnormalities are present, such as meatal or urethral stenosis. Also in those patients with high cervical lesions and nonfunctioning upper extremities, it may be more reasonable to insert a Foley catheter to simplify bladder care for the family.

If none of these problems exist, the intermittent catheterization program may proceed as follows:

The patient's fluid intake is restricted to 1800 to 2000 cc daily and regulated to 400 cc at breakfast, lunch, and dinner; 200 cc at 10 AM, 4 PM, and 8 PM. The patient is given nothing by mouth from 8 PM to 8 AM.

Intermittent sterile catheterization is done every four hours. The time interval is managed according to the residual volumes obtained. The volume should be less than 400 cc; if it is more, the catheterization interval should be decreased to every three hours. Eventually the patient should begin to void spontaneously, although urodynamic testing and pharmacological intervention may still be necessary.

Concomitant with intermittent catheterization is the triggering of reflex bladder activity. Credé maneuvers should not be done prior to specific urodynamic work-up. In spastic bladders affected by upper motor neuron injury, there are trigger areas to stimulate reflex voiding. The most effective trigger area is suprapubic. The application of rhythmic tapping is thought to produce a summation effect on the tension receptors in the bladder wall, and activation of the reflex arc via the afferent discharges produced. The best suprapubic triggering technique is to tap the suprapubic area rapidly seven or eight times, stop three seconds and repeat. This process can be done for one to two minutes. If the patient voids, the volume should be recorded and the patient catheterized for a "post-voiding" residual volume. These two volumes should be specifically identified as the *voiding volume* and the *catheterized volume*. If the patient does not void, he should be catheterized if it is at the proper time interval. As the catheterization interval is decreased because the patient is spontaneously voiding, the triggering of the bladder should continue at intervals of every four hours. If the patient is taught to trigger his own bladder, it is not necessary that he wake during the night to do this if it will not be followed by catheterization.

In the beginning of the reflex stimulation the stimulus needs to be of high intensity and long duration. As the training progresses, the stimulus needed to produce voiding will be more specific, of shorter duration, and less intense. Care should be taken when the triggering technique is performed or directed that the force used to stimulate reflex activity does not cause cutaneous injury. This is especially important in patients receiving anticoagulation therapy. In addition to the suprapubic site, stimulation of other trigger areas includes: stroking the glans penis or vulva, dilating the anus, pulling on pubic hair, and stroking the thighs.

In "lower neuron bladders," Credé techniques are used to aid in opening bladder neck by increasing intravesical pressure. The Credé technique requires that the patient sit erect, draw in the abdomen (against strong thoracic inspiration and against a closed glottis). The patient places four fingers of both hands over suprapubic areas and applies pressure with increasing intensity. Voiding will occur for the length of time the bladder is compressed.

In the hospital environment, intermittent catheterization technique is always done with strict sterile technique. This is true whether a professional staff member, the patient, or a family member is performing the catheterization. In the home, sterile technique should be continued if possible. At times, modifications may occur because of the financial burden of disposable catheter trays. The family practitioner should investigate the possibility of reimbursement for these catheter sets, since many third parties, both public and private, may assume the cost. If "clean" technique is recommended, the patient and family must be fully educated in principles and practice of the technique. For patients who are progressing well through bladder training, intermittent catheterization will not be a continued financial burden, and could be looked upon as a temporary cost factor. For patients who are not progressing well through the program, or who want to remain on intermittent catheterization rather than have permanent catheter drainage or surgical intervention, a clean technique can be established. This should be considered during the rehabilitation and discharge planning period for inclusion in the patient and family education program.

In spite of sterile procedures, 90 per cent of patients will develop a positive urine culture at some point in their program. They may require a short course (seven to ten days) of appropriate antibiotic therapy without interruption of the catheterization program. If the patient is febrile, however, it is best to temporarily discontinue the intermittent catheterization and insert an indwelling catheter while treatment is initiated. When the patient has been afebrile for one or two days, the intermittent catheterization program may be reinstituted. Reinfection with the same or other organisms suggests inadequate treatment or anatomical abnormality in the genitourinary system. Tissue invasion, either in the kidney, deeply in the bladder wall, or in the prostate, may be responsible and require longer antibiotic treatment periods of four to six weeks. When reinfection does occur, it is best to do a complete urological survey.

The type of catheterization tray used will depend primarily on the patient's dexterity and needs, if cost is not a problem. A sterile set in which the catheter is contained in a closed sterile bag allows the C6 quadriplegic independence in self-catheterizing. Since the urine is contained in a closed bag, there is little chance of urine spilling on the bed, chair or clothing. Quadriplegics can also learn to catheterize themselves with straight red rubber catheters contained in sterile trays. Maintaining sterility is difficult because patients with higher lesions cannot put on sterile gloves. If a patient is to go home using such a tray, the nursing staff can put sterile gloves on the patient and demonstrate "clean" technique in a sterile environment.

With any type of bladder program it is important that the patient and family be aware of, and knowledgeable in, every aspect of the program: the

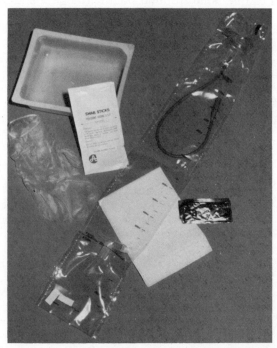

**Figure 22–6.** Catheterization tray with catheter enclosed in a sterile bag to maintain strict sterile technique. The set pictured can be used by a C6 quadriplegic.

goals, principles, procedures, possible complications, and appropriate steps to deal with problems and complications. Patients are responsible for catheterization, performing triggering and Credé techniques, and recording fluid intake and output. By discharge the patient and family should be totally proficient in handling bladder management; if they are not capable, other resources are located to provide for this need, such as community nursing service or attendant care. If the high quadriplegic cannot do his own catheterization, he should be able to totally direct and monitor the program. Intermittent catheterization alone will not always produce a balanced bladder. Pharmacological intervention may be necessary to deal with detrusor-sphincter dysynergia.

Some common problems and the pharmacological intervention employed to achieve a balanced bladder follow.

*PROBLEM*

I. Hypotonic-dysynergic detrusor (with or without increased outflow resistance): Pharmacological intervention is to increase bladder tone and decrease outflow resistance. Suggested drug:

   A. Cholinergic agent–bethanechol chloride (Urecholine) a parasympathomimetic agent. Is cholinesterase resistant, has relatively selective action on smooth muscle of bladder. Dosage: 25 to 50 mg tid. This drug is contraindicated in cases of known bladder outlet obstruction but can be combined with other pharmacological agents (such as phenoxybenzamine) or surgical attempts (external sphincterotomy) to decrease outlet obstruction.

II. Outflow resistance: spasm of the vesical neck and proximal urethral smooth muscle. Pharmacological intervention is aimed at relaxation of urethral smooth muscle. Suggested drug:

   A. Alpha-adrenergic blocker—Phenoxybenzamine. Dosage: 10 mg tid. Patient is started at 10 mg od and blood pressure is monitored for hypotensive effect.

III. Spasm of striated external sphincter: the external sphincter produces obstruction to urine outflow; pharmacological aim is to relax sphincter.

   A. Suggested drugs
      1. Baclofen, a polysynaptic inhibitor—a skeletal muscle relaxant used for general muscle spasticity will also affect external striated sphincter. Dosage: Baclofen can be started at doses of 5 mg qid to produce relaxation.
      2. Diazepam—muscle relaxant with central nervous system effects. Can be used in conjunction with polysynaptic inhibitor to produce desired relaxation effect. Dosage: 1 to 5 mg with doses of baclofen.

IV. Vesical hyperreflexia—in female patients on intermittent catheterization program in whom spontaneous voiding between catheterization is not a goal. Pharmacological aim is to decrease bladder contractility.

   A. Suggested drugs
      1. Anticholinergic—propantheline bromide to block uninhibited bladder contractions. Dosage: 15 mg q 4–6 hours.
      2. Imipramine hydrochloride—increases bladder capacity by decreasing bladder hypertonicity. Dosage: 25 mg qid.
      3. Ephedrine—increases urethral resistance by causing peripheral release of norepinephrine and direct stimulation of alpha and beta receptors. Dosage: 25 mg q 8–12 hours.
      4. Musculotropic relaxants—thought to act directly on smooth muscle at an intracellular site distal to the cholenergic receptor mechanism.
         a. Flavoxate hydrochloride: Dosage: 100 to 200 mg tid, po.
         b. Oxybutynin chloride. Dosage: 5 to 10 mg qid po.

In cases in which pharmacological agents and intermittent catheterization fail to produce a balanced bladder or program acceptable to the patient, other forms of intervention must be used. Intermittent catheterization programs may fail because the patient may not spontaneously void sufficiently, and the frequency of catheterization may be unacceptable or impractical for the patient or family to continue. Drugs that have produced the desired urological effect may produce undesired side effects, making it difficult to intervene pharmacologically. Another problem with bladder training is spontaneous voiding. Some patients will object to or have difficulty using an external collecting device, making spontaneous voiding an undesirable goal. Females, even with appropriate pharmacological intervention, may be incontinent between catheterization times. Female quadriplegics who cannot perform self-catheterization or trigger the bladder and who are frequently wet between catheterizations will find the bladder retraining program inadequate and may elect an alternative method to control the bladder.

## ALTERNATIVE METHODS FOR BLADDER MANAGEMENT

These are external sphincterotomy, Foley catheterization, urinary diversion, and suprapubic cystostomy.

**External Sphincterotomy.** The primary indications for external sphincterotomy are good detrusor contraction and confirmation by urodynamic testing of outlet obstruction at the external sphincter. External sphincterotomy is usually suggested after trials of intermittent catheterization and appropriate pharmacological therapy have proved unsuccessful in emptying the bladder with acceptable residual volumes. External sphincterotomy is accomplished by electrocautery of several layers of external sphincter tissue. These are done at varying positions around the circumference of the sphincter. One complication, temporary loss of erectile ability, has been reported associated with incisional sites at the 9 o'clock and 3 o'clock positions. There does not seem to be an obvious physiological explanation for loss of erection, and in the most recently reported cases return of erection occurred between three days and six months postoperatively. One author has postulated that the cause of loss of erection is in part associated with a loss of stimulation from chronic bladder irritation secondary to infection and high residual urine. With the removal of these sources of irritation the afferent input may be lessened and thereby erectile ability is decreased.

The procedure of sphincterotomy has enabled patients with elevated sphincter resistance to empty their bladders adequately.

**Continuous Catheter Drainage and Urinary Diversion.** There are considerations for continuous catheter drainage and urinary diversion when a balanced bladder is not achieved through the methods discussed previously. These considerations include upper tract deterioration, poor emptying that cannot be reversed or stabilized with pharmacological or surgical therapy, fistulas or abscesses that make the lower urinary tract unusable as a reservoir, and intractable incontinence in the female spinal cord–injured patient.

**Foley Catheters.** Foley catheters are most often used as an alternative drainage method for female spinal cord–injured patients because there are no satisfactory external collecting appliances for females. Foley catheters are not ideal for long-term management of bladder drainage, since they can lead to many complications: small trabeculated bladder; chronic bladder infection; renal and bladder calculi that are associated with infection; deterioration of upper urinary tract; and, in males, penile scrotal abscess secondary to poor catheter positioning. Hospitalized patients with Foley catheters should be maintained on a closed drainage system. With this technique, an antibiotic ointment is used around the meatal opening, the tubes are never detached, irrigation is not done unless blockage occurs, and the drainage bag is always dependent (if a reversal valve is not present). In the hospital, if blockage occurs, the catheter is pulled out and a new one is inserted. At home a leg bag can be worn through the day and closed drainage used at night. Basic guidelines for changing catheters is every two weeks in the hospital and every six weeks at home. Catheters may need to be changed more often if the catheter becomes blocked

frequently. Patients are instructed to check catheters for blockage by rolling the catheter gently between the fingers and noting the presence of grit or hardened materal. If any foreign material is in the catheter lumen, the catheter should be changed.

Catheters are manufactured in several materials: latex, Teflon-coated latex, and silicone. Silicone is recommended for long-term drainage, but Teflon-coated latex is adequate for six-week catheter changes. Results vary in studies of cost effectiveness of an all-silicone catheter as opposed to a Teflon-coated latex catheter. The cost differential is significant, and this should be considered when prescribing catheter type. The all-silicone type is more expensive. Catheter size should be determined by urethra capacity, with a loose fit being desirable. A 5 cc balloon is preferred, with the smallest amount of fluid necessary to retain the catheter. The smaller the surface area of the balloon, the less potential for encrustation and irritation to the bladder.

Foley catheters should be secured in men by taping the catheter to the abdomen. This will prevent constant pressure at the site of the penile-scrotal junction and possible fistula formation. The catheter may also be secured with lengthwise strips of tape from the catheter to the penis (Fig. 22–7). This taping technique prevents the catheter from sliding up and down in the urethra, which some authors believe "pumps" bacteria back up into bladder. This taping technique also prevents constant pressure and pull against the sphincter. Constant pressure on the sphincter mucosa can cause small tears and irritation. While on Foley catheter drainage the patient should be encouraged to drink large amounts

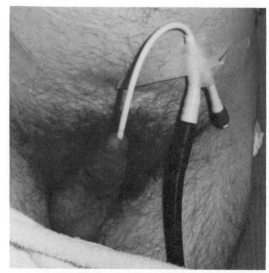

**Figure 22–7.** Indwelling Foley catheter with taping technique to prevent penile-scrotal fistula and abscess.

of fluid—between 3000 to 4000 cc per day. Patients are instructed to report any bleeding or signs of infection to their nurse or doctor.

## URINARY DIVERSIONS

Urinary diversion procedures are recommended (1) when the bladder cannot be used to store urine as in deterioration from-long term catheter placement; (2) when there is inadequate emptying and pharmacological and surgical relief of outlet obstructions are ineffective or unacceptable to the patient; (3) when sepsis recurs; and (4) when there is upper tract deterioration. The most common urinary diversions done today are ileal conduits and ureterostomy. Some patients elect to have these procedures done because they wish freedom from external collecting devices, catheter difficulties, and, possibly, intractable incontinence.

## SUPRAPUBIC CYSTOSTOMY

Suprapubic cystostomy is usually done when other means of bladder management have failed, although there is some controversy about this issue. Proponents of suprapubic cystostomy claim that it preserves the upper urinary tract while eliminating the need for prolonged bladder training, concomitant drug therapy, an external catheter device, and a catheter in the urethra. Antagonists of suprapubic drainage believe that it is a non-physiological method of urinary drainage, and that it can lead to long-term indwelling catheter problems, as with the Foley catheter. Most often, the suprapubic cystostomy is seen as an alternative and not an immediate form of management for the neurogenic bladder.

Use of the suprapubic catheter is supervised in the same manner as indwelling Foley catheters. There should be strict sterile technique in principles of insertion, removal, and connection for drainage. Catheter size is usually 24 to 26 F with 5 cc balloon. The smaller the balloon, the less surface area for foreign material to accumulate and irritate the bladder. The patient should be instructed that if at any time the suprapubic catheter is removed or becomes dislodged and cannot be replaced, a urethral catheter should be inserted. Consultation with a urologist may be necessary for this problem.

The ostomy area can be cleaned with mild soap and water. Patients should observe daily for any signs of purulent drainage or bleeding. Hair growing around the ostomy site can be trimmed or shaved as necessary. A dry dressing can be worn around the suprapubic tube to prevent drainage from soiling clothing.

## EXTERNAL COLLECTING DEVICES

External collecting devices include a multitude of latex condom-type sheaths, fasteners (tapes, glues, straps) and leg bags in which to collect the urine. No one brand or style of external device will work well for every patient. Experimentation is necessary to find the right combination of sheath, fastener, and leg bag to get proper drainage without urine leakage.

Enlisting the help of the community nursing service may assist the family physician in dealing with this problem following discharge. Much of the intervention is based on trial and error and often the nurse must assess the problem in the environment. The main difficulties with external collecting devices are twisting of the sheath inhibiting urine flow, the sheath soaking the patient, kinked tubing causing the sheath to pull off leading to the development of skin breakdown, and inability to correctly fit the penis with a latex sheath (as when the penis is too small or uncircumcised). Some general guidelines for use of external devices for the patient on an intermittent catheterization program are: (1) Do not use adhesives that will irritate the skin. (2) Check penile skin daily for problems. (3) Check the penis 20 minutes after applying adhesive to note for any constriction or swelling. (4) Apply all adhesive tapes and fasteners in a spiral fashion or in a way that will not constrict the penis if swelling or erection occurs.

If small sores develop or the skin of the penis becomes irritated, use of the external sheath should be temporarily discontinued during the night and a urinal propped against the pelvis for urine collec-

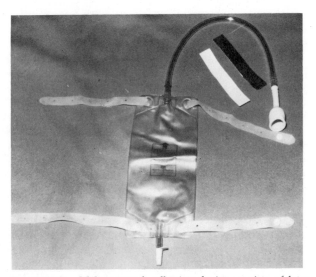

**Figure 22–8.** Male external collecting device consists of latex condom-type sheath, tapes, and collecting bag, which is worn on the leg and held in place with rubber or Velcro straps.

tion. Another alternative is to use a plastic disposable storage bag stuffed with toilet tissue and gently tied to the penis with 1-inch cotton binding. This method works well for patients who have little or no movement at night or when sitting in a wheelchair. One disadvantage is that transfers and turning tend to pull the bag off, causing incontinence. In addition, the bag needs to be replaced with each voiding. One advantage of this technique is that the penis can be cleaned after each voiding and will not be continuously wet. If the external device cannot be discontinued, applying vaseline gauze to the sore will protect it from the latex sheath and urine. Precipitating factors in the development of sores should be discovered and the situation corrected. Sores and irritation are treated by cleansing with peroxide and normal saline or occasionally a mild steroid preparation. Often Vaseline gauze is sufficient to promote skin healing.

## LONG-TERM MEDICAL MANAGEMENT

Once the patient has a balanced bladder or a medically acceptable means of bladder drainage, a urological work-up should be done at least once a year. A complete genitourinary work-up could include urinalysis and culture, postvoiding catheterization for residual urine, intravenous pyelogram, cystometrogram, urethral pressure profile, sphincter electromyogram, and cystoscopy. If the patient becomes symptomatic of urinary tract infection, urine analysis and cultures should be done.

## CLINICAL PROBLEMS

The following are some of the frequently encountered problems in patients with spinal cord dysfuntion: infection, calculi, tumors, urethral lesions, reflux, and renal complications.

**Infection.** Infection often results in a disturbance of micturition caused by mucosa detrusor-pelvic floor reflexes precipitating frequency, urgency, urgency incontinence, and eventually residual urine. Furthermore, infection aggravates bladder dysfunction in patients with a neurogenic disorder and makes treatment more difficult. Bacteriuria most often is caused by the indwelling catheter and may appear as early as 48 hours following introduction of the catheter. The bladder's defense mechanisms have been studied in vivo and in vitro. Of importance are intrinsic biological defenses, adequate hydration, frequent voiding, and total absence of residual urine or presence of minimal amounts. Clinical experience indicates that bacteriuria may subside in normal bladders as well as neurogenic bladders after removal of the indwelling catheter.

The flora cultured from patients with indwelling catheters usually consists of more than one species, with gram-negative organisms predominating. The most common organisms found are Proteus, Pseudomonas, Aerobacter, E. coli, Klebsiella, beta-streptococci and Serratia. Single-organism infection is found most often in the period immediately following introduction of the catheter, whereas mixed infections are the rule in patients with long-term catheters.

**Calculi.** Infection seems to be the culprit in the etiology of urinary calculi in association with a neurogenic bladder. Stones are found in the kidney, ureter, bladder, and urethra. Their growth is facilitated by recumbency, stasis, dehydration, and hypercalciuria as seen during periods of immobilization or in paralysis. Foreign bodies are also important and may include particles of rubber, the Foley bag, and hair.

The incidence of renal stones is variable, ranging from less than 2 per cent to 26 per cent, according to various authors. They occur more frequently in males than in females, one and a half times as frequently in aged patients, and more frequently on the right than the left side. The occurrence is greater with complete lesions as opposed to incomplete lesions, and more frequent among patients with lower motor neuron lesions as opposed to upper motor neuron lesions.

Calculi may be classified as (1) infective, (2) opaque, and (3) metabolic. The former two are most often found in association with neurogenic bladders and consist of phosphates, carbonates, calcium, magnesium, and ammonium. Metabolic stones consisting of cystine or uric acid may be found and provide a matrix for developing opaque stones.

Bladder stones are more common than renal stones. The incidence has been reported by Comarr to be 70 per cent in patients with long-term Foley catheters. The incidence drops precipitously in patients who are catheter-free.

**Tumors.** Benign as well as malignant neoplasms are found in association with infection and indwelling catheters. Benign bladder and urethral polyps occur in approximately 10 per cent of patients. They are usually found in the trigone in areas of contact with the Foley bag. The incidence is three times greater in patients with catheters, compared with catheter-free patients.

Malignancies occur in the kidney, renal pelvis, ureter, bladder, and urethra. The most frequent site is the bladder. The incidence is 50 to 100 times greater in individuals with neurogenic bladders and indwelling catheters or suprapubic tubes than the expected incidence within the entire population.

The role of the catheter in the etiology of neoplasms is indirect. In most reported series patients had infected urine, whereas many patients had been catheter free for years. There is more direct correlation, therefore, with infection than with the catheter, suggesting the catheter's role as the original source of infection.

**Urethral Lesions.** The most common locations for development of urethral lesions are the penoscrotal junction, the perineal urethra, and the vesicourethral junction.

Periurethral abscess most often occurs at the penoscrotal junction resulting from the indwelling catheter compressing the urethra at the point of acute angulation over the pubic bone. Complications include urethritis, fistulas, and diverticula. The incidence of penoscrotal lesions varies from 6 per cent to 30 per cent, depending upon the reported series. The lowest incidence of complications occurs in patients who are catheter-free or those on a program of intermittent catheterization.

**Reflux.** Vesicourethral reflux occurs in 30 to 40 per cent of patients, being more common in the large hypotonic bladder affected by lower motor neuron injuries. Structural changes may not be evident initially; however, eventually upper tract deterioration occurs as a result of chronic infection. Etiologies include local infection, vesicle neck obstruction, and neurogenic factors. Complications include hydroureter, pyelonephritis, hydronephrosis, and renal stone.

**Renal Complications.** The problems are pyelonephritis, hydronephrosis, and stone formation. End-stage complications are renal failure and death.

Pyelonephritis may be caused by blood-borne organisms, lympathic spread, or reflux. Recurring acute episodes are associated with an ominous prognosis.

Hydronephrosis occurs in from 25 to 43 per cent of patients and is related to the neurological deficit, reflux, and infection. Its appearance within the first five years is usually an indication of a poor prognosis. Late-onset hydronephrosis usually is associated with minimal upper tract changes and low mortality rates.

Causes of death have been most accurately defined for those patients with spinal cord dysfunction, especially traumatic spinal cord lesions. Review of the literature indicates the renal mortality to be 36 per cent of all deaths in these patients and 6 per cent of all patients. Early evidence of severe urological morbidity indicates a poor prognosis for life expectancy. Peak mortality rates occur at 10 and 15 years following injury.

Renal death associated with hypertension occurs in 8 per cent to 14 per cent of patients and is a contributory cause of death in 20 per cent of patients.

Amyloidosis accounts for 17 to 40 per cent of deaths. As a cause for renal failure, it has been incriminated in 70 per cent of such cases. The etiology of amyloidosis is chronic sepsis.

Malignancies cause 6 per cent of all deaths in such patients, with 50 per cent of neoplastic deaths caused by primary lesions within the genitourinary system.

# Bowel Function and Control
*by William E. Staas, M.D. and Janet G. LaMantia, R.N., M.A.*

The control of bowel function is a unique problem for the patient with spinal cord injury. Contrary to popular belief, bowel control is usually easier to attain than is bladder control. It is a mistake, however, to assume that this can be achieved by simply writing an order for the laxative of choice as needed.

The mechanisms of continence, the physiology of normal defecation, neurological impairment affecting normal defecation, and a program for bowel control are covered in the following discussion.

## FECAL CONTINENCE

The ileac contents normally pass into the colon, which stores them during active absorption of water and sodium. The colon secretes mucus as well as bicarbonate and potassium into its lumen and propels the modified contents into the rectum. The rectum is normally empty except for the time immediately preceding defecation. The important anatomical structures that contribute to continence include (1) angulations of the rectosigmoid, (2) spiral valves of Houston, (3) the rectal "flap valve," and (4) the anal "flutter valve."

The lateral curves and the anterior and posterior angulations of the sigmoid have been demonstrated to have valve-like action. They do not, however, have sphincteric action. With rectal distention, the valves of Houston become visible. These semilunar folds containing circular muscle fibers serve to prevent movement of the fecal material, which is usually solid.

The 90-degree angulation of the rectum, which produces occlusion above the anal canal, constitutes the rectal "flap valve." During increased intra-abdominal pressure, this angle becomes accentuated and occludes the rectal canal. The anorectal area has a "flutter valve" action that aids in maintaining fecal continence during daily activities associated with increased intra-abdominal pressure. It has been proposed that with increased intra-abdominal pressure, the force is transmitted to the external walls of the anorectal area. This tends to collapse the walls and occlude the lumen. This seems to occur only when intrarectal pressure is not increased.

The distal three centimeters of the rectum comprise the internal anal sphincter, which is composed of circular smooth muscle. Studies have demonstrated this to be an area of high pressure compared to the rectum, suggesting that the internal sphincter is in a constant state of tonic contraction. This acts as a safeguard against loss of small amounts of fecal material that might otherwise enter the anal canal.

Straited muscles of the pelvic diaphragm or anorectal ring include the puborectal, pubococcygeal, iliococcygeal and coccygeal muscles. The puborectal is the strongest of the muscles and most important functionally. It forms a sling which swings around the posterior portion of the rectum and attaches to the pubis. Contraction of this sling pulls the rectum upward, producing a sphincter-like action at the anorectal junction by forming an acute angle between the anus and the rectum.

The external anal sphincter is made up of striated muscle with two deep muscle bundles adjacent to the internal sphincter and a third bundle distal and subcutaneous to the internal sphincter. With distention of the anal canal, this anatomical relationship is accentuated. Electromyographic studies of the external sphincter have demonstrated continuous motor unit activity during the resting state compatible with tonic contraction.

## NERVE PATHWAYS

The rectum is devoid of organized nerve endings. The assumption is that afferent impulses originate in nerve endings that are similar to or the same as endings of the myenteric plexis. The rectum is insensitive except to stretch. Distention proximal to the rectum causes colicky pain, whereas distention of the rectum itself produces the feeling of urgency or need to defecate.

Numerous organized nerve endings are found, however, in the anal canal, including those that respond to touch, cold, pressure, and friction. The perianal skin also has a rich nerve supply. Because of this diversity of nerve endings, the anus is able to distinguish between gas, liquid, and solid matter.

Motor innervation of the rectum and anal sphincters is by sacral roots 2, 3, and 4. The external sphincter is dependent upon its extrinsic nerve supply for tone and contraction. Because of the inherent mechanisms, the internal sphincter can function fully with complete isolation from its extrinsic nerve supply.

## INTEGRATION

Electromyographic studies have documented electrical activity in both anal sphincters during the resting state, indicating muscle contraction. During distention of the rectum there is reflex relaxation of the internal sphincter and increased tone in the external sphincter. These reflexes play a significant role in the maintenance of rectal continence. With distention of the rectum and relaxation of the internal sphincter, descending feces has access to the anal canal, which can discriminate between various states of matter. Simultaneous reflex contraction of the external sphincter obliterates the distal segment of the anal canal, thus maintaining continence.

When afferent impulses produce cortical awareness, this aids the individual in perceiving the nature of material within the anal canal. Voluntary contraction of the external sphincter affords an additional force to prevent incontinence. Although the external anal sphincter rapidly fatigues, a brief period of voluntary contraction is usually sufficient to inhibit rectal contraction. Compliance in the rectum following this permits a larger rectal volume to be accommodated.

The internal anal sphincter is under the influence of the autonomic nervous system and not under voluntary control. Its high resting pressure contributes to constant closure of the anus, thus preventing spillover of small amounts of liquid or gaseous material when such material is present in the rectum in quantities inadequate to cause distention. Thus the internal sphincter is primarily responsible for maintaining continence for liquid and gas.

The external sphincter has an important function in maintaining continence for solid material, since it contracts during rectal distention. This facilitates continence by initiating rectal compliance. Prolonged distention of the rectum produces intermittent short periods of rectal contraction in association with simultaneous contractions of the external sphincter. Sphincter contractions, however, persist for longer periods than rectal contractions, thus deterring the movement of stool. The external sphincter also contracts reflexly when there is an increase in intra-abdominal pressure that could threaten continence.

# DEFECATION

Both the autonomic and somatic systems are involved in the act of defecation. Cortical perception of appropriate stimuli may initiate defecation reflexes through the lumbosacral autonomic nerves. Conditioned reflexes are integrated at a subcortical level.

When feces enter into the descending colon, stretch receptors stimulate nerve impulses that travel over the inferior hypogastric plexis to the spinal cord, where they may initiate a spinal reflex or continue to the cerebral cortex producing awareness of distention. Similar phenomena occur with receptors in the rectum. However, the impulses travel via the inferior mesenteric plexus. When distention is accompanied by contraction, urge to defecate is perceived cortically.

With the entrance of feces into the rectum, the ascending colon contracts. This is the rectocolic reflex. Additionally, there is reflex rectal contraction mediated by the pelvic splanchnic nerves originating from S2 to S4. The center for this rectal reflex is in the sacral cord. Distention of the rectum produces reflex relaxation of the internal sphincter, while the external anal sphincter initially contracts. With prolonged rectal distention, there is inhibition of tone in the external anal sphincter, thus preparing for defecation.

## VOLUNTARY DEFECATION

The act of voluntary defecation begins with closure of the glottis, followed by descent of the diaphragm and contraction of the abdominal muscles, producing increased intra-abdominal pressure. The motor activity of the left colon is inhibited, resulting in flattening of haustrations with elongation and straightening of the colon. Fecal material is propelled into the ampulla. When the bolus arrives at the upper rectum, the pelvic musculature relaxes, the pelvic floor descends, and simultaneously the internal and external anal sphincters relax. With straining, there is complete inhibition of the external anal sphincter documented by electromyographic evidence of electrical silence. When voluntary defecation is completed, the pelvic floor rises until once again the rectal lumen is obliterated and the anal sphincters contract. The sacral parasympathetic nervous system is primarily responsible for the nervous control of defecation. Voluntary straining can be eliminated without impeding normal defecation. Similarly, voluntary inhibition may block the usual sequences and permit the accumulation of feces in the rectum, thus disrupting the normal defecation mechanism.

## BOWEL PROGRAM

A bowel retraining program has the basic objectives of achieving continence and regularity for the patient with spinal cord injury. The goal is to achieve control on a regular basis—defecation every one to three days without the need for laxatives or enemas.

There are many factors that influence a bowel program; these should be considered of equal importance during assessing and planning of a bowel routine for the patient. These factors include level of injury, past bowel routine, future life style, level of independence expected, medications, dietary habits, emotional factors, exercise, and potential level of cooperation by the patient.

**Level of Injury.** SPASTIC, UPPER MOTOR NEURON. Activation of the reflex arc occurs when fecal material moves into the rectum.

FLACCID, LOWER MOTOR NEURON. Damage to the sacral segments or nerve roots destroys simple reflex arc activity, and automatic emptying of bowel is lost. Training with reflex activity at higher level is still possible through peristaltic rushes initiated at a higher level by way of the vagus nerve.

**Past Bowel Conditions.** These may include overuse of laxatives and enemas, and the chronic cycle of constipation and diarrhea. Bowel problems such as ulcerated colitis, diverticulitis, and hemorrhoids may have been present.

**Future Life-Style.** School, work, available assistance, and morning or evening routine will influence the scheduling of the bowel program.

**Level of Independence Expected.** The patient's ability to manage a bowel routine independently will affect planning regarding the use of assistive devices and equipment, and the possible training of another person.

**Medications.** If the patient is on fluid restriction, bulk formers and stool softeners are prescribed. Dioctyl sodium sulfosuccinate (Colace) 100 mg twice to three times per day is started; the dosage is adjusted on the basis of the consistency of the stool. Metamucil will alter the consistency of the stool by forming soft, bulky stools and can be prescribed as an adjunct to diet when hard stools with constipation or frequent soft pasty stools are a problem. Senna tablets and granules are used when a mild laxative is needed. This will assist the stool to move into the lower bowel so that a suppository or digital stimulation can completely empty the bowel. Stronger laxatives are used only when fecal impaction is a problem and is not relieved by stimulation. Laxatives are never routinely prescribed in a bowel program.

Other medications prescribed in addition to medications to assist in the bowel program may have undesired effects: antibiotics can destroy normal bowel flora and cause diarrhea; propantheline and oxybutynin chloride can cause constipation.

**Dietary Habits.** Diets poor in fiber and fluid intake and high in gas-forming foods, and an inconsistent diet, will create problems in regulating routine and consistency of stool. These must be evaluated and changed.

The necessary diet is high in fiber, high in bulk, and high in nutrient value. It should include meat, at least three servings daily of vegetables, fruits, and juices, and granola, wheat germ or bran or all three (1 tablespoon twice a day added to cereal). Raisins and popcorn can be encouraged. White bread should be discouraged, and whole wheat, grain, and rye breads encouraged. One half cup yogurt three times per week helps maintain normal flora of the bowel. Yogurt is especially useful after a course of antibiotics. Raw vegetables, at least two servings daily, are valuable.

If the patient is overweight, caloric consumption can be decreased by decreasing dietary fat and sugar content.

The patient should evaluate different foods carefully as to which are constipating by removing them from the diet, and slowly reintroducing them, noting their effect. Tea, cheese, white rice, and applesauce can be constipating, whereas some fruits, especially cherries, peaches, blueberries, and strawberries, may cause diarrhea. These foods should be carefully added in small amounts to the diet. Patients should be encouraged not to eliminate a large group of foods from the diet because of previous experience of either diarrhea or constipation.

**Emotional Factors.** Stress, depression, and fatigue will influence style of life, possibly altering routine in terms of schedule, diet, and exercise.

**Exercise.** Activity is important—prolonged bed rest will interfere with bowel mobility, whereas daily exercise will increase muscle tone and aid bowel training.

**Patient's Potential for Cooperation.** The bowel program planned should encourage the patient's participation in accordance with the appropriate mental and physical capability. The patient's suggestions and preferences should be included in the program when possible. Cooperation by the patient on a day-to-day basis is essential to regulation of the bowel routine.

After careful history and consideration of these factors, an individual bowel program can be prescribed on the basis of the following guidelines. Prior to starting a new bowel routine, the bowel should be free of impaction. Cleansing enemas can be used if needed. If soapsuds enemas do not relieve impaction, oil retention enemas should be tried. Enemas are not used routinely in bowel programs because they stretch the bowel and cause a loss of its natural elasticity. The bowel will respond poorly to reflex stimulation with continued use of enemas, and a dependence on laxatives and enemas can result.

## TIMING OF BOWEL ROUTINE

A schedule is begun that approximates the patient's previous routine—for example, defecation may be attempted every day in the morning. However, this may have to be re-evaluated to conform more to limitation imposed by the patient's condition and expectations of life style. An every-other-day timing is satisfactory and may allow the patient more "free" time. Some patients have good evacuation on a three-day routine. Generally a program begins every other day in the evening; a more individualized routine will evolve as the patient's pattern emerges.

Gastrocolic reflex activity should be utilized in bowel routine. If it is inconvenient to perform bowel program functions immediately after a meal, a hot cup of tea or coffee or an evening snack will assist in producing the gastrocolic reflex.

## USE OF SUPPOSITORIES

Suppositories are used to initiate reflex activity of the bowel. To act, the suppositories must come into contact with the bowel wall. The bowel should be checked for stool in the lower rectum; if it is present, it should be removed and then the suppository inserted.

The suppository should be at room temperature on insertion. Suppositories melt at 90 degrees. Refrigeration will delay the action of the suppository.

*Bisacodyl* is absorbed into mucous membrane of the bowel and acts by irritating the bowel and initiating reflex peristalsis.

*Vacuetts suppositories* are activated in water before insertion. The suppository releases carbon dioxide and distends the bowel initiating reflex peristalsis.

*Glycerine suppositories* soften the stool and stimulate reflex peristalsis. The action is usually less effective than that of Bisacodyl and Vacuetts.

The rectum should be stimulated with a gloved lubricated finger prior to insertion of a suppository. The tip of a finger is inserted into the rectum and the finger gently rotated 15 to 30 seconds.

## DIGITAL STIMULATION

Digital stimulation is used to induce reflex contraction of the colon. In a successful bowel routine, digital stimulation may replace the suppository. To perform digital stimulation, the patient is instructed to lubricate a gloved finger, insert it into the rectum, and stimulate the inner sphincter by rotating the finger. Reflex activity will cause the sphincter to relax, and the stool will be expelled into the rectum.

## POSITIONING

Whenever possible, the patient should be instructed to sit for the bowel program. This is the normal physiological position: peristalsis is greater and gravity assists stool elimination. An abdominal binder can also be used in this position to increase abdominal pressure. If the patient cannot transfer to a toilet or balance himself, a commode chair is used. These chairs can either be used alone or positioned over the toilet. The chair is constructed to allow the patient or person assisting to insert a suppository while the patient is sitting in the chair and to check the bowel for complete emptying after initial evacuation. Other methods to increase effective emptying include abdominal massage, and consumption of one or two cups of hot liquid 15 minutes before the bowel routine. The patient should be advised not to sit for longer than 45 minutes. Weight shifts should be done every 20 minutes.

### Bed Positioning

If the patient cannot sit for the bowel routine, bowel evacuation can be accomplished in the left sidelying position.

The patient should never be advised to use a bedpan. Even careful padding cannot protect insensate skin. Plastic-backed bed protectors can be used under the patient's hips. Suppository or digital stimulation will aid in complete bowel evacuation in this position.

Table 22–3 lists problems that can complicate the bowel program.

A successful bowel routine will require effort and consistency by both the patient and the physician. It is helpful for the family physician to enlist the aid of community nursing services, especially when assessing patient bowel patterns and ability to carry out the routine. The routine should be carefully planned, well-documented, and consistent. Health care professionals should avoid adding or deleting medications from the routine until each medication has been sufficiently evaluated. The patient should eventually become the expert in regulating the bowel.

## GASTROINTESTINAL PROBLEMS

During the early phases after spinal cord injury, there is a profound catabolic response that may be exaggerated by surgery or other stresses. Weight

**TABLE 22–3.** PROBLEMS ASSOCIATED WITH THE BOWEL PROGRAM

| PROBLEM | MANAGEMENT |
| --- | --- |
| Constipation | . Increase fluids, stool softeners, bulk agent; review diet |
| Diarrhea | Try to eliminate causes: if antibiotic, add yogurt; if secondary to certain food eliminate the irritant; rule out impaction; avoid use of medications to stop diarrhea that may cause cycle of constipation-diarrhea-constipation |
| Suppository does not work for over 1 hour | Make sure suppository is at room temperature prior to insertion; insert 15 minutes before sitting; review and correct diet; add senna 8 hours before bowel routine (2 tabs) |
| Rectum empty—mucous lining dry | Rule out impaction; increase fluids; review diet-correct |
| Small hard stools | Same as above, plus use stool softeners, bulk formers |
| Abdomen distended | Rule out impaction |
| Patient complains of "bloated" feeling | Correct diet |
| Poor results during scheduled bowel routine | Ensure consistency of program (time, day, method); expect change with change in life style, diet, etc.; allow time for routine to become re-established |
| Continued results from suppository through day | Review diet; increase bulk formers; senna can be added to assist stool into lower bowel for complete emptying. If problem continues and diet is well regulated: Dibucaine ointment inserted into lower rectum after completion of bowel routine will counteract continued action of suppository |

loss is to be expected along with hypoproteinemia and possible extensive nutritional problems. It is important to provide adequate nutrition during this phrase through oral or, if necessary, intravenous means. A 30 to 40 calories per kilogram body weight diet, with adequate vitamin coverages, is necessary, especially as the patient begins the therapy program. Monitoring of body weight, complete blood count, and serum proteins is helpful in evaluating nutritional status and the effectiveness of the prescribed diet. Adjustments may be necessary before weight loss becomes profound.

In addition to nutritional difficulty, the stress response may be associated with upper gastrointestinal ulceration. Stress is reported to be present in 5 to 25 per cent of cases of spinal cord injury and is perhaps more common in the quadriplegic than the paraplegic. It is best to watch those patients carefully, checking blood counts and stools for occult blood during the acute and early phase. Most spinal cord injury centers use antiulcer medications, including Cimetidine or antacids or both, to reduce gastric acidity and the incidence of bleeding from ulceration.

# Decubitus Ulcers

by William E. Staas, Jr. M.D. and Janet G. LaMantia, R.N., M.A.

Decubitus ulcers are a major problem among chronically ill and debilitated patients. The literature indicates a close association with central nervous system diseases including stroke and spinal cord injury. The incidence of decubitus ulcers among spinal cord–injured patients varies from 25 per cent to 85 per cent. They account for 7 to 8 per cent of deaths among these patients. With the development of these lesions, the cost of nursing time per patient is increased up to 50 per cent. The dollar cost for treatment is conservatively estimated at 15 thousand dollars per patient, and the insurance industry, based on 1969 figures, sets aside 25 per cent of anticipated expenses for patients with spinal injury for management of decubitus ulcers. Additional cost considerations include time away from family and job. Clearly the morbidity and mortality are significant and prevention is the primary goal. Prevention, however, depends on a thorough understanding of the etiology.

Although still subject to extensive discussion, the etiology of decubitus ulcers appears to be primarily related to pressure. Other possible influences to be considered include time, friction, temperature, moisture, and psychosocial and other factors.

The lesions can be graded. The following classification system is recommended by the National Spinal Cord Injury Data Collection System.

Grade I— limited to superficial epidermis and dermal layers.
Grade II— involving the epidermal and dermal layers and extending into the adipose tissue.
Grade III—extending through superficial structures and adipose tissue down to and including muscle.
Grade IV—destruction of all soft tissue structures down to bone. There is communication with bone or joint structures or both.

## ETIOLOGY

### PRESSURE

Kosiak and Lindan have shown the importance of pressure as a major contributor to the development of decubitus ulcers. Lindan, making direct visual observations on rabbit ears, demonstrated that pressure causes tissue damage by closure of blood vessels resulting in ischemic necrosis. Kosiak, in experiments on rats and dogs, defined the time-pressure relationships as well as the clinical and histological changes occurring throughout the tissues. Seventy millimeters of pressure applied continuously for two hours resulted in pathological changes. He demonstrated an inverse relationship between pressure and duration of pressure in the production of ulcers. Intense pressures applied for short durations can be damaging, just as lesser pressures applied for prolonged periods of time may cause damage to the tissues. Tissue injury results when applied pressure exceeds capillary pressure. Normal capillary pressures are approximately 32 mm on the arterial segment and 13 to 15 mm on the venous side.

The histological changes observed with ischemic

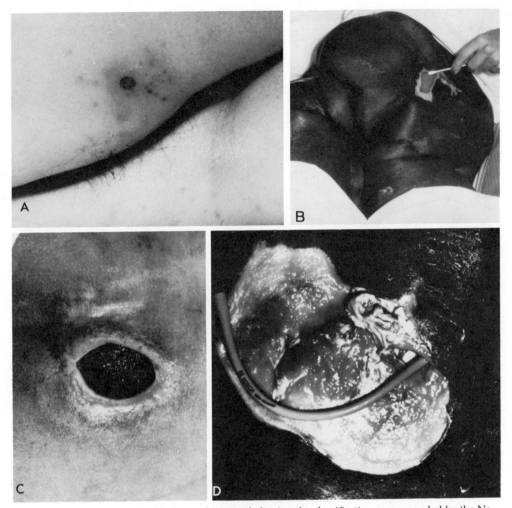

**Figure 22–9.** Pictured are decubitus ulcers graded using the classification recommended by the National Spinal Cord Injury Data Collection System: *A*, Grade 1; *B*, Grade 2; *C*, Grade 3; *D*, Grade 4.

necrosis include venous sludging and thrombosis, edema with cellular extravasation and infiltration, increasing membrane permeability, and pathological changes in muscle fibers. The changes observed in muscle fibers include decrease or loss of cross striations and myofibrils, hyalinization of fibers, neutrophilic infiltration, and phagocytosis by neutrophils and macrophages.

Clinically, reactive hyperemia occurs when pressure is removed. The hyperemic response appears over the compressed skin and subcutaneous tissues and lasts for approximtely 50 per cent of the time the pressure is applied. Within 24 hours, the skin will usually return to normal. The appearance of the ulcer usually is delayed for from three days to up to nine days. Preceding the ulceration by two to four days is the appearance of edema and inflammatory response, which, unlike the initial hyperemia, will not blanche. The initial ulceration

appears to be localized to the skin. However, as time progresses over a period of days or weeks, the full thickness of the lesion can be appreciated as liquefaction occurs. The lesions have been typically described as icebergs, with the skin lesion representing the tip of the iceberg. The skin lesion is usually smaller than the diameter of the deeper lesion, and undermining and fissuring with sinus tract formation is characteristic of the grade IV lesion.

## ALTERED VASOMOTOR PATHWAYS

Loss of vasomotor control affects circulation to the muscles, skin, and mucosa. Pressure that would not compromise circulation under normal conditions produce this effect with the loss of spinal motor pathways. Compromised circulation leads to poor cell nutrition and cell death.

## SENSORY LOSS

With loss of afferent pathways, the patient cannot feel the discomfort resulting from pressure on an area. With paresis there is altered sensory or no sensory input to clue position change. Resulting continued pressure can lead to ischemia and tissue death.

## PARALYSIS

Impaired motor pathways interfere with the ability to change position even when sensory input is intact, and the pressure is not relieved even with impending ischemia. Edema, as a result of paralysis, also contributes to decubitus ulcer formation. Dependent extremities are especially prone to edema. Pressure sores develop more readily when the distance between cells and capillary blood flow is increased by the accumulation of interstitial fluid.

## SHEARING

The physical forces acting in shearing pressure sores are angular forces that slide the upper layers of tissue over lower layers. This action contributes significantly to the size and grade of the resulting ulcer. The continuous rubbing of skin surfaces produces both abraded skin and tissue and compromised circulation with the pressure exerted.

Dinsdale studied the role of pressure and friction in the development of decubitus ulcers. Using normal and paraplegic swine, he demonstrated that friction and pressure as low as 45 mm resulted in skin ulceration. Using an isotope clearance technique, he was able to demonstrate that friction did not produce ulcers by an ischemic mechanism. The results of his investigation suggest that frictioning predisposes to ulceration at pressures less than 500 mm. With pressures in excess of 500 mm, friction does not appear to increase the likelihood of ulceration. Considering that in most clinical settings pressures are less than 500 mm, friction must be considered as a possible etiological factor in the development of tissue necrosis.

Spasticity is the prime cause of shearing: adductor spasms draw knees and ankles together, creating shearing and pressure. Flexor spasms in bed will draw heels across sheets or, in a wheelchair, will pull heels against heel loops, possibly resulting in skin breakdown. Shearing is also seen in poor turning technique in which skin of hips and buttocks is pulled across a surface (bed, wheelchair, transfer board.) Plastizote orthotic jackets and halo vests used in spinal stabilization can set up shearing forces, especially with poor fit and increasing mobility of the patient.

## INFECTION

Local infection of an existing sore contributes to the further development of the sore by extending the size, compromising circulation, and interfering with new tissue growth. Chronic infectious states (urinary tract infection, respiratory tract infection, and existing decubitus ulcers) compromise general health and tissue healing.

## COMMON SITES

Pressure sores are most common over bony prominences. The most prevalent sites are listed with discussion of the forces and activities that contribute to pressure development.

### SACRUM

**Direct Pressure:** in supine position, pressure unrelieved by turning or insufficient time off back; poor wheelchair posture.
**Shearing Forces:** sliding down in bed when head of bed is raised; poor turning technique in bed.
**Maceration:** Prolonged contact with urine, sweat, feces, or all these.

### TROCHANTERS

**Direct Pressure:** prolonged sidelying; trauma during wheelchair transfer when trochanter is hit against wheel of chair; scoliosis causing weight to be shifted to opposite hip; heterotopic ossification; poor wheelchair fit.
**Shearing:** lower extremity spasticity causes heels to be drawn across bedsheets or against heel loops of wheelchair footrests.

### ANKLES

**Direct Pressure:** lateral malleolus—secondary to sidelying and insufficient turning, or trauma during transfer activity. Poor footrest position; medial ankle rests on pins of heel loops.
**Shearing:** medial malleolus—adductor spasms drawing ankles together and across one another.

### ISCHIAL TUBEROSITIES

**Direct Pressure:** insufficient pressure relief in sitting position, poor position of wheelchair footrests (if too high weight is shifted onto ischium).
**Shearing:** poor sliding board transfers; skin and tissue is dragged over board.

### KNEES

**Direct Pressure:** anterior knee secondary to prone position; insufficient pressure relief.
**Lateral Knees:** sidelying with insufficient turning.

### ELBOWS

**Direct Pressure:** leaning, especially in prone position; trauma when elbows are used for leverage and to change position.

### TOES

**Direct Pressure:** trauma from bumping toes when in wheelchair, poor prone position, poorly fitting shoes, tight elastic hose.

### SCAPULAE

**Direct Pressure:** prolonged supine positioning.
**Shearing:** sliding down in bed.

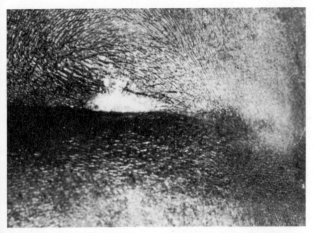

**Figure 22–10.** A common site of decubitus ulcer resulting from temperature or moisture is the inner gluteal fold as pictured.

## TEMPERATURE AND MOISTURE

The significance of temperature and moisture in contributing to ulcer formation has been discussed on the basis of clinical observation. However, detailed studies of these variables are lacking. Clinical experience suggests that some of the lesions observed, especially the grade I and Grade II lesions seen in the inner gluteal fold and other sites not over bony prominences, may be related to temperature and moisture. These lesions can be particularly challenging to manage and frequently are resistive to traditional methods of treatment.

The continuous irritation of skin by sweat, urine, and feces can result in bacterial growth, maceration, and sloughing of skin, especially when in combination with ischemia (secondary to pressure).

## FACTORS ASSOCIATED WITH DECUBITUS ULCERS

### PSYCHOSOCIAL FACTORS

Anderson and Andberg studied the psychosocial factors associated with ulcers. In an earlier study Cull was unable to demonstrate a relationship between numerous psychosocial variables and the incidence of pressure sores except that in this study females had a lower incidence than males. In the study by Anderson and Andberg, the patient's history of pressure sores was first documented. The incidence of skin breakdown was recorded by number of days lost by the individual from normal daily activities and number of days hospitalized. In addition, each patient was questioned concerning his feelings about the measures taken in skin care. Other variables studied included satisfaction with education classes, employment, avocational activi-

ties, organization or group activities, living arrangements, and sexual activities. The final instrument used was a study of self-esteem as measured by the Tennessee Self-Concepts Scale.

The results of the study were most informative. Contrary to popular belief, quadriplegics showed fewer days lost compared with paraplegics. Quadriplegics independent in skin care had the fewest days lost, while paraplegics in need of help to care for their skin experienced the greatest number of days interrupted. Patients with no time lost scored higher on their feelings and attitudes about the practice of skin care and on satisfaction with the six groups of listed activities than individuals who did experience time lost. Interestingly, there was no difference observed on the Tennessee Self-Concepts Scale between these two groups. In general, the satisfaction with life activity was most closely correlated with the presence or absence of disabling skin problems and attitude toward the importance of skin care.

Other factors to be considered include nutrition, anemia, and hypoalbuminemia.

### NUTRITION

The nutritional status of the patient can be affected by numerous variables. Negative nitrogen balance is a major contributor to weight loss and tissue wasting. Anorexia obviously will contribute to or aggravate this problem. Anorexia is commonly observed in depressed patients as well as those with chronic disability. In addition, drugs may cause anorexia, as will excessive cigarette smoking. Adequate protein reserves are necessary in order to maintain the vitality of tissue and to aid in wound healing in the patient with a decubitus ulcer or multiple ulcers. The problem is compounded by the continual loss of protein from the ulcers.

### ANEMIA

Anemia appears to be another contributing factor to the breakdown of tissue. It is also a factor in retarding wound healing. Many spinal cord–injured patients have anemia of chronic disease, while others have iron-deficiency anemia or anemia secondary to blood loss that may be associated with peptic ulcer disease or a decubitus ulcer. Certainly a hemoglobin of 15 gm is more compatible with the preservation and regeneration of healthy tissue, whereas a hemoglobin of 10 gm is not.

### HYPOALBUMINEMIA

Hypoalbuminemia, that is, a serum albumin level under 3.5 gm per dl, is often found in patients with decubitus ulcers, in spite of normal body weight. Hypoalbuminemia and body weight are therefore not directly related. This factor can be influenced by diet as well as disease state. The constant oozing of serum from a decubitus ulcer can deplete the body stores of protein and specifically albumin. The association with tissue necrosis has been demonstrated; however, the specific mechanisms are unclear other than the mechanisms postulated for tissue vitality. Prevention and treatment of these ulcers requires a team effort. Close communication between the physician and the nurse is necessary so that appropriate methods of management can be instituted and maintained without compromising other facets of the patient's care. The cornerstone of management is prevention.

## PREVENTION

All patient educational programs on decubitus ulcers should be directed toward prevention. Pressure sores are easily developed and difficult to heal but are also usually preventable. Prevention is a 24-hour-a-day process. Educational programs should involve physicians, nurses, therapists, attendants, and family. *The patient must be the center of the prevention team*, the most knowledgeable and the directive member of the team.

The educational program is geared to teaching the patient and the family to (1) check the skin for potential pressure problems, (2) use correct pressure relief and cleansing techniques and (3) be aware of potential hazards to the skin.

### INSPECTION AND CLEANSING

Skin care and inspection must be done twice daily (morning and evening), but should be done more often if an area is prone to breakdown, or if a new activity is initiated that might increase pressure or cause shearing. Every attempt should be made to ensure that patients can see and evaluate their own skin. A quadriplegic who cannot hold the inspection mirror can direct another person to position the mirror so that both can inspect the skin. The cleansing program should include washing with mild soap and water to keep the skin free from perspiration, urine, and feces.

### HAZARDS

Safety awareness is also a part of the prevention program. The spinal cord–injured person must be constantly aware of possible hazards to the skin. Prolonged exposure to sun can result in severe burns. Prolonged exposure to cold can cause frostbite of fingers and toes. Bathing water temperature must be carefully regulated to avoid burning insensate areas. Contact of the extremities with radiators, water pipes, car heaters, and metal seat belts (when hot) can cause burns of elbows, toes, calves, soles of feet, and thighs.

### PRESSURE RELIEF

The primary method of relieving pressure is to remove the source of pressure. Correct positioning in bed is important and all bony prominences should be supported. When a patient is turned he must be lifted, not dragged, across the sheets. Foam blocks that support the heels off the mattress should be used. Sheepskin pads do not relieve pressure.

Air and foam mattresses should not be considered as a form of pressure relief. The patient may find them comfortable, but practitioners should caution the patient about feeling "safe" when using them. Some water mattresses when properly inflated will float the patient over the surface with documented mean capillary pressure of 11 mm Hg per square cm of body surface in the supine position. Since all water mattresses will not accomplish these low pressures and some mattresses will not have enough structural capacity to float the patient properly, care should be taken in prescribing the proper mattress. Camper mattresses are not recommended. Waterbeds can cause difficulty in turning and positioning a totally dependent patient.

In the hospital the water mattress may be used when patients have skin breakdown, resist prone positioning, and/or are wearing orthoses such as halo vests or plastic body jackets. In the home the water mattress may be used in the presence of chronic skin breakdown, inability to turn or be turned, or inability to tolerate the prone position.

In the sitting position, weight-bearing areas are confined primarily to the regions of the ischial tuberosity and thighs. Thus there is much less surface area when sitting compared with the supine position. Clearly, pressures will be greater when the patient is sitting and will depend on the posture and the supporting surface. It has been calculated that there are approximately 150 square inches of surface area over which to distribute pressure. Assuming a 75 per cent load, the pressure would exceed 26 mm per square cm if evenly and totally distributed. However, since pressure is concentrated on the ischial tuberosities, the pressures are in excess of what the tissue will tolerate. This has been reaffirmed by studies measuring pressures between the body surface and various supporting cushions. No cushion to date has been found to reduce pressures below capillary pressure. Among the various devices studied are Bio-Flote Gel Pad, Adaptaire, Stryker Flotation Pad, Comfort Cushion, Reston Flotation Pad, Dri-Flote Wheelchair Pad, Latex Foam Rubber Pad, Spenco Skin Care Pad, Bye-Bye Decubiti, Jobst Hydro-Float Pad, and Jobst Hydro-Float Cushion.

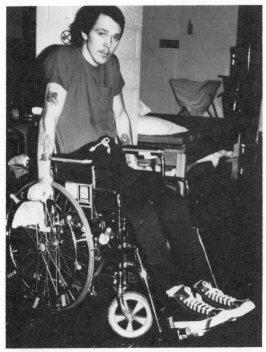

**Figure 22–11.** The wheelchair pushup is the most effective way of relieving pressure in the sitting position.

What this means in practical terms is that the patient must shift body position at regular intervals. No cushion or supporting device commercially available at this time will prevent decubitus ulcers when the patient is in the sitting position. There is a danger that the staff or the patient or both may rely upon a cushion or similar device to prevent decubitus ulcer formation. The only way to prevent decubitus ulcers when sitting is to regularly shift weight. The most effective way to do this is a wheelchair push-up. However, some patients are unable to adequately clear the skin surface or perform a push-up. In these cases, the lateral weight shift can be very effective. Some patients use a special belt adaptation attached to the side arm of the wheelchair that permits them to stabilize and then shift weight. Other patients simply lean forward and then backward. For the C4 or higher quadriplegic, the use of a motorized reclining wheelchair permits the patient to shift position from sitting to supine or semisitting at regular intervals. Weight shifts should be carried out at least every 30 minutes when sitting.

## WOUND MANAGEMENT

Management of the ulcer requires implementation of the same measures recommended for prevention. It is extremely important that pressure relief be accomplished. A decubitus ulcer will not heal with continuous pressure. Adequate nutrition, adequate hemoglobin level, and normal serum protein are prerequisites to healing with or without surgical intervention. Numerous local methods have been described and recommended, suggesting that no single method is a panacea. Local cleansing and debridement of devitalized tissue are important.

Experience has shown that many decubitus ulcers will heal with nonoperative management, given the right circumstances of management. Obviously there must be patient cooperation and willingness to comply with staff recommendations. Generally for grade IV lesions, surgical intervention will be required, especially in the region of the ischial tuberosities. In our experience a grade IV lesion over an ischial tuberosity does not heal with

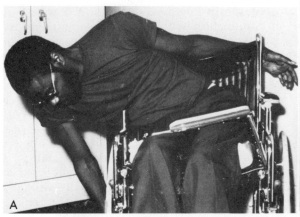
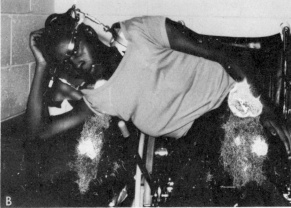

**Figure 22–12.** Lateral weight shift: *A,* Arm is hooked around push handle of wheelchair and patient leans to one side to clear ischeal tuberosity. Process is repeated to the opposite side. *B,* Patient lowers self or is lowered to couch, chair, or other level surface beside wheelchair. This technique is utilized by the patient who is unable to balance or maintain hooked arm position.

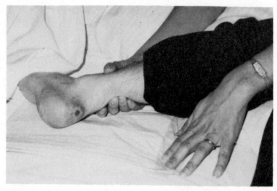

**Figure 22–13.** Good skin closure without surgery.

nonoperative management. Grade IV lesions in other areas may heal without surgical intervention.

Wound care is managed with both local treatment and surgical approaches. The main principle in wound management is to keep the ulcer clean and uninfected. A clean wound free of necrotic tissue should be established as quickly as possible. This will allow for free wound drainage and a decreased number of bacteria in the wound.

An outline of wound management by grade follows:

*Grade I:* Local cleansing, pressure relief program, weekly measurements and grading of ulcer.

*Grade II:* Local cleansing; if wound is draining, gauze packing or Dextranomer to absorb drainage; if wound is necrotic, sharp debridement and enzymatic debridement; and gauze packing; weekly measurements; pressure relief program; and grading of ulcer.

*Grade III and IV:* Local cleansing, removal of necrotic tissue with sharp debridement and enzymatic debridement, gauze packing or Dextranomer, pressure relief program, weekly measurements and grading of ulcer. Referral to spinal cord center or plastic surgeon or both.

## TOPICAL AGENTS

Topical agents applied in local wound treatment are used for their anti-infective properties and to stimulate growth of granulation tissue. A myriad of topical agents are credited with "curing" pressure sores. These preparations range from blood plasma to homemade preparations of honey and sugar. Some of the most commonly used agents reported in the literature are benzoyl peroxide, Gelfoam, Caraya, Dextranomer, and a variety of sugar preparations. Antibiotic agents are most often used in conjunction with topical preparations.

The objective in all stages of ulcer treatment is to keep the wound clean and support tissue healing by relieving pressure and maintaining systemic health. A variety of agents may be used, including hydrogen peroxide 3 per cent, normal saline, povidone iodine, collagenase ointment, neosporin powder, and Dextranomer (see later discussion). Peroxide, normal saline, and collagenase have been discussed previously for their role in wound care.

**Povidone Iodine.** Povidone iodine is an antibacterial agent. It acts as a wound irritant to stimulate granulation tissue. These antibacterial and irritant properties make it a good agent for treating grade I and some grade II ulcers. In grade I and II ulcers, when yellow fibrous tissue covers the wound, povidone iodine will assist in the stimulation of granulation and the sloughing of fibrous tissue. Both the drying effect and antibacterial properties of povidone iodine will decrease wound contamination. Special precautions should be employed when using povidone iodine.

1. The wound should be monitored for signs of irritation and local sensitization. This complication may present with the appearance of bleeding into the wound, causing thrombosis of newly formed capillary buds. The wound may begin to take on a blue-black color. This is especially true in deep wounds; povidone iodine should either be discontinued or cut to at 1:2 solution with normal saline.

2. Iodine should be used only for the length of time its anti-infective or irritant properties are needed. In some cases when superficial grade I ulcers are treated, povidone iodine may act to keep the wound open, thus preventing epithelialization. These superficial healing ulcers may be kept clean with peroxide and normal saline instead of povidone iodine.

3. Povidone iodine should be applied directly to the open wound and not the surrounding tissue. Povidone iodine is drying and irritating to good skin. In addition, the drying effect of the iodine can cause fissuring of wound edges and possible extension of the wound.

**Neosporin Powder.** Neosporin powder is used in conjunction with collagenase ointment. When collagenolytic enzymes are used, bacteria proliferate in the liquefaction of necrotic tissue that takes place. The presence of bacteria will delay wound healing even though the wound is sloughing necrotic tissue. Even with the frequent wound cleansing and redressing there is the possibility of absorption of bacteria. Neosporin powder applied to the wound surface prior to collagenase application should sufficiently control bacterial counts. Both neosporin and collagenase are usually used when the wound is at least a grade III with a large amount of necrotic tissue.

## DEBRIDEMENT

There are three methods used to debride wounds: sharp debridement, enzymatic debridement, and mechanical debridement with cleansing and dressing techniques. Local cleansing is accomplished with a wide variety of topical agents. Dressing technique will depend on the agent employed in cleansing or debriding the wound.

If eschar covers the wound, it should be debrided. The eschar does not permit free drainage of infected material.

Necrotic tissue that fills the wound cavity must also be debrided to ensure a clean wound base. This debridement will speed the healing process since the wound must otherwise slough the necrotic tissue prior to granulating.

### Sharp Debridement

Eschar and underlying necrotic tissue are best removed by sharp debridement. Debridement using scissors, forceps, and scalpel can be done at the bedside and should be repeated daily until a clean wound is obtained. Care should be taken in deep wounds not to cause bleeding that cannot be controlled by pressure. The practitioner must be cautious when debriding ulcers of patients on anticoagulant therapy. If excessive bleeding is noted, the wound should be packed with Gelfoam, pressure applied, and the patient evaluated for reversal of anticoagulation.

On successive days after an episode of bleeding the hematocrit and hemoglobin values should be monitored and kept within normal limits. Use of gauze sponges that have cotton lining should be avoided—the cotton will adhere to the wound surface. Using circular motion with friction cleanses the wound from center to periphery. Saline is poured either directly onto the wound to rinse peroxide or onto gauze, and the same cleansing process is followed. The agent used to cleanse the wound is not as important as the mechanical action employed in removing bacteria and dead tissue. Hydrogen peroxide and saline are economical, easily used, and easily rinsed from the wound surface. Soap and water, although economical, may sometimes be difficult to remove from deeper wounds.

### Enzymatic Debridement

In deep wounds, when sharp debridement is difficult secondary to sinus formation and the depth of the wound, enzymatic preparations should be used. Enzymatic debriding agents fall into two categories: fibrinolytic and collagenolytic. Collagenolytic agents are preferable since in our experience there is less local wound irritation than with fibrinolytic preparations. These enzymatic preparations do not penetrate eschar, and it must either be removed or scored with a scalpel before application of the enzyme. Enzymatic agents are not used in place of sharp debridement but in conjunction with it. The liquefaction of necrotic tissue makes its removal easier with sharp and mechanical debridement. When patients are not hospitalized and seen only once or twice a week for wound care, the enzyme preparations assist with daily debridement.

### Mechanical Debridement

Mechanical debridement is done by local cleansing and dressing techniques. The actions of flushing the wound with solution, wiping it with gauze, and removing gauze packing that has adhered to wound surface, mechanically remove dead tissues and bacteria. Mechanical debridement is done several times daily in conjunction with wound dressing.

### WOUND CLEANSING

Many topical agents are available to cleanse a wound. Some of the agents most often employed are soap and water, hydrogen peroxide and saline, povidone iodine solutions, Dakin's solution and Burow's solution. We use hydrogen peroxide 3 per cent to cleanse the wound and normal saline to rinse the peroxide from the wound. In deeper wounds in which the oxidizing action of peroxide produces a large amount of "foam," we use peroxide and normal saline in a 1:3 ratio. This dilution of hydrogen peroxide makes its removal from the wound easier. Hydrogen peroxide should be poured onto a sterile all-gauze sponge.

### DEXTRANOMER

Dextranomer, a granular powder composed of large dextran molecules, is used to treat open draining ulcers that are free of necrotic tissue. The hydrophilic action of the Dextranomer molecule draws fluid up to four times the weight of a single bead. The extremely high force of the capillary pull reduces surrounding tissue edema and removes bacteria and byproducts of tissue necrosis. Since Dextranomer draws exudates into the beads and away from the wound bed, it increases tissue granulation and decreases the chance of a wound developing sinuses secondary to fluid accumulation. If it is used in wounds with deep sinus tracts, care must be taken to remove all the beads to avoid entrapment of the beads. Dextranomer has been found extremely effective in containing wound drainage and creating a clean, well-granulated wound bed. However, there has been some occurrence of local wound irritation with its use. The irritation seems to be related to beads of Dextranomer escaping and contacting surrounding good skin. This problem can be controlled by putting a thin layer of petroleum jelly around the periphery of the wound. The jelly will not be absorbed into the beads and the underlying tissue will be protected. When the ulcer is no longer secreting, Dextranomer should be discontinued.

A special consideration when prescribing Dextranomer is cost. It is an expensive topical agent, but it has been found to be cost-effective in that a clean, well-granulated wound is quickly established. Deep wounds that are packed with gauze and an array of topical agents are prone to infection, delay of granulation, and accumulation of fluid that may cause development of sinus tracts. Dextranomer limits the possibility of these complications, making wound repair less time-consuming and costly.

### DRESSING TECHNIQUES

**Grades I and II Ulcers.** In grade I and II ulcers, the wound is simply cleansed with peroxide and normal saline. In some cases the area of nonepithelial tissue is "painted" with povidone iodine. The areas of pink, healthy epithelial tissue are not painted to avoid irritation. In grade II ulcers when the edges are thickened with fibrous tissue, the edges should be irritated daily to prevent this accumulation of tissue. The end of a sterile cotton swab or forceps may be used. Two layers of an all-gauze type of sponge are used to cover the wound. (A gauze sponge with cotton lining adheres to the wound). Dressing changes should be carried out twice daily and done more frequently if drainage is soaking through the gauze. If drainage soaks through the gauze, the entire dressing should be removed and the wound cleansed and redressed. The dressing should not be reinforced with more gauze when drainage is seeping through. The additional gauze will add bulk and therefore pressure to the wound site. A wet dressing against a wound is also a medium for bacterial growth.

**Grades III and IV Ulcers.** In cases in which necrotic tissue is present, the wound should be dressed with a wet-to-dry technique. This is done whether or not an enzymatic debridement agent such as collagenase is used. The purpose of this dressing technique is for the basic gauze to dry and adhere to the surface necrotic tissue in the wound. When the dressing is changed and the gauze removed, the dead tissue will be pulled off with the gauze. The dressing to be applied in using this technique should be wet with normal saline and then excess saline should be squeezed out. The damp gauze will then dry adhering to the wound and when removed, will aid in debridement of the wound as described.

### Packing the Wound

Rolled gauze is preferred to a gauze sponge when large, deep wounds are packed, because the coarse weave of the gauze will adhere better to necrotic tissue. In addition, a gauze sponge may be "lost" in a sinus of a deep wound. If the wound to be packed is large enough to accommodate more than one length of rolled gauze, the ends should be tied together. In smaller wounds either a strip type of packing (plain) or "fluffs" made from a gauze sponge may be used. These "fluffs" will allow more contact of gauze with the wound surface resulting in increased debridement. Two layers of a dry gauze sponge should be sufficient to cover packing.

### Dressing Intervals

The basic rule for dressing changes is to allow enough time for the damp gauze to dry and adhere to the wound but not allow the packing to become totally saturated with wound drainage. Dressing changes should be done at least twice daily and more often if drainage soaks through the packing. When drainage soaks through the packing, the dressing should be changed and the wound thoroughly cleansed. Reinforcing the outside layers with more gauze or sponge is not adequate. Leaving soaked packing in the wound will lead to increased bacterial growth and possible development of wound sinuses.

The program of local treatment involves simple cleansing, frequent debridement, and frequent dressing changes. The less complicated the dressing techniques, the more often they can and will be done. Involved dressing techniques of mixing pastes or wrapping with Saran wrap can take many hours of time, and the benefits of a clean wound have not been demonstrated to be superior to simple wound cleansing. A consistent program that the patient and family can learn and apply when needed at home is essential.

## SURGICAL INTERVENTION

Not all decubitus ulcers will close spontaneously. Depending on the depth of the ulcer, the area will heal free of hair follicles and sweat glands. Epithelial tissue will be thin and without the normal dermal papillae seen in normal skin. The scar tissue that closes the wound may adhere to the underlying bone. The inflexibility of this tissue will leave it more susceptible to forces of friction and pressure.

Grade III and IV ulcers over the trochanters, ischia, and sacrum most often require skin grafting, although occasionally a grade II ulcer will not form epithelium and may require surgery. The longer any wound remains open the more difficult it will be to close secondary to fibrous tissue forming around the edges, holding the wound open in a

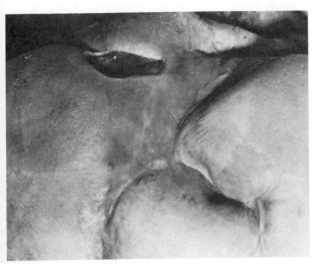

**Figure 22-14.** Poor wound healing with scar tissue adhering to underlying bone.

primarily avascular wound bed. Grades III and IV ulcers and ulcers resistant to closure should be referred to a plastic surgeon and spinal cord injury center.

The process prior to surgical intervention includes diagnostic work-up, presurgical management of spasticity and contractures, and the conditioning of the patient to tolerate postsurgical positioning. This process is best accomplished at an established spinal cord–injury center, in which staff is available and knowledgeable in this pro-

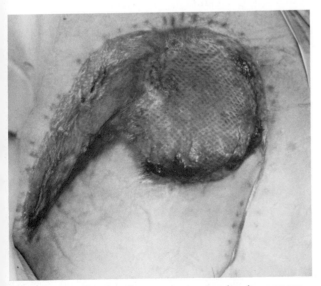

**Figure 22-15.** Rotation flap as seen two weeks after surgery.

cess. Skin grafts and rotational flaps may fail from lack of attention to pre- and postsurgical intervention.

Diagnostic work-up prior to surgery on decubitus ulcers should include a detailed medical evaluation, monitoring of serum protein, hematocrit and hemoglobin levels, and serial x-rays of decubitus ulcers to define wound depth and communications and to rule out the presence of heterotopic ossification. If protein and hematocrit and hemoglobin levels are not within normal limits, blood transfusions and hyperalimentation may be necessary.

Management of heterotopic ossification, spasticity, and contractures is discussed in detail in another section. These complications must be managed prior to surgery if a flap or graft is to be successful. Contractures will interfere with positioning the patient postoperatively and spasticity will create shear stresses that may cause the flap to be displaced. Heterotopic ossification should be mature prior to any surgical intervention. If a decubitus ulcer is repaired over active heterotopic ossification failure may occur with the continued presence of new bone forming beneath the area of repair secondary to stress and pressure over an already tenuous site.

Conditioning the patient to tolerate postsurgical positioning will ensure that the wound will not have to endure undo stress with frequent turning and repositioning secondary to patient discomfort. The most commonly used postsurgical position is the prone position. Patients can be conditioned to tolerate this position comfortably, but it is important to do this prior to surgery so that problems with comfort and patient compliance can be dealt with.

The approach to pressure sore management is complex and should be targeted to the prevention of ulcer development. Many factors influence both the development and the healing of pressure sores. These factors range from the physiological to the sociological. The approach of the family physician must be to review all the contributing factors to pressure sore development and to translate these into an education and treatment program. The treatment program should be based on physiological principles but should take in account the whole patient with his psychosocial and emotional needs.

As with nonoperative management, patient cooperation is of the utmost importance if plastic surgery is performed. With good care and patient cooperation, management of this problem can achieve a healed wound and a restored patient. If either is lacking, the complications include chronic local infection with abscess formation, osteomyelitis, sepsis, amyloidosis, and death.

# Hypercalcemia

*by Jay D Roberts, M.D.*

Hypercalcemia in spinal cord injury is seen more commonly in the younger age group, especially in the preadolescent. Hypercalciuria is common after acute paralysis, probably related to the lack of stimulus of contracting muscle across bones with resultant decreased deposition of matrix and calcium. In spite of this, elevations of serum calcium do not usually occur except in the young, in whom bone metabolism is active with significant osteoblastic activity. One should have a high index of suspicion for this problem in the young spinal cord–injured group, especially if the patient develops vague gastrointestinal symptoms such as anorexia and nausea or abdominal discomfort and vomiting of unknown etiology. Along with these presenting symptoms and signs, constipation, polyuria, and polydipsia may also occur. In those cases in which the syndrome is progressive or severe, the patients may develop dehydration, psychotic behavior, lethargy, and finally, coma. It must be kept in mind that the complete quadriplegic patient may not present with all these findings because of the lack of sensation.

A baseline metabolic survey including calcium balance studies (calcium, phosphorus, alkaline phosphatase, and 24-hour excretion of calcium) should be obtained on all acute spinal cord–injured patients. A weekly calcium balance study should be done thereafter in the preadolescent age group. If acute hypercalcemia does occur (above 11 mg per cent), initiation of immediate treatment should be carried out:

1. Hydration: infusions of half normal saline, alternated with normal saline, should be given. A central venous pressure line may be inserted to better evaluate the state of hydration and give clues to the treatment program. Ordinarily, an end point of 10 to 12 cm of water, venous pressure, is considered ideal.
2. Diuresis: furosemide or other appropriate parenteral diuretic agent is given to augment calcium excretion and prevent volume overload. Subsequent intravenous infusion of electrolytes and water should be guided by the venous pressure and the quantities of sodium and potassium in the urine.
3. Persistent hypercalcemia: other modes of therapy may be indicated such as rapid infusions of corticosteroids, calcitonin, EDTA, and finally, mithramycin.
4. Diet: once the calcium level has approached normal values, the patient may be placed on a diet that is in the low calcium range (400 mg per 24 hours).
5. Calcium balance studies should be done on a daily basis until safe levels have been reached; at this time, return to weekly studies is indicated.

If there is little response to these steps, oral phosphate supplementation should be considered.

The long-term management of hypercalcemia includes a low calcium diet, maintenance of hydration and mobilization, a salt intake of 8 to 10 gm per day, and phosphate supplementation. Monthly calcium balance studies may be necessary in order to follow the effectiveness of the long-term management.

# Heterotopic Ossification

*by Jay D Roberts, M.D.*

In acute spinal cord injury, para-articular deposition of bone occurs in 10 to 50 per cent of the cases, usually within the first six months of injury. The cause is unknown, although trauma, edema, and vascular changes, among others, have been suggested as etiological factors. It is most often found around the hips, although other joints below the level of the injury may be affected. Characteristically, the earliest suspicion of its presence is the slightest decrease in range of motion noticed frequently by the physical therapist. At about the same time, local swelling and warmth may be present. The presentation may be very similar to deep vein thrombophlebitis except that the swelling in

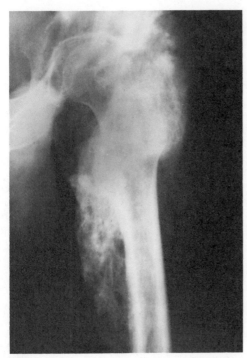

**Figure 22–16.** Heterotopic ossification about hip demonstrating joint fusion.

heterotopic ossification is more often localized, although edema of the entire extremity may be present.

An elevated alkaline phosphatase level is suggestive, but a bone scan is more diagnostic, demonstrating increased uptake in the suspicious area. In early cases, x-rays may be negative even when limitation of motion is present in the affected joint. In a perplexing situation in which phlebitis is still a consideration, a venogram is mandatory to solve the dilemna.

The major problem with heterotopic ossification is the restricted range of motion that will result if immobilization occurs. It is not uncommon to see a paraplegic with an ankylosed hip resulting from heterotopic ossification who has lain supine for four weeks during the postoperative phase of decubitus ulcer surgical repair. Passive range of motion, therefore, is essential to prevent incapacitating joint contractures.

When a surgical procedure contraindicates motion during the acute phase of the postoperative period, exercises should begin as soon as possible. The rehabilitation team should be in contact with the surgeon so as to identify a safe period for the exercises. Aggressive range of motion exercises may be dangerous if the joint is fused, since fracture may occur quite easily, especially in the presence of the common problem of osteoporosis. Diphosphonates may be used early in the process but are of no help in the progression of heterotopic ossification when x-rays have become positive. Occasionally, surgery may be necessary when all other means have failed. Surgery is necessary only when the limitation of motion has further impaired function or presents a problem with nursing care. The indication for surgery must be carefully weighed against the problems of the procedure itself with the attendant massive bleeding that occurs and the increased tendency to infection. Furthermore, ossification may continue after surgery, especially if the bone has not attained maturity. Bone scans are critical, indicating prognosis after surgical removal, since prognosis is better when there is little or no uptake at the area.

# Spasticity

*by William E. Staas, M.D., Frank Naso, M.D.*
*and Jay D Roberts, M.D.*

Spasticity is a common problem in the spinal cord–injured patient and can result in alteration in function from the uncontrolled activity and contractures. Additionally, because of sometimes-bizarre positioning, patients may have difficulty with their personal care along with the development of decubitus ulceration. The changes in tone that come about in the spinal cord–injured patient are related to the loss of controlling impulses from the higher centers of the cord to the alpha motor neuron. This results in increase in sensitivity of the muscle spindle and increase in the activity of the gamma efferent and a continued cycle that results in the increased tone. Spasticity is obviously not a problem with those patients who have lower motor neuron disease that occurs in conus or cauda equina lesions. The problem, however, can be intense in lesions in the high paraplegic and in the quadriplegic. It usually appears earlier in incomplete lesions, occasionally at the time of the injury, whereas in complete transection it follows the stage of spinal shock. The loss of reflexes of the latter phase is replaced first by increase in the deep tendon reflexes, to be followed by increase in resistance of passive stretch, and finally, paroxysms of flexor or extensor spasms with no obvious initiating event. When these are intense, the slightest stimuli will elicit a response that occasionally is uncomfortable if not painful.

It must be kept in mind that spasticity need not necessarily require treatment. Indeed, some patients are able to function at a higher level and use the sudden changes in tone to improve their functional independence. However, when the spasticity interferes with the patient's life style or is a problem to medical or surgical management, treatment should be considered.

Three major approaches are available for treatment of the spasticity of the spinal cord–injured patient, including pharmacological agents, selective neurolytic procedures, and destructive surgical intervention.

Drug management involves the use of agents that are effective at various levels of the central and peripheral nervous system. Diazepam and its analogs are examples of drugs that act at the higher centers of the nervous system. The sedative effect may result in a calming effect in the patient, and this may be the only mode of action. As an isolated modality of treatment, however, it is ineffective because of the intense sedation that occurs. Occasionally, the patient who is in need of minimal therapy will do well with small doses of 2 to 5 mg three to four times a day. More often, however, this agent and its analogs are more helpful in combination with drugs such as dantrolene sodium and baclofen. Another problem which results from the isolated use of diazepam is its potential for abuse.

Baclofen is a new agent that is capable of inhibiting monosynaptic and polysynaptic reflexes at the spinal level, but it may also have supraspinal effects. It is best to begin with 5 to 10 mg twice daily and gradually increase the dose according to the patient's response. Although the manufacturer's recommended maximum dose is 80 mg per day, many patients do not respond until that dose level has been exceeded. The patient's clinical response should be carefully monitored, and this should be weighed against the side effects, which include weakness and lethargy. At excessively high or toxic doses, depression of the central nervous system may occur manifested by somnolence, respiratory or cardiovascular signs, or ataxia and nystagmus. Since the drug is excreted primarily by the kidney, it should be used cautiously if there is impaired renal function. Additionally, it has been observed that abrupt withdrawal can be associated with bizarre mental behavior, including hallucinations and psychosis. Therefore, if the drug is to be discontinued for any reason, it should be tapered slowly rather than stopped abruptly.

For the patient who does not respond to maximal doses of baclofen, it is suggested that diazepam be added to the regimen, in titrated doses to achieve the desired effect.

Another drug that has been used in this situation is dantrolene sodium, which apparently produces musculoskeletal relaxation by affecting the release of calcium from the contractile elements. As is the case of the other agents, side effects such as drowsiness, vague dizziness, and generalized weakness are common. The drug has recently received less than overwhelming acceptance, primarily because of possible hepatotoxicity. Since the drug is detoxified by the liver, there have been reported cases of both nonfatal and fatal abnormalities in liver function. If baseline liver function tests are abnormal, the drug should be omitted from the medical regimen. In the absence of abnormalities, the drug should be used in titrated doses, beginning with 25 mg once daily and increasing this to two, three, and four times a day and thereafter by 25 mg increments until a dosage of 100 mg four times a day has been achieved. SGOT, SGPT, alkaline phosphatase, and total bilirubin levels should be monitored frequently, probably on a weekly basis, at the outset of therapy. If no changes have occurred, the tests should be repeated on a monthly basis and thereafter less often as the maintenance program has been achieved.

Selective blocking of the motor points or peripheral nerves has been of value in decreasing local spasticity and improving function (see Chapter 24). In motor point block, a small amount of 5 per cent phenol is injected to temporarily inactivate the electrical activity of the motor unit. Motor point area is located by evaluating the area that requires the smallest electrical stimulus to produce a maximal response. It is best to first use an anesthetic agent such as procaine so as to evaluate the improvement in function before the more permanent phenol is injected. The most common muscles used are the gastrocnemius in cases of intense equinus spasticity and the iliopsoas muscle in flexor spasms. Usually, repeated blocks are necessary, since the procedure lasts for varying periods up to six months.

Such nerves as the obturator can be easily blocked in cases of adductor spasticity, particularly when that interferes with personal hygiene or sexual function.

Various procedures of a destructive nature have been used to control spasticity dating back to 1908, when Forster introduced posterior rhizotomy. Other procedures have been added over the years, including anterior rhizotomy, subarachnoid injection, chordectomy, and myelotomy. Selective motor rhizotomy, in which the anterior root is cut, effectively controls spasticity, but at the same time produces marked muscle wasting and atrophy and with this a tendency for decreased tolerance to pressure over bony prominences and increased risk of decubitus ulcers. More recently, posterior sensory radio frequency rhizotomies have been advocated by some, since surgery is not necessary. Unfortunately, with the alternation in sensation that follows there is an added tendency for development of for decubitus ulcers for a further impairment in function of the patient.

Chemical destruction of the spinal cord and chordectomy will also relieve spasticity by interfering with monosynaptic and polysynaptic reflexes. Unfortunately, this may result in further alteration of bowel, bladder, and sexual functions.

In 1951, Bischof reported on the value of longitudinal myelotomy and over the years the technique has been refined. The original lateral/longitudinal myelotomy produced flaccid lower extremities. However, in 1976, Yamada reported a modification in technique in which intermittent dorsal midline incisions in the gray matter are made lateral to the central canal under operative microscopy at the L1 to S1 levels. In this procedure, relief of spasticity was noted but postural re-

flexes were preserved and there was no compromise in the remaining voluntary motor function. In general, sensation was preserved, as was bladder and bowel function and capacity for penile erection; however, the procedure necessitates a laminectomy from T10 to T12.

Relief of disabling spasticity is of critical importance to the patient and every effort should be made to control the problem with minimal morbidity. At the outset, simple reassurance is necessary since the patient does not understand the paroxysms of involuntary activity that occur in the presence of paralysis. With understanding occasionally comes some degree of control and, finally, the ability to use the activity in some instances. Nonetheless, in many cases spasticity does deserve treatment as indicated. It is best to use drug management because most patients do respond adequately if the dose is carefully adjusted to their needs and combinations of drugs are used when appropriate. If indeed this does not produce effective control, then selective motor point blocks or, rarely, destructive procedures can be used.

# Pain

*by William E. Staas, Jr., M.D.*

Pain lasting more than six months is usually referred to as *chronic pain*. Three types of chronic pain are recognized in spinal injured patients. *Type A* pain is associated with damage to the bony spine and surrounding soft tissues. The discomfort is usually described as throbbing or aching in nature and localized to the region of the injured site. *Type B* pain is caused by damaged nerve roots and is described as sharp or lancinating or like an electric shock. It classically radiates into involved dermatomes. *Type C* pain is also referred to as *central pain, referred pain,* or *phantom pain.* This is found in association with damage to the spinal cord itself. It is described as sharp, burning, or like an electric shock or a feeling of expanding tissues. Its location is typically perineal or lower extremity.

The incidence of pain in spinal cord–injured patients varies from 5 per cent to 100 per cent. The incidence of severe pain is reported to be from 5 per cent to 30 per cent. Onset varies from within the first six months after injury to more than four years following injury. Most patients, however, note the onset within the first six months. There is a lower incidence of severe pain among patients with cervical lesions and a higher incidence in those with lumbosacral or cauda equina lesions.

Type A pain seems most responsive to transcutaneous nerve stimulation (TENS), while types B and C are often poorly responsive to this modality. Interestingly enough, cervical lesions are less responsive to TENS, while thoracic and cauda equina lesions are more responsive.

The psychophysiology of pain has been thoroughly researched by Sternback. The factors that influence pain and the pain state are varied and complex.

The pain *threshold,* or level at which a stimulus is perceived as painful, is reasonably constant for each individual and does not appear to vary with the psychological state. Pain *tolerance* is the maximum pain tolerated by an individual. This variable is closely correlated with the psychological state of the individual and can be altered by drugs. Tolerance may be increased by decreasing anxiety, by increasing sensory input (distraction), and by motivation. It can be decreased by sensory deprivation and increased anxiety.

The expression of pain may be confused with pain tolerance or pain threshold. The stoic individual may have a pain threshold and tolerance similar to the patient who is acting out his pain behaviors. Pain expression seems to be related to two major determinants. One is cultural and the other relates to the degree of individual introversion or extroversion. Extroversion commonly is associated with expression of pain, while introversion is often associated with absence of pain expression. Pain complaints have also been correlated with social factors, including lower socioeconomic status and class, large family size, history of previous pain experiences, history of relatives with pain experinece, poor marital adjustment, and poor sexual adjustment. Studies have shown that complaints of pain are significantly correlated with degree of neuroticism. Studies in groups of pain patients reveal that patients with acute pain demonstrate normal personality profiles. However, the degree of pain experienced by the patient can be related to the degree of anxiety present. On the contrary, chronic pain patients demonstrate somatic preoccupations and reactive depression. Some authors have concluded that pain may be substituted for anxiety or depression, suggesting that the experience of pain may be less disturbing than other feelings.

The phantom body pain experienced by spinal cord–injured patients is perhaps the most mysterious and challenging of the pain syndromes. The perception of severe and chronic pain from body parts that are insensate is difficult to understand and manage. The patient's discomfort often leads to multiple operative procedures such as neurectomy, rhizotomy, cordotomy, and on rare occasions lobotomy. Although these procedures may offer varying success, in most instances lasting relief is not achieved.

In view of the failure of anatomically discrete destruction procedures, Melzack has proposed that the physiological mechanism underlying these pains must be rostral to the level of spinal cord transection and the loss of sensory input to the central nervous system must play a role in producing the phantom pain. This suggests that pain is not merely a projection of inputs from the periphery to the brain. He proposes a neuronal pool at multiple levels in the spinal cord and brain, which initiate a "pattern-generating mechanism." These neuronal pools are presumed to include the dorsal horns of the spinal cord and interacting systems associated with cranial nerves. Other nuclei along the course of somatosensory projections are also thought to be involved. With deafferentation, the cells of these pools fire spontaneously and in abnormal bursts for excessive periods of time. It is assumed that the pattern generations are projected to the brain to regions that localize sensory inputs as well as those that perceive the experience of pain.

The bursting activity may be influenced by somatic, autonomic, and visceral impulses in addition to cortical influences associated with person-

ality and emotions. Inhibitory centers in the brain stem are also capable of influencing the activity from the neuronal pool. Loss of input from body segments would therefore decrease input to the brain stem inhibitory mechanisms that normally affect the sensory transmission. With loss of brain stem inhibition, noxious stimuli may precipitate bursting patterns. Bursting activity may be unchecked as a result of lack of inhibition, resulting in pain that persists for prolonged periods of time.

The central pattern-generating mechanism concept, therefore, reduces the significance of peripheral input to a minor role. Peripheral inputs may modulate activity in the pattern-generating mechanism. However, their removal may not influence pain once it has been established. The pain mechanisms that are triggered and modified by multiple inputs have therapeutic implications. The use of several procedures or approaches simultaneously may be more successful in managing the pain problem than the use of a single modality. Electrical stimulation may aid in "closing the gate" to pain signals, thus affording relief. Psychotropic drugs, particularly tricyclic antidepressants alone or in combination with phenothiazines, often are effective in increasing pain tolerance and reducing need for analgesics. Relaxation techniques have been reported to be of value, and operant conditiong with biofeedback (see Chapter 4) may reduce pain behaviors and offer good long-term results.

It is imperative that the spinal cord–injured patient suffering pain undergo a thorough evaluation of the problem before a management plan is implemented. To commit the patient to take narcotic drugs should be discouraged, as should reinforcement of pain behaviors. The patient already committed to narcotics should participate in a frank and open discussion of the problem, including the known factors of incidence, physiological mechanisms, management alternatives, and outcomes. Every effort should be made to withdraw the patient from narcotics using an appropriate withdrawal plan agreed to by the patient. During narcotic withdrawal, alternative methods should be used to achieve pain relief. In our experience, the use of tricyclic antidepressants has been most beneficial. A single dose is given at bedtime and then adjusted according to the patient's tolerance and response. The major side effects of the drug are anticholinergic action and sedation; close observation for urinary retention must be kept in mind. Complementing the antidepressant medication, the use of non-narcotic analgesics given at regularly prescribed intervals rather than as needed has been a successful means of management. Narcotic analgesics are not recommended or prescribed for this problem. Results are usually favorable if the patient is motivated to achieve pain relief.

# Neurological Evaluation and Functional Assessment

*by William E. Staas, Jr., M.D.*

From time of entry into the center, the patient should have frequent neurological and functional examinations. This is particularly important during the early phase of management but just as important during ongoing rehabilitation and when the patient is seen for follow-up after discharge. The only method of accurately assessing improvement or deterioration is to accurately perform and record these evaluations. The major components include motor evaluation, sensory examination, and examination of reflexes.

The motor examination should include major muscle groups from proximal to distal in the upper extremities, thorax, abdomen, and lower extremities. Table 22–4 highlights the major roots and their respective muscles. These muscles can be examined without compromising the stability of the patient's spine.

The sensory examination should include all dermatomes from C2 to S5, including use of pin and brush. In addition, joint position sense should be tested in both upper and lower extremities. The examination should include testing with the patient's eyes covered so that the objectivity of the examination is maximized. If this is not done, inaccurate assessment may be the result.

Deep tendon reflexes, including biceps, triceps, knee, and ankle, should be tested and recorded. In addition, the plantar reflex should be tested, and recordings should indicate upgoing, downgoing, or absent response. Finally, the bulbocavernosus (S2 to S4) and the anocutaneous (S5) reflexes should be tested and recorded. The bulbocavernosus reflex is elicited by squeezing the glans penis or clitoris or gently tugging on the indwelling Foley catheter and observing for contraction of the anus. The anocutaneous reflex is tested by gently touching the perianal region with a pin and observing for contraction of the anus. This testing should be done bilaterally. To complete the assessment, the presence or absence of spasticity and clonus should be recorded.

With the information obtained on the neurological examination and functional assessment, the type and level of lesion can be accurately determined. By repetitive evaluation of the patient, change in neurological status and function can be recognized. The areflexic state of spinal shock, in which all reflexes are absent, including those elicited perirectally (anocutaneous and bulbocavernous), may last only a matter of hours.

If sensation is preserved in the perianal area, the deeper layers of the spinal cord may have escaped complete destruction. "Sacral sparing" can signal future motor return at associated cord levels in the lower extremities and possible ambulation potential. The presence of some sensation and/or persistent volitional control of any muscle groups below

**TABLE 22–4.** NEUROLOGICAL EXAMINATION

| ROOT | MUSCLE |
|------|--------|
| C5 | Deltoid |
| | Biceps |
| C6 | Extensor carpi radialis longus |
| | Pronator teres |
| C7 | Triceps |
| | Extensor indicis |
| C8 | Flexor carpi ulnaris |
| | Flexor digitorum superficialis |
| T1 | Opponens pollicis |
| | Abductor digiti minimi |
| T8–T10 | Upper abdominals |
| T10–T12 | Lower abdominals |
| L2 | Iliopsoas |
| L3 | Quadriceps |
| L4 | Anterior tibialis |
| L5 | Extensor hallucis longus |
| S1 | Gastrocnemius |

the lesion characterizes "partial lesions." In cases in which no evidence of motor or sensory function is present below the lesion, prognosis for further return is poor.

It is extremely important to give patients and families a reasonable functional prognosis outlining, with the information at hand, self-care and ambulation potential and bowel, bladder, and sex-

ual function. In complete lesions, functional ambulation is unlikely for T2 to T8 levels but is possible with long leg braces and spinal attachments. For T8 to L1 levels, ambulation with long or short leg braces may be possible.

An understanding of the neurological level and functioning muscles will permit the clinician to estimate the functional potential of the patient.

# Rehabilitation

by Judith M. Perinchief, O.T.R., Gail Miller, B.S., L.P.T.,
Thomas L. Ashcom, Jr., O.T.R., C.R.C., Deborah McMurdo, O.T.R.,
Robert L. Heineman, L.P.T., Lorraine E. Buchanan, R.N., M.S.N.,
Margaret Reddy, R.N., M.A. and Janis Quinn, L.P.T.

The occupational and physical therapist interact closely with physicians, nurses, respiratory therapy personnel, psychologists, social workers, and vocational staff people in evaluation, goal setting, program implementation and reassessment of the patient and his problems. These persons comprise the "functional team." Goals and program are problem oriented and are specific to each individual patient.

## ACUTE CARE PHASE

The importance of early therapy intervention cannot be overstressed. Therapy plays an important role in prevention of complications such as contractures, decubitus ulcers, and upper respiratory difficulties, all of which result in decreased function as well as extending hospitalization. Therapy involvement within the first few days of admission to the hospital, via physician referral, consists of an introduction and description of the therapy program, socialization to ease the patient's anxiety, an introduction to equipment and procedures that will be unique to the patient, initiation of the respiratory program, and assessment of the patient's functional level, including passive range of motion, sensation, and muscle power. Emphasis in the intensive care unit (ICU) continues in monitoring neurological status, increasing respiratory capacity, maintaining range of motion within precautions related to spinal instability, and maintaining proper posture in bed. The occupational therapist provides upper extremity orthoses necessary at this time to maintain proper alignment and position of the wrist and hand.

## INTERMEDIATE CARE PHASE

During this phase the programs are expanded to include initial mobility activities, self-care activities, and strengthening exercises. Most spinal cord patients experience orthostatic hypotension during this process. Normal sitting blood pressure for a quadriplegic is approximately 90/60. In order to minimize this shock to the vascular system, venous pressure stockings and abdominal binders are utilized.

Mobility encompasses the following:

1. Proper fit and application of external spinal mobilization appliances.

2. Gradual elevation of patient's head and trunk in bed.

3. Pressure relief techniques and timing schedules with weight shifts.

4. Stable transfer and bed mobility techniques.

Self-care activities are intiated as tolerance to the upright position increases and upper extremity endurance is sufficient. Paraplegics are expected to take an active role in their daily care. With the use of adaptive equipment, as necessary, quadriplegics can begin learning self-feeding and light hygiene techniques. Those patients with certain types of halo traction devices encounter difficulty with these activities because of positioning and interference of the uprights of the halo device. In such cases, feeding training is deferred until the halo device is removed.

The respiratory program is of primary concern during this phase because respiratory complications are a major cause of death. Deep breathing,

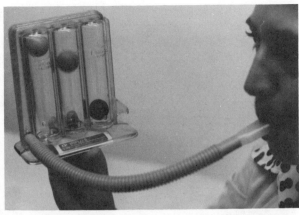

**Figure 22–17.** Patient breathes into incentive spirometer elevating plastic balls to top of cylinders. This provides visual feedback for patient in monitoring respiratory status.

effective coughing, and proper body positioning are taught and reinforced. The use of an incentive spirometer, which gives visual feedback, is beneficial in encouraging deep breathing and strengthening of respiratory musculature. An aggressive program of strengthening primary and accessory respiratory musculature is undertaken and continued throughout the entire rehabilitation program.

The patient and family are trained in techniques of assisted coughing when the level of the lesion is T9 or above. In assisted coughing (quadriplegic) the use of the patient's or family member's hand is substituted for the absent abdominals and low back musculature and intercostals.

The patient is also trained to monitor his respiratory status using an incentive spirometer on a daily basis following discharge. This enables him to detect early signs of an upper respiratory complication and take the appropriate preventive measures.

## REHABILITATION PHASE

The emphasis of the program is now on strengthening of all available musculature, passive range of motion, and training in techniques to improve level of function. Training in physical therapy includes transfer and wheelchair skills. The occupational therapy program also incorporates constructive activities designed and adapted by the therapist to provide range of motion, strengthening of remaining musculature, increasing endurance, sitting and standing balance, and mobility. As expected, stabilization devices slow the program progression and limit the achievement of functional goals. The program can become more intense as the patient's strength, endurance, and emotional balance become stronger. Throughout the entire rehabilitation phase, weekly reassessments are performed in order to match patient progress with projected patient-team goals.

## MOBILITY

Whether the patient is paraplegic or quadriplegic, full passive range in all extremity joints is necessary for the achievement of function. Additionally, some joints require greater than normal flexibility and are therefore selectively stretched. A minimum of 110-degree hip flexion is needed to achieve and maintain the long sitting position required during dressing and self-ranging exercises. Other areas require that specific amounts of tightness in muscles be allowed; for example, if upper back extensors are not allowed to tighten somewhat, sitting posture, respiratory function, and transfers may become compromised. Also in C5 and C6 quadriplegics the finger flexors are allowed to tighten so that when the wrist is extended the fingers will passively form a gross grasp (called *tenodesis action*). For all spinal cord–injured patients, gaining maximum strength is necessary so that physical activities can be performed. What musculature remains must have sufficient strength and endurance to lift all or most of the body weight, often from positions of poor mechanical advantage. With the C5 and C6 quadriplegic, use of substitute muscular movements is taught to compensate for muscles with strength grades below poor. In the C6 quadriplegic, forward humeral flexion combined with external rotation substitutes for absent triceps, thus producing the ability to push the weight up for transfers and pressure relief activities.

Transfer training instruction continues until the patient is independent or has reached the level of least-needed assistance, and the family member or attendant demonstrates the ability to assist appropriately. When indicated, the following wheelchair transfers are taught: bed, chair, toilet or commode, shower chair and tub seat, car, and floor. Putting the wheelchair into the car is taught to paraplegics and lower level quadriplegics only.

Equally as important as transfers are bed activities; i.e., positioning, rolling, coming to sitting. Since truncal and upper extremity strength is limited except in the T10 and lower paraplegic, these activities must be taught by breaking them down into component parts and finally recombining them into the proper sequence as the individual's strength and ability improve.

For almost all complete cord injuries the wheelchair is the primary mode of mobility. Special attention is given to the individual's ability to propel and manage the accessories of the chair. After proper selection of chair and its components, training is instituted that includes positioning and movement around in the chair; pressure relief methods; management of accessories; propulsion on level, uneven, rough, and carpeted surfaces; activities to improve mobility in bending and balancing for retrieval of objects within the environment and transporting objects in the wheelchair. For individuals with hand function (C8 and below) "wheelies" are taught so that curbs do not present an obstacle to the individual's movement around in the community or on the job. High-level quadriplegics require power wheelchairs, frequently with a power recline feature so that the individual can independently relieve pressure. Evaluation for a proper chair and training in its use is a combined functional team activity.

## SELF-CARE

The paraplegic and lower quadriplegic (C6 to T1) receive extensive training in daily living skills including grooming, bathing, and dressing from a wheelchair or bed level. Unless the patient is limited in mobility by spasticity or heterotopic ossification of the hips and knees, independence in self-care activities should be accomplished. Reinforcement of these activities is important because they provide secondary gains of daily range of motion, balance, and coordination exercises.

For the higher quadriplegic (C5 and above), adaptive equipment is required for compensation of decreased motion, balance, and locomotion or reach. These include deltoid assist slings or counterbalance overhead slings, balanced forearm orthoses, or mobile arm supports. Assistive devices are used to help the patient achieve independence in specific self-care activities such as feeding, brushing teeth, and washing the face. These devices might be used by a high-level quadriplegic, but as the level of lesion descends the amount of equipment needed lessens.

It should be noted that the C7 to T1 quadriplegic usually functions independently with hands and does not require assistive devices. The patient must have input in the design and prescription of this equipment as acceptance of these devices is a determining factor in their use. Training of the quadriplegic patient in communication skills includes those that are appropriate to the patient's needs. For example, the high quadriplegic who is a student will have emphasis on typing skills and use of an adapted tape recorder for school.

The higher quadriplegic frequently requires specialized environmental control systems to allow independence within the home or work environment. These may be simple wired switches to operate a lock or door, or they may be very elaborate devices that perform as many as 16 to 20 functions electronically through pneumatic control by

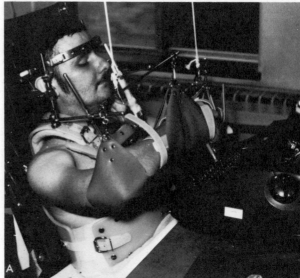

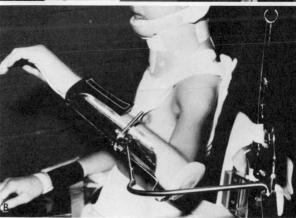

**Figure 22–18.** *A,* Use of counterbalanced overhead slings with quadriplegic patient for training in functional activities. *B,* Balanced forearm orthoses is attached to the back upright of the wheelchair by a bracket, making this the more portable device and therefore the choice for long-term usage.

the patient. Evaluation and training with this equipment is included in the occupational therapy program as appropriate.

## HOMEMAKING

If the patient is the primary homemaker, training to the maximum functional level is included in the occupational therapy program. This training encompasses all aspects of homemaking (cleaning, cooking, laundry, marketing, and child care). Special adaptations or assistive devices may facilitate independence. It is not unreasonable to expect the C6 quadriplegic to be able to perform some homemaking activities and to direct others in the management of the household. In this way the patient can become a contributing member of the family.

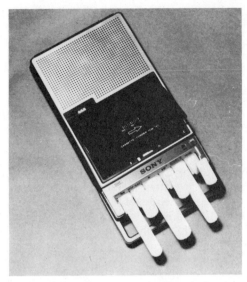

**Figure 22–19.** Adapted tape recorder for use by the quadriplegic student in school or for avocational purposes.

## ORTHOTICS

One of the most controversial issues in the management of the spinal cord–injured patient is bracing and ambulation. Almost all paraplegics and some quadriplegics desire to ambulate again and request bracing. Much care should be taken in determining if a patient should be braced. Those with incomplete injuries frequently ambulate depending on the remaining muscle strength and amount of spasticity. However, complete injuries present a different set of problems. Because energy requirements can easily exceed four times normal, careful consideration should be given to the patient's motivation, the past and present performance in maintaining functional level and freedom from pressure sores, the level of injury, and the purpose ambulation will serve. Until only two below-knee orthoses or one above-knee orthosis (L2, L3) is needed, ambulation seldom becomes the primary mode of mobility. If more than this amount of bracing is necessary, generally ambulation will be for short distances only and requires another person for balance assistance and transfer to standing. This can only be considered therapeutic ambulation—that is, for exercise and psychological purposes. Since training takes many hours daily, ambulation training should be undertaken only if the patient is independent at the wheelchair level and while an inpatient. If the paraplegic patient is being trained with lower extremity orthoses, a standing program is pursued in occupational therapy, which includes performing activities to facilitate balance while functioning with upper extremities. This is of particular importance if the patient is expected to achieve functional ambulation.

The quadriplegic patient receives intensive training in strengthening remaining muscles of the upper extremities and in patterns of substitution for zero- or trace-graded muscles. Training in coordination and endurance is equally important. At this point upper extremity orthoses are used to position the hand for greatest level of function and substitute for weakened or absent grasp. These orthoses may be static or dynamic (movable parts). Some may be quite elaborate in design and sophisticated in the control achieved. The patient must have a complete understanding of the function and purpose of the orthotic device before it is prescribed. As with other adaptive equipment, the patient's acceptance and motivation for use of the orthosis are of utmost importance, as the training program is an involved process and success comes only through practice and perseverance.

Throughout the rehabilitation phase the functional team is involved with teaching of patient and family. Elaborate teaching materials are utilized to help the patient and family become familiar with every detail of care and every technique that leads to independent function. Discharge planning, which includes home modifications and equipment prescriptions, is the responsibility of functional team members and is an ongoing process. Home evaluations are done early in the rehabilitation phase by the functional team. On the basis of the findings, realistic equipment needs can be identified.

## EQUIPMENT

### BEDS

With the exception of the very high quadriplegic, it is advisable for the patient to sleep in a regular bed of double or queen-size width. This allows for ease of bed positioning and movement, adequate space for dressing the lower extremities, and more normal sexual relationships. The electrically powered beds that are commercially advertised are highly satisfactory for many patients with good transfer skills. The fact that the entire bed cannot be raised and lowered from the floor makes it difficult for a family member or attendant to bathe, dress, and position the dependent individual. In these cases, electric high-and-low hospital beds with side rails are more appropriate.

### BATHROOM EQUIPMENT

To permit routine thorough cleansing regimens, a tub or shower seat may be necessary. The styles vary from stationary benches or chairs to self-propelled wheelchairs with built-in commode features. It is paramount that adequate support be provided,

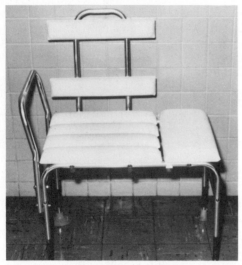

**Figure 22–20.** Park bench tub transfer seat has sturdy legs with suction cups, a padded seat, and back with spaces for water drainage. The extension protrudes over the edge of the tub to facilitate transfers.

and a nonskid surface and an unobstructed, safe transfer area be available. It is often wise to have as few pieces of equipment as possible, so combining features is sensible. Tub railings or grab bars are often used by the individual as an additional safety factor for transfer in the bathroom area. These should be securely fixed to the walls and should not interfere with the transfer area. In our experience the most appropriate tub bench is as il-

lustrated in Figure 22–20. The self-propelling shower and commode chair is used by the patient whose bathroom has been modified to include a drive-in shower.

## HYDRAULIC PATIENT LIFTER

This enables one person to transfer a totally dependent patient to and from wheelchair, tub, bed, car, or commode. There are various models available: free-standing, mobile, or those attached directly to tub or car. Considerations in prescribing the appropriate lifter include style, type of sling, type of straps, height of sling, and height of base of lifter. The safest and most often recommended slings are the all-in-one style.

## TRANSFER BOARDS

These are used to bridge the gap between the wheelchair and the bed, commode, or car. Additionally, they are used to ease the transfer between equipment of uneven height. The patient either slides across independently or with assistance, or if strength is insufficient to bridge the gap in one move, the patient may stop partway, rest, and reposition. Since most individuals who use such boards lack grasp, hand-holds of various sizes and placements are made in order to facilitate board placement.

## CUSHIONS

According to current literature, no wheelchair cushion will prevent sitting pressure sores. Cushions are, however, useful for height adjustment, providing sitting comfort where needed, and some (air-filled types) facilitate the patient's position changes for pressure relief. A multitude of cushions are available and care should be exercised in prescribing them. Factors to be taken into account are:

1. Composition: air, foam, gel, water, combined water and foam

2. Covering material: nylon, cloth, vinyl, rubber

3. Thickness: variations possible from 1 to 4 inches

4. Weight: variations possible between several ounces and 20 pounds

5. Expense: $30 to $300

6. Patient's sitting posture

7. Subjective comfort: judged by trial of various cushions

8. Need to reduce shear force when chair is reclined

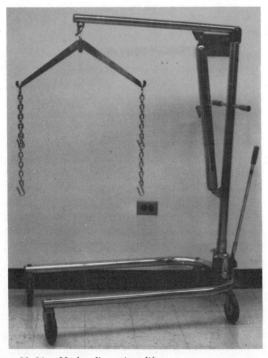

**Figure 22–21.** Hydraulic patient lifter.

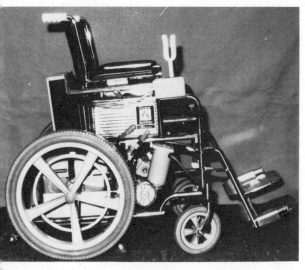

**Figure 22–22.** Proportional drive motorized wheelchair for C5 or C6 quadriplegic. Note adaptation to hand control.

## WHEELCHAIRS

These are chosen to meet the patient's functional abilities as well as social, vocational, and environmental needs. Therefore, they should be prescribed by experienced functional team members. There are several common types of wheelchairs: manual, sports, and power (motorized) (see Chapter 25). Factors to be considered are:

1. Seat depth and width

2. Back height

3. Reclining or standard frame

4. Overall width of chair

5. Total weight of chair

6. Weight of patient

7. Function chair must serve

8. Special accessories

Motorized wheelchairs are indicated as the primary mode of mobility for the higher quadriplegic (C5 and above). The lower quadriplegic may require a motorized wheelchair for use in selective environments (school, college, or work). Prescription of the motorized wheelchair is similar to that of the manual wheelchair in consideration of weight and height factors and in addition of accessories. The type of driving control must be consistent with the patient's capabilities. The conventional motorized wheelchair is hand operated. However, various control options are available. These include:

1. Chin control

2. Head control built into headrest

3. Pneumatic (Sip 'n Puff)

4. Tongue control

5. Voice control

Major considerations in selecting the type of control are mobility required, fatigability, and medical and financial considerations. Other factors used in considering options on motorized wheelchairs are portability, power reclining features, postural control options, and environmental needs.

### AMBULATION AIDS

The choice of the proper ambulation aid rests upon many variables: the amount of support necessary, the strength and build of the individual, the level of the spinal cord lesion, the intended

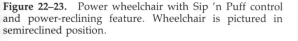

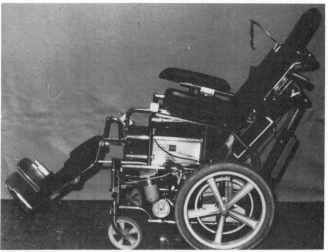

**Figure 22–23.** Power wheelchair with Sip 'n Puff control and power-reclining feature. Wheelchair is pictured in semireclined position.

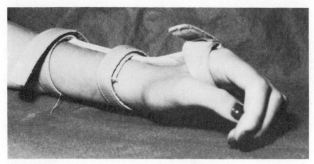

**Figure 22–24.** Dorsal wrist cockup splint.

type of ambulation (therapeutic or functional), patient preference, and occasionally, cost. Ambulation equipment provides varying amounts of support and stability. Listed in order from greatest amount of support and stability to the least are: (1) stationary standing frames, (2) walkers (with and without front wheels), (3) axillary crutches, (4) forearm or platform crutches, (5) three- and four-pointed canes, and (6) standard canes. For rare occasions specialized wheelchairs with standing features are even available. The less bulky the device, the more mobility the patient has.

### UPPER EXTREMITY ORTHOSES

**Static Orthoses.** To maintain proper positioning in the weak or absent wrist musculature of the quadriplegic, a static wrist orthosis may be provided. There are essentially two types of static wrist orthoses. Initially, the patient is issued a dorsal wrist cockup splint, which positions the wrist in slight extension. Later, a simple palmar wrist cockup splint is used. This latter type is indicated for use with the patient who has adequate wrist

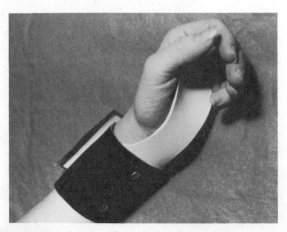

**Figure 22–25.** Simple palmar wrist cockup splint.

strength to functionally use tenodesis of the wrist and simply prevents overstretching of the wrist extensors when the wrist is relaxed.

**Dynamic Orthoses.** There are basically two types of orthoses used to substitute for loss of grasp. The tenodesis splint is wrist-driven by the extensor carpi radialis. This muscle must have active extension against gravity and tolerate minimal resistance. The splint may be fabricated by the occupational therapist or the orthotist from thermoplastic or metal materials. As strength and substitute motions become stronger through training and daily repetition, the wrist-driven orthosis may eventually be discarded.

The outside-powered orthosis is activated by carbon dioxide or electronic control, and, once activated, provides static prehension. Elaborate control harnesses are worn by the patient to initiate the controls. This device is usually fabricated by an orthotist and the training is done by the occupational therapist. The patient's motivation for and acceptance of this type of orthosis is vital because of cosmesis and patience required in training.

### LOWER EXTREMITY ORTHOSES

The exact type of orthosis prescribed is determined by the muscle function remaining in the lower extremities as well as their intended purpose (functional ambulation, therapeutic ambulation, or standing only). In general, braces fall into two groups:

1. Below-the-knee orthoses (ankle-foot orthoses, or below-knee orthoses) that stabilize the foot and ankle and have some effect at the knee and hip, depending on the type and setting of the ankle joint. Most common are the molded plastic (MAFO) and the double metal upright attached to the shoe.

2. Above-the-knee orthoses (knee-ankle-foot orthoses) provide stabilization at the foot, ankle, and knee.
    A. The Scott-Craig orthosis, which has a solid ankle and bale lock release system at the knee.
    B. The more conventional metal with leather cuff or the metal with plastic cuff supports.

### ENVIRONMENTAL CONTROL UNITS

An ECU is an electronic device enabling the high-level quadriplegic to operate appliances, lights, and other equipment in his environment. The type of control is dependent upon the patient's motor power and finances. Types of controls include rocking lever switches, chin switches, and pneu-

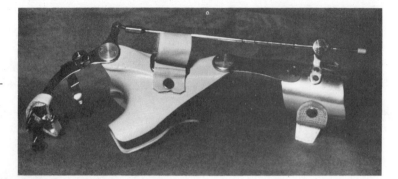

**Figure 22–26.** Wrist-driven tenodesis splint (Engen hand orthosis).

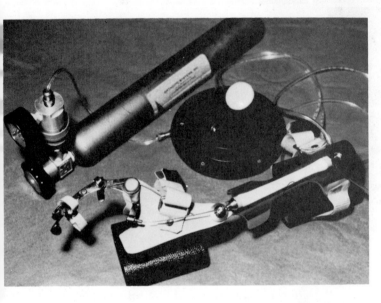

**Figure 22–27.** $CO_2$ powered (McKibben muscle) wrist flexor hinge orthosis. (Orthotic Systems, Inc. Houston, TX)

**Figure 22–28.** Lower extremity orthoses. *A*, Molded ankle foot orthosis (MAFO). *B*, Scott Craig knee-ankle-foot orthoses. *C*, Conventional metal knee ankle foot orthoses.

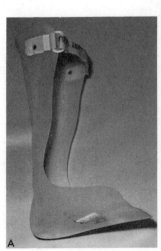

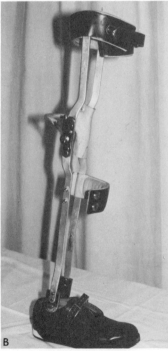

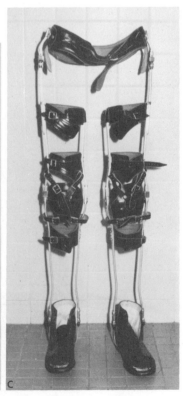

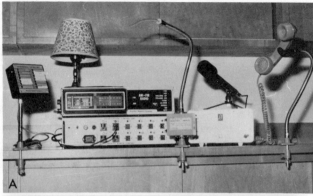
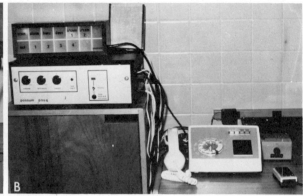
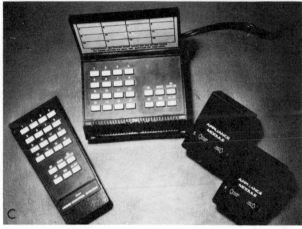

**Figure 22–29.** Three of the most commonly used environmental control units are *A*, Prentke Romich ECU, *B*, Possum–PSU4, *C*, BSR Home Control Unit with adapters.

matic and tongue switches. Examples of equipment that can be operated by an ECU are:

1. Lamps
2. Radios
3. Door locks
4. Call bells
5. Television sets
6. Telephones
7. Electric beds
8. Intercom systems
9. Tape recorders
10. Typewriters

There are several systems marketed that cost in the neighborhood of $2500. These elaborate units offer a wide variety of control switches and appliances. Several companies offer units for approximately $100 to $200 that enable the quadriplegic to control on-and-off functions of several appliances.

### ACTIVITIES OF DAILY LIVING EQUIPMENT

Table 22–5 is a partial list of adaptive equipment used to increase the independence of the spinal cord–injured patient. The type and number of devices depend on the individual patient's condition—level of lesion, complications, and strength. For further information on these devices consult the list at the end of Chapter 3.

**TABLE 22–5.** ACTIVITIES OF DAILY LIVING EQUIPMENT

| FEEDING DEVICES | DRESSING DEVICES | MISCELLANEOUS |
|---|---|---|
| Palmar C-clip | Reachers | Wheelchair gloves |
| Universal holders | Stocking donners | Adapted catheter clamps |
| Vertical holders | Friction cuffs | Suppository inserters |
| Built-up handles | Button hooks | Typing sticks |
| Long straws | Zipper pulls | Telephone holders |
| Plate guards | Dressing sticks | Writing aids |

**Table 22–6.** COMPLICATIONS THAT COMPROMISE FUNCTIONAL ABILITY OF THE SPINAL CORD–INJURED PERSON

| COMPLICATION | EVIDENCED BY | MANAGEMENT APPROACH |
| --- | --- | --- |
| Respiratory | Diminishing vital capacity, increased secretions, diminishing endurance | Referral to physical or respiratory therapist for deep breathing exercises, strengthening of respiratory musculature, postural drainage with or without percussion and vibration, patient/family education |
| Skin | Pressure areas, healing decubitus ulcers, healing graft, abrasions | Referral to occupational/physical therapist for retraining in proper positioning and weight shifting, proper transfer techniques, patient/family teaching in protective techniques |
| Joint/soft tissue laxity or tightening | Increased or decreased range of motion beyond normal, increased heat or edema, increased skeletal abnormality, increased skin problems, spasticity | Referral to occupational/physical therapist for range of motion exercises, selective stretching, positioning appliances for the trunk or extremity, patient/family education in proper positioning |
| Skeletal deformities | Muscle imbalance, scoliosis, kyphosis, gibbus formation, extremity fractures, decreasing range of motion, spasticity, prolonged immobilization | Referral to occupational/physical therapist for range of motion exercises, selective stretching, strengthening, general conditioning and mobilization, patient/family education |
| Prolonged immobilization (i.e. bedrest, casting, etc.) | Skeletal deformities, change in muscle tone, skin breakdown, decreased endurance, muscle atrophy/decreased strength, osteoporosis, loss of range of motion, decreased respiratory capacity, orthostatic hypotension, deep vein thrombosis/pulmonary embolism, psychological complications | Referral to occupational/physical therapist for program of range of motion and general mobilization, selective stretching, strengthening, proper positioning, instruction in weight shifting, instruction in pulmonary hygiene, instruction in mobilization techniques, orthotic devices and adapted equipment, endurance training |
| Diminished integration into community | Breakdown of/or inappropriateness of equipment, architectural barriers within environment, inaccessibility of transportation, lack of recreational opportunities | Referral to professionals at regional spinal cord injury center or a center for independent living |

**TABLE 22–7.** COMPLICATIONS: STANDARD INTERVENTION

| PROBLEM AREA | STANDARD INTERVENTION | COMPLICATIONS | MANAGEMENT APPROACH |
|---|---|---|---|
| Surgical-orthotic stabilization 1. Halo | Inspect sites prior to cleansing; cleanse pin site twice daily with half strength peroxide and saline, paint with Betadine ointment, checking screws daily for security and checking skin at buckle sites of jacket | Loosening of screws, cellulitis of pin sites | Securing of screws; culture and sensitivity of site, more frequent cleansing of pin site if necessary |
| 2. Body jacket | Skin checks daily after removal of jacket | Skin breakdown | Modification of jacket by original vendor; calorie count to prevent weight gain; local care to skin (refer to section on skin) |
| 3. Rods and pins | Instruction to patient: body jacket for activities at all times until removed by physician order; no bending from waist, no diving or contact sports after discharge | Infection; displacement of rods | Refer back to orthopedist for management |
| Pulmonary | Postural drainage and percussion; assisted cough; deep inspiration exercises | Congestion | Prompt intervention with assisted cough and bronchial drainage; tracheal suction if needed. |
| | Glossapharyngeal breathing; use of Triflow 4x daily | Hypoventilation | Summed breathing, IPPB, spirometry |
| Diet | High residue and bulk | Constipation | Increase bulk in diet; high colonic enema or rectal wash; addition of mild laxative eight hrs prior to suppository |
| | High protein, high caloric with vitamin supplement; limit calcium and gas-forming foods | Weight loss | Thirty calories/kg of body weight with vitamin supplement and supplementary feedings |
| Circulatory | Antiembolism thigh-high stockings; inspect legs daily for redness, swelling, tenderness; measure thighs and calves daily; passive range of motion exercises | Pulmonary embolism thrombophlebitis | Bed rest, anticoagulation, hemoculture of stools and urine, frequent vital signs |
| Postural hypotention | Elastic hose or Ace wraps to thigh; abdominal binder; gradual elevation of head of bed to promote tolerance of upright position; monitoring of blood pressure during elevation as well as pre- and post-transfer. | Severe hypotension | In bed: return to supine position; monitor blood pressure until stable. In wheelchair: elevate legs and tilt chair until symptoms cease |
| Contractures | Range of motion two times daily; careful positioning with foot supports and body alignment | | |

In considering the potential of any spinal cord–injured person, there are psychological, motivational, and supportive factors that cannot be overlooked. These may be the most significant factors in achieving independence in functional skills.

## FOLLOW-UP PHASE

During the follow-up phase, occupational and physical therapy concentrate on the following areas: (1) Maintenance of maximum level of function. If the patient has lost function, which areas have been compromised and reasons for this are determined. (2) Condition of durable medical equipment, particularly wheelchair, environmental control runits, and shower chairs. (3) Degree of use of orthotic devices and self-help devices prescribed at the time of discharge. If the patient is not using these devices, which areas have been compromised and reasons for this are determined.

On a long-term basis, complications to various systems can compromise the functional ability of the spinal cord–injured person. At such times the patient will require the services of an occupational or physical therapist. Tables 22–6 and 22–7 serve as guidelines for intervention by these professionals.

# Psychological, Social, and Vocational Considerations

*by Judith Hirschwald, M.S.W., Melania M. Liberto, M.S., Daniel C. Sullivan, C.R.C., Thomas L. Ashcom, Jr., O.T.R. C.R.C., Karen Lucas, B.S., and Carl H. Marquette, Ph.D.*

As medical science makes advances in life-prolonging treatment for the spinal cord–injured, this catastrophic disability must be viewed in terms of psychological and social problems with medical complications. In other words, there is responsibility on the part of health care providers to consider the quality of life of the disabled individual, not just the increased longevity made available by more sophisticated medical procedures. The impact of this type of injury is felt in every area of the person's life—from self-esteem, body image, interpersonal relations, and sexuality to vocational opportunities, housing, and recreation. The rehabilitation process in its broadest sense involves relearning, a process that touches on every aspect of a person's life. He must relearn how to function as a total human being, working, playing, and finding satisfaction in relationships in an environment designed for able-bodied people. Some of the issues addressed in this part of the chapter are applicable to any individual with a physical disability, and some are specific to the spinal cord–injured population. However, the principles and concepts presented are critical to incorporate into an attitude and frame of reference as ongoing care and support are provided to newly injured spinal cord patients and their families.

## THEORIES OF ADJUSTMENT

There are various theories of the so-called "adjustment process," which describe stages of shock, denial, depression, anger, and acceptance. Although these concepts are useful when looking at the rehabilitation process in general, on an individual basis they are often misleading. Suffice it to say that the disabled person is as unique in his coping mechanisms as any of the able-bodied population, bringing to this traumatic situation the personality characteristics and coping devices that worked effectively or ineffectively prior to the injury.

One of the more common misconceptions is that there exists a moment in time when the person with a spinal cord injury suddenly "accepts" or "adjusts" to his disability—with no clear definition yet developed of what "accept" or "adjust" actually mean. Learning to live with a disability is a process that continues throughout the persons's lifetime. In fact, our experience suggests that disabled persons never relinquish that last spark of hope that someday, sometime they will walk again. This hope may be the core that enables them to continue to rebuild their lives, in whatever way is satisfying and productive for them.

Therefore, rather than building on a stage theory model of adjustment, three components of the process are discussed as crucial to consider in the individual's process of adaptation to a catastrophic disability: (1) the individual's depression or the behavior labeled as such by family or professional staff, (2) the individual's use of denial of objective reality of the disability, and (3) the level of motivation of the disabled person to participate in rehabilitation or life activities or both.

In the acute care phase of injury the individual is subjected to extreme sensory and cognitive deprivation, restricted mobility, and social isolation. Many if not all of these initial experiences will continue in varying degrees throughout the disabled person's lifetime, some as direct ramifications of the organic nature of the injury, such as impaired tactile sensation, and others as a result of environmental and attitudinal barriers, such as inaccessible office buildings. It is impossible to totally separate the emotional and psychological aspects of learning to live with a dsiability and the social and attitudinal aspects. It is this concept, among others, that makes the use of the team approach to adjustment to disability a necessity. However, to simplify the understanding of the process of "adjustment," individual issues are dealt with first and social, sexual, and vocational aspects explored more fully later in this section.

## INDIVIDUAL ISSUES

The depressive reactions observed, particularly during the early stages of the injury, are often ascribed to mourning over loss of bodily functions. According to Eisenberg and Falconer, this reaction may actually be due in part to sensory deprivation and restricted environmental stimulation, factors that may also account for the body image distortion frequently observed among spinal cord–injured persons. In other words, the problems encountered may be the result of sensory and social isolation and not necessarily the product of psychological adaptation. Although mourning is obviously a normal and adaptive response to a catastrophic loss, it is important to recognize other significant factors at work and, more importantly, to realize that a traumatic disability does not necessarily produce serious psychological effects on the injured person. George Hohmann, a paraplegic himself, described this process as the "normal reaction to an abnormal situation."

More specifically, from the point of injury the disabled person has lost significant control of his environment as well as of simple bodily functions that we all take for granted on a daily basis. It is this overwhelming sense of helplessness that raises the issue of suicide as the ultimate control over one's life. The option of suicide may be crucial to one's ability to continue to learn to live with the disability. Although this is the extreme of having a choice, the concept of learning to control one's environment to get one's needs met constructively must be a central focus in the relearning process.

## DENIAL

Even though a person may be continuing to live with the disability, this does not imply that the person has accepted the permanence of a disability. The hope of return will always continue, as was stated earlier, but this sense of hope must be distinguished from that defense mechanism called denial. Denial is a normal reaction to overwhelming stress and is typically seen in full force in the early stage of the rehabilitation process. This is a protective device for the individual who is attempting to deal with a major blow to his sense of self and should be respected as such. Direct confrontation of this denial with repeated explanations of the physiological reality is rarely effective, and is generally greeted with anger and more rebuttals. More effective and perhaps more realistic intervention is to focus on the immediate limits of the physical disability and the methods to deal with them in the "here and now," leaving the hope for future gains intact. When this denial of objective reality interferes with crucial aspects of self-care such as skin, bladder, or mobility, more definitive professional intervention is required.

## MOTIVATION

A professional person or family member may view the patient's unwillingness to assume responsibility for his own care as "lack of motivation." However, what is motivation? Is it a dynamic force within the individual or is it those rewards in the environment for which the person will work? We believe motivation is probably a combination of both. It is more the interaction of the person's psychodynamic functioning and his interaction with environmental rewards, e.g., what Rotter calls his "locus of control." With this concept, intervention strategies may be more appropriately chosen, rather than labeling an individual as "poorly motivated." For example, a person who tends to have an external locus of control may need a structured environment with more concrete goals and external reinforcement for appropriate behavior. The congruence of goals between the disabled person and those persons interacting with him is crucial to the individual's ability to comply with desired behavior. Broad rehabilitation strategies should be directed toward decreasing positive consequences of successful avoidance or escape behavior.

While the phenomena of depression, denial, and lack of motivation are inherent in the process of adaptation, each person is unique with his own sense of time and of readiness. A time to mourn for one person is a time for anger for another. A time to learn wheelchair activities for one might be a time to learn to relate to a loved one for someone else. We as professionals need to sharpen our sensitivities to allow for the unique coping methods of individuals within their own time framework.

## COPING ISSUES

For all individuals, change evokes feelings of anxiety and fear. The first major drastic change for the individual who is newly disabled is the move from the rehabilitation center back into the community. During months of confinement for the spinal cord–injured patient, the rehabilitation center often becomes a protective friendly cocoon. Even though forays are made into the community, to home, and to planned recreational and sporting events, the cocoon is always there. A rapport exists between staff and patients, and a peer group is there for the patient, who understand and whose members are available 24 hours a day. Staff people are knowledgeable about spinal cord injury, and are avilable for questions and monitoring even if they do not need to directly perform care. These same staff members provide an atmosphere of acceptance for individuals with a disability and, in general, relate to them as "normal people." A communication, both humorous and serious, exists among patients and between staff and patients that would not be understood in the larger society. Many patients have said that they did not really begin to deal with their disability until they were discharged and had to try to cope in a world that erects many attitudinal and societal barriers (see Chapter 29). Rehabilitation centers struggle to develop strategies to ease the transition between the center and home, but for most patients and families this move is extremely traumatic.

Consequently, individuals with a recent spinal cord injury, newly discharged from a rehabilitation center, are as a group at a most vulnerable point. In our opinion, this critical traumatic period of relearning to live in the outside world continues six months to a year after discharge. Ignoring, for a moment, all the fears, anxieties, and uncertainties the individual patient brings to the situation, a close look at the social realities confronting him seems critical to obtain some understanding of this next step in the coping process.

The disability, per se, makes the performance of daily activities more difficult. For instance, before the injury a shower may have consumed 15 minutes of the day from start to finish and was accomplished at will with no prior planning. Now the process may take an hour and a half, may involve considerable preplanning, and may be accomplished only when someone is available to assist. The loss of control felt by the individual over this one formerly simple task can only be imagined by one who has never had the experience. Larger tasks present larger obstacles. Going out to dinner can no longer be a spur-of-the-moment decision. Several questions have to be answered first: Is there parking close to the restaurant? Is the restaurant accessible to a wheelchair, including the bath-

room? Am I ready to handle the stares, comments, and perhaps questions that may come from the personnel and patrons at the restaurant? In short, society presents significant barriers both architecturally and attitudinally for the individual with a disability. The first few times the patient decides to risk confronting these barriers and the consequences of this risk are critical in shaping his feeling about his ability to cope with the outside world.

In the larger sphere of life, the disabled individual now discharged is confronted directly with other limitations to his choice of life style, which he probably dealt with on only a theoretical level while still hospitalized. Where he and his family live and how they live will probably be altered substantially. If their former home or apartment can be modified for wheelchair accessibility, it is unlikely that the ideal modifications have been completed as of this point. In fact, for some patients the ideal or even minimum modifications will never be made, because funding is not available. The independence in some activities gained in the rehabilitation center may not be possible because ramps are not completed or money is not available to build them. Now, a wife and children may sleep upstairs, but the patient husband must sleep downstairs because they cannot afford to move from their two-story or split-level home. This arrangement is hardly conducive to normal family relationships and certainly serves to heighten a patient's feeling of isolation and difference. A housewife may not be able to resume normal homemaking activities for her family, not because of her physical capabilities but because of inaccessibility of the kitchen. Adults may have had no choice but to return to the home of their parents, even though they were previously living on their own.

The patient's life style can also be altered significantly by the amount of assistance the individual requires and who is available to provide this care. Adults become dependent on parents, and husbands on wives for basic day-to-day needs: dressing, bathing, bowel and bladder care. The adult often feels he has returned to the status of a two- or three-year-old in his relationship with his parents, and the wife feels she has become a nurse or has acquired a second or third young child to add to her responsibilities as a mother. Individuals with a disability have lost much freedom to determine when they will get up in the morning and when they will go to bed at night, because their schedule must now be adapted to the other responsibilities of the caretaker.

The readjustment and redefinition of relationships and roles that must occur during this initial discharge phase are understandably overwhelming to many individuals and their families. The sheer physical energy that must be expended on the labor involved is enormous, in addition to that required in trying to mesh schedules, routines, and responsibilities. Parents often have difficulty remembering that their son or daughter is still an adult in ability and has the right to make independent decisions, when the physical care needed reminds the parents of the care they gave the child as an infant. The wife may have considerable difficulty relating to her husband as a capable, responsible, mature individual when she cares for him physically much as she does her two-year-old.

Recreational and social outlets previously open to and enjoyed by the individual with the disability may now be closed, with other alternatives not readily definable nor accessible. Transportation is generally a major problem, particularly if the family does not own a car or if the cost of a van is prohibitive. Public transportation usually is only minimally accessible, so "going out" for an evening may be impossible, even if the restaurant, theater, sports arena, or friend's home is architecturally accessible. Important recreational outlets, as sources for enjoyment and a release of tensions, may no longer be available. If hitting a tennis ball or cleaning out the closets was a mechanism previously used for releasing tensions or dealing with frustration, alternative methods must now be developed. Walking away from an argument or removing oneself from an unpleasant or uncomfortable situation may no longer be an alternative; the patient and family must develop new ways of handling stressful situations.

These common social factors are critical to understanding some of the reality with which a newly disabled person and family are faced immediately upon reentry into the community. Consequently the depression, frustrations, and anxieties seen by a family physician at this time may relate only minimally to the psychological and internal adjustment to the actual physical limitations.

Perhaps the most useful empirical measure of a patient's feelings about his disability lies in the exploration of his day-to-day behaviors, his goals for the future, and his degree of self-satisfaction with his daily life and goals. An exploration in this area will quickly identify a constructive or destructive life pattern and provide significant clues to the coping ability of that patient at that point in time.

Another extremely significant set of information for the family physician to know is the life style of the individual prior to the onset of his disability. Patterns of behavior after the disability gain significance only as related to patterns of behavior before the disability. An individual whose previous life style included minimal social activity outside the home will probably not become a "social butterfly" now that he is disabled. Therefore, for this given individual, frequent social interaction outside the home is not a valid behavioral measure of his current ability to cope with a disability.

A third common and understandable "trap" for the able-bodied lay person or professional is to view the individual with a disability as a disabled person, as a paraplegic, or as a quadriplegic. The danger of using this stereotype is failure to recognize that the person sitting in the office is an individual first, with all the same feelings and life concerns as the able-bodied. The disability is perhaps the first and most outstanding clinically observable fact about him. To most of us, as able-bodied individuals, the disability is overwhelming, and we feel that we would not be able to handle such a devastating physical insult. Consequently, we become too ready to attribute and to accept certain behaviors and certain feelings as a natural product of the disability, and are reluctant to explore other causations, as we would with an able-bodied patient. Severe depression with all its potential self-destructive components may be exhibited by the individual with a disability because of his disability. However, we are often too quick to make and act on the assumption that this is the cause of his depression, telling ourselves that he is entitled to be depressed, since anyone would be depressed in the same situation. Our assumption may be correct—the disability per se may be the cause of the situation, but we risk missing a critical clinical diagnosis if we do not go further. Perhaps the depression is related to a poor marital relationship, to a parent-child problem, to just being fired from a job, or to a myriad of other reasons common to the able-bodied as well. The disability cannot be cured, but help for the other problems of life is available to the individual with a disability as well as to the able-bodied.

Some of these reality factors can and are being changed, thus making the adjustment to the community slightly easier for the disabled person and family. The Disabled Rights Movement, begun in the early 1970s by a group of disabled persons in Berkeley, California, is finally beginning to have an impact across the country (see Chapter 29). Legislation in the form of the 1978 Amendments to the 1973 Rehabilitation Act addresses the issues of housing, attendant care, and other basic living problems of the severely physically disabled. Sections 503 and 504 of the Rehabilitation Act address the civil rights of the physically disabled, mandate accessibility, and support the concept of "mainstreaming" the disabled individual into the larger society at all levels. The basic aim of the disabled rights movement and the subsequent legislation is to begin to allow disabled people the same life choices as are afforded to the able-bodied population. Independent living centers can provide either actual living accommodations or act as resources for locating accessible, affordable housing. Attendant care can allow the adult a choice of living with his parents or resuming a separate living arrangement; it also can provide for the physical and personal care needs of the husband so the wife can more easily relate again to her husband as a wife and not as a wife-nurse. In the 1970s transportation systems in some areas became more accessible and in other areas special services began to be developed. New construction, mandated in the public sector and lobbied for in the private sector, has been made accessible for the wheelchair user. Public attitudes have been changing, and as the individual with a disability is able to become more visable in society at large, attitudes should alter even further.

The stagnant economic environment of the early 1980s has produced a slowing of the independent living movement, but significant gains have been made that will have far-reaching effects. Certainly these changes will not eliminate the tremendous adjustment and relearning process that must be faced by the spinal cord–injured person, but they will certainly increase his ability to maintain control over his life and assist him in resuming as much of his former life style as is compatible with his real physical limitations.

## SEXUALITY

As noted previously, spinal cord–injured persons face many challenges physically, psychologically, and socially. Their bodily functioning has been altered in many areas. A decrease in physical ability has often brought about a devaluating of sense of self and a change in interpersonal and social relationships. In other words, disabled people may now view themselves as less of a man or woman. They may now view themselves as "asexual" in that part of the definition of self includes a concept of adequate sexual performance. Unfortunately, the spinal cord–injured individual is often given the overt or covert message of no longer being sexual. This view is not only psychologically devastating but also functionally incorrect (see Chapter 28).

### MALES

Studies have shown that with upper motor neuron lesions approximately 90 per cent of males can have reflexogenic erections. About 70 per cent of the 90 per cent will be able to have sufficient erection to allow successful sexual intercourse. However, the vast majority will not be able to ejaculate or have orgasm. Individuals with lower motor neuron lesions have psychogenic erections with a success rate for coitus between 24 and 50 per cent. The possibility of ejaculation is higher than with upper motor neuron involvement. An individual with a partial cord lesion has a greater chance of physiological sexual function than the individual with a complete transection at both the upper and lower motor neuron levels.

The percentages related to the ability to sire children are very low with spinal cord–injured males. The lowest percentage is 1 per cent for complete upper motor neuron lesions and the highest is approximately 10 per cent for males with incomplete lower motor neuron lesions. The difficulty in achieving fertilization is related to many factors. The two obvious factors are related to problems in having erection and ejaculation. The sperm may also be impaired as a result of unsuitable temperature regulation, urinary tract infections, testicular atrophy, and hormonal imbalance. There may also be scarring and blockage of the seminal passages as a result of infections. In addition, retrograde ejaculation may occur. Although siring children through intercourse is difficult for spinal cord–injured males, many couples have raised families by adoption or artificial insemination.

At times it may be difficult to differentiate between organic and psychological erectile impotence. This differentiation is important because different treatment modalities are utilized on the basis of the cause of the impotence. Psychogenic problems can be worked with in a counseling framework, while an organic condition may best be treated with a penile prosthesis. The two major types used in surgical treatment are the Small-Carrion prosthesis and the Scott-Bradley prosthesis. The most common complication with the Scott-Bradley is mechanical failure. Psychological complications such as depression have been reported with both prostheses. Therefore, counseling should include both the patient and his partner. It is not uncommon that males will have the unrealistic expectation that the surgical procedure will return orgasm and ejaculation.

### FEMALES

Less information is available for females, but it has been noted that there is an increase of sexual sensation and activity for injured females. Frequently following the onset of spinal cord injury, females experience amenorrhea for a period of several months. The exact cause is unknown, but is probably related to stress or to a disturbance in pituitary-ovarian function.

However, females with spinal cord injury are still fertile and able to become pregnant. There is an increased incidence of bladder infection and increased risk of autonomic hyperflexia during delivery and labor. In addition, lack of feeling can cause labor to be undetected, and it is recommended that the woman be admitted to the hospital prior to due date. It is also quite important that her physician be knowledgeable about spinal cord injury.

Since women can become pregnant after a spinal cord injury, a discussion concerning alternative contraceptive means is crucial. Oral contraceptives increase the chances of thrombophlebitis and subsequent pulmonary emboli. Intrauterine devices can be problematic if the individual cannot feel if it becomes loose or penetrates the wall of the uterus. Women with limited hand function may have difficulty manipulating the diaphragm or using foam or jelly. In spite of the possible problems, a diaphragm is probably the most feasible and safe method. A physician knowledgeable in the area of spinal cord injury should help the patient choose the most appropriate contraceptive technique considering her particular circumstances.

## COUNSELING CONSIDERATIONS

Although spinal cord–injured individuals may have difficulty with sexual function, the sex drive can remain strong. This can lead to frustration if they view sexuality in terms of normal functions. They need to understand that sexual expression is more than just coitus. They need to know their limitations but also what they can still do. All areas of sexual activity should be reviewed with them, including the gamut of sexual expression from holding hands to oral sex.

In talking to or counseling a spinal cord–injured person on sexual functioning, one has to remember that some forms of sexual expression may be taboo to the individual. Religious, moral, and esthetic considerations cannot be ignored. Individuals should be educated as to all forms of sexual functioning but with no pressure to perform in any particular manner. They have to be in touch with their own feelings and decide what is acceptable for them. According to recent information from the National Spinal Cord Injury Data Research Center, 50 per cent of spinal cord injuries occur in the 15- to 25-year age group. Related to the young age range, a little over half the spinal cord–injured patients are single. For the individual who was sexually inexperienced at the time of injury, providing general sex education is crucial, in addition to information concerning changes relative to the spinal cord involvement.

The effects of spinal cord injury on marriage have been investigated by several researchers. Although this is a very complex issue, some assumptions about the role of sexuality as one of many variables affecting the marital relationship may be addressed. One study ascertained that infertility rather than changed sexual functioning was a major concern to females married to injured males. There is some evidence that marriages contracted after injury are much more stable than those existing prior to injury. In the sample of males matched by Crew et al. according to level of disability, 11 of 35 preinjury marriages failed in comparison to 4 of 35 postinjury marriages. It should be noted, however, that sexuality is only one of several factors possibly involved.

Both males and females need help in developing a positive self-image and body image. One element of this help is given when health professionals treat them as competent sexual human beings. They have the need for and the right to acquire accurate sexual knowledge and counseling. At the present time the best source for this service is a regional spinal cord injury center.

Spinal cord–injured individuals need to experiment sexually to find out what they can do and what is pleasurable both to them and their partners. This requires communication and a desire to be sexual. To find partners, they must get out and meet people and become active in all spheres of life. The more productive their life in all areas, including the sexual, the less chance of self-pity and depression.

## VOCATIONAL ISSUES

Until recently, the ability to work was based largely on the spinal injury level, but current thinking views the level of injury purely as an early predictor for the start of vocational planning. Now, careful consideration is given at the start of the vocational planning process to an evaluation of the individual's observable work characteristics and job readiness. This process begins when the individual has arrived at the point of overt demonstration of behaviors that are necessitated by or seen in a work environment.

Initiative, perseverance, interest, and sense of responsibility are some of the factors that should be considered at the start of vocational planning. These facets of behavior are readily discernible as the individual moves through a program of physical restoration and into the community.

Today, as job modification is better understood, as help with home renovations is possible, and as rehabilitation engineering is producing adaptive devices that compensate for the loss of physical function, job opportunities are becoming more readily available and the possibilities for competitive employment can now be seen on a much broader scale.

Employers are becoming increasingly aware of their responsibilities to the disabled within the community and have begun to institute programs of job modification. A review of current job analyses may lead an interested employer to consider a change in work procedure and work environment directed toward increasing the capabilities of the disabled.

While it is true that more is being done today because of affirmative action programs, a large portion of job modification is done by individual employers who, for one reason or another, have become sensitive to the potential productivity of disabled workers.

Presently, most comprehensive rehabilitation facilities are augmenting their programs with the inclusion of vocational evaluation services. As individuals evidence interest, it is now possible to assist them in making appropriate vocational choices. A vocational assessment should include a vocational evaluation in which work activities, real or simulated, are used as the basis for assessment. Vocational evaluation using work sample systems assist the individual in matching his potential, interests, and capabilities with various vocational options. In essence, this approach is primarily designed to evaluate the person's present skills, his learning potential, his need for job training, and his job performance factors. With certain populations, the work sample approach as described is felt by many to be more informative than other traditional assessment methods. Many patients who have limited reading skills and who fear standard testing procedures do not seem to have as much anxiety in a work sample evaluation. Then, too, work sample programs are often conducted in environments that are less threatening, where peer relationships are developed, and where performance behavior and worker traits can be more successfully evaluated. It should be noted that, although a large percentage of success in many occupations has been secured by completion of high school, college, and advanced degree programs, not everyone needs to return to school, because work opportunities have also been documented in selected jobs that require only a limited general education. Various opportunities are available in which physical qualifications are at a minimum, as in certain aspects of computer sciences, the transportation industry, the optical industry, and in sales and other personal service jobs.

Expanded vocational opportunities and new assessment tools are now increasing the communication among the rehabilitation facility, the employer, and the prospective employee. In addition, vocational evaluators are continuing to assess employer response and job accessibility following the disabled employee's return to gainful employment.

To further assist disabled individuals who wish to explore vocational opportunities, state governments offer vocational rehabilitation services administered by state vocational rehabiitation programs. An individual can apply for these services through the local office of the state vocational rehabilitation agency.

Among the services provided by the state vocational rehabilitation agencies are:

Evaluations including medical examination and such other examinations as orthopedic, neurologic, psychological as might be necessary to help the individual to determine the nature and extent of his disability, his abilities, interests, and his need for other rehabilitation services.

Medical, surgical, psychiatric, or other allied services which can assist the individual in substantially reducing the impact of his disability on his ability to function. Also included are equipment and devices such as wheelchairs, artificial limbs, and hearing aids, counseling and vocational guidance to assist the individual in adjusting to his disability and in developing a vocational plan.

Job training in a trade or technical school or college, or on-the-job training, or work adjustment training, and assistance with transportation, books, special licenses and occupational tools and equipment.

Assistance with job placement, so that the individual can find a job which will utilize his skill and capability, and follow-up after he begins to work to assist with adjustments to the job or work situation.

Services provided, which may vary from one state to another, are often provided in conjunction with an individual's rehabilitation program in a hospital or rehabilitation center, but many patients are not ready to begin active vocational planning until they have returned to their home and community. An individual may be referred to the state agency at any time these services are needed. Disabled individuals who are already employed but who require certain services to make it possible to continue to work are also eligible. In many states homemaking is an eligible occupation for vocational rehabilitation assistance to a housewife without required outside employment.

For individuals whose primary rehabilitation is being coordinated through a workman's compensation program or through a private insurance carrier, referral may also be made to the state vocational rehabilitation agency for additional services that may be needed. Most regional spinal cord injury centers have a representative from the state vocational rehabilitation agency who participates in the psychological, social, and vocational evaluation of the patient during initial rehabilitation and who continues to be available to the patient after he has been discharged to his home for continuing vocational planning services.

## RESOURCES OF A REGIONAL SPINAL CORD INJURY CENTER

Certainly, no one resource can begin to meet all the needs of the spinal cord–injured patient relative to his adjustment to disability. However, expertise and resource referral information relative to the psychological, social, and vocational needs of this special group of patients is available through the regional spinal cord center system. The several programs outlined are peculiar in their modeling to the Regional Spinal Cord Injury Center of the Delaware Valley, Philadelphia, Pennsylvania, but similar resources could be anticipated in all centers.

(1) *Psychological, social, and vocational team.* Within the center and available to each patient on an individual basis are psychologists, social workers, vocational counselors, and vocational evaluators.

In addition to individual counseling with patients and families, this staff forms a team that meets with each patient to offer their combined expertise in solving problems of formulating and implementing independent living or vocational goals or both. This process can begin at any point and serves as an excellent problem-identification and problem-solving vehicle for the patient in the community who needs assistance with social, psychological, or vocational concerns. In addition to these core members, other individuals often join the team as appropriate to a given patient's needs: representatives from insurance companies or private rehabilitation agencies, employers, family members, counselors from state rehabilitation agencies, and so forth. Close working relationships are maintained with medical and nursing personnel, the staff on the functional team, and other appropriate community persons, such as family physicians and community agency representatives.

To date, this team approach has proven to be a viable model in working with patients to achieve their vocational and educational potential.

(2) *Social skills and assertiveness training.* The purpose of this training is to attempt to help spinal cord–injured patients learn or relearn those skills necessary to appropriately communicate their needs within and outside the rehabilitation center and to develop the new skills they will require in interpersonal relationships. This training offered as an educational course is available at any time to individuals with a disability who have an interest in improving their skills in this area.

(3) *Peer relationships.* Individuals with spinal cord injury and their families often feel isolated in a community where they have no access to other spinal cord–injured patients and their families. Such contact can often provide critical emotional support as well as an opportunity to share experiences and expertise in dealing with day-to-day concerns. A regional spinal cord injury center can often provide a resource for this critical peer support in several ways. In some centers, an outpatient group exists for this purpose, and would be available and appropriate for those patients or families or both who are able to come to the center.

Other types of groups offer similar peer support systems and may be more easily available to patients who are not with the geographic area of a regional spinal cord injury center. One such group is the National Spinal Cord Injury Foundation, with headquarters in Newton, Massachusetts. Its national organizational goals are CARE (peer counseling and outreach), CURE (research), and COPING (legislative and political concerns). Local and state chapters reflect these national goals to a greater or lesser extent, depending on upon local issues and concerns. Another organization is the National Wheelchair Athletic Association, which offers the disabled individual participation in a wide variety of athletic activities on a competitive level.

(4) *Equipment and environmental modifications.* Within each regional spinal cord injury center there exists a team of professionals with knowledge concerning specialized equipment and adaptations. These professionals can assist in matching equipment to the individual's needs. Expertise is also available in the identification and modification of architectural barriers in the home and work environment. Resources as to potential funding and technical expertise within the community can also be provided.

(5) *Transportation training programs.* Driver training programs for disabled persons are available. Following initial assessment of the patient's capabilities, instruction can be given in the safe and efficient operation of a motor vehicle (car or adapted van) using the necessary equipment tailored to the patient's needs.

(6) *Sexuality.* Specialized programs, audiovisual materials, and journals on sexuality issues for spinal cord–injured individuals and their families are available as resources.

(7) *Recreation.* Potential recreational outlets are as broad in scope for the individual with a disability as for the able-bodied population. Through the contributions of professional persons such as rehabilitation engineers, occupational therapists, recreational therapists, and the disabled population, attitudinal and physical barriers to the participation of the disabled person in athletics and other leisure activities have been decreased. The regional spinal cord injury system can serve as an information center in the identification of specially adapted equipment and potential programmatic resources.

# Discharge Planning and Lifetime Follow-up

*by William E. Staas, Jr., M.D.*

---

Discharge planning begins at the time of entry into the acute care hospital. The initial interview with the patient and family should provide sufficient information so that an initial plan for discharge to home and return to community can be initiated. Obviously there are many contingencies and complexities that will affect the plan. The major strengths and weaknesses of the family and community structure must be identified early. By this we refer to the functional, psychosocial, and vocational issues. The primary responsibility for development and implementation of the plan rests with the managing physician and the social worker, in addition to the patient and family. Numerous meetings and discussions must occur throughout the patient's hospitalization, during the acute phase as well as the ongoing rehabilitation phase. Discharge represents one segment in the process the patient goes through.

At the time of initial examination, a diagnosis and prognosis should be established. This encompasses not only the neurological but also the functional prognosis. A thorough understanding of the functional significance of the level of spinal injury aids in projecting the expected outcome. An understanding of spinal stability or lack of stability and the required orthopedic management aids in planning an appropriate rehabilitation program as well as affecting expected length of stay in hospital. Medical management needs should be estimated, as well as the functional retraining program and adaptive equipment needs. Prognosis for further improvement and improved neurological function can usually be estimated. The literature strongly indicates that the condition of a patient who sustains a complete traumatic spinal cord injury and demonstrates no motor or sensory change within 24 hours will usually not change significantly. Patients with incomplete injuries may demonstrate improved neurological function. However, the longer the time period without significant improvement, the less the likelihood of significant improvement.

As the patient progresses through his management program, weekly patient and staff conferences should be held to define problems and establish goals and document progress. With this information at hand, the physiatrist can project reasonably accurately the expected outcome and time for discharge. As the expected date of discharge is established, specific supports must be identified and procured. Included are purchases of durable equipment, modification of the environment to meet patient needs, teaching of patient and family, provision for appropriate transportation, and identification of appropriate community resources, including family physician. It is imperative that the managing physician be contacted and included in the management program. Similar communication must be established with agencies working with the patient in the home environment, such as community nursing services. On the day the patient returns home, all communications should have been established, appropriate equipment obtained, environmental modifications accomplished, patient and family teaching accomplished, and an appointment made for follow-up care by the rehabilitation team with a commitment to lifetime follow-up at regularly scheduled intervals.

In our lifetime follow-up system, the patient is seen 1 month following discharge, and then again at 3 months, 6 months, 12 months and yearly thereafter. The patient and the managing family physician are instructed to contact us any time an acute problem or question arises. If the patient requires intervention beyond the skills of the managing physician, we prefer to admit the patient to our center until the acute problems are solved. The patient is then returned home to the care of his family physician with our continued availability as an ongoing resource.

At each follow-up visit the patient is seen by the physiatrist, the nurse clinician, and the patient systems coordinator. As needed, the patient may also be seen by a social worker, a psychologist, a rehabilitation counselor, a vocational evaluator, a physical therapist, and an occupational or recreational therapist. At the one-month evaluation after discharge, the patient has a CBC, urinalysis, and culture, and a postvoiding catheterization specimen for residual urine is obtained. Other studies are performed as indicated.

At the three-month evaluation the patient has the same studies performed as were done on the one-month evaluation, in addition to a SMA 6 and 12. At the 12-month and subsequent yearly evaluations the patient has the same studies performed as were done at the six-month evaluation in addition to an intravenous pyelogram, creatinine clearance, cystogram, cystometrogram with urethral

**TABLE 22–8.** DATA OF FOLLOW-UP SYSTEM, REGIONAL SPINAL CORD INJURY CENTER OF DELAWARE VALLEY (November, 1979 through November, 1980)

I. Statistics
51 clinics held

| | DATA | NON DATA | NEW EVALUATIONS | TOTAL |
|---|---|---|---|---|
| No. patients seen | 58 | 43 | 7 | 108 |
| No. clinic visits | 100 | 68 | 8 | 176 |
| No. nonclinic visits | 89 | 45 | 0 | 134 |
| No. cancellations/no-shows | 35 | 45 | 2 | 82 |

II. Patient Problems Presented
  A. Medical/nursing
    1. Genitourinary system (Total no. of problems 154)
      a. Bladder routine: includes problems with all types of bladder training and urinary drainage — 57
      b. Urinary tract infection: patients presented with an infection that necessitated treatment — 93
      c. Complications: hematuria (2), urethral diverticulum (2) — 4
    2. Musculo skeletal system (Total no. of problems 93)
      a. Spasticity (presented as a problem, i.e., interfering with sleep or activities of daily living) — 43
      b. Spinal stabilization orthosis (required adjustment, orthopedic consult) — 25
      c. Contractures — 9
      d. Heterotopic ossification — 6
      e. Scoliosis (noted as a problem that required monitoring/intervention) — 6
      f. Subluxed shoulder — 4
    3. Skin (Total no. of problems 76)
      a. Decubutus ulcers: Grade I (21), Grade II (20), Grade III (10), Grade IV (16)
      b. Rashes — 6
      c. Ingrown toenails — 3
    4. Gastrointestinal system (Total no. of problems 66)
      a. Bowel routine: includes nonfunctional routines, diarrhea, constipation — 34
      b. GI disturbances: burning pain, gastritis, nausea, vomiting, hiatal hernia, abdominal distention, bleeding — 9
      c. Nutritional: overweight, underweight, fluid intake problems, dietary education — 20
      d. Complications: perianal abscess, hemorrhoids — 3
    5. Education (Total no. of problems 51)
      Problems presented as demonstrated through lack of understanding of disability. Spinal cord injury follow-up system, need for family, physician, etc. No family physician, lack of knowledge of disability and self-care demonstrated by development of problem and patient's inability to relate it to cause/prevention. — 35
    6. Medication/management (Total no. of problems 50)
      a. Includes bowel, bladder, blood pressure, pain, infection (urinary and respiratory); spasticity — 37
      b. Anticoagulation therapy — 11
      c. Allergic reaction to medication — 2
    7. Neurosensory (Total no. of problems 34)
      a. Pain (patients presented pain as a major complaint, unrelated to new injury or trauma) — 26
      b. Autonomic complications: sweating (3), temperature regulation (2), dysreflexia (3) — 8
    8. Cardiovascular system (Total no. of problems 33)
      a. Blood pressure regulation — 15
      b. Edema — 11
      c. Thrombophlebitis — 5
      d. Right-sided heart failure — 1
      e. Intramuscular bleeding to muscle strain while on anticoagulants — 1

*Table continues on opposite page.*

TABLE 22–8    (Continued)

|  |  |  |  |  |
|---|---|---|---|---|
| 9. | Respiratory (Total no. of problems 20) | | | |
|  | Problems include chest congestion, inadequate vital capacity, pneumonia, pulmonary failure, asthma | | | |
| 10. | Other (Total no. of problems 9) | | | |
|  | a. | Anemia | | 2 |
|  | b. | Hearing loss | | 1 |
|  | c. | Insomnia | | 2 |
|  | d. | Swelling right groin | | 1 |
|  | e. | Lethargy | | 2 |
|  | f. | Mandibular abscess | | 1 |

B. Functional
1. Mobility — 47
2. ADL — 23
3. Equipment
  a. Inability to use equipment — 2
  b. Does not have equipment — 32
  c. Equipment breakdown — 22
  d. Evaluation for new equipment — 27

C. Psychological, social, vocational
1. Inability to cope with disability — 32
2. Difficulty with family relationships — 51
3. Significant architectural barriers in home — 60
4. Financial problems — 55
5. Difficulty in formulating vocational/educational plan — 74
6. Lack of adequate transportation — 63
7. Inability to afford or establish independent housing — 19
8. Needs attendant care — 40
9. Inadequate recreational and social outlets — 56
10. Needs referral to BVR or other rehabilitation agency — 16
11. Needs driver evaluation and training — 36
12. Sexual counseling — 39
13. Excessive alcohol or drug abuse — 11

III. Referrals made from clinic
  A. Within system
    1. Physical therapy — 22
    2. Occupational therapy — 3
    3. Physical and occupational therapy — 6
    4. Volunteer within system — 4
    5. Counseling — 5
    6. Work tolerance program — 1
    7. Consultation with specialists
      a. Urologist — 9
      b. Orthopedist — 7
      c. Plastic surgeon — 6
      d. Surgeon — 1
      e. Neurologist — 1
      f. Physiatrist (special problem) — 2
      g. Gastroenterologist — 1
    8. Family medicine clinic — 7
    9. Home visits — 8
    10. Driving evaluations — 5
  B. To outside community
    1. Physical therapy — 5
    2. Physical, occupational therapy — 5
    3. Community nursing service — 14
    4. Counseling services — 3
    5. Recreational swimming — 1
    6. Attendant care pilot program — 6

IV. Hospital readmissions or admissions
  A. Within system — 41
  B. Outside system — 9

V. Patient deaths — 2

TABLE 22–9. LIFE EXPECTANCIES FOR FEMALE SPINAL CORD INJURY VICTIMS BY AGE AT TIME OF INJURY AND IMPAIRMENT CATEGORY*

| AGE AT HOSPITAL DISCHARGE | GENERAL POPULATION | LIFE EXPECTANCY (YEARS) | | | |
| --- | --- | --- | --- | --- | --- |
| | | Paraplegia | | Quadriplegia | |
| | | INCOMPLETE | COMPLETE | INCOMPLETE | COMPLETE |
| 10 | 65.59 | 64.09 | 50.94 | 58.05 | 37.81 |
| 20 | 55.85 | 54.41 | 41.75 | 48.55 | 29.56 |
| 30 | 46.24 | 44.82 | 32.85 | 39.24 | 21.83 |
| 40 | 36.80 | 35.47 | 24.40 | 30.27 | 14.77 |
| 50 | 27.84 | 26.64 | 17.03 | 22.06 | 9.29 |
| 60 | 19.50 | 18.52 | 10.94 | 14.86 | 5.37 |
| 70 | 11.84 | 11.15 | 6.02 | 8.68 | 2.55 |

*From Young, J. S. and Northrup, N. E.: Statistical information pertaining to some of the most commonly asked questions about spinal cord injury. SCI Dig. 1:11–32, Spring 1979.

pressure profile, and, if indicated, cystoscopy. Other studies are carried out as deemed appropriate. For the latter set of evaluations, the patient may require a brief readmission to the hospital. At that time a thorough functional assessment is performed in addition to an analysis of the patient's equipment needs and the status of his equipment. Recommendations are made with regard to changes in rehabilitation program, procurement of new or additional equipment, and renovation or maintenance of equipment as needed.

Table 22–8 is a summary of a 12-month experience with the lifetime follow-up program. Of interest is the fact that approximately 50 per cent of patients did not arrive on the day scheduled. All patients are contacted by telephone as well as by mail as part of our routine scheduling process. Prior to discharge, the patient and family are informed of the lifetime follow-up program and offered the opportunity to participate. When a patient does not keep a scheduled appointment, he is contacted for another appointment. Every effort is made to prevent patients from "dropping out." Patients relocating to another region are referred to another designated spinal injury center.

The patient problems identified are grouped under medical and nursing, functional, and psychological, social, and vocational (PSV). The problems we have identified are those that were anticipated; our experience to date reinforces the need for close and continuous monitoring by the rehabilitation team. Problem identification and problem solving is a continuous and dynamic process.

Because of improved health care, the life expectancy of spinal cord–injured patients has improved significantly. Tables 22–9 and 22–10 highlight life expectancies for male and female spinal cord–injured victims. Paraplegics tend to live longer than quadriplegics and patients with incomplete lesions tend to live longer than patients with complete lesions. Thus the "incomplete quad" has a greater life expectancy than the "complete para."

TABLE 22–10. LIFE EXPECTANCIES FOR MALE SPINAL CORD INJURY VICTIMS BY AGE AT TIME OF INJURY AND IMPAIRMENT CATEGORY*

| AGE AT HOSPITAL DISCHARGE | GENERAL POPULATION | LIFE EXPECTANCY (YEARS) | | | |
| --- | --- | --- | --- | --- | --- |
| | | Paraplegia | | Quadriplegia | |
| | | INCOMPLETE | COMPLETE | INCOMPLETE | COMPLETE |
| 10 | 59.09 | 57.22 | 42.20 | 49.88 | 28.60 |
| 20 | 49.65 | 47.85 | 33.73 | 40.88 | 21.57 |
| 30 | 40.61 | 38.95 | 26.29 | 32.57 | 16.45 |
| 40 | 31.53 | 29.98 | 18.55 | 24.13 | 10.49 |
| 50 | 23.08 | 21.70 | 11.96 | 16.61 | 5.90 |
| 60 | 15.75 | 14.65 | 7.08 | 10.61 | 2.97 |
| 70 | 9.72 | 9.00 | 3.93 | 6.29 | 1.50 |

*From Young, J. S. and Northrup, N. E.: Statistical information pertaining to some of the most commonly asked questions about spinal cord injury. SCI Dig. 1:11–32, Spring 1979.

**TABLE 22–11.** DAYS HOSPITALIZED: FOLLOW-UP YEARS TWO AND THREE FOR ALL CASES (N = 384)*

| | DAYS HOSPITALIZED | | | | | |
| | Year 2 | | | Year 3 | | |
| NEUROLOGICAL CATEGORY | No. Cases (N) | $\bar{X}$ (DAYS) | SD | No. Cases (N) | $\bar{X}$ (DAYS) | SD |
|---|---|---|---|---|---|---|
| Paraplegics | | | | | | |
| Incomplete | 65 | 12 | 28 | 62 | 8 | 23 |
| Complete | 120 | 15 | 34 | 122 | 11 | 33 |
| All | 185 | 14 | 32 | 184 | 10 | 30 |
| Quadriplegics | | | | | | |
| Incomplete | 99 | 14 | 28 | 100 | 8 | 21 |
| Complete | 99 | 26 | 37 | 92 | 17 | 34 |
| All | 198 | 20 | 34 | 192 | 12 | 28 |
| All cases† | 383 | 17 | 33 | 376 | 11 | 29 |

*From Young, J. S. and Northrup, N. E.: Statistical information pertaining to some of the most commonly asked questions about spinal cord injury. SCI Dig. 1:11–32, Spring 1979.
†Includes 8 cases for which the number of days hospitalized was known but the category of neurological impairment was unknown.

These figures reinforce the need for lifetime follow-up and for management directed not just toward survival but toward improving the quality of life.

John S. Young, Director of the National Spinal Cord Injury Data Research Center and Executive Editor of the *Spinal Cord Injury Digest*, has analyzed national data on rehospitalization in the second and third years following spinal injury. Table 22–11 lists mean hospital days. For all patients, the mean was 17 days in the second year and 11 days in the third year. Complete quadriplegics experienced the greatest number of days hospitalized.

Table 22–12 highlights days hospitalized for hospitalized patients only. There is little difference based on neurological category. However, fewer days were required in the third year compared with the second year, and the greatest reduction in number of days occurred among those with incomplete injuries as compared with those with complete injuries.

Looking more specifically at the upper 20 per cent of patients using total accumulated hospital days, we see that 20 per cent of patients used 82 per cent of hospital days (Table 22–13). Among the

**TABLE 22–12.** DAYS HOSPITALIZED IN YEARS TWO AND THREE FOR 2 HOSPITALIZED CASES ONLY*

| | DAYS HOSPITALIZED | | | | | | | |
| | Year 2 | | | | Year 3 | | | |
| NEUROLOGICAL CATEGORY | Total Cases (N) | $\bar{X}$ (DAYS) | SD | Med | Total Cases (N) | $\bar{X}$ (DAYS) | SD | Med |
|---|---|---|---|---|---|---|---|---|
| Paralegics | | | | | | | | |
| Incomplete | 23 | 33 | 39 | 13 | 15 | 27 | 38 | 9 |
| Complete | 53 | 34 | 44 | 18 | 45 | 32 | 48 | 11 |
| All | 76 | 33 | 42 | 17 | 60 | 31 | 46 | 10 |
| Quadriglegics | | | | | | | | |
| Incomplete | 44 | 32 | 36 | 18 | 29 | 27 | 34 | 11 |
| Complete | 72 | 35 | 40 | 21 | 52 | 30 | 40 | 13 |
| All | 116 | 34 | 38 | 20 | 81 | 29 | 38 | 13 |
| All cases | 192 | 34 | 40 | 19 | 141 | 30 | 41 | 13 |

*From Young, J. S. and Northrup, N. E.: Statistical information pertaining to some of the most commonly asked questions about spinal cord injury. SCI Dig. 1:11–32, Spring 1979.

**TABLE 22–13.** DAYS HOSPITALIZED IN POST-INJURY YEARS TWO AND THREE AND PERCENT OF TOTAL DAYS FOR THE UPPER 20 PERCENT OF ALL CASES*

| | | | | | | ALL CASES: DAYS HOSPITALIZED | | | | |
| | | Year Two | | | | | | Year Three | | |
| Neurological Category | No. Of Cases | Total Days | Upper 20 Percent | | | Total Days | | Upper 20 Percent | | |
| | | | Days | % | | | | Days | % | |
|---|---|---|---|---|---|---|---|---|---|---|
| Paraplegia | | | | | | | | | | |
| Incomplete | 64 | 750 | 713 | 95 | | 399 | | 398 | 99 | |
| Complete | 122 | 1794 | 1578 | 88 | | 1447 | | 1369 | 95 | |
| All | 185 | 2544 | 2285 | 90 | | 1846 | | 1782 | 97 | |
| Quadriplegia | | | | | | | | | | |
| Incomplete | 97 | 1416 | 1211 | 86 | | 792 | | 760 | 96 | |
| Complete | 100 | 2541 | 1759 | 69 | | 1573 | | 1320 | 84 | |
| All | 197 | 3957 | 3048 | 77 | | 2385 | | 2121 | 90 | |
| All Cases | 383 | 6501 | 5357 | 82 | | 4211 | | 3930 | 93 | |

*From Young, J. S. and Northrup, N. E.: Statistical information pertaining to some of the most commonly asked questions about spinal cord injury. SCI Dig. 1:11–32, Spring 1979.

**TABLE 22–14.** DAYS HOSPITALIZED IN YEARS TWO AND THREE AND PERCENT OF TOTAL DAYS FOR THE UPPER 20 PERCENT OF HOSPITALIZED CASES ONLY*

| | DAYS HOSPITALIZED | | | | | | | |
| | Year Two | | | | Year Three | | | |
| NEUROLOGICAL CATEGORY | No. Cases N | Total Days | Upper 20 Percent Days | Upper 20 Percent % | No. Cases N | Total Days | Upper 20 Percent Days | Upper 20 Percent % |
|---|---|---|---|---|---|---|---|---|
| Paraplegics | | | | | | | | |
| Incomplete | 23 | 750 | 469 | 63 | 15 | 399 | 320 | 80 |
| Complete | 53 | 1794 | 1169 | 62 | 45 | 1447 | 1061 | 73 |
| All | 76 | 2544 | 1551 | 61 | 60 | 1846 | 0000 | 73 |
| Quadriplegics | | | | | | | | |
| Incomplete | 44 | 1416 | 903 | 64 | 29 | 792 | 529 | 67 |
| Complete | 72 | 2541 | 1471 | 58 | 52 | 1573 | 1015 | 65 |
| All | 116 | 3957 | 2325 | 59 | 81 | 2365 | 1544 | 65 |
| All Cases | 192 | 6501 | 3824 | 59 | 141 | 4211 | 2894 | 69 |

*From Young, J. S. and Northrup, N. E.: Statistical information pertaining to some of the most commonly asked questions about spinal cord injury. SCI Dig. 1:11–32, Spring 1979.

**TABLE 22–15. DIFFERENTIAL DIAGNOSIS AND MANAGEMENT**

| PROBLEM | DIAGNOSTIC EVALUATION | INITIAL TREATMENT | MANAGEMENT | PAGE REFERENCE |
|---|---|---|---|---|
| **Fever** | | | | |
| 1. urinary tract infection | Urine culture positive | Appropriate antibiotic | If not improved within 24–48 hours, consider admission or referral | 404 |
| 2. Pulmonary infection | | | | |
| a. High quad | Cough, wheezing, sputum positive, findings on auscultation or chest x-ray | Consider admission or referral | | 386–393, Table 22–7 |
| b. Low quad/High para | Same | Appropriate antibiotic, monitor vital capacity or ABG, chest physical therapy | If not improved within 24–48 hours, consider admission or referral | 386–393, Table 22–7 |
| 3. Deep vein thrombosis | Urine–negative Chest–negative Consider $I_{125}$IPG or venogram | Start heparin, do not range LE, later change to Coumadin | May require admission for work-up and treatment | 395–396 |
| **Bladder** | | | | |
| 1. Increased residual urines | Review fluids and medications; may require urodynamic studies | Modification of drugs | If persists, may require admission | 398 |
| 2. Difficulty with external collective devices | | | Contact center | 403–404 |
| 3. Autonomic hyperflexion | Increased blood pressure with bradycardia and distended bladder or distended bowel | Relieve obstruction, if necessary guanethidine | If persists, refer to center | 401 |
| **Bowel** | | | | |
| 1. Fecal impaction | Diarrhea, distended abdomen and possible large impaction | Cleansing or oil retention enema | Review diet, drugs, and program | 408 |
| 2. Ileus | Temperature elevation, distended abdomen, no bowel sounds | Consider ruptured viscus and admit to hospital for work-up | | 409 |
| 3. Constipation or diarrhea (mild) | See section Bowel Problems | | | 409 |
| **Skin** | | | | |
| 1. Decubitus ulcers Grade I and II | Ulceration over ischial tuberosity or other site through dermis or to adipose tissue | Keep patient off site completely | Contact center | 410–419 |
| 2. Decubitus ulcers Grade III and IV | Ulceration over ischial tuberosity or other site down to muscle and/or bone and tendon | | Refer to center | 410–419 |
| **Limitation of Motion** | | | | |
| 1. Contractures | LOM that does not release on stretch | Refer to local physical therapist for program | If progressive, refer to center | 59–64, Table 22–7 |
| 2. Spasticity | LOM that does release on stretch | Modify drugs, review exercise program | | 421–423 |

| Problem | Assessment | Action | Referral | Page |
|---|---|---|---|---|
| 3. Heterotopic Ossification | LOM that does not release on stretch and positive x-ray bone scan or elevated alkaline phosphatase | Contact center | Refer for evaluation and treatment | 420–421 |
| **Spasticity** | | | | |
| 1. Increased with low-grade fever | Consider urinary tract infection | See FEVER | | |
| 2. Causes serious functional limitation | | Increase Baclofen | If not adequately controlled, refer to center | 422–423 |
| **Pain** | | | | |
| 1. Radicular | Establish dermatome symptoms and signs, x-ray, EMG | Nerve block TENS | If unsuccessful, do not give narcotics | 423–424 |
| 2. Phantom | By history | Reassurance | Refer to center | 423–424 |
| **Sexual** | If related to altered neurophysiological responses and adaptation | | Refer to center | 423–424 |
| **Mobility** | Determine if there is an objective decrease in mobility and rule out underlying medical illness; Ask visiting PT/OT to confirm findings and assess | Contact center; refer to home care or outpatient therapy in local hospital or rehabilitation center | If patient problem persists, refer to center | 427–428, Table 22–6 |
| **Activities of daily living** | Determine if there is an objective decrease in self-care and rule out underlying medical illness; ask visiting PT/OT to confirm findings and assess | Same | Same | 427–428, Table 22–5 |
| **Equipment** | | | | |
| 1. Equipment repair | Ask visiting therapist to assess | Local vendor or facility may resolve problem | If not, contact center | 437, Table 22–7 |
| 2. New equipment determination | | | Refer to center | |
| **Individual coping** | | | | |
| 1. Denial | Determine neglect of health maintenance; assess patient or family seeking "miracle cure" | Emphasize proper attention to care and review complications; contact center if patient persists | Refer to center | 438 |
| 2. Depression | Assess severity if suicidal | Exercise usual precaution | Refer to center | 439–441 |
| **Family/Attendant** | | | | |
| Loss of family member or attendant | If family member or attendant leave patient, determine if patient can manage alone | Contact center | Refer to center | |
| **Vocational/Recreational** | | | | |
| 1. Change in work status | Any problems related to this area, refer to center | | | 442–443 |
| 2. Change in recreational status | | | | |
| **Transportation** | Determine if problems will result in other problems with any of the above | Contact center | | 444 |

incomplete paraplegics, the upper 20 per cent utilized 95 per cent of hospital days. Further refinement of this analysis is depicted in Table 22–14, which summarizes the utilization for those patients hospitalized. By comparing Tables 22–13 and 22–14, we can appreciate that a core of patients requires many days of hospitalization while the majority of patients require few days in the hospital.

This information obviously has prognostic significance as we begin to translate the group statistics to indiviudal patients. In our own experience, the most frequent causes for readmission are acute urinary tract infection with sepsis and decubitus ulcers requiring medical and surgical management. In addition, patients require readmission for reassessment of their medical and functional status and for retraining to higher levels of function. The first group of patients utilized the greatest number of hospital days.

A list of suppliers of devices and clothing is found at the end of Chapter 3.

## REFERENCES

Alba, A. et al.: Management of respiratory insufficiency in spinal cord lesions. Proceedings of the Seventeenth Veterans Administration Spinal Cord Injury Conference, 1969, pp. 200–214.

Anderson, T. P., Andberg, M. M.: Psychosocial factors associated with pressure sores. Arch. Phys. Med. Rehab. 60:341, 1979.

Becker, D. P., Gluck, H., Nulsen, F. E. and Jane, J. A.: An inquiry into the neurophysiological basis for pain. J. Neurosurg. 30(1):1–13, 1969.

Bischof, W.: Die longitudinale myelotomie. ZBL Neurochir. 11:79–88, 1951.

Bors, E: Neurogenic bladder. Urol. Surv. 7:177–250, 1957.

Bors, E. and Comarr, A. E.: Neurological Urology. Baltimore, University Park Press, 1971.

Bors, E. and Comarr, A. E.: Neurological disturbances of sexual function with special reference to 529 patients with spinal cord injury. Urol. Surv. 10:191–222, 1960.

Bors, E. and Turner, R. D.: History and physical examination in neurological urology. J. Urol. 83:759–767, 1960.

Braddom, R. L. and Johnson, E. W.: Mecamylamine in control of hyperreflexia. Arch. Phys. Med. Rehabil. 50:448–453, 1969.

Bregman, S.: Sexuality and the spinal cord injured woman. Minneapolis, Sister Kenney Institute, 1975.

Carter, E. R.: Medical management of pulmonary complications of spinal cord injury. Adv. Neurol. 22:261–269, 1979.

Cheshire, D. J. F.: Respiratory management in acute trauma tetraplegia. Paraplegia 1:252–261, 1964.

Clingenbeard-Gersten-Haehn: Energy cost of ambulation in traumatic paraplegia. Am. J. Phys. Med. 43:157–163, 1964.

Comarr, A. E.: The practical urological management of the patient with spinal cord injury. Urol. Surv. 7:177–195, 1959.

Comarr, A. E.: Sex classification and expectations among quadriplegics and paraplegics. Sexual Disab. 1(4):252–259, Winter 1978.

Coon, W. W.: Epidemiology of venous thromboembolism. Ann. Surg. 186:149–164, 1976.

Corcoran, P.: Energy expenditures during ambulation. In Dow-

ney, J. A. and Darling, R. C.: Physiological Basis of Rehabilitation Medicine. Philadelphia, W. B. Saunders Company 1971.

Cotton, L. T. and Roberts, V. C.: The prevention of deep vein thrombosis with particular reference to mechanical methods of prevention. Surgery 81:228–235, 1977.

Council on Thrombosis of the American Heart Association: Prevention of venous thromboembolism in surgical patients by low-dose heparin. Circulation 55:423A–426A, 1977.

Crewe, N. J., Athelstan, G. T. and Krumberger, J.: Spinal cord injury: a comparison of pre-injury and post-injury marriages Arch. Phys. Med. Rehabil. 60:252–256, 1979.

David, A., Gur, S. and Rozin, R.: Survival in marriage in the paraplegic couple: psychological study. Paraplegia 15:198–201, 1977–1978.

Davis, R.: Spasticity following spinal cord injury. Clin. Orthop. 112:66–75, 1975.

Davis, R. and Lentini, R.: Transcutaneous nerve stimulation for treatment of pain in spinal cord injured patients. Bull. Prosth. Res. 22:298–301, 1974.

DeBarge, O., Christensen, N. J., Corbett, J. L., Eidelman, B. H., Frankel H. L. and Mathias, C. V.: Plasma catecholamines in tetraplegics. Paraplegia 12:44–49, 1974.

Dembo, J., Leviton, G. and Wright, B.: Adjustment to misfortune—a problem of social-psychological rehabilitation. Rehabil. Psych. 22:1–100, 1975.

DeVino, M. J., Fine, P. R. and Stover, S. L.: The prevalence of SCI: a reestimation based on life tables. Spinal Cord Injury Digest 1:3–11, Winter 1980.

Dinsdale, S. M.: Decubitus ulcers: role of pressure and friction in causation. Arch. Phys. Med. Rehab. 55:147, 1974.

Eisenberg, M. G. and Falconer, J. A.: Treatment of the spinal cord injured. Spingfield, Charles C Thomas, 1978.

Erickson, R. P.: Autonomic hyperreflexia: pathophysiology and medical management.

Fink, S. P.: Crisis and motivation: a theoretical model. Arch. Phys. Med. Rehabil. pp. 592–597, November 1967.

Ford, J. and Duckworth, B.: Physical management of the Quadriplegic. Philadelphia, F. A. Davis Company, 1974.

Fordyce, W. E.: Evaluating and managing chronic pain. Geriatrics 33(1):59–62, 1978.

Frankel, H.: Bowel training. Paraplegia 4:257–258, 1967.

Freehafer, A. A. and Mast, W. A.: Lower extremity fractures in patients with spinal cord injury. J. Bone Joint Surg. 47A683–694, 1965.

Fugel-Meyer, A.: Handbook of neurology. The respiratory system. 335–347.

Furlow, W. L.: Surgical treatment of erectile impotence using the inflatable penile prosthesis. Sexual Disab. 1(4):299–306, Winter 1974.

Goodman, A. A. and Osbourne, M. P.: An experimental model and clinical definition of stress ulceration. Surg. Gynecol. Obstet. 134:563–571, 1972.

Gresiak, R. C.: Relaxation techniques in treatment of chronic pain. Arch. Phys. Med. Rehabil. 58:270–272, 1977.

Grieve, J.: The role of disturbed pressure gradients in recurrent urinary infection. Br. J. Urol. 29:289–295, 1967.

Gross, D., Ladd, H. W., Riley, E. J. et al.: The effect of training on strength and endurance of the diaphragm in quadriplegia. Am. J. Med. 68:27–35, 1980.

Guttmann, L.: Clinical management of spasticity. In Spinal Cord Injuries: comprehensive management and research, ed. 2. Oxford, Blackwell Scientific Publications, pp. 543–557, 1976.

Head, H. and Riddoch, L.: The automatic bladder, excessive sweating and some other reflex conditions in gross injuries of the spinal cord. Brain 40:188–263, 1917.

Hohmann, G.: Psychological aspects of treatment and rehabilitation of the spinal cord injured person. Clin. Orthop. 112:81–88, 1975.

Hull, R. et al.: Combined use of leg scanning and impedence plethysmography in suspected venous thrombosis. N. Engl. J. Med. 296:1497–1500, 1977.

Hussey, R. W. and Stauffer, E.: Community ambulation requirements. Arch. Phys. Med. Rehabil. 54:544–547, 1973.

Ivan, L. P.: Myelotomy in the management of spasticity. Clin. Orthop. 108:52–56, 1975.

Johnson, B., Thomason, R., Pollares, V. and Sadove, M. S.: Autonomic hyperreflexia; a review. Milit. Med. 140:345–349, 1975.

Kewalramini, L. S.: Neurogenic ulceration and bleeding associated with spinal cord injuries. J. Trauma 19:259–265, 1979.

Kewalramini, L. S.: Autonomic dysreflexia in traumatic myelopathy. Am. J. Phys. Med. 59:1–19, 1980.

Khanna, O. P. et al.: Practical urodynamics technique and interpretation. Hahnemann Medical College and Hospital, 1978.

Kisswetter, U. and Schoker W.: Lioresal in the treatment of neurogenic bladder dysfunction. Urol. Int. 30:63, 1975.

Kivilaakso, E. and Silen, W.: Pathogenesis of experimental gastric-mucosal injury. N. Engl. J. Med. 301:364–369, 1979.

Kosiak, M. et al.: Evaluation of pressure as a factor in the productional ischeal ulcers. Arch. Phys. Med. Rehab. 39:628, 1958.

Kosiak, M.: Etiology and pathology of ischemic ulcers. Arch. Phys. Med. Rehab. 40:62, 1959.

Kosiak, M.: Etiology of decubitus ulcers. Arch. Phys. Med. Rehab. 42:19, 1961.

Kosiak, M.: A mechanical resting surface: its effect on pressure distribution. Arch. Phys. Med. Rehab. 57:481, 1976.

Kozial, I. and Machlea, R. N.: Cutaneous ureteroileostomy in spinal cord injured patients; a 15 year experience. J. Urol. 114:709, 1975.

Lange, P. H. and Smith, A. D.: A comparison of the two types of penile prosthesis used in the surgical treatment of male impotence. Sexual Disab. 1(4):307–311, Winter 1978.

Langworthy, O. R., Kolb, L. C. and Lewis, L. G.: Physiology of micturition. Baltimore, Williams and Wilkins Company, 1940.

Lawman, E. and Klinger, J.: Aids to independent living. New York, McGraw-Hill Book Company, 1969.

Lindan, O.: Etiology of decubitus ulcers: experimental study. Arch. Phys. Med. Rehab. 42:774, 1961.

Lipson, A. et al.: Nitroprusside therapy for a patient with pheochromocytoma. JAMA 239:427–428, 1978.

Madersbachen, J.: The twelve o'clock sphincterotomy technique—indications, results. Urol. Int. 30:75, 1975.

Malik, M.: Manual on management of the quadriplegic upper extremity for MD's, OT's, PT's and orthotists. Harmarville Rehabilitation Center Publication, 1979.

McMaster, W. C. and Stauffer, E. S.: The management of long bone fracture in the spinal cord injured patient. Clin. Orthop. 112:44–52, 1975.

Melman, A.: Development of contemporary surgical management for erectile impotence. Sexual Disab. 1(4):272–281, Winter 1978.

Melzack, R. and Loeser, J. D.: Phantom body pain in paraplegics; evidence for a central "pattern generating mechanism" for pain. Pain 4:195–210, 1978.

Miller, S. S., Staas, W. E. and Herbison, G. J.: Abdominal problems in patients with spinal cord lesions. Arch. Phys. Med. Rehabil. 56:405–408, 1975.

Montero, J. C., Feedman, D., and Montero, D.: Effects of glossopharyngeal breathing on respiratory function after cervical cord transsection. Arch. Phys. Med. Rehabil. 48:650–653, 1967.

Mooney, T., Cole, T. M. and Chilgren, R. A.: Sexual options for paraplegics and quadriplegics. Boston: Little, Brown and Company, 1975.

Morales, P. and Golimbu, M.: Colonic urinary diversion: 10 year experience. J. Urol. 113:302, 1975.

Muellner, S. R.: Physiology of micturition. J. Urol. 65:805, May 1951.

Muravchick, S. et al.: Pentolinium for control of reflex hypertension in spinal cord injured patients. Paraplegia 16:350–356, 1978–1979.

Nathan, P. W.: Intrathecal phenol to relieve spasticity in paraplegia. Lancet 2:1099–1102, 1959.

Nepomuceno, C., Fine, P. R., Richards, J. S., Gowens, H., Stoven, S. L., Rantanuabol, U. and Houston, R.: Pain in patients with spinal cord injury. Arch. Phys. Med. Rehabil. 60:605–609, 1979.

Nicholas, J. J.: Ectopic bone formation in patients with spinal cord injury. Arch. Phys. Med. Rehabil. 54:354–359, 1973.

Paeslack, V.: Disorders of bowel function in spinal lesions. Paraplegia 4:250–254, 1967.

Pedersen, E.: Clinical assessment and pharmacologic therapy of spasticity. Arch. Phys. Med. Rehabil. 55:344–354, 1974.

Perkash, I.: Intermittent catheterization and bladder rehabilitation in spinal cord injury patients. J. Urol. 114:230–233, 1975.

Perkash, I.: An attempt to understand and to treat voiding dysfunction during rehabilitation of the bladder in spinal cord injury patients. J. Urol. 115:36, 1976.

Pierce, D. S. and Nickel, V. H.: The Total Care of Spinal Cord Injured. Boston, Little Brown and Company, 1977.

Priebe, H. U. et al.: Antacid versus cimetidine in preventing acute gastrointestinal bleeding. N. Engl. J. Med. 302:426–430, 1980.

Rabin, B. J.: The sensuous wheeler: sexual adjustment for the spinal cord injured. San Francisco, Multimedia Resource Center, 1980.

Rosman, N. and Spira, M.: Paraplegic use of walking braces. Am. J. Rehabil. Med. 55:310–314, 1974.

Rossier, F. et al.: From intermittent catheterization to catheter freedom via urodynamics; a tribute to Sir Ludwig Guttman. Paraplegia 17:73–85, 1979.

Rotter, G.: Generalized expectancies for internal versus external control of reinforcement. Psychological Monographs: General and Applied 80:1–28, 1966.

Roussan, M. S., et al.: Bladder training: its role in evaluating effect of antispasticity drugs on voiding in patients with neurogenic bladder. Arch. Phys. Med. Rehabil. 56:463–468, 1975.

Shaul, S., Bogle, J., Hale, J., and Normal, A. D.: Toward intimacy: family planning and sexuality concerns of physically disabled women. Everett, Washington, Planned parenthood of Snohomish County, 1977.

Sheps, S. G. and Kirkpatrick, R. A.: Subject review: hypertension. Mayo Clin. Proc. 50:709–720, 1975.

Shontz, F.: Physical disability and personality. In Neff, W. (ed.): Rehabilitation Psychology. Washington,: American Psychological Association, 1971.

Simon, R. L., Hyers, T. L., Gaston, J. P. and Harker, L. A.: Heparin pharmacokinetics: increased requirements in pulmonary embolism. Br. J. Haematol. 39:111–120, 1978.

Small, M. P.: The Small-Carrion penile prosthesis: surgical implant for the management of impotence. Sexual Disab. 1(4):272–281, Winter 1978.

Staas, W. E. and Denault, P.: Bowel control. Am. Fam. Phys. 7(1):90–100, 1973.

Sternbach, R. A.: Psychophysiology of pain. Int. J. Psychiatry Med. 6(1/2):63–73, 1975.

Stolov, W. C.: Rehabilitation of the bladder in injuries of the spinal cord. Arch. Phys. Med. Rehabil. pp. 467–474, November 1959.

Stoner, S. Z. et al.: Intermittent catheterization in patients previously on indwelling catheter drainage. Arch. Phys. Med. Rehabil. 54:25–30, 1973.

Stover, S. L., Hataway, C. J. and Zieger, H. E.: Heterotopic ossification in spinal cord injured patients. Arch. Phys. Med. Rehabil. 56:119–204, 1975.

Stover, S. L., Hahn, H. R. and Miller, J. M.: Disodium etidronate in the prevention of heterotopic ossification following spinal cord injury (preliminary report). Paraplegia 14:146–156, 1976.

Tanaka, M. et al.: Gastroduodenal disease in chronic spinal cord injury. Arch. Surg. 114:185–187, 1979.

Tarakulcy, E., et al.: Vesicoureteral reflux in paraplegics; results of various forms of management. Paraplegia 10:44, 1972.

Taylor, N., Benni, R. and Horning, M. R.: Neurogenic bowel management. Am. Fam. Phys. 7(5):126–128, 1973.

Todd, J. W. et al.: Deep venous thrombosis in acute spinal cord injury: a comparison of $I_{125}$ fibrinogen leg scanning, IPG and venography. Paraplegia 14:50–55, 1976–1977.

Trieschmann, R. B.: The psychological, social and vocational adjustment to spinal cord injury: a strategy for future research. Rehabilitation Services Administration Publication, 1978.

Venier, L. and Ditunno, J. F.: Heterotopic ossification in the paraplegic patient. Arch. Phys. Med. Rehabil. 52:475–497, 1971.

Villaverde, M. and McMillan C. W.: Fever, from Symptom to Treatment. New York, Litton Educational Publishing Inc., 1978.

Wharton, G. W. and Morgan, T. H.: Anklosis in the paralyzed patient. J. Bone Joint Surg. 52A:105–112, 1970.

Wheeler, H. B.: A modern approach to diagnosing deep venous thrombosis. J. Cardiovasc. Med. 5:217–231, 1980.

Yamada, S., Perot, P. L., Ducker, T. B. and Lockard, I.: Myelotomy for control of mass spasms in paraplegia. J. Neurosurg. 45:683–691, 1976.

Young, J. S.: Use of guanethidine in control of sympathetic hyperreflexia. Arch. Phys. Med. Rehabil. 44:204–207, 1963.

Young, J. S.: Follow-up care. SCI Dig. 1:2/35/36, Winter 1980.

Young, J. S. and Northrup, N. E.: Statistical information pertaining to some of the most commonly asked questions about SCI. SCI Dig. 1:11–32, Spring 1979.

# 23

# Neurogenic Bladder

*A. S. Abramson, M.D.\* and M. S. Roussan, M.D.*

The condition known as neurogenic bladder occurs most frequently with multiple sclerosis and with injury to or malformation of the neural contents of the spinal canal. There are other, less frequent, causes. Common to the condition in all these patients is the limited number of separate functions that can go awry. The most important among these are expulsion and retention of urine and duration of voiding. Abnormalities of these functions cause deviations from normal storage and emptying, resulting in retention of urine. Residual urine can be eliminated with appropriate management, and complications stemming from this problem can be avoided. In view of our inability to do much about reversing pathology, management must be directed toward the functional improvement of the process of voiding itself. Complications are more likely to be avoided if management techniques are applied early and in response to an orderly evaluation.

The process of voiding can be expressed as follows:

$$(P - R) \, T \text{ determines } V$$

when   $P$ = urine expulsion pressure (intracystic pressure)
   $R$ = urethral pressure causing resistance to urinary outflow
   $T$ = duration of voiding
   $V$ = percentage of bladder capacity voided

Although this is not a mathematical formulation, its symbolism can be recognized as a universal expression of both normal and disordered voiding. On the one hand, the formula tells us that, in the normal individual, pressure is created to expel urine from the bladder that is greater than pressure to retain urine in the bladder. The pressure to expel exists long enough to allow complete emptying. On the other hand, it tells

us that, in the individual with neurogenic bladder or with mechanical obstruction to outflow, the pressures of expulsion may become too weak, or the pressures of retention may become too strong, or both these problems may be present. Thus, the result of the pressures and resistance acting simultaneously and against one another may not be a positive quantity or, if positive, it may not last long enough. Urine will be left behind.

Ideally, the goal of management of the neurogenic bladder is to simulate normality—complete emptying at regular intervals throughout the day. This gives full play to the natural tendency of the bladder to resist invasion by and growth of pathogens.

Besides expressing a synthesis of the voiding process, the formula allows for an orderly analysis of the variables of expulsion, retention, duration of voiding, and volume. The patient with a neurogenic bladder requires such an analysis to determine how the variables have contributed to the voiding disorder and also to guide orderly management.

## EXPULSION PRESSURES

Intracystic pressure (ICP) is one factor among others that affects voiding. It is the result of the addition of intra-abdominal pressure (Pa) to pressure created by detrusor muscle contraction (Pd).

Therefore:   $ICP = Pd + Pa$

Normally, most if not all of the pressure (ICP) is generated by the detrusor (Pd). When the detrusor begins to fail, intra-abdominal pressure is brought into play. Detrusor pressure tends to be lower when the bladder is hypotonic as occurs in lower motor neuron lesions (of the conus and cauda equina). Since the bladder is a vesicoelastic organ, the detrusor may also be weakened by repeated overstretching of its wall. This can occur over time with outlet obstruction resulting from a spastic external urinary sphincter as occurs in upper motor neuron lesions. In this case, the bladder becomes enlarged and hypotonic even though it may originally have been hyperactive and of smaller than normal capacity.

## RESISTANCES TO OUTFLOW

A second factor that determines whether the outflow of urine will be satisfactory or unsatisfactory is the resistance offered by the urethra and its component parts. There is an inherent resistance of the urethral tube itself that is determined by its length and cross-sectional area as well as by the number and angles of bends in the tube. With a longer, more flexible urethra and a smaller cross-sectional area in the male, the tubal resistance ($Ru$) is greater than in the female. It may be enough to prevent complete emptying from a bladder whose detrusor cannot generate enough intracystic pressure. If there are no other obstructing elements such as an hypertrophied bladder neck ($Rn$), a spastic external urinary sphincter, or a denervated contractured sphincter ($Rs$), the increasing and sustaining of intra-abdominal pressure should easily overcome the tubal resistance ($Ru$) to achieve complete emptying.

Therefore:    $R = Ru + Rs + Rn$

## DURATIONS OF VOIDING

Expulsion and resistance are interdependent.[1] In the normal individual the sphincter maintains a modest state of tonic contraction as the bladder gradually fills. At times the tone may be extremely slight, probably because tubal resistance is adequate for the individual to remain continent. When the emptying detrusor contraction occurs, the tone of the sphincter is inhibited to allow free voiding (Fig. 23–1). The emptying contraction is characterized by rapid elevation of intracystic pressure followed by a slower decline. Detrusor contraction must generate a fairly high pressure before voiding begins simply to overcome tubal resistance. Voiding will continue in an unbroken stream to a lower pressure during relaxation of the bladder because the urethra had been distended previously by the stream. All the pressure above these opening and closing pressures is effective in expelling urine. If the effective pressure is at a low level, the stream is weak; if at a high level, the stream is strong. Therefore, completeness of emptying is dependent upon the length of time that the effective pressure is operative. In the normal individual, the time span and the effective pressure are usually enough to empty the bladder completely.

The same principles apply to the individual with neurogenic bladder. For example, excessive urinary sphincter tone may occur in the spastic individual, and it may not become inhibited during emptying detrusor contraction. Instead, there may be heightened tonic or phasic sphincter contractions or both, thus increasing the sphincteric resis-

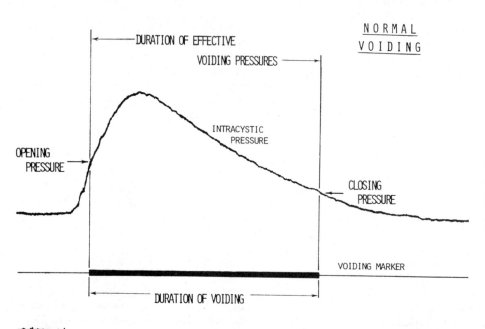

**Figure 23–1.** Definition of opening, closing, and effective voiding pressures. (From Abramson, A.: Neurogenic bladder: a guide to evaluation and management. Arch. Phys. Med. Rehab. 64:6, 1983.)

tance. The relationship between smooth (detrusor) and striate (external urinary sphincter) muscle becomes dyssynergic. In addition, the central excitatory state that is being facilitated increasingly by a rapidly increasing tempo of stimuli generated by bladder stretch during filling creates a small, hyperactive bladder subject to high pressure and short-duration uninhibited detrusor contractions.[2] Duration of effective pressure will be short, and it will be irregularly repeated and will permit only spurting or dribbling of small amounts of urine. On the other hand, an upper motor neuron bladder that has become overstretched and hypoactive because of persistent outlet obstruction will generate a lower detrusor pressure, which may not be able to overcome the heightened sphincteric resistance. Voiding will be largely interdicted except for overflow. A lower motor neuron bladder may also be incapable of developing a high enough pressure for a long enough time to overcome tubal resistance plus sphincteric resistance caused by shrinkage of the denervated sphincter. In all of these cases, substantial residual urine is the usual result. These foregoing are only a few examples illustrating that frequently duration of effective intracystic pressure is not enough to achieve complete bladder evacuation. When duration must be lengthened, the best way of doing so is for the patient to voluntarily develop adequate and prolonged intra-abdominal pressure, but the stress of maintaining such increased pressure may not be sustainable for very long. For that reason, multiple consecutive attempts at increasing intra-abdominal pressure are indicated, since total effective emptying time is what counts.

Therefore: $T = T_1 + T_2 + T_3 - - - - -$

## URINE VOLUMES

The amount of urine that is expelled has little meaning without consideration of the amount left behind. It is the residual urine volume (Vr) that does the damage. The total bladder capacity may be excessively large. It may expel a large volume (Ve) and yet leave a large residual urine volume (Vr), or the capacity may be small so that the bladder may expel a small volume (Ve) and leave a small residual (Vr) that is proportionately large in relation to the capacity. It is well known that a residual urine volume of 50 ml or less is acceptable even in the normal person. This is a good general rule, but it has become almost customary to accept a larger residual volume provided that the urine is free of pathogens. However, there must be a limit. Rapidity of fluid exchange in the bladder is an important factor in the bladder's ability to cleanse itself. Therefore, it is logical to emphasize the rela-

tionship between expelled volume (Ve) and residual volume (Vr). Some investigators have chosen a residual of 10 per cent of capacity as representing a balanced bladder because, in that case, it does not stray far from the norm of 50 ml except in the exceedingly large bladder. Others have accepted 15 per cent and still others 20 per cent. These are empirical and probably represent extensive clinical experiences with acceptable levels of safety. For all, the goal must be the lowest possible residual.

Therefore: V can be expressed as $\dfrac{Ve}{Vr + Ve} \times 100\%$

and represents the percentage of bladder capacity voided, which according to various authorities should be 80 to 90 per cent at a minimum.

The formula can now be expressed in its analytical form as follows:

$$\dfrac{[(Pa + Pd) - (Ru + Rs + Rn)] \, (T_1 + T_2 + T_3 - - - - - -)}{\text{determines } \dfrac{Ve}{Vr + Ve} \times 100\%}$$

All the factors in this formula are operative at one time or another. It may seem useful to have a detailed knowledge of all of them, but such an exhaustive analysis is not entirely necessary. As we shall see, some of these factors, when known, provide adequate indirect information about others. The formula is now ready to be used as a guide to the orderly evaluation and management of the neurogenic bladder.

## EVALUATION

Much can be determined from history, physical examination, and measurement of residual urine, and often management is based on these determinations alone. Such evaluation, which tends to be qualitative except for the residual urine determination, may lead to forms of management that are somewhat less than optimal. A consideration of all pertinent quantitive factors outlined in the analytic formula adds much to the process for the specific patient. It is for that reason that urodynamic studies have been developed,

Urodynamic studies have tended to become increasingly complex. Starting with retrograde cystometry, which measures intracystic pressure, measurements of related phenomena have been added from time to time. Cystometry tells us something about the action of bladder but not about other essential factors in voiding. With the understanding that there is a synergistic relationship between the actions of the bladder and the sphincter, simultaneous recording of the changing intracystic pressure and electrical activity of the external urinary sphincter has been developed.[3] However, this has created a number of problems, since instrumentation per se can alter the phenomena under observation. Normally, the bladder is filled with fluid in an antegrade fashion and at a certain rate. Retrograde filling of the bladder with fluid or with gas (carbon dioxide) at a rapid rate may be overstimulating and therefore is not comparable. Excretory cystometry is more physiological and is likely to provide information that is closer to what actually happens. The presence by itself of a catheter in the highly sensitive urethra may produce excessive stimulation.[4] Some investigators try to circumvent the introduction of a foreign body into the urethra by determining intracystic pressure through a suprapubic route, but even this may cause aberrant stimulation because the abdominal wall must be acutely punctured. For want of a method without instrumentation, the less the interference with the natural process, the more accurate the information will be.

Cystometry does not discriminate between pressures produced by the detrusor and the abdomen. For that reason, intrarectal pressure is often measured by the means of an intrarectal balloon in the belief that this reflects abdominal pressure. The assumption is that subtraction of this pressure from intracystic pressure will clearly delineate the pressure produced by detrusor contraction. Unfortunately, the rectum is a contractile viscus along which gas and the fecal bolus may be propelled. Therefore, the best that can be said is that this determination measures intrarectal pressure, which has a doubtful relationship to intracystic pressure. In most cases, however, cystometry largely measures detrusor pressure. Abdominal pressure becomes important only when the detrusor fails to generate enough pressure even with the use of cholinergic drugs. In that case, enhancing intra-abdominal pressure through training may elevate intracystic pressure sufficiently to initiate and maintain the urinary stream. In most cases, measurement of intracystic pressure is probably enough to determine the management method to be employed.

Simultaneous recording of the activity of the external urinary sphincter poses other problems. It is not difficult to insert electromyographic recording electrodes at or near the sphincter,[5, 6, 7] but occasionally such invasion of tissue provides still another focus of irritative feedback. Autonomic crises that develop with distention of the bladder in patients with high cord lesions usually abate when the bladder is emptied. We have seen episodes of crises that have been maintained until the electrodes had been removed (Fig. 23–2). An alternative method is to do surface recording from the rectal sphincter. The rectal and urinary sphincters, being embryologically of cloacal derivation, have common innervations and respond similarly in

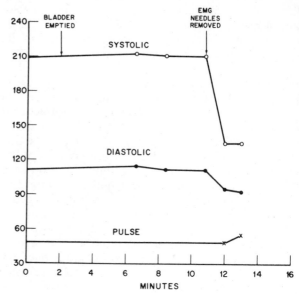

**Figure 23–2.** Example of perineal EMG electrodes sustaining autonomic crisis. (From Abramson, A.: Neurogenic bladder: a guide to evaluation and management. Arch. Phys. Med. Rehab. 64:6, 1983.)

cases of transverse myelopathy. This method is minimally invasive.

Electromyography of the sphincter gives only a semiquantitative impression of its activity and does not tell anything about other components of the urethra that may play a role in obstructing outflow. Urethrometry is required to elicit all obstructive elements and to quantify them. It can provide a urethral pressure profile when a special catheter equipped with a pressure-sensitive balloon is slowly withdrawn along the urethra from the bladder to the meatus. The catheter is length-calibrated so that the sites of pressure changes can be determined. The most frequent site of excessive pressure is at the level of the sphincter and tends to reflect its degree of spasticity in an upper motor neuron lesion (Fig. 23–3) or the degree of contracture of the denervated sphincter in a lower motor lesion. The second most frequent site is at the bladder neck, which may have become hypertrophied because of the prolonged use of a Foley catheter or because of benign prostatic hypertrophy, an uncommon condition in the age groupings under consideration. Urethrometry can also detect and place the occasional stricture. While tubal resistance is rarely a problem that needs elaborate management, the sphincter or the bladder neck or both frequently are problems, and their localization gives direction to the management process.

Flowmetry is another technique used in urodynamic studies. It determines the changing rate of urine flow. Although it has the merit of not being an invasive technique, there is not a fundamental need for its use. It is not how the urine flows that

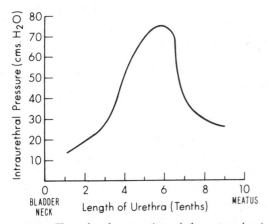

**Figure 23–3.** The role of contraction of the external urinary sphincter in obstructing urine outflow. (From Abramson, A.: Neurogenic bladder: a guide to evaluation and management. Arch. Phys. Med. Rehab. 64:6, 1983.)

is important but how much. Determination of the volume expelled and of the residual volume gives that information.

Frequent monitoring of the blood pressure throughout bladder filling is essential in the individual with high transverse myelopathy who is prone to develop autonomic crises. It is less necessary when the transverse lesion is below the midthoracic level or in patients with multiple sclerosis.

In summary, combined excretory cystometry and rectal sphincter electromyography are minimal requirements in evaluating function of the neurogenic bladder. Urethrometry gives added valuable information as does monitoring of the blood pressure in selected patients. Determinations of expelled volume and residual volume are essential. Finally, in the patient who has had repeated urinary infections, the intravenous urogram and the cystogram will determine whether reflux and deterioration of the upper urinary tract have become problems, but these need not occur with early and appropriate management as will be outlined.

## MANAGEMENT

Intermittent catheterization II has become the method of choice for immediate management when the onset of neurogenic bladder is sudden as in trauma to the contents of the spinal canal. It allows the bladder to intermittently fill and empty, it prevents overstretching or shrinkage, and it allows the system to remain closed most of the time and thus minimizes the risk of infection. It simulates the normal physiological action of the bladder until the individual passes out of the state of spinal shock without providing noxious afferent feedback to the spinal cord during its period of reorganization. The

central excitatory state in the isolated spinal cord is allowed in this way to develop and establish itself without having an excessive tendency to facilitation.[2] At the appropriate time, as determined by urodynamic studies and with suitable training, a satisfactory process of voiding can be established in the majority of patients. Occasionally, cholinergic drugs will be helpful when the bladder is hypoactive, as will anticholinergic drugs when the bladder is hyperactive. In addition, hyperactivity of the sphincter can be suppressed by the judicious use of an antispasticity agent. However, pharmacological agents should not be used as a substitute for but rather as an aid to bladder training and only when monitoring of residual urine has indicated that such agents may be of some help.

Complete emptying of the neurogenic bladder is only occasionally a completely spontaneous occurrence. It needs active participation by the patient, which is rarely self-taught and is seldom developed as a result of verbal explanation alone. Bladder training is required that is closely monitored by the therapeutic team until the patient is able to achieve the desired result (Fig. 23–4).

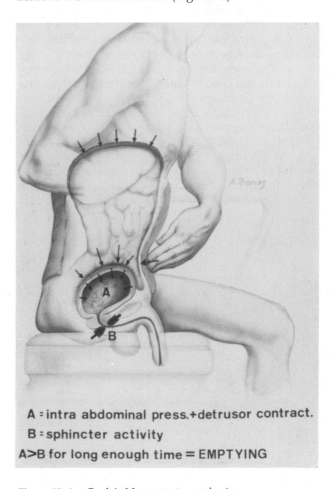

A = intra abdominal press.+detrusor contract.

B = sphincter activity

A>B for long enough time = EMPTYING

**Figure 23–4.** Crede's Maneuver to expel urine

Certain principles must be observed in bladder training. It should be done on a toilet seat to allow unhindered lowering of the pelvic floor, which has been shown to precede voiding.[8] Voiding in a chair, no matter how soft the cushion, not only interferes with the fall of the pelvic floor but also produces some pressure on the posterior urethra, especially in the individual with atrophic buttocks.

A bladder that is sensitive to reflex stimulation may contract in response to suprapubic tapping or other reflex stimulation (Fig. 23–5). However, the sphincter may undergo dyssynergic action at the same time so that only a small amount of urine is expelled in spurts or dribbles. When that occurs, the use of an antispasticity drug or stretching of the rectal sphincter or both may help to improve urine outflow. The principle underlying this method is that although effective voiding in each response to tapping is of short duration, the cumulative effect of as many responses as are needed until no urine flows may empty the bladder. This is only one kind of split voiding. Another technique is used after repeated reflex stimulation leaves an unacceptable residual amount, or when the bladder is hypoactive, enlarged, and unresponsive to reflex stimulation. In that case, there is need to enhance intracystic pressure by increasing intra-abdominal pressure. This can be done by applying the Valsalva maneuver repeatedly until no more urine flows. The maneuver may be reinforced by an elastic abdominal binder when the abdominal wall is not under voluntary control.

Some individuals are not able to empty the bladder despite appropriate physical and pharmacological management. Also, some are not physically able to participate in management of their own condition. There are at least two approaches to these problems. First, intermittent catheterization can be carried on indefinitely, and some patients do well on such a regimen. Second, persistent obstruction can be relieved by means of sphincterotomy or transurethral resection or both depending on indications for either or both as determined by urethrometry and cystoscopy.[9, 10] Even though major obstruction is relieved, voiding may still have to be assisted by sustained suprapubic pressure. In the case of contracture of a denervated sphincter, periodic dilatation of the urethra is indicated as if the sphincter were a stricture.

The onset of a neurogenic bladder can be more gradual and subtle in patients with multiple sclerosis. Complaints of urgency, frequency, nocturia, hesitation, and incontinence in any combination should not be long neglected. These symptoms occur when the bladder is either hyperactive or hypoactive and when the sphincter is spastic. Most often, they tell us that the patient is not emptying the bladder and are signals that intervention is necessary. On occasion, the basic problem is not that the bladder is being incompletely emptied but that it is too active to permit storage of adequate amounts of urine. In that case, anticholinergic drugs can improve urine storage, lengthen the time between voidings, and thus reduce frequency, nocturia, and incontinence. There is always the danger that increasing residual urine will be retained with their use. If so, the symptoms may not be relieved. Antispasticity agents and bladder training are essential to balance the bladder. When the bladder is hypoactive, the management regimen should also be the same except that cholinergic drugs are indicated.

Incontinence is a difficult problem, not only in the patient with multiple sclerosis. Pharmacological agents together with training can reduce its frequency, but balancing the bladder by these

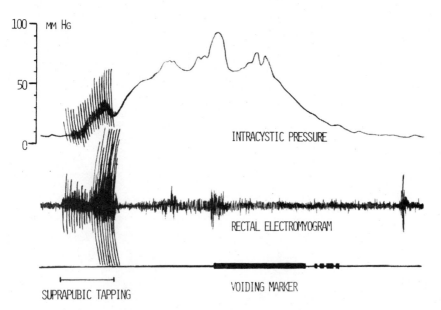

**Figure 23–5.** Effect of suprapubic tapping in stimulating detrusor contraction. Because of dyssynergic sphincter, only spurting and dribbling occurred. Lioresal reduced the number of maneuvers required from 11 to 4 to completely empty the bladder. (From Abramson, A.: Neurogenic bladder: a guide to evaluation and management. Arch. Phys. Med. Rehab. 64:6, 1983.)

means may not eliminate it entirely. If the patient cannot sense the full bladder or even if the full bladder is sensed, the capacity to inhibit urine flow temporarily may be absent so that incontinence is bound to occur, even if less frequently. In the male, this contingency can be managed with an external collecting device, but there are no good collecting devices for females. Besides, the incidence of urinary infection with such devices is greater than without them. More appropriately, the patient should learn to anticipate the full bladder and make a deliberate effort to void before it becomes full. This would require a method of even fluid intake during the day, consideration of the ambient temperature and humidity, and accurate timing of elimination based upon these factors.

If the multiple sclerosis patient develops a markedly overstretched, poorly contracting bladder as a result of prolonged obstruction by a spastic sphincter, decompression by means of intermittent catheterization is the method of choice. Catheterization should be frequent enough to take care of a large fluid intake and yet not to allow more than a modest accumulation of urine (less than 500 ml). This regimen should include bladder training with an antispasticity agent. Residural urine should be measured after each catheterization after an attempt has been made to empty the bladder according to the principles previously outlined. With this regimen, the residual volume often tends to decrease gradually until almost normal function is restored. At this time, intermittent catheterization is discontinued. Because of the unpredictability of effects of multiple sclerosis, periodic re-evaluation is called for, especially when symptoms change.

# REFERENCES

1. Abramson, A. S., Roussan, M. S. and Feibel, A.: Pathophysiology of the neurogenic bladder. Bull. N. Y. Acad. Med. 49:775–785, 1973.
2. Abramson, A. S. and Roussan, M. S.: The role of spinal cord facilitation in neurogenic bladder function. Paraplegia 11:125–131, 1973.
3. Abramson, A. S., Roussan, M. S. and D'Oronzio, G.: Method for evaluating function of the neurogenic bladder. J.A.M.A. 195:554–558, 1966.
4. Abramson, A. S. and Feibel, A.: The effects of urethral catheterization in the patient with "neurogenic" bladder. Bull. N. Y. Acad. Med. 50:580–588, 1974.
5. Giovine, G. P.: Premesse al Trattamento Neurochirurgico Delle Disfunzione Vesciali Neurogene: I. Studi Salla Funzione Dello Sfintere Striato Dell'uretra, L'elettrofinterografia. Chirurgia 14:39–62, 1958.
6. Ruskin, A. P.: Anal sphincter electromyography. Electromyography 4:425–428, 1970.
7. Ruskin, A. P. and Davis, T. E.: A new urethroanal reflex revealed by sphincter electromyography. Arch. Phys. Med. Rehab., 56:218–220, 1975.
8. Muellner, S. R.: The voluntary control of micturition in man. J. Urol. 80:493–478, 1958
9. Ross, J. C., Damanski, M. and Gibbon, N.: Resection of external urinary sphincter in the paraplegic: preliminary report. Trans. Am. Assoc. Genitur. Surg. 49:193–198, 1957.
10. Emmet, J. L.: Transurethral resection in treatment of true and pseudo cord bladder. J. Urol. 53:545–564, 1945.
11. Newman, E. and Price, M.: External catheters: a review of their use with spinal cord lesion patients (Abstrt). Arch. Phys. Med. Rehab. 60:535–536, 1979.

# 24

# Physiatric Management of Spasticity by Phenol Nerve and Motor Point Block

*by Ali A. Khalili, M.D.*

## INTRODUCTION TO THE PHYSIOLOGY OF SPASTICITY

Normally the net effect of all afferent and descending impulses in alpha and gamma motor fibers is inhibitory (Fig. 24–1A). When, because of release from the net inhibition, gamma motor activity is increased, the afferent discharge from muscle spindles in response to stretch becomes out of proportion to the stimulus, and an increased stretch reflex, or spasticity, results (Fig. 24–1B). Generally, gamma fibers control the afferent volley from muscle spindles by controlling the tone of intrafusal muscle fibers. Impulses from other receptors in capsule or subcutaneous tissue may facilitate or inhibit motor neurons depending on the location and the extent of the stimulus. Therefore, delicate manipulation of the peripheral input to the central nervous system may change the extent of spasticity; it may facilitate or even provoke movement. This physiological principle has been widely used by some therapists, particularly in the management of children with spastic cerebral palsy.

One should be aware that spasticity reduction by this method is of brief duration, and an evoked movement does not become a voluntary purposeful one. Application of this principle is justified if it is used to diminish spasticity in order to perform range of motion exercises to prevent contractures. However, with today's knowledge and experience I see no reason to spend much time and effort in a clinical setting on "peripheral neuromuscular facilitation" with the hope that evoked movements will become volitional ones. An intensive investigation in this area might be worthwhile by a group interested in the problem in a facility whose aim is discovery of knowledge rather than acquisition of grants-in-aid for institutional or personal glory.

In the central nervous system various centers have an inhibitory or facilitory effort at different synapses through descending impulses by way of rubrospinal, reticulospinal, tectospinal, and vestibulospinal tracts and corticofugal fibers, depending on the somatotropical localization. There are also poorly defined neurons besides Renshaw cells at the anterior horn column with inhibitory functions.

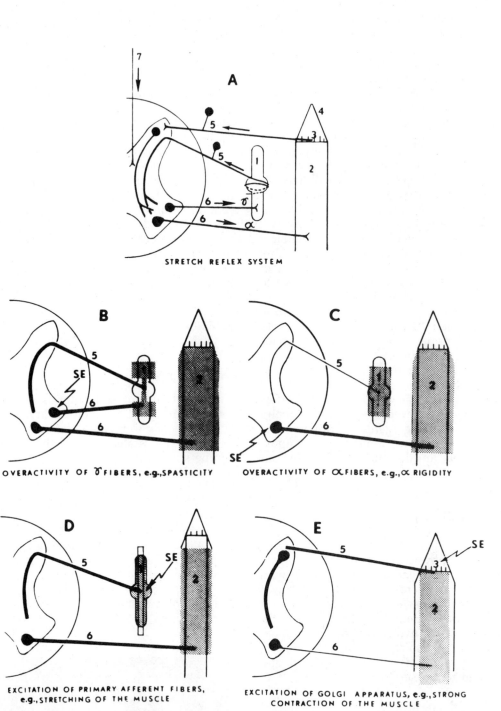

**Figure 24–1.** Diagram showing regulation of stretch reflex: The thickness of the afferent and the efferent fibers shows the frequency of firing. The muscle spindle and the extrafusal muscle fibers are shown by the solid black line. Dotted line patterns show the muscle after stimulation of the nerve. (1) Muscle spindle, (2) extrafusal muscle fibers, (3) tendon organs, (4) tendon, (5) afferent fibers, (6) efferent fibers: alpha fibers, gamma fibers, (7) decending fibers, (SE) start of excitation. (From Khalili, A. A. and Benton, J. G.: A physiologic approach to the evaluation and arrangement of spasticity with procaine and phenol nerve block including a review of the physiology of the stretch reflex. Clin. Orthop. Med. July–Aug. 1966.)

## PROSPECTIVE VIEW OF THE MANAGEMENT OF SPASTICITY

In a spastic patient usually the spasticity is more pronounced in one muscle or group of muscles in different segments of the limb or body. Clinically the physician prefers to diminish or relieve spasticity in only one muscle or group of muscles, depending on the functional goal to be achieved, rather than reduce spasticity in the entire paralytic or paretic extremity. Considering that any pharmaceutical agent used systemically will have a nondifferentiating effect, with present state of art and science, it is inconceivable to believe that patients with severe and complicated spasticity will be helped by systemic medications. The management of these patients will remain a major clinical problem until we know definitively the effect of nuclei in the central nervous system that have to do with facilitation and/or inhibition and, most important, are able to map clearly their somatotropical relationship. Then we will need improved technology, such as the use of laser beams, to attack microscopic points in inhibitory or facilitory areas of the muscle or muscle groups in which we wish to diminish spasticity. Until such knowledge of histology and physiology is acquired and such perfection in technology is achieved, we have to acquaint ourselves with all existing agents, techniques and modalities, their scope and limitations, to apply them appropriately in the management of our spastic patients.

## PHYSIATRIC MANAGEMENT OF SPASTICITY

A physiatrist—a physician specializing in physical medicine and rehabilitation or a physician with similar training and interest—is often called as a consultant for the management of spasticity in a patient with central nervous system involvement, or he might be directly involved in the comprehensive rehabilitation of such a patient.

The following questions should be raised and answered intelligently in the management of spasticity:

1. Why diminish spasticity?
2. Where should the spasticity be diminished and how?
3. What is the goal to be achieved?
4. Will the reduction of spasticity in the desired area have a deleterious effect in the same or other areas, either functionally or otherwise?

If a procedure is to be carried out, one should answer the following questions:

1. When should it be done?
2. Who is the best trained and most experienced person to do it?

After these questions have been raised, they should be answered intelligently, discussed with the patient or the family or both, and a conclusion reached. The patient has to be treated appropriately with pharmaceutical agents, therapeutic exercises, modalities, appliances or surgical procedures or both. Often in conjunction with these procedures, a physiatrist will be in charge of the comprehensive rehabilitation of the patient, including prescription of physical modalities, therapeutic exercises, braces, an appropriate wheelchair, various utensils, and modification of living environment, as well as recommendations for job modification or training, and supervision of psychosocial counseling and planning. As a rule, it is better to clarify long-term rehabilitation goals and then to manage spasticity to match these goals rather than vice versa. In some patients, management of spasticity might be the early step in total care.

## PHENOL NERVE AND MOTOR POINT BLOCK OF SPASTICITY 2–19

### APPARATUS

A direct current stimulator is used, which consists essentially of a 90-volt battery, a manually operated rheostat to regulate the current, an ammeter with multiple scale to show the range from milliampers to microampers, and a foot switch. The foot switch gives the operator freedom of both hands during the block. The stimulator is connected to an active and a dispersive electrode. The active electrode, connected to the negative pole of the stimulator, is usually a 22-gauge spinal needle 2 or 3 inches in length whose entire shaft, except at the bevel, is insulated with Teflon coating (Fig. 24–2). As the friction coefficient of Teflon is very low, the needle electrode may move easily during isolation of the fibers. To prevent this, the surface of the coating should be relatively rough for better

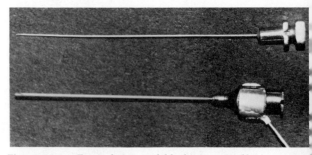

**Figure 24–2.** For isolating and blocking nerve fibers, a spinal needle with Teflon coating on its entire shaft except at the bevel is used. (From Khalili, A. A. and Betts, H. B.: Management of spasticity with phenol nerve block. Final Report RD-2529-M, Washington, D.C., U.S. Dept. of Health, Education, and Welfare, Social and Rehabilitation Service, 1970.)

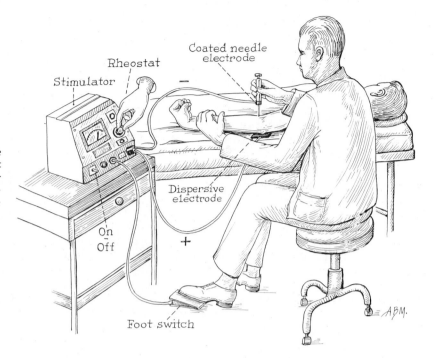

**Figure 24–3.** Appartus and procedure used for peripheral nerve and motor point phenol block. (From Khalili, A. A.: Peripheral phenol block for spasticity: In Roge, D. (ed.): Spinal Cord Injuries. Springfield, Charles C Thomas, 1969.)

stabilization. The dispersive electrode, connected to the positive pole of the stimulator, is usually placed opposite the active electrode on the same limb (Fig. 24–3).

## Phenol Solutions

A solution of 2 or 3 per cent phenol in distilled water is used. Phenol crystals are dissolved in sterile distilled water (warm, if necessary). Then the solution is passed through a Millipore filter, filtered into sterile serum vials, then stoppered, sealed with sterile technique, and labeled.

## General Technique of Block

The nerve is approached with an active coated needle using the usual technique employed for nerve blocking, with some modification at times, and stimulated by turning the foot switch on briefly. As the tip of the coated needle approaches the nerve, less current is required to elicit the maximal contraction. The needle is in the desired location when the least intensity elicits the maximum contraction in the muscle fibers in which the spasticity is to be relieved or alleviated. In this manner, the entire nerve trunk or only the nerve fibers to a muscle or a portion of a muscle can be isolated and blocked. When isolation is perfect, the phenol solution is injected. If isolation of the nerve and injection of phenol are properly performed, there should be immediate relief of spasticity in the related muscles.

If a more localized blocking is desired, the nerve can be approached with similar technique at a mo-

tor point. In such a case, the motor point is localized as described for chronaximetry by percutaneous stimulation with a square wave current of indefinite duration, after which a coated needle electrode is used for accurate isolation and injection of the blocking agent.

## MANAGEMENT OF VARIOUS CLINICAL PICTURES OF SPASTICITY BY SELECTIVE PHENOL NERVE BLOCK

### Upper Extremity Spasticity

**Finger and Wrist Flexor Spasticity.** Flexor digitorum profundus is the only flexor of the last four distal phalanges, and flexor digitorum sublimis is the prime flexor of the last four midphalanges. The former muscle cooperates with the latter in producing flexion of the last four proximal interphalangeal and metacarpophalangeal joints and wrist. These muscles also have a pronatory effect in the forearm. Normally synergistic contraction of wrist extensors not only prevents the wrist from going into flexion when the fingers are flexed but creates some mechanical advantages in grasp when the wrist goes into about 30 degrees of extension. The prime flexors of the last four metacarpophalangeal joints are dorsal and volar interossei and the lumbricales. These muscles are also the extensors of the last four proximal and distal interphalangeal joints. The palmaris longus, a frequently absent muscle, is also an accessory flexor of the last four metacarpophalangeal joints. Flexor digiti minimi also produces flexion at the fifth metacarpophalangeal joint. Flexor carpi radialis and ulnaris and palmaris longus are the prime flexors of the wrist. These muscles also have pronatory effect in the forearm. The flexor effect of flexor digitorum sublimis and profundus in the wrist has already been stated. Flexor pollicis longus is the primary flexor of the interphalangeal joint of the thumb and also produces flexion at the metacarpophalangeal joint and to a slight degree also at the carpometacarpal joint. Flexor pollicis brevis flexes the thumb at the metacarpophalangeal joint and produces a slight degree of flexion at the carpometacarpal joint.

The median nerve innervates flexor digitorum sublimis, flexor carpi radialis, palmaris longus, flexor pollicis longus, superficial head of flexor pollicis brevis, first and second lumbricales, and flexor digitorum profundus to index and middle fingers. The ulnar nerve innervates flexor carpi ulnaris, all interosseous muscles, third and fourth lumbricales, median head of flexor pollicis brevis, flexor digiti quinti, and flexor digitorum profundus to the ring and little fingers (Fig. 24–4A).

The prime pronators of the forearm are pronator quadratus and pronator teres, which are innervated by the median nerve; however, flexors of the wrist and the long flexors of the fingers have also a pronator effect.

There might be indication for median or ulnar nerve block or both types.

MEDIAN NERVE BLOCK. The median nerve is approached in the antecubital fossa at the level of the medial epicondyle where the nerve is medial to the brachial artery. If for some pathological reason the artery cannot be palpated, percutaneous stimulation of the nerve is used to determine its location. A coated needle electrode then is used to isolate the desired fibers. Depending on the clinical picture, the primary goal might be to block flexor digitorum sublimis or related wrist flexors of flexor digitorum profundus (Fig. 24–4B).

The nerve fibers to pronator teres, which is a strong pronator, should usually not be blocked. This is because, following the block, it is desirable for the hand to remain in semipronation, which is a more functional position for most patients with paresis and is more acceptable cosmetically. When there is spasticity in the elbow flexors, particularly the biceps brachialis, relief of spasticity in the pronators would result in a semi-flexed elbow, supinated forearm, and open-hand "begger's hand," which is very unsatisfactory cosmetically. When the nerve is approached at the medial epicondyle level, the fibers to pronator teres have usually already branched out from the median nerve; however, the physician should avoid the fibers to pronator teres as much as possible in case there is more distal branching off of these fibers.

In some persons the nerve is very superficial. In such a case the nerve usually should be approached in an oblique fashion rather than vertically as is done when the nerve is embedded in a mass of fatty tissue in an obese patient, and isolation of the nerve usually is very difficult. In such cases, after the tip of the coated needle electrode is in the vicinity of the nerve, probing should be brisk in order to catch the nerve (like catching a fish in the water with a stick).

ULNAR NERVE BLOCK. The ulnar nerve is approached about one fingerbreadth proximal to the medial epicondyle, at the medial aspect of the distal part of the biceps, medial to the median nerve. Depending on the clinical picture, the desired fibers of the nerve are searched for after the coated needle electrode has passed through the medial intermuscular septum. Patients with a spastic upper extremity usually cannot be placed prone (as is normally done for an ulnar nerve block) for a longer period of time due to spastic elbow flexors, shoulder adductors, and internal rotators. Therefore, approaching the nerve from the volar aspect of the arm is advantageous because it enables these patients to be placed in a comfortable supine position making it possible for the physician to take his time to search for and isolate the desired fibers.

Depending on the clinical picture, the fibers to flexor carpi ulnaris or flexor digitorum profundus to the fourth and fifth digits or to the interosseous muscles innervated by the ulnar nerve could be isolated and blocked (Fig. 24–4C).

To prevent compression neuropathy or paresis, the solution should not be injected into the fibroosseous canal where the nerve passes through at the medial aspect of the elbow.

In a severely spastic hand one usually plans a block of median and ulnar nerve; however, after the block of one nerve there is, in most cases, enough relief of spasticity in the territory of the other nerve to eliminate the need for a further block. Therefore, as a rule of thumb, the nerve with the maximum spastic territory should be approached first, and generally about a week later a decision should be made as to whether a further block is needed.

**Elbow Flexor Spasticity.** The prime flexors of the elbow are brachialis anticus and biceps brachialis, which are innervated by the musculocutaneous nerve. The auxiliary flexors of the elbow are the brachioradialis and extensor carpi radialis longus, which are innervated by the radial nerve. The block of the musculocutaneous nerve is usually sufficient to overcome a flexed position of the elbow due to spasticity. Gravity, when the patient is in an upright position, and slight spasticity of the elbow extensors tend to extend the elbow. Preservation of spasticity in the auxiliary muscles and part of the brachialis anticus, which is sometimes innervated by the radial nerve, helps to prevent

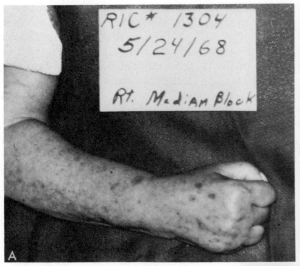
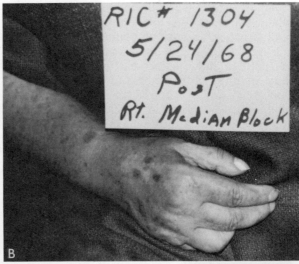
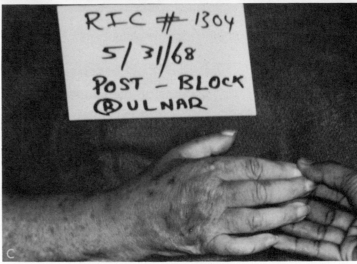

**Figure 24–4.** *A,* Finger flexors spasticity commonly occurs in spastic hemiplegic. Not only does it interfere with function, in severe cases maintaining hygiene of the palm of the hand becomes a major problem. *B,* Spasticity is relieved in median nerve territory, immediately following median nerve block with 3% of distilled phenol solution. *C,* Complete relief of spasticity has occurred in all fingers and wrist flexors after ulnar phenol nerve block in addition to the median nerve block.

full extension of the elbow, whereby the extremity assumes a rather normal and cosmetic position.

MUSCULOCUTANEOUS NERVE BLOCK. The nerve is approached within the longhead of the biceps laterally, and the shorthead of the biceps and the coracobrachialis medially, immediately below the lower edge of pectoralis major, while the extremity is placed in about 70 degrees abduction with the elbow extended as much as possible. In this area where the musculocutaneous nerve crosses over the brachialis anticus obliquely, the nerve should be searched for with a coated needle and the fibers to brachialis anticus and/or biceps, depending on the clinical picture, isolated and blocked.

**Unusual Clinical Pictures.** Sometimes some unusual clinical picture is seen, such as spasticity in triceps, shoulder abductor, shoulder adductor, internal and/or external rotators, or spasticity in a patient with a spastic paresis who had a muscle transplant. Depending on the clinical picture, motor point phenol blocks or partial phenol block of various nerve fibers has to be done. Kinesiological electromyography might be indicated prior to the block, particularly in a patient with a tendon transplant who requires selective relief of spasticity in various muscles.

## LOWER EXTREMITY SPASTICITY

**Plantar Flexor Spasticity.** Plantar flexor spasticity is the most commonly seen manifestation of central nervous system involvement with spasticity. The plantar flexors are gastrosoleus, plantaris, flexor digitorum longus, flexor hallucis longus, tibialis posterior, and peroneus longus. Spasticity in gastrosoleus causes the most problems.

Plantar flexor spasticity may cause plantar flexion during swing phase in an ambulatory patient. As such a patient usually is unable to compensate for this spasticity by flexing the knee or hip-hiking, swing phase becomes cumbersome or impossible. In a wheelchair-bound patient plantar flexor spasticity creates difficulty in transfer. Clonus of the ankle usually occurs while the patient is sitting in the wheelchair with the foot on the pedal. In a bed-bound patient clonus of plantar flexors may cause a friction sore at the dorsal aspect of the heel or heel cord. Plantar flexor spasticity may cause difficulty in putting the shoes on or in keeping them on.

Prolonged spasticity in the muscles results in the development of contracture, which is often seen in the gastrocnemius rather than soleus. Inappropriate stretching of the gastrosoleus may cause subluxation of Chopart's joint.

The spasticity can be managed either by motor point block or medial popliteal nerve block (Fig. 24–5A, B). Motor point blocks require multiple needling. For instance, the gastrosoleus has six motor points; frequently, besides reduction or relief of spasticity in the gastrosoleus, some reduction in spasticity in other flexors is also required. Therefore, a block of the medial popliteal nerve is usually indicated with fibers to the gastrosoleus being the prime target.

After the popliteal artery is palpated, the nerve is approached lateral to the artery in the upper portion of the popliteal fossa, just distal to the bifurcation of the sciatic nerve, into the medial and lateral popliteal nerve—approximately 4 fingerbreadths above the popliteal crease.

If the artery cannot be palpated, the nerve is isolated first by percutaneous stimulation. Approaching the nerve at the proximal part of the popliteal fossa has the following advantages: (1) It prevents inadvertent injection of phenol solution into the knee joint. (2) If the tip of the needle is too lateral during stimulation, contraction in the territory of the common peroneal nerve is observed, thereby indicating that the tip of the needle should be deviated medially. (3) If the needle electrode is too proximal, it will go through the hamstring muscles; consequently, during stimulation, while the nerve is approached, movement of the needle can be observed because it causes contraction of the related muscle. To support the medial arch of the foot and prevent calcaneal navicular ligament sprain, some spasticity should be maintained in the long toe flexors, particularly in the patient with long-standing spasticity.

A block of the peroneus longus is not usually needed since this muscle is a plantar flexor and evertor, and the evertor action of this muscle is beneficial in counteracting the invertor spasticity, particularly that of tibialis posticus.

**Foot Invertor Spasticity.** The prime invertor of the foot is tibialis posterior (Fig. 24–6). Flexor digitorum longus and flexor hallucis longus are accessory invertors. Tibialis anterior is an invertor in the supinated foot, and its spasticity may aggravate the severity of inversion in the foot. Inversion occurs most frequently during swing phase, and in the ambulatory patient this is dangerous because of the possibility of sprain or fracture of the ankle or a fall or both. In a nonambulatory bed-bound patient, invertor spasticity usually is not a problem; however, it may be disabling in a patient who is independent in transfer activities.

If inversion is primarily caused by tibialis posterior spasticity, motor point block of this muscle is indicated. However, as spasticity in invertors usually is concomitant with plantar flexor spasticity, a medial popliteal nerve block is indicated, with the primary target being fibers to the gastrosoleus and the secondary target tibialis posticus. If tibialis an-

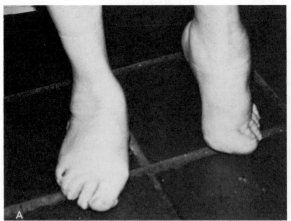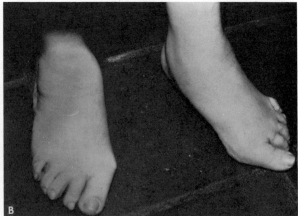

**Figure 24–5.** *A,* Plantar flexors spasticity is often seen in spastic hemiplegia, paraplegia, and quadriplegia. It interferes with ambulation and promotes contracture formation. This hemiplegic patient has pre-existing contracture, the residual effect of a previous case of polio, besides the spasticity. *B,* The spasticity is relieved and the heel reaches the floor on weight bearing following medial popliteal phenol nerve block. There is no sensory impairment; voluntary plantar flexion is preserved and dorsi-flexion is increased.

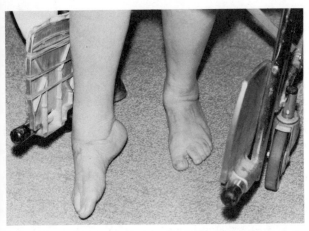

**Figure 24–6.** Invertors spasticity is most hazardous in ambulatory and wheelchair bound patients. It may cause sprain of the ankle and/or fall and fracture.

terior spasticity would still cause significant inversion, a supplementary motor point block of the tibialis anterior should be done.

**Toe Flexor Spasticity.** Flexor digitorum longus acts mainly as a flexor of terminal joints of the last four toes. In the absence of spasticity in lumbricals and interossei, which are flexors at the metatarsophalangeal joints, and flexor digitorum brevis, which primarily flexes the proximal interphalangeal joints, severe curling of the toes may take place. When this occurs the tips of the toes and sometimes the distal parts of the nails become weight-bearing areas making ambulation painful. If significant spasticity is present also in the lumbricals, interossei, and flexor digitorum brevis, various degrees of flexion occur in metacarpophalangeals and proximal and distal interphalangeal joints, depending on the extent of spasticity in these muscles. Therefore, on ambulation, increased anteroposterior and mediolateral arching of the foot takes place causing the tip of the toes to become an increased weight-bearing area, with resulting pain. Sometimes spasticity and pain in these muscles occurs only after some ambulation. Because the pain is relieved after a short rest, it may be mistaken for intermittent claudication. At times spastic contraction in flexor digitorum longus takes place while the patient is trying to put his shoes on, making the task impossible because of curling of the toes.

In isolated flexor digitorum longus spasticity, motor point block of this muscle is indicated. Use of plantar, tibialis posterior, or medial popliteal nerve and/or various motor point blocks might be indicated, depending on distribution of spasticity.

**Toe Extensor Spasticity.** The main extensors are extensor pollicis longus, extensor digitorum longus, and extensor digitorum brevis. In contrast to the hand, the insertion of pedal interossei does not extend beyond the proximal phalanx of each digit. Consequently, they take no part in the extension of distal joints.

Toe extensor spasticity causes hyperextension of the toes, which usually occurs at the beginning of swing phase of the gait contrary to flexor spasticity, which often occurs at the end of swing phase. Extension of the toe, particularly the first one, may cause pain and toenail problems. A tight toebox is a precipitating factor in the development of problems. If spasticity in the extensors of toes is severe, subluxation of the metatarsophalangeal joint may occur gradually. This may occur during recovery from spinal shock or after the central nervous system injury has reached a stable stage.

Depending on the muscles involved and the extent of spasticity, a motor point block or a block of related fibers of the common peroneal nerve is indicated. The extent of spasticity in antagonistic muscles should be evaluated prior to such a block to prevent severe flexor spasticity.

**Knee Flexor Spasticity.** The knee flexors are the hamstring muscles (semimembranosus, semitendinosus, long and shorthead of the biceps), gracilis, gastrocnemius, plantaris, and popliteus. Hamstring muscles are the prime flexors of the knee. Semimembranosus, semitendinosus, and longhead of the biceps are biarticular; they are knee flexors as well as hip extensors. Therefore, spastic flexion of the hip and extension of the knee may be exaggerated if a significant degree of spasticity in hip flexors and knee extensors exists prior to the relief of spasticity in the hamstring muscles. Before attempting to relieve spasticity in the hamstrings, one has to be willing to perform a block of L2 and L3 and possibly L1 and L4 spinal nerves to overcome such a problem. When the sole of the foot is supported, hamstring and soleus muscles extend the knee. Therefore, before spasticity in these muscles is relieved, the knee-extending effect on the weight-bearing extremity of voluntary and/or spastic contraction of these muscles has to be carefully evaluated.

A block of sciatic nerve fibers to the hamstring muscles or a motor point block of individual muscles will relieve the spasticity. If, in addition to spasticity of the hamstrings, plantar flexor spasticity exists, sciatic nerve block is the procedure of choice. The nerve is usually approached at the gluteal fold. In this location an early branching of the sciatic nerve sometimes exists, and these individual branches should be searched for and blocked.

**Knee Extensor Spasticity.** The quadriceps is the prime knee extensor. When the foot is supported, the hamstring and soleus muscles become knee extensors also. Often some spasticity in knee extensors is desirable. Extensor spasticity on weight bearing might be the main or the sole source of energy to bring the knee into extension. Once the knee has reached full extension, some patients have learned to shift the line of gravity in front of the knee axis and thus prevent the knee from buckling, even though at this stage relaxation in the quadriceps occurs. At times severe spasticity of quadriceps prevents knee flexion in swing phase of the gait in the patient with spastic paresis. Often clonus of the quadriceps, involuntary extension of the knee while the patient is sitting, and inability of the patient to bend his knee actively or passively are the main disturbing problems.

In no patient is complete relief of spasticity in quadriceps indicated, especially in the presence of some spasticity in the knee flexors, and a balance should be established between flexors and extensors depending upon the functional goal to be achieved. Partial block of femoral nerve or limited motor point block of quadriceps will relieve spasticity. The nerve is approached at the proximal part of the thigh lateral to the femoral artery. It is advisable to approach the nerve about two fingerbreadths distal to the inguinal ligament in view of the difficulty in diagnosing a hernia or detecting an inadvertent intestinal perforation by the needle electrode in patients with sensory and motor impairment.

**Hip Adductor Spasticity.** The hip adductors are adductor longus, brevis, and magnus, the gracilis, and the pectineus. The adductor longus and brevis and the gracilis are innervated by the anterior branch of the obturator nerve. The adductor magnus is innervated by the posterior branch of the obturator and a branch of the sciatic nerve. The femoral nerve innervates the pectineus.

Bilateral adductor spasticity causes scissor gait in ambulation and makes perineal hygiene difficult, particularly in the female. Adductor spasticity also causes flexion of the hips with undersirable consequences. Unilateral hip adductor spasticity results in pelvic obliquity and pseudoshortening of the spastic side when the muscles go into spastic contraction.

Partial obturator nerve block is indicated and usually is sufficient. Enough spasticity should be left in adductors to overcome the spasticity in hip abductors and to prevent abduction deformity, which often is seen after obturator neurectomy.

Because of severe adductor spasticity the legs usually cannot be abducted; therefore, the obturator nerve in its canal is usually inaccessible. The two branches of the nerve are approached and blocked at the proximal part of the thigh medial to the femoral vein. Sometimes, due to early division, the branches to various muscles cannot be isolated. In such cases a motor point block of spastic muscles should be performed as a supplementary procedure. A block of the pectineus muscle is seldom needed.

**Hip Internal Rotator Spasticity.** The principal internal rotators are adductor magnus, tensor fasciae, and the anterior portion of gluteus minimus and medius. The foremost fibers of gluteus maximus also can produce internal rotation when the hip is markedly flexed. A mild degree of internal rotation of the extremity causes abnormal gait in the ambulatory patient. A severe degree of internal rotation causes the tip of the foot, on swing phase, to hit the weight-bearing extremity, which frequently causes the patient to fall. In a growing child spastic internal rotation of the hip often causes progressive deformities, particularly in the distal part of the extremity.

Prior to any block the effect of each muscle on internal rotation should be accurately evaluated. At times a kinesiologic electromyographic study of spastic muscles should be carried out before a motor point block of the muscle is performed. An obturator nerve block with a block of fibers to adductor magnus should be tried first if adductor and internal rotator spasticity coexist.

**Hip External Rotator Spasticity.** The principal external rotators are gluteus maximus, piriformis, obturator internus, obturator externus, quadratus, femoris, and gemelli. These muscles, except gluteus maximus, are inaccessible for phenol block of peripheral nerve and motor point because of their anatomical position and innervation. At times a block of gluteus maximus may be indicated. Hip external rotator spasticity often causes a more stable knee by externally rotating the axis of the knee joint from the frontal plane. However, in the acceleration stage of swing phase, the heel of the swinging foot may hit the weight-bearing extremity, in which case a block of the hamstrings might be helpful.

**Hip Flexor Spasticity.** The prime hip flexor is the iliopsoas. Tensor fascia lata, rectus femoris, and sartorius are accessory hip flexors. Adductor longus is an adductor in all positions and a flexor up to 70 degrees of flexion; adductor brevis and magnus are adductors and also hip flexors up to 50 degrees of flexion. Gracilis, besides being an adductor in all positions, is a hip flexor up to 20 to 40 degrees of flexion. The pectineus is a weak flexor. Hip flexor spasticity often causes positioning problems in a bedridden or wheelchair-bound patient with the resulting complications. Flexed position of the hip causes development of flexion contracture, which significantly interferes with erect ambulation. Spasticity or contracture or both usually cause increased lumbar lordosis, especially in a growing patient. Ambulation without appropriate means to reduce hip flexor spasticity or contracture or both may aggravate the deformity, because the line of gravity is passing in front of the axis of the hip joint and exaggerates hip flexion.

To determine hip flexor spasticity, the patient should be in a supine position with the legs hanging freely away from the examining table. In this position flexion of the hips secondary to spastic contraction of the hamstrings can be ruled out.

An appropriate partial nerve block or motor point block is indicated if spastic hip flexion is caused by spasticity in an accessory hip flexor. To relieve prime hip flexor (iliopsoas) spasticity, a block of L1, L2, or L3 or all three spinal nerves at the paravertebral area is indicated. The iliopsoas muscle is deeply located and perfect isolation of nerve fibers to this muscle is practically impossible; therefore, the real indication for spinal nerve block is relief of spasticity in the hip flexors, hip adductors, and the knee extensors. In the presence of knee flexor spasticity, such a block may aggravate the knee flexion, thus requiring a further block to relieve this spasticity.

The indication for lumbar spine nerve block in hemiplegic patients is very limited. In my experience it has been limited to patients with spinal cord injury and multiple sclerosis.

## REVIEW OF THE FINDINGS

For the management of spasticity of various etiologies, 495 phenol nerve blocks were done with 267 blocks under a strict research protocol to determine the clinical and physiological effects. Since termination of the study the procedure has been used widely in the management of spastic patients. The findings were:

1. In 94 phenol nerve blocks with completed follow-up study, it was demonstrated that the duration of effectiveness of block ranged from 10 to 850 days, with an average duration of 317 days.

2. Paresthesia developed in 13 per cent of patients undergoing a total of 267 peripheral phenol nerve blocks. It was managed by reassurance or a simple analgesic or both. A tight and heavy woolen stocking for paresthesia of the distal lower extremity and a tight and heavy woolen glove for distal upper extremity paresthesia were effective in eliminating the discomfort of light touch, particularly when it occurred at night from movement of the sheet. It is my impression that paresthesia to a great extent is related to traumatic neuritis rather than chemical neuritis.

3. Immediate pre- and post-block amplitude ratio study of Achilles tendon–evoked potentials, M-response distal and proximal, and H-reflex distal and proximal were done following nine medial popliteal phenol nerve blocks with 2 and 3 per cent phenol solutions in eight patients. It was concluded that phenol solutions of these dilutions relieve spasticity primarily by blocking gamma motor fibers and, to a certain degree, I-A afferent and small alpha motor fibers. Preservation of at least some of alpha motor function has been demonstrated clinically and electromyographically.

**Case 1.** A 19-year-old patient with diagnosis of dystonia musculorum deformans, following cryo-surgery of thalamus developed spastic right hemiplegia. At the time of referral to me the patient had severe spasticity with sustained clonus in addition to dystonic contractions in plantar flexors. Right medial popliteal phenol nerve block with 3 per cent phenol solution relieved spasticity in plantar flexors and abolished clonus and ankle jerk. Voluntary plantar flexion and dystonic contractures persisted in the plantar flexors.

Relief of spasticity primarily was related to gamma motor block, and preservation of voluntary and dystonic contractions was related to the preservation of at least some of the alpha motor neurons. Also, it was concluded that gamma loop had no direct contributing effect on dystonic contraction in dystonia musculorum deformans.

**Case 2.** A 33-year-old patient developed a state of hypertonia of unknown etiology in left plantar flexors. At the time of referral there was severe spasticity with sustained clonus in plantar flexors. This was relieved by 3 per cent phenol solution block of the medial popliteal nerve. Ankle jerk and clonus were relieved, but the hypertonic state, particularly in the gastrosoleus, persisted. Electromyography showed rather persistent action potential at rest related to alpha rigidity[3] and was managed with 7 per cent phenol solution motor point block of the gastrosoleus (Fig. 24–1C).

4. Histologically, within the nerve trunk, I-A and gamma motor fibers to a muscle are in the same vicinity as alpha-motor fibers.

## REFERENCES

1. Khalili, A. A. and Benton, J. G.: A physiologic approach to the evaluation and management of spasticity with procaine and phenol nerve block including a review of the physiology of the stretch reflex. Clin. Orthopaed. (July-Aug.) 1966, pp. 97–104.
2. Khalili, A. A. and Harmel, M. H.: Preliminary report on the management of spasticity by selective peripheral nerve block with dilute phenol solutions. Am. Cong. Phys. Med. Rehabil., Saratoga Springs, N. Y., 1963.
3. Khalili, A. A., Harmel, M. H., Forster, S. and Benton, J. G.: Management of spasticity by selective peripheral nerve block with dilute phenol solutions in clinical rehabilitation. Presented before the Am. Cong. Phys. Med. Rehabil., Dallas, Tex., 1963.
4. Khalili, A. A., Harmel, M. H., Forster, S. and Benton, J. G.: Management of spasticity by selective peripheral nerve block with dilute phenol solutions in clinical rehabilitation. Arch. Phys. Med. 45:513–519, 1964.
5. Katz, J., Feldman, D. J. Knott, L. and Russell, A. J.: Peripheral nerve blocks with dilute phenol solution in the treatment of spasticity. Anesthesiology 26:254, 1965.
6. Halpern, D. and Meelhuysen, F. E.: Phenol motor point block in the management of muscular hypertonia. Arch. Phys. Med. Rehabil. 47:659–664, 1966.
7. Glass, A., Liebgold, H. and Mead, S.: Peripheral phenol blocks in the treatment of spasticity in children. 20th Annual Meeting of Am. Acad. Cerebral Palsy, New Orleans, La., 1966.
8. Khalili, A. A. and Betts, H. B.: Isolated block of musculocutaneous and perineal nerves in the management of spasticity with special reference to the use of a nerve stimulator. Anesthesiology 28:219–222, 1967.
9. Katz, J., Knott, L. and Feldman, D. J.: Peripheral nerve in-

jections with phenol in the management of spastic patients. Arch. Phys. Med. 48:97–99, 1967.

10. Halpern, D. and Meelhuysen, F. E.: Duration of relaxation after intramuscular neurolysis with phenol. J.A.M.A. 200:1152–1154, 1967.

11. Knott, L., Katz, J. and Rubinstein, L. J.: Separate and combined effects of phenol, hyaluronidase and dimethyl sulfoxide on the sciatic nerve of the rat. I. Acute studies. Arch. Phys. Med. 49:100–104, 1968.

12. Fusfeld, R. D.: Electromyopgraphic findings after phenol block. Arch. Phys. Med. 49:217–220, 1968.

13. Glass, A., Cain, H. D., Liebgold, H. and Mead, S.: Electromyographic and evoked potential responses after phenol blocks of peripheral nerves. Arch. Phys. Med. 49:455–459, 1968.

14. Moritz, B. M. and Svantesson, G.: Electromyographic studies of peripheral nerve block with phenol. 5th International Cong. Phys. Med, Montrael, 1968.

15. Mooney, V. Frykman, G. and McLamb, J.: Current status of intraneural phenol injections. Clin. Orthop. 63:122–131, 1969.

16. Khalili, A. A. and Betts, H. B.: Conduction velocity, electromyography and amplitude ratio studies after phenol nerve block for the management of spasticity. 7th International Cong. Electroencephal. Clin. Neurophysiol. San Diego, Calif., 1969.

17. Khalili, A. A.: Peripheral phenol block for spasticity. In Ruge, D. (ed.): Spinal Cord Injuries. Springfield, Charles C Thomas, 1969, pp. 153–160.

18. Burkel, W. E. and McPhee, M.: Effect of phenol injection into peripheral nerve of rat: electron microscope studies. Arch. Phys. Med. 51:391–397, 1970.

19. Khalili, A. A.: Pathophysiology, clinical picture and management of spasticity. In Harmel, (ed.): Clinical Anesthesia. Neurologic Consideration. Phildelphia, F. A. Davis Co., 1967, pp. 112–136.

20. Khalili, A. A. and Betts, H. B.: Management of Spasticity with Phenol Nerve Block. Final Report RD-2529-M, Washington, D.C., U.S. Dept. of Health, Education and Welfare, Social and Rehabilitation Service, 1970.

# Wheelchair Prescription

*by Dorothy Pezenik, O.T.R. Masayoshi Itoh, M.D., M.P.H., and Mathew Lee, M.D., M.P.H., F.A.C.P.*

## WHY A WHEELCHAIR?

The chair has been defined as a seat for one person, with four legs and a backrest. The wheelchair, possibly because of its name and predecessors, has become one of the most frequently misunderstood and misused medical appliances.

Historically, the wheelchair was not invented to provide a seat or even a seat with wheels, the latter being the ancestor of a variety of industrial seats and office chairs. The fundamental principle of the wheelchair is to substitute moving wheels for lower extremities in order to provide mobility for those deprived of ambulation. In a wheelchair, the seat is to the wheels as the saddle is to the horse or the driver's seat is to the car; and neither car nor horse was improvised to go with seat or saddle.

"Wheeled chair" has become the accepted concept, but a more accurate and appropriate concept would be "chaired wheels." Chaired wheels is undoubtedly awkward to pronounce, so the word wheelchair entered both the medical nomenclature and the lay vocabulary.

The word wheelchair lacks scientific medical aura and tone; the object it refers to looks like a chair on wheels and thus, without hesitation, the public assumes it to be one. Today, at least 1 million persons in the United States are confined to wheelchairs. Thousands upon thousands more are temporary wheelchair users, and it has been estimated that 80 to 95 per cent of the wheelchairs sold are obtained without professional guidance or prescription.

A person in a wheelchair in a supermarket, department store, or on a street is no longer an unusual sight in American communities. The symbol of accessibility (Fig. 25–1), which depicts a man in a wheelchair, has gained international acceptance to signify the existence of special accommodation for the disabled.

Obviously, not all victims of chronic disease will become disabled, nor will they require wheelchairs. Currently, the prevalence of wheelchair users is 3 in 1000 people in this country. However, chronic disease accompanied by aging can be expected to increase the incidence of disabilities that necessitate the use of a wheelchair. Thus, it is germane and prudent to prepare for a commensurate rise in need.

The unprescribed wheelchair is potentially as harmful and hazardous as the self-prescribed drug. It can cause trauma, secondary deformities and disabilities, and other complications that may be irreversible. On the other hand, a correctly prescribed chair will enable some people to continue productivity and many to regain or maintain their functional capacities.

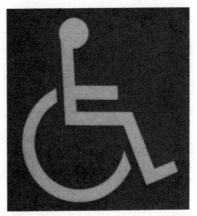

**Figure 25–1.** Symbol of accessibility.

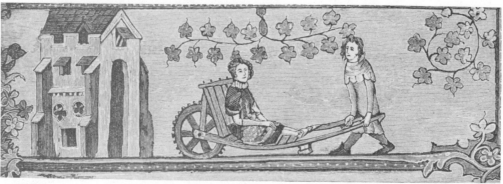

**Figure 25–2.** The lady of the manor, A.D. 1338–1344.

## WHEELING THROUGH THE AGES

For centuries, humans have sought means of transporting themselves over long distances and have sought relief from carrying heavy burdens. In the search, people have been carried on all kinds of litters and chairs, with every animal utilized from dog to reindeer. Since the invention of the wheel about 3500 B.C., people have devised countless vehicles, from chariots to carriages and covered wagons to convertibles, in order to avoid the hardships of travel by foot. However, until the late 19th century, little attention was devoted to providing conveyance or mobility for those who could not walk.

Periods of splendor came and went, civilizations rose and fell, and yet, as late as the 16th century, the sick and lame who wished to move from place to place still had to be carried. The wealthy and the nobility moved elegantly about their palaces and estates, borne on elaborate, well-cushioned litters by servants. The litters were also practical for short-distance town travel and they could be gently eased over the bumpy unpaved streets of that day. Ornate carriages provided the rich with long-distance transportation, and coachmen and body servants assisted invalids during a trip. One such example is shown in a picture from the 14th century entitled "The Lady of the Manor" (Fig. 25–2). A close examination of the woman in this print reveals maldevelopment of her lower extremities.

The poor, lacking resources and luxury and dependent on family or friends, were usually transported on a strong man's back or in a sling. Wheelbarrows were pressed into service for long journeys. However, even royalty did not enjoy complete convenience, as litters were not adaptable to small areas. Philip II of Spain, possessor of the mighty 130-ship Spanish Armada, became ill and infirm in his last years and had no convenient or comfortable invalid chair. In 1595, three years before his death at age 71, a chair with wheels was made for

him with gatched back and gatched legrest panel. This allowed the king to recline and be pushed by his manservant from place to place (Fig. 25–3).

Decades passed and invalids remained dependent, needing others to push, pull, or carry them. Then came the breakthrough: Stefan Farffler built the first self-propelled wheelchair some time between 1650 and 1665. Farffler was crippled and desired a vehicle that he could operate by himself to use to travel to and from church. However, the lo-

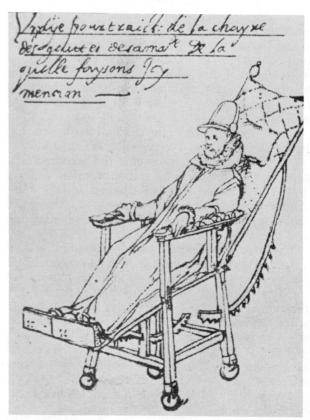

**Figure 25–3.** Sketch of a wheelchair for Philip II made by his valet, Jehan Lhermite, 1595.

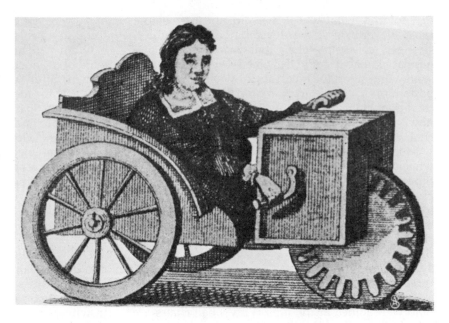

**Figure 25–4.** Farffler's Invalid Chair, 1650.

cal church proved so skeptical of the contrivance that he had to obtain special dispensation from the Bishop of Altdorf to gain admission to the church in his chair (Fig. 25–4). It resembled a tricycle and moved by means of a gear-driven front wheel located beneath the boxed front where his legs rested. This chair, considered one of the oldest handdriven chairs in the world, is now in the Nürnberg Germanic Museum.

By the 18th century, wheelchairs were generally available to the affluent. They were fitted with small wheels on each leg, with propelling rods, and with removable footrests. Often, they were elaborately carved and richly upholstered for both comfort and display.

In the 1800s, captain's chairs and bath chairs with step plates for the feet and wheels with handrims were being produced. Using the handrims, the patient could operate the chair independently or guide it as it was pushed (Fig. 25–5).

A wicker invalid self-propelled chair appeared about 1870. Less expensive and less heavy, this chair was the first conveyance available for common usage, and it remained popular until the 1930s.

Chain-driven chairs using either rotary or lever action came into existence about the early 1900s. Although machine-age science and technology had revolutionized industry decades earlier, few benefits resulted for the disabled until chain-driven chairs were mass produced for disabled veterans following World War II.

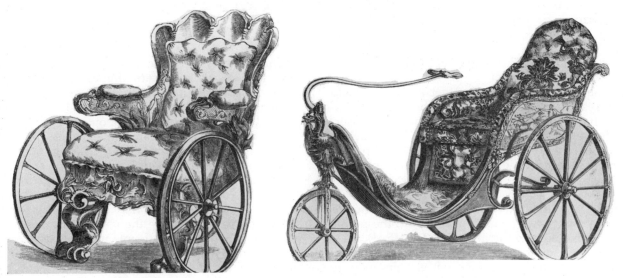

**Figure 25–5.** Wheelchairs of the 1800s. The model at right has a hand control device.

A folding metal wheelchair did not exist before 1933. Nevertheless, the development of a lighter, stronger, collapsible chair that was so easily manipulated that it could be taken anywhere represented an important milestone in wheelchair transportation. A decade later, World War II provided the impetus for many innovations and refinements now commonly found in the contemporary metal chair.

Today, given the required specifications, metal wheelchairs can be constructed to fit almost any type of disability or meet the most unusual needs. Hydraulic seats can be installed for people unable to achieve the standing position from normal seat levels. Exceptionally sturdy chairs have been designed for the extremely obese who cannot support their own body weight. One chair, constructed for a 500-pound patient, was wide enough to seat three normal persons easily. A unique chair was skillfully designed and executed for Siamese twins who were joined at the hips. Very small chairs are now built for little children.

In special and unusual circumstances, chairs have been thickly padded and upholstered in costly fabrics to resemble luxurious armchairs, thus serving to camouflage their real purpose and the user's disability. Chairs have been fitted with a variety of accessories, including umbrella canopies, to protect the users from sun or rain. Most powered wheelchairs now in common use are controlled by hand or chin movements. Others may use puff-and-sip breath control, voice commands and even eye movements.

Looking backward in time, it is clear that the collapsible metal wheelchair of 1933 represented a major step toward emancipation and independence for the disabled, enabling the chairbound at last to keep pace with others. The wheel of progress continues to turn and there is no doubt that the dreams of today will provide the chairs of tomorrow.

## PSYCHOLOGY OF THE WHEELCHAIR

The wheelchair, like any other prosthetic device, evokes feelings and attitudes when used. It also has functional and symbolic meaning to the user.

Some patients accept and tolerate the wheelchair as a necessity to meet a physical need; others become attached to it because its use is less taxing, easier, and more comfortable than walking. Thus, even when such patients regain ambulation, it is difficult for them to relinquish the chair. Some feel it represents a secondary punishment, the primary punishment being the disability. These patients believe their disablement has resulted from sin. In fact, at one time in Europe wheelchairs were frequently made of black metal and black upholstery

and were morbidly considered to be "the next thing to a hearse."

Often patients consider the wheelchair as status symbol in much the same way as the automobile is valued. Shiny chrome, upholstery colors, "custom jobs" with motors or hydraulic seats, plus the number of extra gadgets establish one chair's superiority over another. Most superior of all are the "recliners," which are a class apart, considered to be comparable to a large, expensive automobile. Patients have been known to match chair upholstery to their cars, and many young men install signal horns. The phenomenon is unique among those who must use visible medical appliances, for the majority of those who have to wear a prosthesis or brace prefer to conceal their appliance.

The wheelchair, like the car, is an aid to recreation and socialization. Those who are skillful operators of their chairs participate in wheelchair sports, square dancing, and dramatic productions. In wheelchair sports, scheduled games and a Para-Olympics are attended by the chairbound and the public.

Large, impersonal wards in institutions afford little privacy, but the patient with a wheelchair has an individual "home." Some of these patients carry their treasured belongings in bright-colored cloth bags hung on the back of the chair. An ashtray, urinal, transistor radio, plastic drinking cup, and other accoutrements convert the chair into a one-room efficiency apartment.

Business and industry have become increasingly aware of the potentials of the disabled employee. Airline companies and other distance transportation organizations and taxidrivers now rarely differentiate between the able and disabled. Consequently, the collapsible wheelchair represents the means of attaining a normal life pattern. It is possible to travel to job, to friends, and to educational and recreational facilities.

## RESEARCH

Those involved in the design, production, and prescription of wheelchairs—the engineers, manufacturers, physicians, and those in medical teaching and research centers—are not satisfied with the limited information available about wheelchairs or the patients who use them. Physical and psychological factors in relation to the wheelchair, and the wheelchair itself, are being studied and evaluated.

The distance an average wheelchair user travels in a day is of particular interest. A pilot study was made at Goldwater Memorial Hospital, New York, New York, to determine the distance traveled per day by patients to treatment, meals, wards, and recreation. An odometer attached to the chairs measured the number of feet traveled. Some patients traveled as much as 4½ miles and others only a half mile a day. Of course, those with powered wheelchairs may double or even triple these distance.

Wheelchair users sitting daily hour after hour have problems involving skin tolerance. Much has been done to alleviate the problems, and many cushions of varying thicknesses, materials and design are now available. Air, gel and water as well as different foam densities are all in use.

As has been previously stated, the psychology involved with wheelchair use is in many aspects unique. A psychological study using a semantic differential scale has been conducted at Goldwater Memorial Hospital to determine and evaluate patient reaction to the wheelchair.

Additional studies are being conducted on other physical and psychological aspects and various social and vocational factors. Many institutions are engaging in structural and dynamic engineering and metallurgical research in relation to wheelchairs.

## WHEELCHAIR PRESCRIPTION

### PRELUDE TO PRESCRIPTION

Today, a good wheelchair is like a good compact car, highly maneuverable but still possessing every feature necessary for the driver's activity, comfort, and safety. The disabled no longer depend upon an inventive craftsman, relative, or friend to devise a mode of personal transportation for them. Modern wheelchairs are made up of scientifically designed components that, when variably combined, can provide any patient with unique, custom-designed locomotion. Inherent in the prescription of a wheelchair of today is a thorough knowledge of these many components and of the patient and his needs. As a car is purchased with factors in mind relative to future needs for maximum performance and suitability, so is a wheelchair prescribed.

The patient plus the wheelchair equals a functional member of society. The chair in essence becomes a part of the individual. If the chair does not meet present and future physical and psychological needs or environmental and vocational requirements, the patient obviously cannot perform maximally.

The wheelchair prescription should not be limited to locomotion, safety, and comfort but should reflect consideration of the individual's ability to cope with cultural and home environment and vocational and avocational activity. Wheelchair components may be utilized in myriad ways to fulfill different needs of different patients. The junior-size chair prescribed for a teenager might also be advisable for a petite woman living in a cramped furnished room. A man requires a tray to perform manual precision work on his job. A woman may psychologically need the same tray for makeup.

The wheelchair prescription, concerned with the physical needs of today, must include consideration of the changing needs of tomorrow. Projected complications, precautions, and contraindications can be determined by careful examination of the patient. The diabetic unilateral amputee manages well in a standard chair, but if the prognosis for the remaining limb is questionable, the choice should be an amputee chair for both present and future use. Prescription of both wheelchair and prosthesis for the elderly unilateral traumatic amputee is not inconsistent with efforts to encourage ambulation. The elderly, usually insecure and inept on crutches and one leg, need a wheelchair for use when the prosthesis is removed at night, when dressing in the morning, or when the prosthesis is being repaired.

Functional prognosis virtually dictates the prescription of wheelchairs for patients with progressive neuromuscular diseases. A wheelchair quite adequate for present usage may, in a short time, be useless because of rapid progression of the illness. Hence, it is desirable to prescribe a reclining mechanism for use when sitting balance fails, elevating legrests to prevent knee contractures when leg function declines, and removable armrests to facilitate transfer with or without assistance. Thus, the chair becomes increasingly more serviceable as the patient's functions regress.

The wisdom of an individualized wheelchair prescription for each patient cannot be overemphasized. The initial investment in each chair may be greater, but a carefully prescribed wheelchair has a prolonged and useful life and pays large dividends by promoting maximum physical independence.

### TYPES OF WHEELCHAIRS

The wheelchair has two sizes of wheels—a large wheel always referred to as a wheel and a small wheel called a caster. There are three basic types of modern wheelchairs: (1) indoor, (2) outdoor, and (3) amputee. The position of the wheels distinguishes the indoor and outdoor types of chair. The indoor chair has the wheels in front and has the shortest turning radius, making it highly maneuverable in narrow spaces. The outdoor chair has the wheels in the rear and is more easily propelled on all types of surface. Amputee wheelchairs have wheels in the rear and characteristically have a much longer base than other types. (The principle of longer base with wheels in the rear is always applied to a chair with reclining back. This permits the axles of the rear wheels to be placed much farther back. Such placement moves the center of gravity toward the rear to counterbalance the body weight and compensates for the absence of weight of the limbs, thus decreasing the possibility of tipping backward.)

Choice of a type of chair involves many factors, so none of these chairs should be automatically selected by reason of the name. The medical condition and physical limitation of each patient must guide selection. The outdoor chair may be easier to propel, but the arthritic, with limited shoulder or elbow extension, may not find this to be true. An indoor chair may be more satisfactory for this patient as it eliminates straining to reach backward.

The emphysema patient, on the other hand, should not have an indoor model. Self-operation of an indoor type of chair may cause the body to slump forward; this inhibits thoracic movement. Whenever the patient's physical condition mandates erect sitting posture, the wheels should be placed at the rear. Likewise, paraplegics and quadriplegics should always have the outdoor wheelchair to eliminate forward slump and a resultant jackknifing.

Choice of a type of chair for hemiplegics depends on their physical and mental capacity to use the propelling mechanism. Therefore, selection of types of chairs for hemiplegics will be discussed in the section on handrims.

### CONSTRUCTION AND SIZE

Standard construction refers to chairs whose metal frame, wheels, casters, seat, and back have been fabricated to withstand normal usage and body weight up to approximately 180 pounds. Heavy-duty construction is fabricated to bear much more weight and to withstand rugged use. This chair has a stronger frame and reinforced wheels, casters, seat, and back.

The size of a wheelchair is determined by the width and height of the seat. Seats range in width from 10 to 24 inches; height ranges from 17 to 23½ inches.

An "adult chair" usually is one that has a seat 18 inches wide and 20 inches from the floor, and that will pass through a 25-inch door opening. Narrow adult size is the designation for an adult chair having a 16-inch seat width. Junior chairs have a seat width of 16 inches and height of less than 18 inches. Extra width sizes are adult chairs with either 20- or 22-inch seats. Chairs less than 16 inches wide are considered children's models. Custom-made chairs do not always follow these specifications. There may be fractional variations from the quoted dimensions in chairs from different manufacturers.

The average adult will fit comfortably in an adult-size chair. Smaller adults have excess room at the sides of the seat, and will strain or sit unnaturally in order to reach the wheels. In addition to suffering discomfort, they may develop skin abrasions from friction against the armrests. Narrow

adult or junior-size chairs are more suitable for these patients. Above-knee amputees wearing prostheses may need chairs wider than hip measurement would indicate in order to accommodate the hip section of the prosthesis.

Environmental factors such as living space, working space, and the width of doorways used by the patient influence the choice of size. To be useful, chairs must fit in these areas, and the 2-inch difference in the width between chair sizes can sometimes be a critical factor. When a particular size is mandatory and found to be comfortable but armrests interfere with rising, special arms may eliminate the need for a larger chair. Offset arms, which clear the seat area, give almost 2 inches of additional space without adding to the overall width of the chair.

### WHEELS

The standard wheel is 24 inches in diameter, has 36 spokes and unless otherwise specified, is supplied with the chair. Most patients who do a side transfer from the chair have little difficulty in clearing the 24-inch wheel or sliding forward to avoid it.

Wheels are fitted with either standard or pneumatic tires. The standard tire is solid rubber and provides a comfortable ride on most surfaces. It is durable and most frequently used. The pneumatic tire gives a softer ride and is advantageous for outdoor use on rugged surfaces. The tire may be smooth or treaded, the former rolling well on soft surfaces, while the treaded tire is best on grass or uneven terrain. Because of increased traction, due to the treaded surface, propelling may be more difficult. Both tires must be properly inflated at all times.

Wheels may vary with different brands and information can be found in the catalogues or supplied by the vendor.

Heavy-duty wheels, constructed with oversized bearings and bushings and sturdier axles and reinforced with 36 spokes, are utilized primarily for the heavy-duty chair.

### CASTERS

Casters are the small wheels of the chairs, and come in two sizes, 5 and 8 inches in diameter. The 8-inch caster may be spoked or solid; the 5-inch caster is always solid. The 8-inch caster makes the chair easier to propel and enables it to move over cracks in floors and sidewalks and over doorjambs, rugs, and other uneven surfaces commonly found indoors and outdoors. Therefore, the 8-inch spoked caster is generally preferred. A solid 8-inch caster is available for heavy duty. The 5-inch caster is not recommended for general use and is used mainly with Tiny Tot models and as part of the Sportsman wheelchair package for basketball.

## HANDRIMS

Handrims, attached to the outer side of the wheels, are usually made of steel tubing and are slightly smaller in diameter than the wheel itself. They are grasped by the patient, one in each hand, and pushed forward or pulled backward; these motions rotate the wheels and propel the chair. These rims are desirable even if the patient cannot operate them because they protect the spokes and help to maintain alignment of the wheels.

Handrims may be equipped with knobs or pegs for use by those with poor hand-grasp. The upright peg, attached to the outer circumference of the rim, does not add to the overall width of the chair. The knob, somewhat larger, or the oblique peg, does increase the overall width. Both prevent the weak hand from slipping and can be effectively held by a weak grasp or can be pushed with the palm of the hand.

Knobs or pegs are not always required, and increasing the friction on the surface of the handrim often will be sufficient to provide a better grip. A snap-on rubber handrim cover, or plastic coated handrims or friction tape wrapped around the rim should be considered. These modifications for handrims should be considered for patients with arthritis, quadriparesis, and other neuromuscular disturbances.

As noted previously, there are several types of chairs that are suitable for hemiplegics. An outdoor type with handrims is one choice. With this, the patient operates one handrim with the hand on the unaffected side and uses the sound foot to help push the chair along.

An outdoor chair with a handrim modification that adds approximately 2 inches to the width of the chair is another choice. This modification, called a one-arm drive, consists of two handrims, both attached to the wheel on the patient's unaffected side. One is a normal-size rim and operates the wheel to which it is attached. The second rim is smaller in diameter and operates the wheel on the opposite side of the chair. Simultaneous manipulation of large and small handrims with one hand propels the chair forward or backward. A separate skillful manipulation of one rim or the other is required for directional curves and turns. Consequently, the one-arm drive chair demands good muscles in the sound arm, good coordination, and good learning ability.

The hemiplegic wheelchair is another alternative. It is an adult width wheelchair with the seat height 2 inches lower than standard. This allows the shorter legged patient to reach the floor more easily and use the unaffected foot more effectively for pushing.

It is evident that the functional capacity of each individual hemiplegic influences selection. Variations in functional capacity of hemiplegics are so extensive that testing and evaluation of each patient's performance in each of these three chairs is recommended as judicious procedure prior to prescription.

## LOCKS

Locks are as indispensable to a wheelchair as they are to all other vehicles. They prevent movement of the chair whenever the user stands up, sits down, or transfers. They also may help to retard a rapid descend down a ramp or incline, and are considered part of the standard equipment of every chair.

Locks are located either in front of or behind the wheels, depending on the type of chair. On the outdoor chair the lock is in front of the wheel, and on the indoor type it is behind. Braking action or holding is produced by friction between the tires of the wheels and the locks. A lock is located on each wheel.

There are two types of locks, lever and toggle. The lever provides varying degrees of holding power that can be used as needed, while the toggle has preset holding power that is not variable. However, the toggle lock is simpler and easier to manage than the lever.

The handles on the standard locks are approximately at seat level. A person with nonimpaired upper extremities and trunk balance can easily reach them. However, patients with limited use of one arm, such as hemiplegics, find it difficult to reach with their good hand the lock situated on their involved side. A modified extended handle called a lock extension solves this problem. Bilateral lock extensions may be installed for those who have limitation of motion in both upper extremities, such as arthritics, or for those who have poor trunk balance, such as quadriplegics.

## BACK

The standard back on all chairs except the children's models is approximately 16½ inches high from seat level and on the average adult reaches about to midscapula. Made of a leather-like plastic material with a heavy duty Nylon or duck canvas lining, the standard back gives adequate support to the average patient.

Some paraplegic and quadriplegic patients find

toilet transfer is easier through the back of the chair. A back may be equipped with screw studs or zipper on one side that allows it to be opened and swung out of the way when the chair is backed up to the toilet.

A solid insert back fabricated of padded fiberboard or solid plastic material may be ordered for patients who require extra support to the back. It can be flat or contoured and may be cut out to prevent undue pressure on the sacrum.

For those patients who lean heavily against the top of the back leather, or who hook one arm around a push handle for trunk balance, again putting heavy strain on the back leather and screws, a piece of leather 3 inches deep should be put over the top edge for additional strength.

There are two types of reclining backs for use by arthritics, quadriplegics, paraplegics, and other patients with limited hip flexion. Such factors as poor trunk balance due to muscle weakness, and the need to relieve and change pressure on the buttocks are among factors to be considered. They are also important for respiratory patients, who may need to recline for part of the day.

The semireclining back, at least 22 inches high, either by back leather or by addition of a headrest extension, lowers through 30 degrees from 90 to 60 degrees. In some chairs with removable armrests, a stationary upright at 90 degrees is attached to the side of the chair. This may be an obstacle to a side transfer, unless the patient can move forward enough to avoid it.

The full reclining back is more versatile. It has a 2-inch higher back and may be reclined from 90 degrees to between 20 to 0 degrees and adjusted at any position in between. Since the reclining mechanism is on the rear of the chair, the sides are unobstructed, making a side tranfer easier. It should be noted that this chair may have a 1-inch deeper seat. In this case, a thick back cushion may be used to bring the body forward so that there is adequate space between the edge of the seat leather and the popliteal area.

The back may be modified without structural changes to any desired height. Sectional height upright backs are available from 12½ to 20½ inches. A person with a standard 16½ inch back chair needing a higher back, can add a headrest extension. Two steel posts attached next to the uprights of the chair, with leather stretched between, and the desired height. The whole unit is detachable. Lack of support to trunk muscles causes fatigue and slumping. These effect balance and may cause seat pressure problems as well as respiratory complications.

At the same time consideration should be given to whether the patient needs to be transported in his wheelchair. If very tall or unable to bend forward at the hips and waist, the patient may need to be reclined to enter the van doorway and may need to remain reclined because of the van interior height. Although used in the upright position, the reclining back chair may be needed to give flexibility to the patient's life style.

## SEAT

Unless it is otherwise specified, wheelchairs have sling seats (hammock seat) of the same fabric as the back. Seat width and height were discussed in the section on size; depth is usually 16 inches except in some reclining chairs, children's models, and especially modified chairs. The sling is functional for most patients.

The sling seat is not advocated for patients with tight adductors, a condition prevalent in neurological disorders, or for spastic paraplegics and quadriplegics and cerebral palsy patients. Instead, a solid seat may be indicated. Made of plywood, padded and covered with leather, it is inserted in the chair, resting on the seat rails. The seat board is preferred because these patients have a tendency to be in a position of internal rotation at the hip joint, and the sling seat aggravates this condition. Boards are also suggested for hemiplegics who may find it easier to rise from a seat that is both solid and higher.

Solid insert seats will raise the sitting height of the patient from the floor. This may make it difficult for a patient to stand up. In this case, a solid folding seat may be ordered in place of the sling seat. This seat board drops level with the seat rail. It should be noted that when using either an insert or solid folding seat with more than a 1-inch cushion, the back height and the armrest height may be too low and must be altered. Also, the solid folding seat, when the chair is folded, rises higher than the push handles. This may present problems in getting the chair into the back seat or trunk of a car.

Commode seats serve the incontinent patient and offer a solution to individuals who cannot enter home bathrooms because of chair size or the arrangement of the bath fixtures. Designed like a toilet seat and lightly padded, the commode seat has a seat board as a cover for regular sitting purposes. When it is used by the incontinent, extra padding should be placed on the commode portion to prevent skin irritation or numbness of the buttocks.

## CUSHIONS

Back and seat cushions made for wheelchairs are of foam rubber covered with durable cotton fabric or the same fabric used in the seat and back. The seat cushion most often prescribed is 2 inches thick and can be used with sling seat or seat board. A 3-inch cushion is advisable for heavier patients. The 3- or 4-inch foam cushion often can be used by patients with decubitus ulcers by cutting out areas on the underside of the cushion, thus relieving pressure. Many other cushions of various materials are manufactured, as well as specially formed seats to help ease poor positioning and pressure.

Back cushions are usually 1 inch thick, but a 2-inch cushion may be more comfortable for a patient with bony or protruding scapulae, or one requiring a cut out for the sacral area. It may also be useful to shorten the seat depth. The cotton covered cushion is recommended for patients with decubitus ulcers or sensitive skin, or patients who perspire profusely. It is also more comfortable in hot climates.

## ARMRESTS

The armrest of a wheelchair has a leather-covered padded armpad and protective side panel. The armrest may be nonremovable—that is, fixed. The front post of the fixed arm becomes the front upright of the chair and space between the two uprights decreases to 2 inches less than the seat width; that is, an 18 inch seat width chair has only 16 inches between the uprights.

If the armrest must be fixed for stability, but extra width between the upright posts is needed because of transfer with braces or prostheses, offset arms can be ordered. They are attached to the outer side of the front chair frame and allow the same space between the uprights as the seat leather. This is available only on a chair with an upright back.

Removable armrests may be full length; that is, equal in length to the depth of the chair, or desk length. These have a cutout section at the front so that the chair can roll close to a table or desk. The desk arm may be reversed for the patient who would have difficulty reaching the rear wheels, such as those with limited shoulder abduction or limited elbow flexion and extension. It can also be used by the patient who uses the desk arm to get close to a table and then reverses the arm to obtain higher front support in order to stand up.

Both of these armrests are available with height adjustment feature that allows the armrest top to be raised 5 inches in 1 inch increments.

The armrest height is important to posture, and a tall patient or one sitting on a high cushion will need higher armrests to prevent slumping.

Removable armrests, because the attachment is at the side of the chair, add approximately 1½ inches to the overall width of the chair. If this width must be kept to a minimum because of a narrow doorway, an armrest that wraps around and inserts behind the back upright can be ordered. It will narrow the chair approximately 1½ inches less than the conventional detachable armrest model. It can only be used on an upright back wheelchair.

## FOOTRESTS AND LEGRESTS

The footrest supports just the foot, while the legrest can be raised or lowered as needed, and supports the calf of the leg as well as the foot. Both may be swinging, indicating that they can be swung out of the way, are detachable and are adjustable for leg length.

The swinging, detachable footrest, or elevating legrest, may be used by patients to get as close as possible to bed, toilet or automobile in order to transfer from the chair. The swinging detachable elevating legrest should be prescribed for prevention of knee contractures, for all reclining wheelchairs to allow for changes in body position, and for all patients with circulatory disturbances of the lower extremities.

Footrests or legrests should be used by amputees with prostheses or pylons. The swinging detachable footrest is used to support the above-knee prosthesis and can be removed when it is not worn. The swinging detachable elevating legrest is suggested for the below-knee amputee to elevate the leg and stretch the knee to prevent contractures.

Footrests or legrests should be kept in mind when prescribing the chair for the amputee who may be considered for prostheses in the future.

Heel loops are used to prevent the foot from sliding backward off the pedals. They are most frequently used on the footrest and may be used on legrests in some cases of knee tightness, as they grasp the heel of the shoe and prevent full pressure on the calf. If the foot has a tendency to slide forward because of spasticity, toe loops are used to hold the foot in place.

## ACCESSORIES

There are almost as many accessories for wheelchairs as there are for automobiles. The following are mentioned because of their convenience, safety features, or ability to aid independent function. The wheelchair tray, which clips to the armrests, allows the individual to engage in all activities normally performed at a table. It is shaped to fit around the patient's body and is most helpful to those with limited arm function. A cane and crutch holder attached to the back of the chair is recommended for all patients who ambulate or transfer with cane or crutches. The auto-type safety belt is suggested for patients with poor sitting balance, because a sudden stop or slight tipping on an incline or curb may cause the patient to slide out of the chair.

## POWER

Battery-powered wheelchairs need to be prescribed in consultation with qualified therapists who can properly assess the patient's potential. There are many variations of chairs, controls and placement of controls and these must be evaluated with the patient's physical and mental capabilities.

## SELECTION OF WHEELCHAIR COMPONENTS

While a wheelchair seems to be a simple locomotive device for a physically disabled person, there are numerous components and many variations in each component. Describing all variations is beyond the scope of this chapter. The following descriptions of components are the most funda-

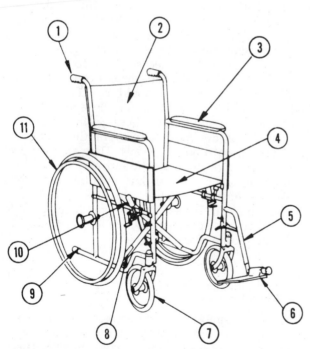

1. Handgrips/Push Handles
2. Back Upholstery
3. Armrests
4. Seat Upholstery
5. Front Rigging
6. Footplate
7. Casters
8. Crossbraces (Serial No.)
9. Tipping Lever
10. Wheel Locks
11. Wheel and Handrim

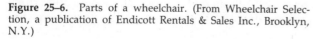

**Figure 25–6.** Parts of a wheelchair. (From Wheelchair Selection, a publication of Endicott Rentals & Sales Inc., Brooklyn, N.Y.)

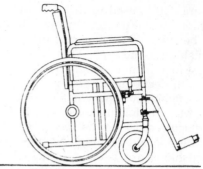

**Figure 25–7.** Outdoor model. (From Wheelchair Selection, a publication of Endicott Rentals & Sales Inc., Brooklyn, N.Y.)

mental for consideration in the prescribing of a wheelchair (Fig. 25–6) and will be found in the wheelchair prescription at the end of this chapter (see Fig. 25–45).

## I. STYLE

*Outdoor*—large wheels in rear (Fig. 25–7)

*Indoor*—large wheels in front, shorter turning radius helps to maneuver in confined areas; difficult for outside driving (Fig. 25–8)

*Amputee*—recommended for bilateral lower extremity amputees; rear wheels are set back approximately 1½ inches to compensate for the change in the rider's center of gravity (Fig. 25–9)

*Sportsman*—lighter weight construction and special design provide greater speed and maneuverability for participation in wheelchair sports; size specifications and standard accessories differ from other types of wheelchairs—check manufacturer's brochures for specifics

*Prone Cart*—self-propelled stretcher

*Posture 90*—14-degree backward cant and solid seat with fixed side; prevents user from sliding forward and helps to improve patient's posture (Fig. 25–10)

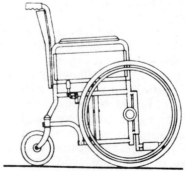

**Figure 25–8.** Indoor model. (From Wheelchair Selection, a publication of Endicott Rentals & Sales Inc., Brooklyn, N.Y.)

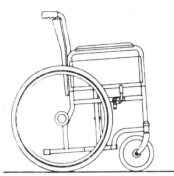

**Figure 25–9.** Model adapted for amputees. (From Wheelchair Selection, a publication of Endicott Rentals & Sales Inc., Brooklyn, N.Y.)

## II. CONSTRUCTION

*Heavy Duty*—rear axles are welded behind back post for greater stability; seat and back upholstery are reinforced; no significant weight increase over standard construction

*Lightweight*—lighter upholstery and frame; wheel and handrim are one piece; reduces chair weight approximately 13½ lbs.

*Active Duty–Lightweight*—frame tubing made of strong but light metal alloy; reduces chair weight approximately 10 lbs while maintaining durability.

## III. SIZE (Table 25–1)

*Adult*—18 inches of seat leather width, 16 depth and 19½ seat height (from floor to the top of the seat rail)

*Narrow Adult*—16 inches of seat leather width; other measurements are the same as *Adult*

*Low or Hemi*—17½ inches seat height; other measurements are same as *Adult*; this is for a patient needing to have one or both feet on the floor for propulsion or a short patient to come to a standing position

*Tall*—the seat is deeper than *Adult*; the seat height and back height may be greater than *Adult*; this is for a taller patient

*Junior*—16 inches seat width, 17½ seat height; this is for a small patient

## IV. FRAME

*Fowler Back*—gatched back, found on stretcher; inclines in 10-degree increments to elevate the head

*Goldwater (Nonfolding)*—motorized units only; solid frame with cross bracing eliminated; allows room for a full tray (containing batteries, module, charger, etc.) to extend from front to back of wheelchair

*Reduce-A-Width (Narrowmatic)*—detachable device attached to the wheelchair seat and armrest; manually cranked to narrow the width of the wheelchair; most frequently used to allow passage through narrow doorways (Fig. 25–11)

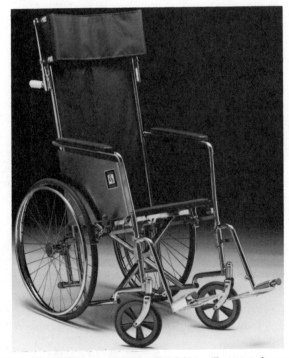

**Figure 25–10.** The Posture 90 Wheelchair. (From catalogue of Everest & Jennings. Camarillo, Ca.)

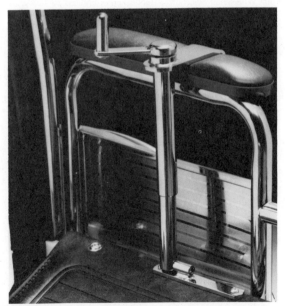

**Figure 25–11.** Reduce-A-Width, a detachable device attached to the wheelchair seat and armrest. (From catalogue of Everest & Jennings, Camarillo, Ca.)

**TABLE 25–1.** STANDARD WHEELCHAIR DIMENSIONS

| STANDARD DIMENSIONS | SEAT WIDTH | SEAT DEPTH | SEAT HEIGHT | ARM HEIGHT | BACK HEIGHT |
|---|---|---|---|---|---|
| **Adult** | 18″ | 16″ | 20″ | 10″ | 16½″ |
| Designed for full-grown adults of average size and build | 45.72 cm | 40.64 cm | 50.80 cm | 25.40 cm | 41.91 cm |
| **Narrow Adult** | 16″ | 16 | 20″ | 10″ | 16½″ |
| For relatively slender full-grown adults; combines dimensions of both Adult and Junior models | 40.64 cm | 40.64 cm | 50.80 cm | 25.40 cm | 41.91 cm |
| **Tall Adult** | 18″ | 17″ | 20″ | 10″ | 18″ |
| For tall, full grown adults | 45.72 cm | 43.18 cm | 50.80 cm | 25.40 cm | 45.72 cm |
| **Tall Narrow Adult** | 16″ | 17″ | 20″ | 10″ | 18″ |
| For tall, slender full-grown adults | 40.64 cm | 43.18 cm | 50.80 cm | 25.40 cm | 45.72 cm |
| **Slim Adult** | 14″ | 16″ | 20″ | 10″ | 16½″ |
| For thin, tall adult or youth | 35.56 cm | 40.64 cm | 50.80 cm | 25.40 cm | 41.91 cm |
| **Junior*** | 16″ | 16″ | 18½″ | 10″ | 16½″ |
| For full-grown adults with smaller than average body size | 40.64 cm | 40.64 cm | 46.99 cm | 25.40 cm | 41.91 cm |
| **Low Seat** | 18″ | 16″ | 17½″ | 10″ | 16½″ |
| For persons who desire a lower seat height or who propel chair with foot | 45.72 cm | 40.64 cm | 44.45 cm | 25.40 cm | 41.91 cm |
| **Kid or 13″ Junior** | 16″ | 13″ | 18½″ | 8½″ | 16″ |
| For children between ages 9–12 | 40.64 cm | 33.02 cm | 46.99 cm | 21.59 cm | 40.64 cm |
| **Growing Chair*** | 14″ | 11½″ | 20″ | 6½″ | 14½″ |
| For children between ages 6–8; A 13″ Junior model with special features; upholstery and footrest can be changed as the child grows | 35.56 cm | 29.21 cm | 50.80 cm | 16.51 cm | 36.83 cm |
| **Child's Chair** | 14″ | 11½″ | 18¾″ | 8½″ | 16½″ |
| All features of adult models but specially scaled down for children | 35.56 cm | 29.21 cm | 47.62 cm | 21.59 cm | 41.91 cm |
| **Tiny Tot-Hi** | 12″ | 11½″ | 19½″ | 6″ | 17½″ |
| **Tiny Tot-Lo** | 12″ | 11½″ | 17″ | 6″ | 17½″ |
| For children between ages 4–6; scaled to size, the "Hi" and "Lo" feature determines the seat height most functional for either attendant or patient | 30.48 cm | 29.21 cm | 49.53 cm | 15.24 cm | 44.45 cm |
| | 30.48 cm | 29.21 cm | 43.18 cm | 15.24 cm | 44.45 cm |
| **Pre-School Pediatric** | 10″ | 8″ | 19½″ | 5″ | 15″ |
| For children between ages 2–4 | 25.40 cm | 20.32 cm | 49.53 cm | 12.70 cm | 38.10 cm |

*Dimensions are for detachable arm chairs. Refer to Catalog for complete dimensions.
Note: Heavy-duty chairs of extra width are available up to 24″ (60.00 cm) and will still fold. Caution should be taken to evaluate seat height for this type of chair.
(From Wheelchair Selection, a publication of Endicott Rentals & Sales, Inc., Brooklyn, N.Y.)

## V. WHEELS

*1-inch Solid Rubber*—most common type; tire is mounted on a 22- or 24-inch spoked rim (Fig. 25–12)

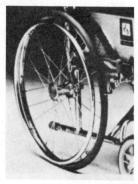

**Figure 25–12.** Standard tire. (From Wheelchair Selection, a publication of Endicott Rentals & Sales Inc., Brooklyn, N.Y.)

*Treaded Pneumatic*—air filled, tubed tire (bicycle tire), absorbs shocks and adds traction on soft, sandy, and rough ground; available in 1¼ or 1¾ inch tire width; more difficult to propel due to added surface tension of tire (Fig. 25–13)

*Slick Pneumatic*—air-filled tubed tire without tread, available in 1¼- or 1¾-inch tire width, provides cushioned ride but is more difficult to propel due to added surface tension of tire

*Cast Aluminum*—tubed pneumatic 2-inch treaded tire with cast aluminum spokes; used on motorized wheelchairs carrying excessive weights and travelling outdoors. (Available from Everest and Jennings only.)

*Endurance*—magnesium die cast in web design with 1-inch solid rubber tire (Invacare) 24-inch wheel

*Handrim Projections (pegs)*—8 rubber-tipped projections welded onto handrims; recommended

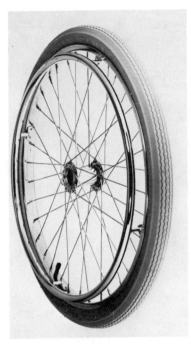

Figure 25–13. Treaded pneumatic tire. (From catalogue of Everest & Jennings, Camarillo, Ca.)

for those who have difficulty grasping standard handrims; may be horizontal, vertical, or oblique; horizontal and oblique increase the overall width of the chair; 12 pegs available on special order (Fig. 25–14)

*One-Arm Drive*—both handrims are on the same side of the wheelchair; the larger, inner handrim drives the wheel to which it is attached and the smaller, outer handrim controls the opposite wheel (Fig. 25–15)

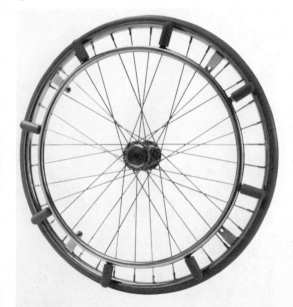

Figure 25–14. Special-purpose handrims. (From catalogue of Everest & Jennings, Camarillo, Ca.)

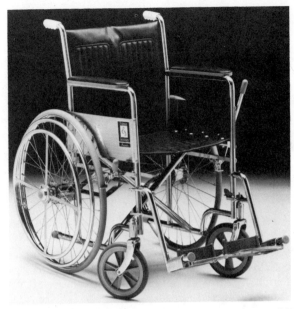

Figure 25–15. One-arm drive control. (From catalogue of Everest & Jennings, Camarillo, Ca.)

## VI. CASTERS

*Casters*—small steering wheel usually in front of chair; available in 8 or 5 inches (Fig. 25–16)

*Caster Housing*—metal socket into which the caster fits; containing bearings that allow the caster to rotate freely

*5-inch Solid*—solid rubber wheel; 5-inch diameter; used on children's wheelchairs, on sports models to decrease turning radius; more difficult to maneuver outdoors

*8-inch Solid*—solid rubber tire with metal Delrin or magnesium spokes.

*8-inch Semipneumatic*—2-inch wide solid rubber wheel. Advantages: provides cushioned ride; is puncture proof; decreased problem of casters be-

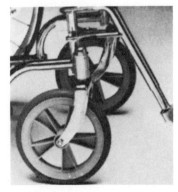

Figure 25–16. Cushioned casters. (From Wheelchair Selection, a publication of Endicott Rentals & Sales Inc., Brooklyn, N.Y.)

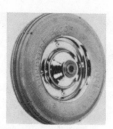

**Figure 25–17.** Eight-inch semipneumatic caster. (From catalogue of Everest & Jennings, Camarillo, Ca.)

coming caught in elevator spaces or sidewalk cracks; disadvantage: harder to push (Fig. 25–17)

*8-inch Pneumatic*—air-filled tire; provides a cushioned ride but is easily punctured; disadvantage: harder to push (Fig. 25–18)

*82 Position*—caster housing is set forward ¾ of an inch for greater forward stability; special anti-flutter bearings are used

*Caster Locks*—pins locking the casters in the forward position prevent the chair from turning (Fig. 25–19)

## VII. LOCKS

*Toggle*—push or pull locking device; standard equipment on all wheelchair models; normally comes as a pushing lock device but may be specially ordered as a pulling device (Fig. 25–20)

*Lever*—long-handled levers used with notched plate; may be used as a braking mechanism for descending ramps (Fig. 25–21)

*Grade-Aid*—incorporated with toggle lock to assist ascent and prevent chair rollback on inclines (Fig. 25–22)

*Lock Extension*—a long hollow tube added to the lock handle; may be used by hemiplegics on the affected side; the longer length makes it easier to be reached by the unaffected hand (Fig. 25–23)

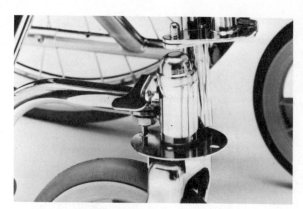

**Figure 25–19.** Caster pin lock. (From catalogue of Everest & Jennings, Camarillo, Ca.)

## VIII. BACK

*Upright*—straight back; seat and back angle is approximately 90 degrees; standard back height is 16½ inches

*Semirecliner*—reclines 30 degrees from 90 to 60 degrees; back held in any position with screw knobs at each side; bilateral extra posts next to arm rests take up some back and seat space in the chair, 16-inch standard seat depth is unchanged (Fig. 25–24)

*Full-Recliner*—back reclines from 90 degrees to within approximately 20 to 0 degrees supine position (Fig. 25–25)

*Detachable*—upholstery can be opened by means of swivel locks, zippers or Velcro; for patients who perform back transfers; when ordering, specify if opening should be on right or left side (Fig. 25–26)

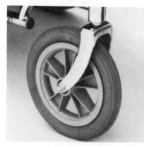

**Figure 25–18.** Eight-inch pneumatic tubed tire. (From catalogue of Everest & Jennings, Camarillo, Ca.)

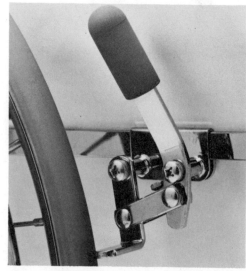

**Figure 25–20.** Toggle locking device. (From catalogue of Everest & Jennings, Camarillo, Ca.)

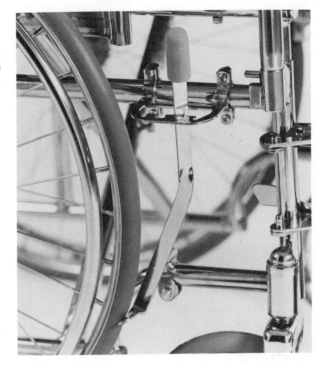

**Figure 25–21 (right).** Lever type lock. (From catalogue of Everest & Jennings, Camarillo, Ca.)

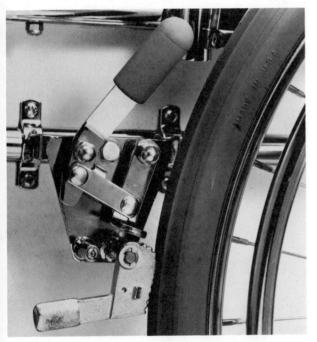

**Figure 25–22 (left).** The Grade-Aid, a device to assist ascent and prevent rollback on inclines. (From catalogue of Everest & Jennings, Camarillo, Ca.)

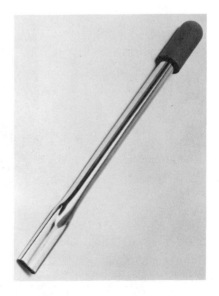

**Figure 25–23 (right).** Lock handle extension. (From catalogue of Everest & Jennings, Camarillo, Ca.)

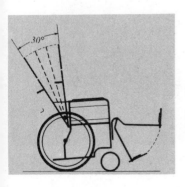

**Figure 25–24 (left).** Semirecliner. (From catalogue of Everest & Jennings, Camarillo, Ca.)

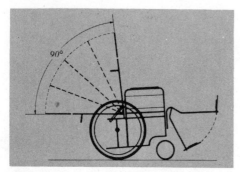

**Figure 25–25.** Full recliner. (From catalogue of Everest & Jennings, Camarillo, Ca.)

*Sectional Height*—available only on active-duty lightweight models with detachable or wrap around arms; accommodates to the individual's changing condition or activities; back heights of 12½ to 20½" with 2-inch increments may be ordered and easily attached to back posts (Fig. 25–27)

*Head Extension*—removable head rest; attaches to back of chair by means of hooks or fitting into back post tubing

*Spreader Bar*—adds stability to frame between back posts; always found on recliners but should be used on any back higher than 22 inches

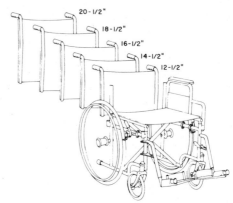

**Figure 25–27.** Sectional height backs. (From Wheelchair Selection, a publication of Endicott Rentals & Sales Inc., Brooklyn, N.Y.)

*Self-Centering*—head rest with high sides so that the head is centered on leather and cannot drop to the side and off the headrest (Fig. 25–28)

*Goldwater*—head rest with 2-inch cushion with Velcro strap fastening to allow for raising or lowering cushion

*Upholstery 3-inch Cap*—an additional piece of leather covering the top edge of upholstery; this should be considered for the heavy patient who leans excessively against the backrest or for a patient who hooks his arm over the back and around the push handle for trunk balance

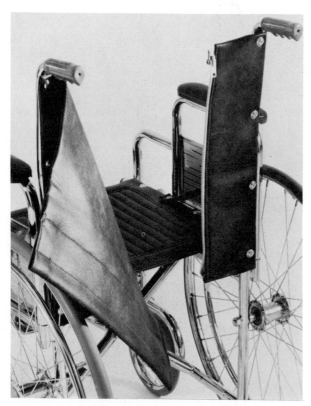

**Figure 25–26.** Detachable back upholstery. (From catalogue of Everest & Jennings, Camarillo, Ca.)

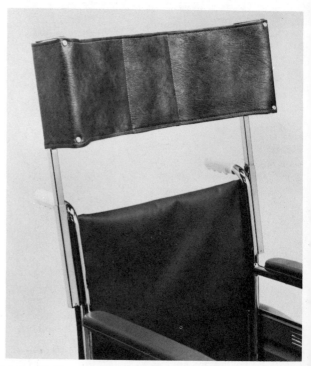

**Figure 25–28.** Self-Centering headrest. (From catalogue of Everest & Jennings, Camarillo, Ca.)

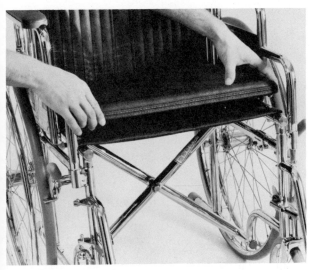

**Figure 25–29.** Solid insert seat. (From catalogue of Everest & Jennings, Camarillo, Ca.)

## IX. SEAT

*Sling*—found in all wheelchairs unless otherwise specified; seat upholstery is suspended between seat rails, allows for wheelchair to fold

*Solid Insert*—foam and Naugahyde–covered board; placed upon seat rails of a sling seat to provide firmer support and improved posture; raises the sitting height (Fig. 25–29)

*Commode*—solid padded board with opening for commode; rests on seat rails with hooks (Fig. 25–30)

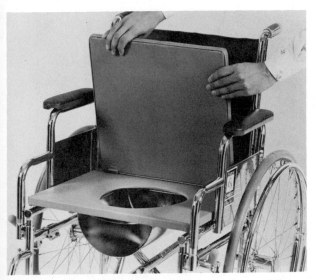

**Figure 25–30.** Commode opening. (From catalogue of Everest & Jennings, Camarillo, Ca.)

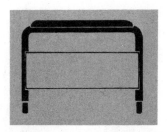

**Figure 25–31.** Full-length armrest. (From catalogue of Everest & Jennings, Camarillo, Ca.)

## X. ARMRESTS

*Armpad*—attaches to armrest to provide comfort and additional arm support; either upholstered or plastic

*Full Length*—extends from rear upright to front upright (Fig. 25–31)

*Desk Length*—cut away in front to allow wheelchair to fit under tables (Fig. 25–32)

*Fixed*—one solid, continuous piece of tubing incorporated directly into the frame and not removable

*Removable (Detachable)*—armrest detaches to permit side transfers; increases overall width of wheelchair 1 to 1½ inches because clearance must be allowed between the wheel and the rear arm socket

*Wraparound/Space-saver*—removable armrest designed with rear arm socket mounted at the rear of armpost and the armpad rail curved around the back upright; this keeps the overall width to fixed armrest width; available on upright back only (Fig. 25–33)

*Variable Height*—removable armrest, either full or desk length; height can be adjusted in 1-inch increments from 9 to 13 inches; available in wraparound or space-saver (Fig. 25–34)

*Offset-Fixed*—rear of armrest is welded onto back post of wheelchair; allows for increased width between front uprights without increasing the overall width of the chair; available for upright backs only (Fig. 25–35)

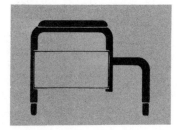

**Figure 25–32.** Desk-length armrest. (From catalogue of Everest & Jennings, Camarillo, Ca.)

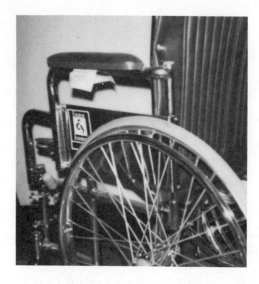

**Figure 25–33 (left).** Wraparound/Spacesaver removable armrest.

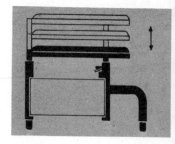

**Figure 25–34 (right).** Removable armrest with variable height. (From catalogue of Everest & Jennings, Camarillo, Ca.)

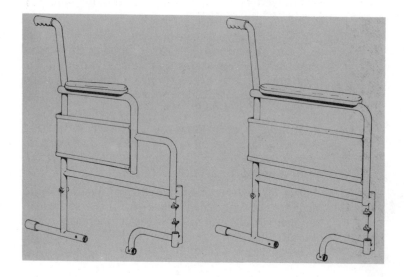

**Figure 25–35 (left).** Rear of armrest is fixed to back post of wheelchair. (From catalogue of Everest & Jennings, Camarillo, Ca.)

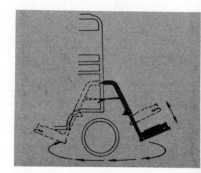

**Figure 25–36 (right).** Footrest. (From catalogue of Everest & Jennings, Camarillo, Ca.)

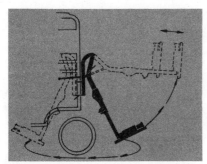

**Figure 25–37.** Legrest. (From catalogue of Everest & Jennings, Camarillo, Ca.)

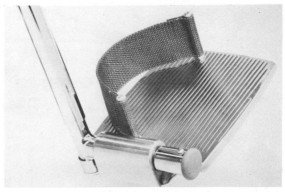

**Figure 25–39.** Heel loop. (From catalogue of Everest & Jennings, Camarillo, Ca.)

## XI. FOOTRESTS AND LEGRESTS

*Footrest*—supports only the feet (has no calf board); cannot elevate; may be swinging; detachable or fixed; includes No. 1 footplace unless specified (Fig. 25–36)

*Legrest*—includes a calf board and No. 2 footplate, may be swinging, detachable elevating or fixed elevating (Fig. 25–37)

*Cam Lock*—spring-type latch to lock and release swinging detachable footrest or legrest

*Pin Lock*—pin-type latch to lock and release swinging, detachable legrest or footrest; pin must be raised before the legrest can be swung outward

*Footplate*—metal piece that supports the foot (Fig. 25–38); available in three sizes:

No. 1—smaller size; standard for footrests; must be ordered specially for legrests

No. 2—larger size; standard for legrests; must be ordered specially for footrests

No. 3—large foot plate with additional length of plate toward rear, has cutout for caster clearance

*Heel Loop*—strap of webbing attached to footplate to prevent feet from slipping backward (Fig. 25–39)

*One-Piece Parallel Foot Assembly*—one continuous board used instead of two separate footplates;

one side of the board is detachable to allow for folding the wheelchair; board is parallel to floor (Fig. 25–40)

## XII. ACCESSORIES

*Anti-tips*—extension of tipping lever bent at 90-degree angle to the ground with rubber stopper or wheel at the tip; prevents backward tipping; may be turned up or removed when not in use (Fig. 25–41)

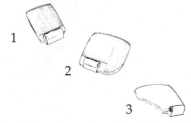

**Figure 25–38.** Footplates. (From Wheelchair Selection, a publication of Endicott Rentals & Sales Inc., Brooklyn, N.Y.)

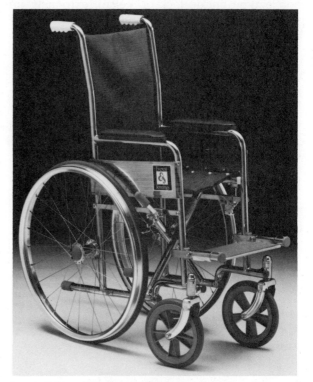

**Figure 25–40.** One-piece parallel foot assembly. (From catalogue of Everest & Jennings, Camarillo, Ca.)

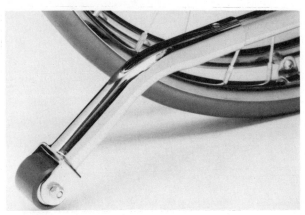

**Figure 25–41.** Antitipping device. (From catalogue of Everest & Jennings, Camarillo, Ca.)

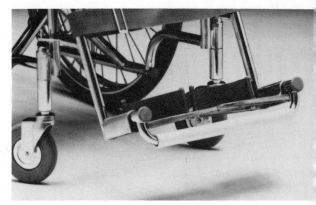

**Figure 25–43.** Roller bar. (From catalogue of Everest & Jennings, Camarillo, Ca.)

*Forward Stabilizers*—attached to front of frame to prevent forward tipping (Fig. 25–42)

*Roller Bar*—attached to footplates on sportsman model to prevent forward tipping; must be ordered with sportsman model footplate (Fig. 25–43)

*Cushion-Seat*—may be ordered in various thicknesses with or without cutout for sacral area; many types of seat cushions available to meet different needs

*Safety Belt*—2-inch-wide nylon material strap attached to the back posts of the wheelchair, usually at waist or stomach level; fastened either by automobile type buckle lock or Velcro; extremely important for prevention of falling accidents (Fig. 25–44)

## XIII. MOTORIZED WHEELCHAIRS

### *Batteries and plugs*

*Battery Tray*—metal tray mounted onto wheelchair frame underneath and behind the seat; holds wheelchair or respirator batteries

*Battery Charger Cable with Screw-Type Terminals*—two wires fastened to the battery terminals with screw clamps rather than clips, with a plug on the other end; the plug accepts the charger plug for charging batteries

*Cinch Jones Plug*—plug between two points in the wiring to connect or disconnect motor, control box, or batteries

### *Controls*

*Joystick*—steering stick; part of the control box

*Junction Box*—distributor box; contains all speed adjustments, fuses, and "on-off" switch in Series 34 wheelchairs

*Control Box*—holds joystick for steering wheelchair; may be mounted in various positions; houses mechanism and switches for operating wheelchair

*Featherweight Switch*—extremely sensitive microswitch used in a 34 or control box; must be ordered specially

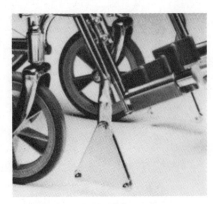

**Figure 25–42.** Forward stabilizers. (From catalogue of Everest & Jennings, Camarillo, Ca.)

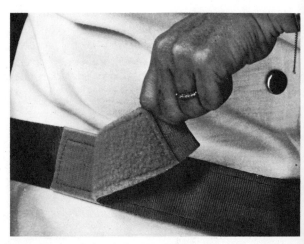

**Figure 25–44.** Safety belt. (From catalogue of Everest & Jennings, Camarillo, Ca.)

GOLDWATER MEMORIAL HOSPITAL

DEPARTMENT OF REHABILITATION MEDICINE

WHEELCHAIR PRESCRIPTION FORM

NAME _____ WARD_____ AGE_____ HGT_____ WGT_____

DIAGNOSIS_____ONSET_____

DISABILITY_____

AMBULATION_____TRANSFER_____

DISPOSITION - HOME/VOCATION_____

_____

SERIAL #_____

PURCHASED BY_____

DEALER _____

DATE OF RX _____

DATE OF APPROVAL_____

MEASUREMENTS:

ACROSS HIPS_____

ACROSS SHOULDERS_____

SEAT TO MID-SCAPULA_____

BACK OF BUTTOCK TO
BACK OF KNEE_____

### 1. BRAND

- [ ] E&J Premier
- [ ] E&J Universal
- [ ] Rolls 400
- [ ] Rolls Elite
- [ ] Stainless Catalina
- [ ] Stainless Newporter
- [ ] Other
- [ ] _____
- [ ] _____

### 2. TYPE

- [ ] Manual
- [ ] Motorized
- [ ] _____
- [ ] _____

### 3. STYLE

- [ ] Outdoor
- [ ] Indoor
- [ ] Amputee
- [ ] Multi-Position (E&J)
- [ ] Multicare (E&J)
- [ ] Posture 90 (E&J)
- [ ] Postura (E&J)
- [ ] Sportsman
- [ ] Prone-Cart
- [ ] _____
- [ ] _____

### 4. CONSTRUCTION

- [ ] Standard
- [ ] Heavy Duty
- [ ] Light Weight
- [ ] Active Duty-Lightweight
- [ ] _____
- [ ] _____

### 5. SIZE

- [ ] Adult 18" wide
- [ ] Narrow Adult 16" wide
- [ ] Hemi Adult 18"
- [ ] Hemi Narrow Adult 16"
- [ ] Tall Chair 18" wide
- [ ] Narrow Adult-Tall Chair 16" wide
- [ ] *Sportsman   Adult
- [ ] *Sportsman Narrow Adult

  * NOTE: Check catalogue for seat
    width, depth and height

- [ ] Extra width _____ "
    (NOTE: E&J seat height varies
    with width)
- [ ] Junior
- [ ] Junior 13 (E&J)
- [ ] Growing Child
- [ ] *Child
  * NOTE: Check width and seat height
- [ ] _____
- [ ] _____

### 6. WHEELS

- [ ] Standard - 1" solid rubber
- [ ] Treaded Pneumatic
- [ ] Slick Pneumatic
- [ ] 24" x _____ "
- [ ] 20" x _____ "
- [ ] .120" Gauge Spokes
- [ ] Cast Aluminum (E&J)
- [ ] Endurance-Magnesium (Rolls)
- [ ] _____
- [ ] _____

### 7. CASTERS

- [ ] 8" Spoke
- [ ] 8" Solid Delrin (E&J)
- [ ] 8" Mag-type (Rolls)
- [ ] 8" Pneumatic
- [ ] 8" Semi-Pneumatic
- [ ] 5" Solid
- [ ] Caster Locks
  - [ ] Extensions
- [ ] Double Weld
- [ ] 82 Position
- [ ] _____

### 8. LOCKS

- [ ] Toggle [ ] Push [ ] Pull
- [ ] Lever
- [ ] Right extension
- [ ] Left extension
- [ ] Bilateral extensions
- [ ] Grade-Aid

**Figure 25–45.** Wheelchair prescription form.

*Figure continues on following page*

-2-

PATIENT:

**9. HANDRIMS**

- ☐ Standard
- ☐ Rubber handrim covers
- ☐ Plastic coated
- ☐ *Left one-arm drive
- ☐ *Right one-arm drive

  Projections

- ☐ Vertical
- ☐ *Horizontal
- ☐ *Oblique
- ☐ *Knobs

  *Check overall width

- ☐ _____

**10. BACK**

- ☐ Upright
- ☐ Special Height_____"
- ☐ Spreader bar (if back is over 22" high)
- ☐ Special hgt. push handles___"
- ☐ Sectional Height (ADL only)
  - ☐ 12½" ☐ 14½"
  - ☐ 16½" ☐ 18½" ☐ 20½"
- ☐ Detachable
  - ☐ Right ☐ Left
  - ☐ Zipper w/o Velcro flap
  - ☐ Swivel lock
  - ☐ Zipper with Velcro flap
  - ☐ Velcro
- ☐ 3" Heavy Duty Cap
- ☐ Semi-Recliner
- ☐ Full Recliner
- ☐ Postura Back #_____(E&J)
- ☐ _____
- ☐ _____

**11. UPHOLSTERY**

- ☐ Standard weight
- ☐ Heavy Duty
- ☐ 3" Cap
- ☐ Color _____

**12. HEAD EXTENSION**

- ☐ Telescopic
- ☐ Hook-on
- ☐ Goldwater
- ☐ Adjustable Angle
- ☐ Postura #_____ (E&J)
- ☐ Self centering
- ☐ _____

**13. SEAT**

- ☐ Sling
- ☐ Solid Insert
- ☐ Special Depth _____"
- ☐ Commode
- ☐ Solid Folding
- ☐ Hook-on Solid
- ☐ Postura #_____ (E&J)
- ☐ Special Upholstery
- ☐ _____

**14. CUSHIONS**

- ☐ Seat _____ "
- ☐ Back _____ "
- ☐ Head _____ "
- ☐ Cloth covered
- ☐ Leatherette covered
- ☐ Other _____
- ☐ Snaps
- ☐ Ties
- ☐ Velcro
- ☐ _____

**15. ARMS**

- ☐ Full Removable
- ☐ Desk Removable
- ☐ Wraparound (upright back only)
- ☐ Variable-Height
- ☐ Standard-fixed (full arm)
- ☐ Offset-Fixed (upright back only)
  - ☐ Full ☐ Desk
- ☐ Special length armpad _____" total
  - _____" extra length to front
  - _____" extra length to rear
- ☐ Multicare (E&J)
- ☐ Sportsman
- ☐ Retractable arm (Rolls 400 Series)
- ☐ _____

**16. FOOTRESTS**

- ☐ Detachable swinging footrest
- ☐ Non-detachable footrests
- ☐ Telescopic footrests-Rolls 400 series

  LEGRESTS

- ☐ Detachable swinging elevating legrests
- ☐ Detach. swing. elev. legrests with below seat height pivot
- ☐ Non-detach. elev. legrest
- ☐ Telescopic elev. legrests-Rolls 400 series
- ☐ Telescopic elev. swingaway legrests-Rolls 400 series
- ☐ Goldwater elevating legrests (45° above seat level) E&J

  ACCESSORIES AND MODIFICATIONS

- ☐ Multicare rigging (E&J)
- ☐ Special length from knee to bottom of heel _____"
- ☐ Reinforced gusset on mounting bracket
- ☐ No mounting bracket
- ☐ Special length calfboard _____"
- ☐ Quad Release
- ☐ Fabric legrest panel _____"
- ☐ H-strap
- ☐ Buckle on strap
- ☐ Hook on strap

  Footplates

- ☐ Change Footplates ☐ #1 ☐ #2 ☐ #3
- ☐ Vinyl coated
- ☐ Adjustable angle (E&J)
- ☐ Sportsman footplate with roller bar
- ☐ One-piece footboard
- ☐ One-piece parallel foot assembly
- ☐ Heel loops
  - ☐ with ankle strap
- ☐ Toe Loops
- ☐ Metal ☐ Leather
- ☐ _____
- ☐ _____

_____
Physician's Authorization

**Figure 25-45** Continued

*Figure continues on opposite page*

PATIENT: _____                    -3-

---

**17.     ACCESSORIES**

☐ Safety Belt

☐ Auto-type          ☐ Velcro

☐ Extra length total _____"

☐ 2nd belt at chest level

☐ Crutch Holder

   ☐ Left          ☐ Right

☐ Reduce a-width

☐ Anti-Tip

   ☐ Front          ☐ Rear

   ☐ Wheels          ☐ Tip

☐ Sportsman footplates with roller bar

☐ Lateral Positioners

   ☐ Right          ☐ Left

   ☐ Bilateral

☐ Other_____

_____

---

**18.  ACCESSORIES FOR RESPIRATORY
            EQUIPMENT**

☐ Bantam Rack

☐ Battery Tray

☐ Charger Tray

☐ 6 amp Charger

☐ 10 amp Charger

☐ Battery Cable Jack with
   Screw Terminals

☐ Battery

---

**19.     MOTORIZED COMPONENTS
                FRAME STYLE**

☐ Standard (with X-brace)

☐ Goldwater (non-fold., no X-brace)

☐ *Stretcher

   ☐ Hgt.____" ☐ Fowler back

---

**20.     METHOD OF CONTROL**

☐ Hand

☐ Breath

☐ Chin

☐ Tongue

☐ Finger

☐ Other

---

**21.     TYPE OF CONTROL**

☐ 3P

☐ 34A 4-speed two 6-volt

☐ 34B 2-speed one 12-volt or two
   6's in series

☐ 3N Lightweight

☐ Other

---

**22.  JOYSTICK AND MOUNTING**

☐ Joystick

   ☐ Cup          ☐ Stick

   Joystick, height _____"

   Joystick, diameter _____"

   ☐ VAPC Bracket

   ☐ VAPC  " 2088-heavy duty

   ☐ Other

   ☐ Extra Rod Length _____"

   ☐ Extra wire _____" total

☐ Mounting

   ☐ Right          ☐ Left

   ☐ Mounted          ☐ Unmounted

   ☐ *Caster End

   ☐ *Above motors

---

**23.     SWITCHES**

☐ Feather-Weight #34

☐ Extra Heavy #34

---

**24.     POSITION OF ON-OFF SWITCH**

☐ On top of Control Box #3P #34

☐ At back of Control Box #3P

☐ At side of Chin Cup #3P #34

☐ Separate Speed Reduction and On-Off
   Switch (3P)

---

**25.     CINCH JONES PLUGS**

☐ Between Module and Control Box (3P)

☐ Between Junction Box and Control Box #34

---

**26.     CHARGERS**

☐ 6 amp ___1 ___2

☐ 8 amp

☐ 10 amp ___1 ___2

☐ Unmounted

☐ Mounted in front of X-brace

☐ Battery cable jack with screw terminals

---

**27.     TRAYS**

☐ Battery (tray to fit batteries and mounted
   not to extend beyond tipping lever)

☐ Bantam rack (14⅛' x 7-5/8") (cannot be used
   with 3P or 3N unless Goldwater frame)

☐ Goldwater

☐ Charger

☐ Other_____

---

**28. BATTERIES (Golfcart or deep cycling only)**

☐ ___ 6-V 134 AH _____

☐ ___ 6-V 225 AH _____

☐ ___ 12-V 45 AH _____

☐ ___ 12-V 85 AH _____

☐ ___ 12-V 95 AH _____

---

NOTE:  *Stretcher Control - when prone, controls should be at caster end; when supine, use
      Fowler back, and controls should be mounted at appropriate height above motor.

COMMENTS:

_____
Physician's Authorization

**Figure 25–45**   continued

*VAPC Bracket*—metal rod bent at 90-degree angle to hold control box on chin control units; bracket mounts on wheelchair back post; can be easily rotated away from the driver's face when the control is not being used

## Basic Information Necessary for Wheelchair Prescription

### I. MEDICAL INFORMATION

A. Diagnosis and Prognosis: A wheelchair must be prescribed with the future of the patient in mind. If the patient's balance, respiratory status or cardiac condition is expected to deteriorate, he may need a semi- or full-reclining wheelchair

B. Surgical procedure in the past and planned: for example, if surgical correction for scoliosis is planned, chair size and accessories may need to be changed

C. Disabilities: Physical, respiratory, or cardiac limitations

### II. PHYSICAL INFORMATION

A. Age

B. Height and weight

C. Body distribution: Weight and length in body and legs

D. Measurement: Across hips, across shoulders, seat to midscapula, back of buttocks to back of knee

E. Limitation of range of joint motion

F. Muscle strength, particularly in upper extremities and trunk

### III. INFORMATION CONCERNING ACTIVITIES OF DAILY LIVING

A. Mode of transfer from and to bed and wheelchair: Standing, lifter, sliding forward, backward or sideways

B. Ambulation ability: Distance and coordination

C. Method of propelling wheelchair: Two hands, one hand, one foot, feet only, none, etc.

D. Feeding: A patient who eats in a wheelchair may need a lapboard

E. Leisure activities: Sports, hobbies, etc.; if a patient travels, the mode of transportation should be investigated

### IV. SOCIAL INFORMATION

A. Where the patient will go: Home, school, work

B. Members of the family: Note particularly those with any medical or other problems

C. Attendant: Who will work directly with the patient, family member or aide

### V. ENVIRONMENTAL INFORMATION

A. Living accommodations: Living in an apartment building or a house

B. Elevator: Size; ability to take a wheelchair

C. Number of steps inside and outside: Height and depth of steps

D. Number of rooms

E. Width of doorways and halls

F. Is carpeting used and where?

G. Furniture placement: Can a patient reach his bedside for transfer? Is there room for a lifter, if used? Is there room for bedside or overbed table? Height of bed, bathtub, toilet, etc.

### WHEELCHAIR PRESCRIPTION

In prescribing a wheelchair, all needs of a patient—physical, emotional, occupational, recreational, and safety—must be met. After such needs are identified, each component should be carefully selected.

In most cases, wheelchair components are standardized by the same manufacturer. According to the patient's needs, these components are put together to make a wheelchair. Since there are so many varieties and variations in each component, a prescription form set up as a check list is useful to make a complete and inclusive specification. The prescription form shown in Figure 25–45 has proven to be extremely useful for this purpose.

It is often impractical for a practicing physician to spend time learning about and memorizing every minor detail and variation of components. Therefore, it is advisable to utilize a consultant who is extremely knowledgeable and experienced in this field. Such an expert may be an occupational therapist, physical therapist, or rehabilitation nurse. A wheelchair dealer or sales representative may or may not have such expertise.

Even these experts may not be able to advise a total wheelchair prescription unless they test a patient on a similar wheelchair that seems to be suitable for this patient. This problem is more critical for a severely disabled patient such as a high quadriplegic who requires a portable respirator.

A wheelchair appears to be a rather simple piece of equipment. However, as previously described, it is a combination of various components to meet the needs of a patient. The notion of "standard wheelchair" should be abandoned. A poorly prescribed wheelchair not only interferes with a patient's function but is also a financial burden to the patient or the community.

# PEDIATRIC HABILITATION

# 26

# Topics in Pediatric Habilitation

*by Hersch Sachs, M.D.*

This chapter will cover cerebral palsy and spina bifida, disorders that are commonly encountered in the care of the growing child. An attempt will be made to discuss some of the newer aspects of treatment and present material usually not covered in a textbook. The discussion will not completely cover each subject.

## CEREBRAL PALSY

Of all the neuromuscular disorders, cerebral palsy is the most common and may serve as a model. Cerebral palsy is a persistent but not unchanging disorder of posture and movement caused by a dysfunction of the brain that occurred before its growth and development were completed. Many other features may be part of the picture. Its main characteristic is that it is a static encephalopathy.

Historically, Little[1] described children with spastic rigidity of the limbs with an impairment of intellectual powers that he considered secondary to asphyxia, prematurity, and difficult birth. Phelps[2] was responsible in the United States for the early interest shown in cerebral palsy.

The incidence of cerebral palsy is difficult to assess because many cases are not reported, but the incidence varies between 1.5 to 2 per thousand in schoolchildren below the age of 21. Etiologically, injury to the brain can occur prenatally, perinatally, or postnatally and may be caused by anoxia, metabolic disturbances, isoimmunization, and other factors. Congenitally acquired cerebral palsy may be caused by infection, maternal anoxia, cerebral

hemorrhage, lack of oxygen supply to the fetus, and numerous toxins, drugs, and metabolic disorders. In the perinatal period, prematurity, smallness for age, mechanical anoxia, trauma, complications of birth, isoimmunization, breech presentation, maternal drug addiction, and hypoglycemia are among the most frequent causes. Many factors may be involved and children who have had intrauterine damage are more likely to have perinatal complications.

Postnatally, infection, trauma, vascular accidents, anoxia, and neoplastic disorders as well as developmental disorders are incriminated. This does not include all causes of cerebral palsy, because in many cases no precise etiological factor can be found. With the refinement of investigative tools, clues may be found that some incident was overlooked by the mother, or a genetically predisposing factor could be discovered that might be related to the later development of cerebral palsy. Prematurity is the factor for 20 to 30 per cent of cases. Prenatal and perinatal complications account for more than two thirds of all cases. The mechanisms by which brain damage occurs are ill defined and not characteristic and cannot be correlated with clinical symptoms.

Fetal or neonatal hypoxia causes a majority of the clinical disorders. According to the severity of the insult, the gamut of lesions may be present, from porencephaly and hydrocephalus to scarring and cystic damage, all of which can cause cerebral palsy. It is possible that milder degrees of anoxia are responsible for the symptoms of minimal brain dysfunction. The area involved by the anoxia determines symptoms of spasticity, blindness or visual perceptual defects, dyskinesia, or athetosis. The degree of hypoxia determines the extent of the lesion; in mild cases only subtle clinical signs may indicate some correlation between symptomatology and pathologic involvement.

In upper motor neuron disease spasticity is predominent. Cerebellar involvement produces ataxia, loss of muscle tone, and dysmetria. Injury to the basal nuclei results in dyskinesia with tremors, poor co-ordination, grimacing, and speech involvement.

Cerebellar hypoplasia has been found by pneumonencephalography in several cases of ataxia. Neonatal convulsions secondary to hypoglycemia have also been ascribed to cases of cerebral palsy.

Numerous etiologies have been ascribed to cerebral palsy, but mechanisms by which they interfere with normal development are probably mediated most commonly by anoxia, hypoxia, or hemorrhage. Less frequently other mechanisms can be involved such as toxins, occlusive vascular disease, or trauma. It is difficult to correlate etiological or pathological factors with the actual clinical picture; therefore, classification of cerebral palsy is based on clinical description.

## CLASSIFICATION

Classification is mainly based on the quality of the disordered movement. Three main classes are described—the *spastic*, the *hypotonic*, and the *dyskinetic*. Spasticity is characterized by increased deep tendon reflexes, increased tone, clonus, and increased resistance to elongation of the muscle with what is called *clasp knife phenomenon*. When the muscle is elongated, there is a resistance that suddenly gives way. Ataxia is characterized by hypotonia and dysmetria. Dyskinesia is characterized by involuntary movements accentuated by emotional stress and uncontrollable jerky movements that usually disappear during sleep. The most common is the spastic type of cerebral palsy, which represents 50 to 60 per cent of cases. The dyskinetic represents between 20 and 25 per cent. Reports of the incidence of ataxia vary widely according to different investigators, from 1 to 10 per cent. Mixed types are quite common and the atonic type is rare; often the condition changes as the child grows.

The number of cases of cerebral palsy has decreased in recent years, probably as a result of better prenatal and perinatal care.

It should be noted that, as a result of earlier treatment and diagnosis, incidence of the classifications of cerebral palsy has changed in the last decade. Spasticity accounts now for about 73 per cent of cases of cerebral palsy. Athetosis, which contributed 38 per cent of cases in the early fifties, does not account for more than 4 per cent now.

Ataxics are constant at about 5 per cent. In the case of spastic patients, there has been an increase in the combined group of paraplegics and quadriplegics from 38 to 53 per cent. The hemiplegic group has decreased from over 50 to 35 per cent. A topographic classification exists also. The various classes are as follows: hemiplegia, which is localized to one half of the body; diplegias, in which the legs are more involved than the upper extremities; and quadriplegias, in which all four extremities are equally impaired. Others are the paraplegic form, in which there is practically no involvement of the upper extremities, monoplegic forms, triplegic forms (which are quite rare), and double hemiplegic forms, in which both halves of the body are involved. Often there are differences in the severity of involvement, and the muscle tone may also vary. Associated disabilities are quite frequent. Some disabilities may not be related to cerebral palsy, but quite a number are probably of the same origin. The diagnosis of cerebral palsy is based on a complete physical and neurological examination as well as a birth history. Laboratory findings may be helpful. Diagnosis of cerebral palsy in early infancy is still very unsure. Suspicion may be aroused by difficulty in pregnancy, delivery, and a neonatal course that places the child in jeopardy. It might be possible to select the newborns who are at increased risk, but many of them will not develop cerebral palsy despite the cluster of signs.

It is well known that the children at high risk are those with a low Apgar score at five minutes, and neonatal seizures as well as intracranial hemorrhage. Hyperactive babies, listless babies, and those who do not demonstrate a Moro reflex have to be followed. Increased tone is expected from the newborn and a few definite neurological abnormalities can be assessed at that time. Even the most experienced observers fail to make definite diagnosis of cerebral palsy in the first four months of life.

Cortical control of the neuromuscular system develops slowly during the first three or four months of life, and impairment of volitional motions is not easy to recognize. One of the exceptions to this dictum is early signs of hemiplegia. As the child grows, some developmental delays may be the first signs of abnormality of the nervous system. First delays to be noted are those of gross motor development. The attention of the physician is often brought to these by the mother, who compares her present child's development with that of a previous child. Medical suspicion is rarely aroused before the mother becomes worried because of the child's delay in sitting. At that time a neurological examination is in order and should be done as described by André-Thomas[3] and with the Brazelton Scale.[4]

Early diagnosis of cerebral palsy is quite difficult

and the disease may only be suspected. Diagnosis is fraught with uncertainties, but it is mainly based on these three symptoms: persistence of primitive reflexes, abnormal tone, and hyperreflexia and persistence of response to repetitive stimuli. Primitive reflexes are unreliable and not detectable at all times. They depend on the state of the infant—crying, quiet, or asleep. Persistence of primitive reflexes may have some predictability for motor deficits, but their relationship to cognitive ability is more difficult to establish. Two reflexes are easiest to investigate—first is *persistence of the asymmetrical tonic neck reflex,* which is significant after six months of age and is also a high risk sign for motor deficit. The *cross extensor reflex* is pathological only when present up to four months of age. Tone may be either increased or decreased. There are only poor parameters to judge muscle tone, which may also be increased by labyrinthine reflexes. When the child is supine and when crying, the extensor tone is increased and when he is prone, the flexor tone is increased. In vertical suspension one should look for scissoring; after two months of age this is a very suspicious sign. If the normal dorsiflexion of the foot is resisted before the age of four months, this might also be a significant sign. Hypotonus is not a reliable sign. It is not indicative of upper motor neuron disease and may be seen in peripheral nerve diseases as well as in some collagen diseases. The two easiest signs to elicit are the anterior SCARF sign and the possibility to abduct the hip with the knees extended beyond 60 degrees with the knees fully extended. Pathologically increased tremors are only significant if there is a widely increased reflexogenic zone. This might be significant and pathological.

The static posture in the supine position is noted first, then resistance to range of motion and the extremities can be compared to one another or to what one expects as a result of experience in such cases. The child is then examined while he performs actively. Hand function and dominance are early signs of weakness in one extremity. Abnormal tone can also be noticed. Often in severe involvement of all four extremities, the child does not even develop crawling. Persistent head lag can be one of the first signs of hypertonicity of the posterior neck muscles. Abnormal hyperextension of both lower extremities, back, and head may be noted when the child is stood up with support under the axillae.

Evaluation for normal muscle tone in children is very important. Hypotonicity may be normal at an early stage or may be prolonged. Most cases of hypotonicity will either become hypertonic or dyskinetic and later may develop into either the athetosic or the ataxic type. Hypertonicity may be manifested when the child is attempting movements, which may be jerky and generalized.

As the infant grows, there is marked spasticity in the adductor muscles, and this often is reflected in difficulty in diapering. The infant feels stiff when being dressed, and this becomes a problem. On examination, often it is hard to bring the child to a sitting position, and he becomes stiff as a board and moves as one solid mass. When attempts are made to stand up the seriously spastic child, he will go into a position of hypertonus—head and trunk fully extended, upper extremities flexed, and lower extremities going into scissoring and crossing over, with the knees fully extended and the ankles in equinovarus. Reciprocal movements and pedaling of the lower extremities may be delayed. The deep tendon reflexes may become hyperactive, with clonus of the ankles. Babinski's sign is of no help in this early diagnosis. The child who may develop athetosis, chorea, or ataxia does not show any definite symptomatology in the first year or two of life. The most prevalent symptom at that time is hypotonicity.

Spasticity is characterized by continuous contraction of the muscles, which are weakened, with elongation of the antagonists. This finally leads to deformities of the joints that are affected by those muscles and contractures of the ligaments and soft tissues surrounding the joints, which will permanently fix the deformity. In addition, the unbalanced pull around the joints may also result in deformities of the bony structures.

Most cases of cerebral palsy begin with a stage of hypotonia of varying length, usually lasting one to three months and then giving way to increasing signs of spasticity. Exceptionally, the period of hypotonia may be prolonged as much as a year.

Hemiplegia, while not recognized at birth, is the earliest indication of cerebral palsy to be diagnosed, and usually this can be done before the age of six months. It is characterized by one-sided weakness. Most often the upper extremity is more affected than the lower. By the age of six months, the child's affected side still shows some fisting and equinus. In less severe cases, this can be recognized by the fact that the child has difficulty in crawling and uses one side more than the other. The early maturational signs are delayed, and some of these children will not have started to stand and ambulate between 12 and 18 months. The parietal syndrome may also be detected in these children, but at a later age when the sensory system can be explored. The deficit is in proprioception; often there may be neglect and impaired awareness of the affected limbs. The hemisensory defect contributes to the movement disorder and is often due to parietal involvement. This results in retarded growth of the affected extremities, and the involved side shows bony muscular underdevelopment with discrepancy in size of both extremities. The discrepancy increases as time elapses and is usually noted between two and three years of age. This adds a cosmetic problem to the sensory deficit. In postnatally acquired hemiplegias, the same symptoms may be found, but depending on the age of onset of the hemiplegia the leg length discrepancy might be different.

The spastic quadriplegic group is the most common and has the greatest number of severely affected children. Clinically, they are characterized by more involvement of the lower extremities and an equal involvement of both sides of the body. Occasionally, one of the upper extremities is much less involved than the rest of the body. In the case of double hemiplegics, the upper extremities are much more involved than the lower extremities.

## SPASTIC PARAPLEGIA

This is often described as diplegia; the lower extremities are much more involved than the upper extremities. It also starts by a period of hypotonia of the lower extremities, which is then replaced by spasticity.

If a thorough neurological examination is made, some hyper-reflexia in the upper extremities is also noted. Delay in development of motor skills of the lower extremities means that standing and walking are delayed proportionately to the amount of brain damage.

## DYSKINETIC CEREBRAL PALSY

The most common is the athetoid type, which is usually no longer the result of neonatal hyperbilirubinemia. The characteristic syndrome of basal ganglionic involvement by hyperbilirubinemia was athetosis, high frequency hearing loss or deafness, and conjugate upper gaze palsy. Intelligence was much less affected. Most cases seen now result from paranatal anoxia, which causes much more diffused brain lesions, and intelligence is commonly affected. In these cases, hypotonia is an early symptom. Persistence of primitive reflexes such as the asymmetrical tonic neck and the Moro reflex are seen in the beginning, and then writhing, involuntary movements develop that are more common in the distal joints. In severe cases, these movements can spread and involve the entire extremity. These characteristics may change, and often other types of involuntary movements (dystonic or choreiform) may appear. They are increased by emotional stress and usually disappear when the child sleeps.

The face or pharyngeal muscles are involved, and the child may have severe dysarthria, drooling, and dysphagia. The upper extremities are often severely involved.

Ataxic cerebral palsy is the least common form and usually less than 10 per cent of cerebral palsy cases can be assigned to this class. Hypotonic features and motor delay are more severe and last much longer. Tone remains diminished throughout life. As these children grow, they will learn to take clues from their surroundings and will better coordinate their movements so that they can usually walk. Tendon reflexes are pendular. Coordination of the upper extremities will also improve.

## DIAGNOSIS

The experienced physician is alert to early findings that may aid in establishing the diagnosis. In the neonatal period, signs likely to predict a later neurological handicap are a low Apgar score 15 to 20 minutes after birth, neonatal seizures, jitteriness, or tremulousness of moderate or marked character, decrease in stable temperature, and occurrence of several apneic episodes. These clusters of signs can help to identify the new-born at increased risk for cerebral palsy. Fortunately, the great majority of newborns with signs predictive of later neurological involvement fail to develop it. The newborn may appear quite normal at birth, but as development proceeds, some signs may be noticed early. Infants with uncleft toes, high-arched palates, microcephaly, hydrocephaly, and those suffering problems of early fetal development may also have brain damage. Infants of diabetic mothers or those who have the appearance of immaturity or postmaturity are at higher risk.

The study plan for these infants should include a thorough history and investigation whenever genetic factors are suspected. Delay in motor development and assessment of tone in the young infant are important to consider. A neurological examination, including assessment of the persistence of primitive reflex, is in order.

In the early months it is hard to attempt to define spasticity in a child. Scissoring is one of the important early clues. Delay in hallmarks of development should also be watched for carefully; clusters of signs must be present before a diagnosis can be made. Among the most important is head erection from the prone position, which should be present from the second month. Head lag when a child is brought from the supine to the sitting position usually disappears before the age of four months. Reaching for nearby objects should be present at the age of five months. Sitting without support is usually attained by the age of eight months. Belly crawling is attained by seven to eight months, and delay beyond this period indicates a potential disability. The first words are usually said at about the age of 12 months. Most children are able to stand alone by the age of 12 or 13 months, and ambulation is expected, independently, by 15 months of age. Additional problems may arise in the developing child. These include feeding difficulties, frequent colic and irritability, and more than normal crying. Others are difficulty in sucking, difficulty with the introduction of solid food, frequent choking, and tongue thrust, making swallowing and sucking much harder. The persistence of strabismus, different gaze disturbances in looking either up or down, and nystagmus are also important signs. As the child becomes older, the diagnosis is usually easier to make.

In the child, spasticity is easy to recognize. In the hemiplegic form it typically involves the upper and lower extremities and the thumb-in-palm deformity under a clenched fist. In milder cases, the sign of value is that when the child tries to reach for an object, his fingers hyperextend and abduct with rotation of the wrist. His leg might also be involved, with flexion of hip and knee and either an equinovarus or equinovalgus foot placement. The typical quadriparetic walks with both hips and knees flexed and with a tendency to scissoring when one leg overshoots the midline and crosses over in the path of the other. Balance in these cases is poor and gait has a jerky appearance. In mild cases, the child may only ambulate with arms extended on a wide base. Additional signs may be drooling and strabismus.

In the dyskinetic type, special attention should be paid to the athetosis of the fingers. They are in motion all the time, with practically no rest. There is toeing in of both lower extremities, with hyperextension of the head and back. Drooling is usually marked. Attempts at speaking or making any effort generates grimacing of the face. Under stress, all these symptoms become definitely worse. One additional sign to distinguish spasticity from rigidity is that rigidity may be shaken out; spasticity remains unaffected.

Ataxic children usually start to walk later than others. They have a high steppage gait with marked flexion of the hips. Their gait is dysrhythmic and usually with flat foot placement on a wide base. There is marked dysmetria, which is characterized by overshooting when they try to grab an object. Prognosis in cases of ataxic cerebral palsy is usually favorable for ambulation, although it is attained at a later age.

In the mixed type of cerebral palsy elements of all three types may be found, with one form occasionally more dominant than another. The prognosis of the different types is very unpredictable. Pathological signs either will become more marked or will be tempered by growth and maturation. Prognosis in the extremely mild or severe case is easy to predict, but it is in the intermediate case that the difficulties arise. The severity of the prognosis often differs according to the type of cerebral palsy. The spastic hemiplegic usually has a more favorable outcome, and most will be able to ambulate.

As noted by several authors, children with spasticity have a tendency to develop fixed deformities and contractures. If certain therapeutic measures are not taken and the follow-up is not continuous, they will functionally become worse although the disease is nonprogressive. In others, because of increased weight, ambulation will stop after it has already started. An athetoid will frequently improve. The dyskinesia will not diminish and mental ability is hard to assess, but usually during the second decade of life these patients will make gains that were judged impossible. It should be kept in mind that we cannot be as rigid as we were in the past when predicting ambulation, but any child who cannot sit beyond the fourth birthday has a seriously diminished potential. The persistence of primitive reflexes—the tonic neck, labyrinthine reflexes, and the Moro reflex—indicates a poor prognosis.

## ASSOCIATED DISORDERS

Associated disorders of cerebral palsy may compound the signs of dysfunction and physical handicaps, changing the entire outcome of rehabilitation. The disrupting impact of those disorders in behavioral as well as motor functions is not fully established. Perceptual, sensory, cognitive, and learning potential of the infant having cerebral palsy has not been as fully studied as it has in the normal child. We do not know whether some of those disorders are reversible and if they are modified by early intervention procedures. About 40 to 50 per cent of these children have convulsive disorders that may interfere with the learning process. Their control is of great importance. They may be of a genetic or familial nature or secondary to the same trauma that resulted in cerebral palsy. The spastic child has a greater tendency to seizures than the athetoid. In the spastic child most seizures are of the major focal type, but minor seizures are not uncommon.

Mental retardation is one of the most severe associated handicaps. One third of cerebral palsy children are of normal intelligence, one third have mild retardation and are in the educable range of intellectual functioning, and one third are usually below the level of moderate retardation. In cases in which severe neuromuscular involvement, microcephaly, and seizures are present, the likelihood of an associated intellectual deficit is increased. Statistically, athetoids have a lesser degree of intellectual limitation than those with other neurological conditions. Spastic quadriparetics are those at greatest risk of retardation. In general, the hemiplegic and quite often the diplegic have mild intellectual involvement. Those with rigid, the atonic, and the quadriparetic forms have the greatest degree of limitation.

Evaluation of intelligence in children with cerebral palsy is fraught with difficulty. Most intelligence tests contain items that are inappropriate to cerebral palsy children or are beyond their physical capacity. Appropriate testing evaluates the areas of strength and weakness of the individual so that specific remedial learning can be tailored to that child.

Behavioral problems have two causes: some of them are due to organic lesions and others are due to complications of emotional development by neurophysiological problems as well as by the reaction of a society that still poorly accepts the handicapped child. Behavioral problems can also interfere with the adjustment of the individual child. These children have a more isolated life and can become dependent. Children with higher intelligence seem to be at higher risk for psychological reactions.

Hearing loss in cerebral palsy affects approximately 20 per cent of patients. Sensory and perceptual disorders as well as dysarthria probably have a disrupting affect on behavioral development. Drooling becomes an embarrassment as the child grows.

Visual disorders are more common in these children than in the rest of the population; the spastic has the highest frequency of visual disorders. The athetoid group seems to have a greater degree of hyperopia. Strabismus, if left uncorrected, will often be complicated by ambliopia and by loss of stereoscopy.

Prognosis in cerebral palsy varies from one case to the other and from one classification to another. Maturation sometimes may be helpful to overcome the handicap to some degree, although cerebral palsy is a static condition. There is a continuous imbalance of muscle pull that contributes to deformities.

A large group of children will have no firm clues for predicting prognosis of development. Prognosis for ambulation is usually good for ataxic and hemiplegic types. In the group delineated by athetosis, spasticity as clinically demonstrated by quadriparesis or diplegia, a good prognostic sign is the ability to sit by two years, but it has been shown that the fact that these children do not sit by the age of two does not eliminate the possibility of walking later.

Persistence of the Moro reflex, asymmetrical tonic neck reflex, or inability to sit by the age of four suggests a poor prognosis.

Hyperkinesis or its correlates, such as short attention span, distractability, poor impulse control or other disorders of behavior and personality, will greatly change the functional outcome.

## TREATMENT

The cornerstone of therapy depends on the patient's processing information derived both internally and externally. Sensory information is organized within the central nervous system. Sensorimotor circuits allow for smooth control of movement and for motor learning. Effective function of the nervous system depends on normal integration of internal and environmental experience.

Treatment requires some knowledge of normal and abnormal development combined with a detailed evaluation. Therapy is based on the integration of sensory input before or during an activity. Motor development usually occurs sequentially and in predetermined stages. Usually, mass total patterns of movements are developed before fine motions. The development of motor activity proceeds from head to extremities and from proximal to distal. Movements are thus encouraged by following the same developmental schedules. The motor development often correlates with developmental maturity of language, social skills, cognition, and emotional development. Rehabilitation of handicapped children is complex, with the goal being realization of maximal functional potential. Involvement of the parents in the program is of prime importance because they should carry over its principles at home. On the other hand, parents should not be placed in a position in which they become excessively controlling, as this might destroy the normal interaction of mother and child. It is important to foster an environment in which the child and parents will improve their relationship.

EARLY INTERVENTION. In long-term studies of retarded children, a marked improvement in their performance and IQ was noted after an early and intensive stimulation program. Many advantages can be derived from this approach if therapy is provided immediately after the diagnosis is made. Some of the mother's anger might be directed toward constructive management techniques. It is important to teach the parents how to manage the child and inform them that professional advice is available. A balance has to be established between encouraging the child's independence and not frustrating him by making unreasonable demands.

As stated, sensorimotor integration and experiences seem to be very important for the development of cognition and behavior. Exploration by the child of his environment is usually limited by his handicapping condition, and this deprivation may aggravate the effect of an existing disability. A multisensory stimulation program is supposed to alleviate some of these shortcomings. In addition, abnormal movements can be controlled by stabilization of certain key joints, and the child can be encouraged to move properly and functionally.

Early use of feeding techniques allow him better access to food and prepare him for linguistic activities.

The treatment of the neuromuscular dysfunction has to be well-timed and selected according to the ability of the child. A plan must be formulated with goals that can be attained without frustrating the child. There are immediate goals that are geared to the functioning of the child and long-term goals that can be established but modified continuously as the child makes gains and matures. The associated dysfunctions will set some limits to his personal and social as well as his cognitive development.

Physical and occupational therapy are the most frequently used conservative treatments. Therapists have gone from working only with specific muscle groups and joints to much broader activities that involve treating deranged movements. These two types of treatment have produced numerous techniques. The classical and traditional method consisted of stretching and passive and active or resistive movements. All the therapy was directed to muscle groups in order to maintain range of motion and to encourage gross motor skills appropriate to the functional level of the child. At the present time, especially with neurodevelopmental techniques, therapy is mainly directed toward management of tonus and facilitation of movements; therefore, techniques differ according to whether the child has hypertonicity, hyperkinesis, or hypotonicity. Grading of the therapeutic experience is according to the degree of sensory input, the use of activities and play, and the role of the parents in the treatment process.

Several techniques have been derived from this philosophy. One of the most popular is the Bobath method,[5] which utilizes inhibition and facilitation of movements and inhibition of postural reflexes. Kabat and Knott[6] and Voss use total body patterns with emphasis on spiral and diagonal resistive movements. Brunstrom promoted movement therapy with increasing control over posture and movement. This technique can be used for goal-directed activities. Rood uses proprioceptive and tactile stimulation to influence tone. She utilizes synergestic reflexes until they can be controlled voluntarily. Fay's method[7] had suggested that ontogeny repeated philogeny, and the outgrowth of this idea is the controversial patterning exercises of the Dolman-Delacato technique.

### Combination Therapy

In the early intervention program there is only a fine line of demarcation between physical and occupational therapy. Goals are identical in both—mainly, the effort of the child is channeled toward goal-directed activity and not in the different patterns of better movement. Training for increased strength and gait is more in line with physical therapy, whereas finer skills of the upper extremities, posture control, and feeding habits are more in line with occupational therapy. New goals have to be defined and other skills learned to master the new activities. In general, rehabilitation works toward two types of goals. One is to give these patients as much independence in activities of daily living as is compatible with their handicap and the second is to utilize their functional skills toward a vocational activity. Perceptual motor impairment plays a large role and must be treated concomitantly in the rehabilitation process. Short-term and long-term goals will have to be adjusted and reassessed according to the child's progress, as he grows.

Myoneural blocks for the relief of spasticity can be used either to judge the possible effect of surgical treatment or to temporarily remove the spasticity in a definite group of muscles. The agents that are commonly used are phenol, alcohol, and lidocaine. They can be injected either at motor points or into the belly of the muscles. The most commonly used agent is phenol for motor point injection or alcohol injected directly into the muscle bellies to reduce stretch reflex activity. It is evident that if a contracture of the muscle is present, this will not be effective. Phenol block of motor nerve points gives selective effects and may relieve spasticity from six months to one year.

Plaster casting to reduce spasticity of the lower extremities is used in patients with equinus deformity. Bilateral short leg walking plaster casts are used, but before applying them one has to make sure that the ankles can be dorsiflexed to neutral. A special technique is used with pressure applied under the metatarsal heads and extension of the toes. A great percentage of patients in whom this method was used had a change in tone and most had improved gait. The explanation for this im-

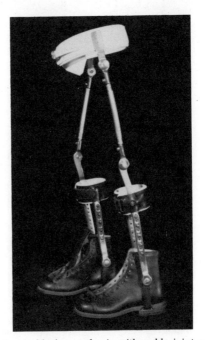

**Figure 26–1.** Ankle-foot orthosis with ankle joint and stirrup attachment with cable twisters connected through knee joints and waist band.

provement is hard to justify; the method is called neurological inhibition.

Bracing in cerebral palsy is a time-honored procedure. The main indications are reduction of axial load, prevention and correction of deformity, and improvement of function. Improvement of function is achieved by stabilizing a limb, diminishing undesired motion, or assisting weak motions. When the axial loading of a lower limb is diminished, the deformity may be reduced. Prevention is best used when the patient is young. Deformity usually results from poorly balanced muscle forces around the joint. If the skeletal deformity has already been fixed, the chances of an orthosis correcting it are minimal. Often the orthoses have to be removed so that the child can exercise the muscles around the joint. Braces to correct the deformities must be applied for long periods of time and can be used in conjunction with wedging of plaster casts. Often a hinge joint is used with adaptable ratchet locks. (One should be careful to apply the supporting devices near the joints to prevent possible subluxations.) The most common brace used is the ankle-foot orthosis, with the knee-ankle-foot orthosis used when the patient's knee flexors are weak (Figs. 26–1 and 26–2). Twister cables attached to a pelvic band may be used either with the knee-ankle-foot orthosis or with an ankle-foot orthosis.

In management of the hemiplegic cerebral palsy, the old type double-bar short leg brace with limited

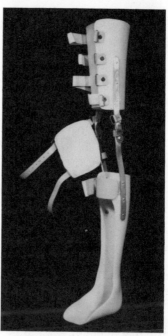

**Figure 26–3.** Plastic laminate knee-ankle-foot orthosis with bilateral knee joints, drop locks, knee cap and solid ankle.

ankle joint is often sufficient, and if additional deformities at the ankles are present, a T strap and shoe modifications may be added. A better correction in mild cases can often be obtained with an ankle-foot orthosis made of polypropylene plastic with a solid ankle. This is often effective in controlling lateral motion of the ankle (Figs. 26–3 and 26–4). The most common deformity at the knee is hyperextension, which will yield to bracing of the ankle. In rare cases the child may have to be braced with a long leg orthosis, which in the majority of cases probably will be discarded for a below-knee orthosis after some training.

In management of the spastic diplegic or quadriparetic, use of bracing is much more controversial. It seems that more and more therapists are abandoning the hip-knee-ankle-foot orthosis attached to a pelvic band. This device is heavy, cumbersome and does not promote earlier ambulation, but it can promote earlier standing by the child. A combination of surgery and bracing may in a great number of cases change a nonambulating to an ambulating patient.

Internal rotation at the hips often can be corrected without a pelvic band just by using steel twister cables. These braces have to be checked frequently; often laxity of the knee joint will contribute to an external tibial torsion deformity.

One of the common deformities seen is a weakened Achilles tendon. Some of those patients have been helped by short leg braces with an anterior stop-and-free plantar flexion. Patients with the

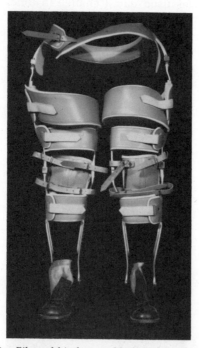

**Figure 26–2.** Bilateral hip-knee-ankle-foot orthosis double bars in duraluminum with provision for extension, ankle joints with stirrup attachment to surgical high-top shoes, knee and hip joints with drop locks, calf and double thigh bands, knee cap and pelvic band.

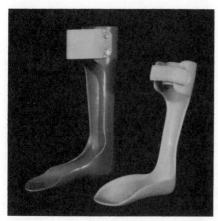

**Figure 26–4.** On the right, an AFO posterior leaf orthosis. On the left an AFO solid ankle orthosis.

dyskinetic types of cerebral palsy often develop functional gaits despite their lack of stability. Bracing is not required in these cases unless some deformity is developing.

In the ataxic type of cerebral palsy it can be beneficial to use weighted shoes. Other types of bracing are not indicated in most of these cases.

### Evaluation of Therapeutic Methods

It is difficult at the present time to evaluate the different therapeutic methods because of overenthusiastic use by professionals and a lack of double-blind studies or long-term evaluation of treated and nontreated children. Nicholson in 1976 and Scherzer in 1973 showed that improvement in motor and social function occurred, but behavior of patients at home showed minimal difference and more studies were necessary before any definite statement could be made. We can conclude that balance training and all motor activities have to be learned and practiced and that postural control is essential in all these activities.

When should therapy be started? By the age of seven or eight years, motor performance attains a plateau. In the normal child, gait pattern is usually established a year to 18 months after walking starts. By seven to eight years the cerebral palsy child's gait patterns are fixed and most probably the adult gait pattern will be the same.

### Drug Therapy of Cerebral Palsy

Diazepam has been used in a variety of dosages to control athetosis as well as spasticity. I have found that this has never given any permanent or even temporary improvement. Dantrolene sodium use is limited and is somewhat complicated by the fact that liver function has to be checked at least every three months. Dosage has to be adapted; starting from one half mg per kg daily, one can increase the dosage to 3 mg per kg 4 times a day. My colleagues and I have not encountered any liver dysfunction in the patients we have treated. In the severely affected child, this drug at times made it easier for the child to be fed. No dramatic results occurred. Some improvement in gait and balance, especially in the spastic, was noted.

### Assistive Devices

For marginal ambulators, assistive devices may make a difference between ambulation and being wheelchair bound. Function of the upper extremities becomes important in these cases. The most prescribed assistive devices are crutches, whether the classical axillary crutches, the Canadian, or the Lofstrand type. Rollators are useful, especially in ambulation at home or in confined areas. Whether a walker is used will depend on the amount of balance that the patient has (Fig. 26–5).

**Figure 26–5.** Rolling walkers. (ConMed Equipment, Westfield, N.J.)

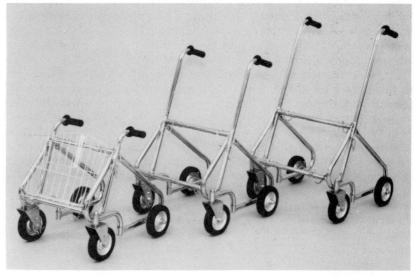

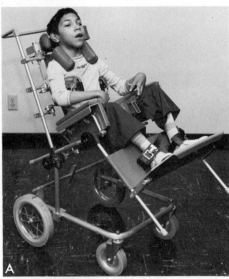

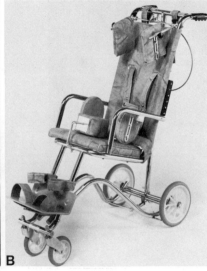

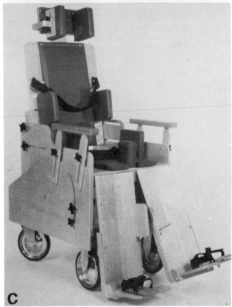

**Figure 26–6.** *A,* Seating system. (L. Mulholland Corp., Santa Paula, Ca.) *B,* Positioning wheelchair. (Stainless Medical Products Inc., San Diego, Ca.) *C,* Eaton Positioning Relaxation Chair.

Wheelchairs by themselves are prescribed both for marginal ambulators and for those who are no longer capable of ambulating independently. There are a variety of chairs, and with modification they can accommodate most patients. They also help children to transfer and to attend school as well as to travel. Modifications include such items as pommels and side wings (Fig. 26–6).

### Surgical Treatment

Orthopedic surgical indications are not the same for the upper extremities and the lower extremities. In the upper extremities, sensory feedback and normal function of hands cannot be obtained by surgery. However, some goals may be reached, including improved function of the hand acting as a stabilizer and sometimes improved gross function and cosmesis.

In the lower extremities, surgery should be performed only after the child has been walking independently for at least a year. There are certain exceptions such as threatened hip subluxation, knee joint contractures, and contractures of the gastrocnemius. In order to avoid psychological problems in the adolescent as a result of orthopedic surgery, it is preferable to try to perform operations when the child is between the ages of four and eight years. The goal of surgical treatment of the lower extremities is functional independence in ambulating. Surgery must be discussed with the parents so that inappropriate hope is not nurtured by them.

Surgery of the upper extremities is mainly for cosmesis and in the lower extremities mainly for ambulation. Lengthening of the Achilles tendon improves the base of weight bearing; release of flexion contracture at the knees prevents knee deformities and promotes more acceptable gait. Adductor release, as well as anterior branch obturator neurectomy, diminishes spasticity of the adductors and prevents subluxations or dislocation of the hips. It also prevents osteoarthritis of the hips that can develop in later life. All types of surgery require immobilization and loss of function. Active periods of therapy are then required, not only to regain lost function but to teach proper gait and to prevent loss of the benefits of the surgical procedure. Neurosurgical management of spasticity has made definite gains in recent years. Chronic cerebellar stimulation by the use of implanted electrodes has produced results in the hands of several neurosurgeons. A new procedure consisting of implantation of the electrodes in the internal capsule is also being tested as of this writing. It is too early to make a final judgment on the procedure, as its effectiveness is still under study.

Treatment would not be complete without placement of the child in an educational facility. The team approach is usually used to determine the most suitable environment. If the child has minimal involvement, a normal school classroom might be recommended; otherwise, special class placement may be more suitable. Part of the treatment also is the carryover of the exercises and physical therapy at home under the supervision of the parents, who become substitute therapists. Families of patients with cerebral palsy will need counseling, and as the child grows the scope of problems to be discussed can vary so that the parents avoid unrealistic expectations.

## SPINA BIFIDA

Spina bifida is probably the most common congenital disease after cerebral palsy. By definition, spina bifida is failure of fusion of the vertebral arches and is subdivided into two classes, *spina bifida occulta* and *meningomyelocele*. Spina bifida occulta is a small lesion usually involving the fifth lumbar and the first sacral vertebrae. The defect is quite common and is found in 25 per cent of children who are in hospitals but probably in no more than 10 per cent of the child population. It is usually asymptomatic and is an incidental finding. Occasionally it may also be associated with other neural tube defects.

Meningomyelocele is a birth defect that takes different clinical forms. Complete neural exposure may be seen, but more often a sac covered by a very thin membrane is seen; this membrane tears easily and some fluid may leak. Meningomyelocele is the protrusion of the meninges through the unfused verebral arches. It can be fully transilluminated. Occasionally, some nerve roots may adhere

to the inner wall of the sac. The incidence of meningomyelocele varies from 1 to 4 per cent, being lowest in oriental and black patients and highest in those of Irish and British ancestry, in whom it affects as many as four per thousand babies.

In the United States about one to two per thousand white babies are affected. The etiology of all neural tube malformations is still obscure. It seems that the predisposition is polygenic and that environmental factors may also play a role. In summary, it may be said that there are many causes, including genetic as well as environmental. There are sex differences and the male-to-female ratio is about 1 to 1.3. There is no definite correlation with marital consanguinity; however, it has been demonstrated that siblings are affected 7 to 15 times more than the general population.

The frequency among different races has been mentioned—blacks are less predisposed, with a very low incidence of spina bifida. Japanese transplanted to Hawaii have a higher incidence than in Japan. Up to now no firm connection has been found between dietary factors and the frequency of the disease.

From a developmental point of view, closure of the tube is completed by 28 or 30 days after conception so that the defect of spina bifida cystica occurs before the 30th day after conception and at a time when the mother is often not aware that she is pregnant. Approximately 80 per cent of meningomyeloceles are localized in the lumbosacral region. When the lesion is below the second lumbar vertebrae, the most affected part is the cauda equina. Thoracic and cervical lesions are distinctly less common and have fewer motor and urinary tract sequelae.

Before aggressive neurosurgical procedures and treatment, the natural history of meningomyelocele resulted in a mortality of 68 per cent of all patients. After development of surgical treatment, this incidence fell and the mortality dropped to about 34 per cent. In Lorber's series 83 per cent of patients had hydrocephaly but not all of them required shunting procedures. Most deaths in the first two years of life had neurological causes. After the age of two years, kidney complications were the leading cause of death. Less than 10 per cent of patients who have had intensive neurosurgical treatment are without any handicaps. In about 40 per cent of the cases the disability is moderately severe; these disabilities are mainly difficulties in ambulation, mental retardation, incontinence of feces and urine, and orthopedic problems.

In other studies in which patients in adult life were surveyed, significant numbers were mentally retarded. Those with lesions at the level of L2 had urinary incontinence, and in a great number of others, urinary problems, including calculi, hydronephrosis and infection, were present. Potential fertility is higher in females, with the total number of patients who are active sexually about 30 per cent. From pathological studies it was found that many defects may be present with meningomyelocele—on autopsy an 18 per cent incidence of urinary tract abnormalities not secondary to neurogenic bladder was noted; for example, horseshoe kidney, cystic lesions, renal agenesis and, much more frequently than in the general population, exstrophy of the bladder. The exact cause of these defects is difficult to assess; incidence may be as high as 10 per cent. Some investigators think that only 3 per cent of patients with meningomyelocele have normal urinary function.

## PROGNOSIS

Untreated children have a mortality of 45 per cent by the age of three months and by two years about 85 per cent will have died. Those patients whose management involved an aggressive neurosurgical approach had a two-year survival of 65 per cent. The quality of life of those surviving who had aggressive neurosurgical procedures is not uniform. A significant number have mental retardation and neurological sequelae. Incidence of those with total flaccid paralysis and incontinence may vary from 30 to 50 per cent. Of the 70 or 80 per cent who develop hydrocephalus, half are educable. Death after the age of two years is due to urinary tract failure or to the consequences of cardiopulmonary disease and kyphoscoliosis.

The hope of improvement in the outlook for all cases will probably involve prevention rather than treatment of the disease itself. Lorber in his review of children with meningomyelocele found that only 41 per cent of children survive. In his studies 7 per cent of the children had an independent earning capacity. Of the survivors only 66 per cent had an IQ less than 80. The survivors were confined to wheelchairs. He advocated criteria for the selection of treatment of newborn with meningomyelocele. He would withhold treatment from those with severe paraplegia, gross head enlargement, and multiple congenital anomalies. In the United States, however, these criteria cannot be applicable as everybody is treated. The legal entanglements that withholding of treatment, even with parental consent, would involve create such problems that selection cannot be applied in this country. Prevention seems to be the most satisfactory way of dealing with this condition, and two tests can be used to predict neural tube defects. One is amniocentesis, done between 14 and 16 weeks of pregnancy in selected patients at high risk. A new test that is not yet in general use evaluates alpha fetoprotein in the mother's blood. Although this is done as a test of the entire population in countries where there is a high incidence of meningomyelocele, this has not been found to be practical in the United States.

A more reliable and accurate test has recently been developed, the choline-esterase test done on amniotic fluid. Precautions have to be made to refrigerate the fluid after withdrawal to preserve the enzymatic potency of the extract.

Ultrasonography should always be used preceding amniocentesis to delineate the fetus, the placenta, and the amniotic sac as well as any neural defect. With the combination of amniocentesis and ultrasonography, more than 90 per cent of spina bifida cases can be recognized.

## MANAGEMENT

The management of children with myelodysplasia must be a team effort as no one professional alone can handle the complexity of the cases. There are three major areas: neurosurgical, urological, and physiatric.

Neurosurgical management begins early after birth. The neurosurgeon usually examines the patient at biweekly intervals for the first three months and then monthly for three or six months. Thereafter, follow-up is at every four months. The head is measured, and if head size increases rapidly, shunting usually is used. Frequent complications may follow placement of a shunt in the peritoneal cavity; shunts are often pinched and with rapid growth only a small length of the shunt remains in the peritoneal cavity. Often, associated spinal anomalies complicate the management. Additional neurological problems can be caused by Arnold-Chiari malformation. Symptoms of cerebellar dysfunction or lower cranial nerve abnormality can indicate this condition. Early diagnosis as well as adequate surgical therapy will prevent greater deterioration. A lesion silent for years may suddenly become symptomatic. The fourth ventricle is usually connected to an intramedullary cyst. The diagnosis is usually established by clinical examination and will be confirmed by computerized tomographic scanning and myelography. Most late complications secondary to myelodysplasia can be discovered only through continuous intellectual and physical function examination.

As stated earlier, only 9 to 10 per cent of patients are without urologic disabilities. Urinary incontinence is common, as are other urinary problems such as infections, calculi, and hydronephrosis. It is well known that children with one apparent congenital defect usually have more than one and this is particularly true in cases of urinary anomalies. On autopsy findings 15 per cent of patients with meningomyelocele had urinary malformations that were not secondary to neurogenic bladder. In a study by Forbes 12 per cent of patients had renal dysplasia, while in controls there were none.[8] It is difficult to gauge the extent of renal impairment at birth. At four years most patients had abnormal cystograms and pathological findings on intravenous pyelograms. If a patulous rectum and anesthesia of the perineal region are found, it can be surmised that bladder function is also impaired. Some patients with only minor motor impairment of the feet can have impaired bladder function. The goals of urological management are to maintain renal function, protect the kidneys from protracted infections, and encourage continence and bowel control.

The American Academy of Pediatrics has recommended that the following tests be done in these patients: in the neonatal period, blood urea nitrogen, serum creatine, urinalysis, culture, and intravenous pyelogram. The urinalysis should be performed at six-month intervals up to the age of three and then yearly, and pyelography should be performed yearly up to age three and then every other year. In management, the Crede method is not universally used because in some patients it may be harmful, especially in those with vesicourethral reflux. Some authors recommend that urinary tract infection be treated aggressively, even asymptomatic bacteriuria. The complications of indwelling catheters are multiple, frequently including nephritis, renal calculi, and increased bladder irritability. Intermittent catheterization seems to be successful with girls; boys are usually fitted with external collecting bags.

Ileal conduits may be recommended when all other measures fail. The conditions for an ileal conduit are urinary incontinence, urinary tract infection, and chemical deterioration. There are frequent complications with ileal conduits—wound dehiscence, infarction of loop, intestinal obstruction, frequent stoma revisions, difficulty with appliances, and renal deterioration. Abnormalities have been seen when the conduit was delayed, and some renal function deterioration and abnormalities of the renal tract have been noted that were present prior to institution of the ileal conduit.

Implantation of an artificial sphincter is theoretically more satisfactory. This consists of an inflatable device with a bulb urethral cuff and reservoir. They work better in those patients with the atonic type of bladder. They are still fraught with numerous problems. In mechanical devices, tubing can split or kink, valves often fail or leak, reservoirs leak, and cuffs rupture. Medical problems are urethral and scrotal erosions as well as vesical neck erosion. Pressure of the cuff can result in necrosis of the urethra. Infections have also been noted. There are some problems inherent in the different plastic materials, but pooled information of several urological centers gave a success rate in pediatric patients of about 75 per cent.

Other main goals of treatment are maintenance of ambulation and locomotion. The level of the cord involvement relates directly to the motor ability of the patient and his prognosis. Involvement at higher levels is evidently much more crippling than at lower levels. The level of involvement also determines the dynamic forces that cause the deformities. In addition, static deformities can result from faulty positioning. Contractures make standing or sitting much more difficult because body alignment is hard to achieve and bracing becomes either impossible or difficult.

PREVENTION OF TROPHIC ULCERS. Pressure on skin that has lost sensation and the covering of bony eminences tends to cause breakdown. The most affected areas are the heel, the malleolar region, the greater trochanters, the ischial tuberosity, and the sacrum. Deformities also contribute to this, as the weight-bearing areas are no longer the physiological areas, and pressure is concentrated on skin that is either not naturally intended to bear it or the pressures may also be concentrated on smaller areas. Poorly fitting shoes on a deformed foot may be an additional cause of irritation. In the perineal area maceration of the skin from urinary incontinence produces excoriations and leads to ulceration. If not treated, the ulcers will extend in dimension and in depth to the point that either periosteitis and eventually osteomyelitis will occur.

Prevention of ulcers is best done by relieving pressure on exposed areas. Use of air mattresses and frequent change of position are important. Heels should be protected from the chafing surfaces of bedspreads. When sitting, a special cutout board, with increased area of contact between the legs and at the weight-bearing points, can be used. The patient should also be trained to change sitting position frequently. Good skin hygiene should be maintained, especially in the perineal area.

Many factors come into account for the remaining adaptability and mobility of the child: intelligence, home environment, and motivation; however, the most important of all factors is the level reached by the neurological lesion. Usually, the level of the lesion is determined by the lowest level at which normal or good power can be found. Lesions are often spotty and there is not a complete loss of power as in transection of the cord. The sensory level often does not correspond to the motor level, but it must be taken into account when prescribing bracing. Often those lesions are affected by other existing lesions, meningitis, neonatal hypoxia, hydrocephalus, and other upper motor neuron lesions that introduce spasticity with a different form of deformity than is present with a pure cord lesion. Involvement at a higher cord level favors static deformities. In the level involving the lower roots, deformities are more dynamic and depend upon the sparing of certain muscles and their unopposed action.

I would like to introduce a classification of different functional levels of walking. Community walkers are those who can walk in the community without any restrictions. They may require crutches or braces, and they can walk on ground and stairs and use public transportation. Household walkers walk only inside the home and outside only on level surfaces. They may require bracing and crutches, and for certain activities they require wheelchairs. Nonfunctional walkers are those who can ambulate only in therapy. Nonwalkers are those who can transfer independently and the rest of the time are in wheelchairs.

Patients with thoracic level involvement have the more severe deformities. They have combinations of kyphosis and different types of scoliosis. The most debilitating combination is fixed lumbar kyphosis with progressive thoracic lordosis and varying degrees of scoliosis. As the hips are flail, the main deforming force is gravity; hips go into flexion, abduction, and external rotation, with varying degrees of knee deformities and equinovarus at the ankles.

The upper lumbar lesions produce the same hip deformities as do the thoracic lesions. With the low level at L3, there is also a tendency to contracture of the knee. Ankles may be either in equinovarus or less frequently in calcaneus. In the lower lumbar level the anterior tibial and the quadriceps are spared. Hips are still in flexion and in external rotation and may sublux. In those cases in which the quadriceps has good power, functional prognosis for long-term independent ambulation is quite favorable. At this level, there are fewer back deformities than in the higher level; nevertheless they should be watched for. Even at L4 level, approximately 50 per cent of patients have spinal deformities and at L5 level, some 25 per cent still may have spinal deformity. Lesions at L4 level have a high propensity for causing dislocation of the hip, which by causing asymmetrical alignment of the hips impairs the stability of the pelvis and predisposes to scoliosis. At the sacral level, where S1 and S2 may be involved, the majority of patients suffer urological problems, and care of the feet becomes essential. There is no weakness around the hips. Some minimal weakness may be present in the hip extensors and rarely deformities of the knees may occur.

At the S1 level the most common deformity is cavus foot and clawing of the toes because of the absence of long toe flexors and intrinsic muscles. These patients have only minimal involvement of the muscles above this level; they are active ambulators and the sensory status of the foot becomes a critical point. If they have no sensory input, the foot deformities with their unbalancing of weight bearing may cause ulceration and other problems. Early surgical intervention in soft tissue lesions may prevent further bony fixed deformities. According to the level of the lesion, a different type of orthosis may be necessary.

## BACK BRACING IN MYELODYSPLASIA

In thoracic lesions the patient needs total support of the lower extremities as well as the thoracic region. Sitting is facilitated if the child is fitted with a corset or a plastic molded jacket. For the simplicity of construction the parapodium (Fig. 26–7) is the easiest to put on and take off and is used for standing. Its different parts ensure stability in the anterior-posterior as well as in the mediolateral direction. Adjustable elements allow for the proper positioning of the lower extremities and the hips. Because of the versatility and adaptability of the device and the capability of interchange of pieces, fitting and adjustment are much easier than with conventional braces. The device can even be used for sitting purposes. Patients who use the device are usually not ambulators, except those with low thoracic lesions involving T11 and below. If the child is older, the conventional hip-knee-ankle-foot orthoses are used, with large thigh and calf bands. Valgus and varus at the knees can be controlled by pullers. Posterior "butterflies" may assist in improving hip extension and decrease lumbar lordosis.

In upper lumbar lesions in which L1 is mainly

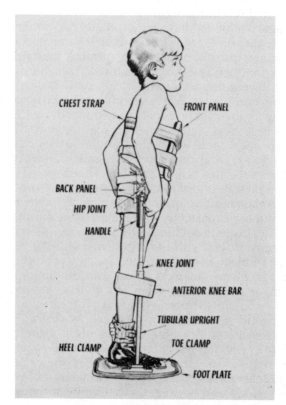

**Figure 26–7.** The parapodium. (From Redford, J.: Orthotics Etcetera, Baltimore, Williams & Wilkins, 1980, p. 349.)

involved, bracing is similar to that described in the thoracic lesions, whether a parapodium or a regular orthosis is prescribed. In a child wtih L2 and L3 involvement, ambulation is started later, and up to the age of two or three years the child can be mobile by crawling or using scooters. Those children having active quadriceps do not need bracing of the hip; therefore, the knee-ankle-foot orthosis will be sufficient. With the use of rollators and later with crutches, these patients can be taught to ambulate. However, frequently these youngsters have weak quadriceps, and knee-ankle-foot orthoses with locked knee joints are needed because of this.

For the first two or three years, the children can be trained in ambulation either by using a rollator or holding onto furniture at home. Usually by about five years they can be taught to ambulate with crutches. Hip subluxation or dislocation is a fact that has to be taken into account because ambulation becomes totally unfeasible when it happens.

In lower lumbar region deformities, bracing depends upon the root that is preserved. If L4 is intact, calcaneovarus deformity of the foot and sometimes knee extension contracture may occur. In the L5 root there is some power in the hip extensors and abductors; there is also some power in the knee flexors. As the anterior musculature of the ankle is also preserved, the most characteristic deformity is a calcaneus foot. In these cases the ankle foot orthoses is recommended. The ankle should have limited dorsiflexion; lateral T straps are added to prevent inversion of the foot. The calcaneus foot deformity frequently requires surgical correction. In a small number of patients in whom there is still a hip dislocation, ambulation will be compromised.

Involvement of the S1 and S2 levels has a much better prognosis. These patients are able to ambulate with only short leg braces, and they are good community ambulators. They might use either a cane or a crutch. At a lower level, only shoe modifications are needed. The shoes can be lined with lamb's wool to reduce discomfort.

## REHABILITATIVE THERAPY

Active rehabilitation measures must be postponed until back surgery has healed. Frequently, the child's hips may be flexed and externally rotated and the knees are flexed. If this position is permitted to prevail for a long time, contractures will occur. At this early stage it is hard to use any rigid constraints. Devices are made to bring the lower extremities into neutral position at the hips by inserting them in long socks and elastics that bring the socks together. In this position, the effect of gravity also extends the knees. To obtain some abduction at the hips, children should be wearing double or triple paper diapers. Mild manipulations can be undertaken at that time by the physical therapist. The parents are instructed to maintain the child in the prone position. This by itself prevents hip flexion contracture and encourages strengthening of the upper back muscles. Rolling can be encouraged after the age of three to four months. This might be a challenge as the lower extremities are usually flail, and unless the child is helped nothing is gained by it.

After the age of six months, these children may be trained to sit. This becomes an important goal as they learn to use their hands to bring them to midline. Special chairs or highchairs can be used. Certain companies produce bean bag chairs. Support is given to the trunk, and if the head is not stable, extensions can be made to include the head also. Reclining chairs might be required in the case of some instability of the back.

The occupational therapist mainly encourages bimanual activities, transfer activities, and early sensory stimulation to improve spatial and perceptual abilities.

An additional benefit is that with the supports the children can be placed in a stroller and pushed around. At this stage, strength of the upper extremities may be increased by providing toys and different materials that the child can reach for and spacing them so that the range of motion and power are increased. The different weights and shapes increase the perceptual training as well as provide exercise in spatial concepts.

Standing is started when the child tries to pull himself up. At that time supporting devices may be tried. Prone standers, standing tables, and appropriate appliances are worn (Fig. 26–10). In higher thoracic lesions, sitting with a corset becomes a reality, although it does not prevent scoliosis and hip flexion contractures, which should be treated. Standing with a parapodium is initiated at around two years. The parapodium can be adapted to the site of the back lesion. It is also possible to adapt a specially molded chest jacket to help in the management of spinal asymmetries. In addition, prone scooters and crawlers help in maintaining mobility.

The child with upper lumbar lesions is able to sit before the age of 18 months with marked lordosis. Bracing is started early to prevent hip contractures and to help in standing. Long leg braces with pelvic band and hip joints may be used initially. These braces can later be cut down to long leg braces. Crutches are used when the child has gained stability after using a rollator. This ability is frequently attained at about five to six years of age. Shoe fittings, inserts, and special linings must be used to prevent pressure sores. If the equinus is slight, it is treated by special heel inserts before surgery is resorted to.

In lower lumbar lesions at the level of L4, knee extension contractures are avoided. Calcaneovarus deformity is treated surgically. In deficit of L5, cal-

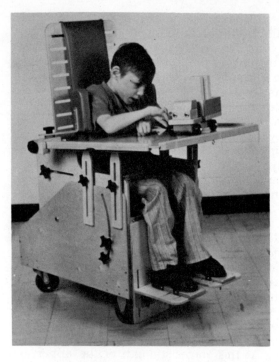

**Figure 26–8.** Specially adapted chair. (Community Playthings, Rifton, N.Y.)

caneus develops. Children only need ankle-foot orthosis with solid ankles or double-bar braces with no dorsiflexion and T straps to correct the varus tendency. Ambulation will be accomplished at two years of age.

### COUNSELING THE PARENTS

This should start shortly after birth at the hospital, with explanations of the nature of the disease and why neurosurgery must be performed. Both parents should be present when the full explanation is given. After neurosurgery the parents should be informed about management of the child and why close supervision by the rehabilitation department is necessary.

Parents' primary reactions are often confusion, disbelief, and anxiety. There can be an attitude of denial with mounting tension in the home. The

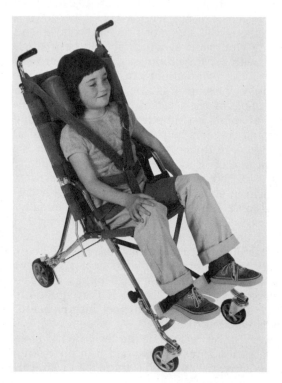

**Figure 26–9.** Specially adapted stroller with adduction straps and head wings.

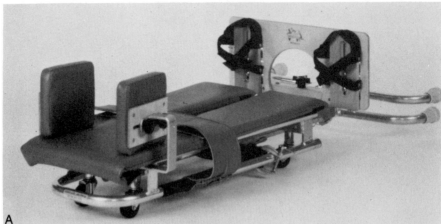

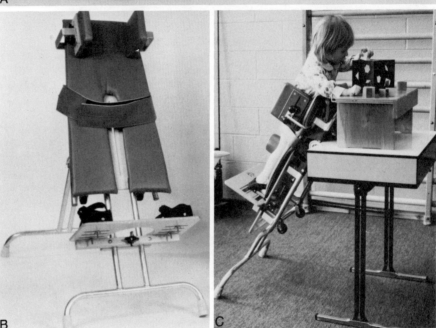

**Figure 26–10.** Prone stander. *A*, Collapsed; *B*, standing; *C*, in use. (Invacare Corp., Elyria, O.)

fact that the parent's expectations of a perfect child are unfulfilled and that they are disappointed must be dealt with. Parents also may feel that the child's disability is their punishment for some wrongdoing.

The Physiatrist must give an exact and objective picture of the disability. This might have to be repeated as it takes time for parents to adjust to the truth. Parents also have to be imbued with the idea that they are responsible for the rearing and the continuous care of their child. Finally, they usually must be referred for genetic counseling.

Help from the hospital social service department can alleviate normal tension in the household; if severe stress is noted one should not hesitate to refer the parents to the psychiatric department. The professional team will help them in making their decisions.

## REFERENCES

1. Little, W. I.: Trans. Obstet. Soc., 3:293, 1862.
2. Phelps, W. M.: Etiology and diagnostic classification of cerebral palsy. Proceedings of the Cerebral Palsy Institute of New York, New York Association for Aid of Crippled Children, 1950.
3. André-Thomas, et al.: The Neurological Examination of the Infant. London, Heineman, 1960.
4. Brazelton, T. B.: Neonatal Behavioral Assessment Scale. Spastic Intl., 1973.
5. Bobath, K., and Bobath, B.: The neuro-developmental treatment of cerebral palsy. Phys. Therap., 47:1039–1041, 1967.
6. Kabat, H., and Knott, M.: Proprioceptive facilitation techniques for treatment of paralysis. Phys. Therap. Rev., 33: 35–64, 1953.
7. Fay, T.: The use of pathological and unlocking reflexes in the rehabilitation of spastics. Am. J. Phys. Med., 33:347, 1954.
8. Forbes, M.: Renal dysplasia in neurospinal dysraphism. (Abstract) Arch. Dis. Child., 46:883, 1971.

# Rehabilitation of Head Injury Patients

*by Professor J. P. Held*
*(Translated from the French by Asa P. Ruskin, M.D.)*\*

The problem of rehabilitation of the head-injured patient can be divided according to the two separate categories of injury: mild and severe. The first involves the effects of minor head injury occurring either without loss of consciousness or with only a brief loss of consciousness. These cases occur quite frequently, especially in the adult, usually as a result of an accident. They result in a postconcussion syndrome that is largely subjective. There is a vast literature devoted to the description and importance of this syndrome, which every year is the subject of innumerable medical-legal depositions.

It would be more useful for the physician to refer these patients in the early post-traumatic period to an appropriate multidisciplinary rehabilitation center rather than simply to wait and eventually try to determine an appropriate degree of permanent partial disability. Early rehabilitation should emphasize the nonmedical aspects of the multidisciplinary approach, utilizing the physical therapist, occupational therapist, physical education instructor, recreation therapist, and psychologist in an effort to de-emphasize medical aspects and lessen the dramatic quality of the event. The patient should be involved in a well-organized program of activities including sports, games, and diversions,

as well as preprofessional or modified work activities. Frequently this type of early rehabilitation program prevents the development of the subjective syndrome or, in a significant number of cases, at least reduces its intensity and permits the patient to return to his normal work at an earlier date without permanent sequelae.[3]

Rehabilitation of patients with severe head injuries is of course the major concern and will be discussed from the standpoint of measures to be taken during the period of coma and after the return of consciousness. Improvement in the techniques of reanimation and intensive care over the past 10 to 15 years has vastly increased the number of individuals who are able to survive severe accidents, particularly traffic injuries—however, often this survival is at the price of severe neurological and psychiatric deficits.

It is frequently very difficult to know exactly the size and number of brain lesions except for those patients who have localized hematoma. This remains true, even though repeated brain scans and similar studies are done. Most severe head injuries result in diffuse cerebral contusions that frequently produce multiple lesions of the hemispheres and involvement of the brain stem. It has always been difficult to define the severity of head injury, and although it is not an absolute criterion, the best measure still seems to be related to the length of coma—in particular, if this lasts one or more weeks.[6, 12]

---

\*Photographs of Dr. Ruskin's Patient by Herbert A. Fischler, M.A., R.B.P., F.R.M.S., Chief, Audiovisual Resources, Kingsbrook Jewish Medical Center.

## COMATOSE PERIOD

It is essential that a rehabilitation plan be initiated during the early stages of coma. A general discussion of the numerous problems involved in intensive care, including orthopedic management, care of the skin, respiratory and excretory management, among others, are beyond the scope of this chapter. It is limited to a few points of particular concern to the rehabilitation team.

Frequently the comatose head-injured patient will have marked hypertonic spasticity. This is particularly significant in patients manifesting decerebration or decortication. Spasticity of this intensity makes any movement, even passive, quite difficult, particularly movement of the extremities. The lower extremities are frequently in hyperextension, with equinovarus deformity of the feet and the upper extremities in extension and hyperpronation. These abnormal postures are frequently not as fixed as might appear; they can be changed with the classical rehabilitation techniques used in the treatment of spasticity that employ the tonic neck reflexes and labyrinthine reflexes described by Magnus and emphasized by Ober. In some cases, unfortunately, even early and repeated therapy does not prevent the development of severe deformities. As soon as feasible—that is to say, as soon as the patient is able to breathe on his own and no longer requires mechanical respiratory assistance—the therapeutic exercises should be carried on outside of the patient's bed, preferably with the patient on an exercise mat or padded exercise table.

There are many who advocate exposing the comatose patient to a diversity of intense stimuli in an effort to produce an effect on the reticular activating system. The use of loud noises, touching with ice, and similar practices are claimed to be of benefit by some, but this is as yet unproved. It has been observed, however, that comatose patients exhibiting mild agitation may respond to the calming effect of music or a soothing human voice reading poetry.

The head injury is frequently accompanied by other severe injuries that might not be noticeable because of the coma. Fractures or dislocations of the extremities can be missed and it is often difficult to diagnose a low cervical fracture (particularly C7), a lumbar fracture, or a fracture of the neck of the femur. All these secondary injuries can greatly complicate the rehabilitation efforts. Conservative surgical management of these conditions is necessary, even though in the instance of fractures they can become complicated by excessive exostosis and periarticular soft tissue calcification. This may make subsequent mobilization of the joint impossible and severely limit the ultimate rehabilitation goals.

The length of coma is obviously quite variable and can range from a few days to several months. There is no absolute parallel between the length of coma and the long-term prognosis; however, it appears that usually there is a definite correlation between the length of coma and the degree of sequelae, with a much worse outlook for those patients in whom the coma has lasted more than two weeks and still worse if it lasts a month or more. I do not believe, however, that the length of post-traumatic amnesia is as reliable a prognostic sign as was reported by Jennett.[7]

### WAKING FROM COMA

Termination of the comatose period frequently occurs progressively. The patient begins by reacting to painful stimuli, first by reflex reaction and later in a more appropriate and adapted response. The eyes open intermittently and react to threat or loud noises and follow a moving light. In the beginning, periods of consciousness are brief and often it takes weeks before the patient regains a normal level of consciousness. It is not unusual in some patients, particularly younger individuals, for a period of relatively prolonged mutism to occur, during which the patient responds to questions only by head or eye movements.

Immediately after a period of coma, characteristic behavior problems can occur. Sometimes patients are very fearful and resist all attempts at rehabilitation and the pain that might be concomitant to these efforts. They are frequently agitated and negativistic and can be violent, striking out at the therapist and others. The majority, however, are passive and tend to immobility, turning in on themselves. They will roll over and turn their backs to the person speaking to them and may assume the fetal position.

This explains some of the difficulties faced by the rehabilitation team. It is necessary for team members to adopt a friendly and caring attitude, while at the same time firmly asserting the rehabilitation process. In this regard it is also important to work with the family to help avoid an overly solicitous attitude and provide a maximally stimulating environment.

The patient's general behavior frequently regresses, with young adults becoming quite infantile. Some will be fixated on an oral level, becoming preoccupied with food and putting everything at hand into their mouth. Various types of stereotypic behavior can be seen.

## EVALUATION AND REHABILITATION

The evaluation can be accomplished little by little as the patient slowly progresses over the days and weeks following coma. A detailed evaluation of the orthopedic sequelae may be done first and subsequently evaluation of sensorimotor deficits can be made. A full evaluation of cognitive deficit is done last, frequently over a period of several weeks, allowing for a precise analysis of the residual deficit symptoms that are extremely complex and interrelated.

*Motor deficits*, which are highly integrated deficits involving all central nervous system motor pathways as well as peripheral nerves, can be extremely difficult to sort out. In *visual deficits*, one must attempt to evaluate and separate true blindness, visual agnosia, Balint's syndrome, extraocular muscle paralysis, as well as visual field defects and hemi-inattention syndrome.

## COGNITIVE DYSFUNCTIONS

These can be extremely complex and require frequent and repeated examination to be understood. Various types of language and communications impairment can include apraxia, different degrees of aphasia, cognitive problems, and difficulties in higher intellectual function, as well as a host of behavioral disorders. All these occurring in different degrees can constitute a mixed syndrome that defies precise categorization.

I will briefly review the various elements of the rehabilitation evaluation and the appropriate therapeutic approach.

## MUSCULOSKELETAL PROBLEMS

Many head-injured patients will have suffered multiple injuries, sometimes with a vertebral fracture that can be missed in the beginning and that obviously presents a serious obstacle to effective rehabilitation. Whenever possible these fractures should be treated orthopedically in a way that permits the earliest possible movement. In many of these injuries healing occurs rapidly, frequently with extensive ectopic calcification (Fig. 27–1). When these injuries occur in the vicinity of joints, calcification can cause severe limatation in range of motion. This type of problem can occur at any articulation, and all manner of limitations have been described.[6, 12]

Joint involvement with ankylosis can result from spastic contractures as well as periarticular ectopic calcification. In the upper extremities, limitation in range of motion is most frequently seen in the shoulder and the hand, and can progress to a painful "shoulder-hand syndrome" with elements of reflex dystrophy. In the lower extremity the most frequent involvement can produce limitation of the hip in flexion and external rotation with flexion contracture of the knee and equinovarus deformity of the foot.

Usually these orthopedic problems will respond

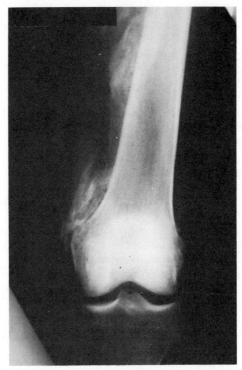

**Figure 27–1.** Soft-tissue calcification near the femur.

to standard physical therapy techniques: positioning, passive mobilization and active assistive therapeutic exercises combined with anti-inflammatory medication and local injection. These methods will usually suffice if the patient is started on a treatment regimen early enough so that the problems of spasticity are not allowed to become irreversible. Unfortunately many patients are not seen until spastic deformities have become established, with a fixed elbow flexion at 90 degrees, knee flexion contracture at 90 degrees or more, and equinovarus of 120 to 130 degrees. Under those circumstances surgical correction is the only efficacious approach (Figs. 27–2 and 27–3).

Ectopic calcifications forming osteomas in the muscles or periarticular areas are nonspecific in nature and occur fairly often following severe head injury. The reported frequency varies considerably with the study being reported, and ranging from 1 in 12 to 1 in 4;[11, 13, 14] calcifications may occur at several sites in the same patient. There is a predilection for proximal articulations, particularly the hip and elbow and less frequently the knee and shoulder. Calcification at other localizations occurs but is most unusual. The symptomatology varies: the first sign frequently is pain or an inflammatory reaction of the joint that is most easily recognized when the elbow or knee is involved. Limitation in range of motion or ankylosis occurs and may not be correctly diagnosed until seen on x-ray. The time of onset of ectopic calcification varies, but may be fairly early in the period after the accident; it matures progressively but usually stabilizes in from 6 to 18 months.

The calcifications themselves are constituted of normal bone formation occurring outside the normal skeleton or joints; radiologically they progress through successive stages. At first indistinct and cottony, they become increasingly dense and well outlined. They can develop as an exostosis of a normal bone and occasionally form a bridge between two bones or remain completely independent with no connection to the normal skeleton. Localization at the hip is usually medial, anterior, or posterior; at the knee it is most often next to the medial condyle; at the elbow it can be either anterior or posterior, limiting pronation and supination.

The pathogenesis of ectopic calcification and osteoma formation has been extensively studied but remains a mystery. Some of the possible causes include problems of calcium metabolism, sympathetic system disturbance, and vascular disorders. Similar osteoma formation is frequently observed in patients with spinal cord injury, tetanus, and severe burns. No effective preventive therapy is known; many investigators have tried different treatments, including corticosteroids and radiotherapy. Diphosphonates utilized in the treatment of Paget's disease have been suggested. Surgical removal cannot be undertaken until the lesion is fully matured—that is, at least 18 months after onset. Surgery is considered at that time only if the osteoma produces a significant functional impairment (hip ankylosed in flexion with external rotation or elbow at 90- to 100-degree extension). Various criteria have been proposed to follow the development of the osteoma and estimate its stability; clinical or x-ray appearance, local temperature, radioisotope bone scan, blood calcium level, blood phosphorus level and urinary hydroxypro-

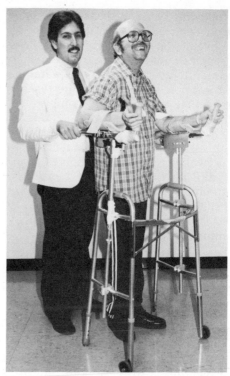

**Figure 27–3.** Specially adapted walker that accommodates 90-degree elbow flexion.

line. None of these tests have a proven value; however, the simultaneous evaluation of several allow one to determine the degree of maturity and stabilization of the lesion. Surgical removal is usually successful and recurrence is rare, provided that the appropriate time frame is respected.

## NEUROMUSCULAR PROBLEMS

The neuromuscular problems are always part of a complex diffuse brain damage syndrome involving to some extent sensory, language, and cognitive functions with behavior disturbances and impairment of perception and sensorimotor integration. For didactic pupuses, the subject matter has been divided into separate categories, but all these elements that coexist to a greater or lesser degree are closely interrelated. (For further discussion, see Chapter 1 on stroke.)

### Hemispheric Motor Syndrome

In the majority of cases, the patient has hemiplegia. Occasionally a more limited monoplegia can be seen or a more diffuse lesion with bilateral involvement, producing double hemiplegia that can be more severe on one side or the other.

When hemiplegia results from a hemispheric lesion, the clinical picture is essentially the same as

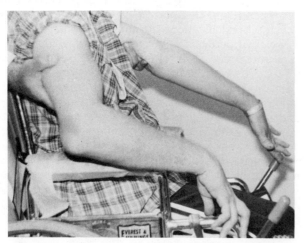

**Figure 27–2.** Right elbow with 90-degree fixed deformity. Note the spastic posturing of the left hand.

in a cerebrovascular accident. It has the same poor prognosis for return of function in the upper extremity. There are similar problems of aphasia with lesions of the dominant hemisphere and problems of spatial orientation and body image that are more easily demonstrated in right hemisphere lesions.

The effects in some patients demonstrating corticospinal tract involvement, especially when bilateral, seem to be the result of brain stem injury rather than diffuse hemispheric damage. In these cases, recovery is frequently better, and although it may be asymmetrical, the overall prognosis is considerably more favorable than when similar motor deficit is the result of cerebrovascular lesions. The patient is more likely to regain voluntary control of motor function and may be left with only a mild residual spasticity. In these cases, even the upper extremity and hand muscles may regain fine motor control, with only some residual diminution of dexterity and speed when rapid alternating movements are performed.

Rehabilitation techniques are in all respects similar to those employed in the treatment of stroke patients.

## Peripheral Nerve Lesions

It is not unusual to find that persons who have suffered prolonged coma develop secondary peripheral nerve involvement as a result of pressure and nerve entrapment. This is more likely to occur if the patient is thin; the involvement is often not noticed during the comatose period because examination is difficult and the clinical signs are masked by the coma itself. Peripheral nerve injury should be thought of when physical examination shows an isolated decreased deep tendon reflex or a localized area of diminished response to pinprick. Several peripheral nerves are commonly involved, in particular the radial, ulnar, median, sciatic, and peroneal.

In most cases the eventual recovery and return of function is satisfactory, but the delay for reinnervation can take a year or longer.

The diagnosis can be confirmed by electromyography and nerve conduction studies. The usual rehabilitation techniques appropriate to peripheral nerve damage can be utilized.

## Cerebellar Syndrome

Cerebellar lesions and tract involvement are fairly common, especially among young individuals with brain stem lesions. The lesions cannot, of course, be diagnosed until sufficient time has passed for some voluntary function to have returned—a period of weeks to months. The first sign might be a difficulty with sitting balance or some degree of ataxia persisting in upper extremity function after satisfactory motor strength has returned. Fortunately, the majority of these patients tend to have a spontaneous recovery; however, this can occur quite slowly, requiring a period of months or even years.

Rehabilitation therapy of these patients is extremely important in order to combat the combination of ataxia and spasticity with concomitant asynergia. The rehabilitation is a very slow and progressive process. I have obtained good results utilizing a technique that is based in part upon the Bobath method. In the first stage, exercises are done with the patient lying supine in a comfortable position. Active exercises are at first localized and slow, with the therapist teaching the patient to voluntarily associate the function of agonist and antagonist muscles. It is important that the patient not try to concentrate on more than one or two muscle groups at a time. These exercises are made progressively more complex by adding additional muscle groups and proceeding from distal to proximal muscle groups of the upper and lower extremities, then attempting to integrate activities involving the proximal portions of the lower and upper extremities working together. This permits progress to exercises of the upper and lower trunk. Training in head and neck stability is done at the same time as the work on the extremities and trunk. Only after the patient is able to perform these exercises well in the supine position can he progress to analogous exercises in a prone position similar to the breast stroke in swimming.

When coordination of the pelvic and shoulder girdle has been achieved, the patient can progress to knee and arm crawling exercises, increasing the complexity by bringing into play two extremities on the same side and then reciprocal use of the extremities. This is followed by "walking" on the knees, holding the torso erect, at first with the patient allowed to rest his weight on his thighs and on the lower portion of the legs and subsequently maintaining vertical alignment of the trunk and upper portions of the legs. This entire process is a lengthy one in severe cerebellar syndromes. It is frequently necessary to spend several months at each level before the patient progresses to the next step, as too rapid a progression will result in a therapeutic failure.

If each step outlined is carefully obtained, it is relatively easy for the patient to progress to standing in parallel bars. It remains, however, difficult to progress from simple standing to ambulation, as any movement, even of small magnitude, requires good standing balance. Exercises progress slowly with the therapist progressively teaching forward and backward movements and then lateral movements of the extremities individually and then reciprocally. The slowness of progress can be discouraging for the patient and therapist alike. However, in a majority of cases, a satisfactory standing balance can be accomplished as can progressively independent ambulation going from parallel bars to walker and then to cane. A year or more might be required for this. It is certainly preferable to make this significant investment in therapeutic effort rather than relegate the patient prematurely to a wheelchair existence.

Rehabilitation and functional use of the upper extremities is rendered more difficult because of the patient's need to utilize two canes or a walker in order to maintain standing balance and ambulation. In occupational and physical therapy of the upper extremities the slowly progressive acquisition of functional activity is emphasized, concentrating at first on isolated muscle groups and only slowly progressing to integrated functions.

The overall prognosis for return of motor function in the head-injured patient is reasonably good; the vast majority achieve the ability to get up and ambulate independently. Those with hemiplegic syndrome might not regain full use of the involved upper extremity, and a few with severe ataxia remain wheelchair bound.

## SENSORY DEFICITS

### Visual Difficulties

A certain number of head injuries are accompanied by trauma to the optic nerve. When this trauma is bilateral, the rehabilitation problem is complicated. Rehabilitation is even more difficult when there is also a hemiplegia with hemisensory defect such that the patient has only one hand, retaining intact sensory perception. Rehabilitation of these patients requires highly specialized techniques, usually available only in institutions for the sightless.

Occipital lobe lesions can result in cortical blindness. In some instances the patients themselves may be unaware of their loss of vision and may confabulate responses when asked what they "see." In other cases, some degree of tubular vision persists and can be utilized even though the patient's function is severely limited. If recovery occurs, it is unpredictable and extremely variable.

Hemispheric lesions, particularly of the right hemisphere, can result in a left hemi-inattention syndrome with problems in spatial orientation and body image. This is in no way different from the syndrome seen in patients following cerebrovascular accidents and is discussed in Chapter 1.

Visual agnosia, which is an inability to recognize objects and understand them when the visual perceptive mechanism is intact, can be so massive in the beginning as to appear to be blindness. This can be complicated by a psychological paralysis of gaze (Balint's syndrome) or a visual motor incoordination resulting in a wandering gaze. The visual agnosia can regress progressively, with the patient first becoming aware of moving lights, then subsequently fixed lights and later images, colors, and faces, with recognition of numbers and letters returning last. Rehabilitaton training includes having the patient follow a moving light and name objects, then pictures and colors, going from brilliant saturated colors to finer differentiation. With a moving light or object, the patient is taught to explore his entire visual field so that objects are not neglected because of hemi-inattention.

Cognitive visual disturbances can be further complicated by the existence of a homonymous hemianopia or other visual field deficit. While the prognosis for recovery of visual field deficit is generally not good, patients can learn to adapt to this in a satisfactory manner.

The perceptual visual disturbances can be further complicated by extraocular muscle paralysis with consequent diplopia.

### Olfactory Deficits

While injury to the olfactory nerve endings is not uncommon in mild head injury, it appears to be rare in severe head injury cases. This may in part be due to a failure in recognition of olfactory disturbance that is masked by problems in communication when the physician's primary attention is directed to other overwhelming problems. When it occurs, it is usually accompanied by problems in perception of taste and should be looked for when the patient's state of consciousness and awareness permits.

### Auditory Deficit

Deafness is extremely rare unless there has been a fracture of the base of the skull. Examination in the early stages should include visualization of the eardrums for retrotympanic hemorrhage or rupture, as well as the presence of Battle's sign (ecchymoses in the mastoid region). Audiometry should be performed when feasible if clinically indicated, and electronystagmography can be useful in evaluating the frequently associated vestibular dysfunction and distinguishing disequilibrium of vestibular origin from that of cerebellar lesions. It is, of course, important to recognize the existence of auditory impairment when evaluating the patient for cognitive deficits or behavioral problems that can be compounded by any significant degree of deafness.

## LANGUAGE DISORDERS

### Mutism

Akinetic mutism is common just following the coma. Communication may be carried out by eliciting eye movements or occasionally head movements. The period of mutism may last for several days or a few weeks and then gives way to a progressive return of speech, beginning with whispering and rapidly increasing to normal talking. This recovery of vocal function takes place spontaneously and there is no specific therapy required.

## Aphasia

All varieties of aphasia can occur in head injury, depending on the site and extent of cerebral damage.[9] The types of aphasia that occur in head-injured patients are similar to those seen in stroke patients, and most frequently involve some combination of the classically described categories including motor aphasia, "sensory" aphasia, jargon aphasia, anomic aphasia, and frontal lobe type diminution in linguistic spontaneity. Treatment by means of speech therapy is discussed in Chapter 1.

## Dysarthria

Dysarthria, sometimes with total anarthria, is much more frequent than aphasia following head injury and is secondary to lesions of the brain stem. Sometimes patients have an almost total lack of breath and cannot make any sounds. There may also be a severe loss of voluntary function of the entire group of facial and laryngeal muscles required for speech. Fortunately, however, the paralysis is rarely total. Significant deficits in ability to control and modulate breath production produces a "pneumophonic dyssynergia."[4]

The dysarthria may be further complicated by various combinations of vocal cord paralysis, cerebellar dysfunction, and spasticity (Fig. 27–4). The resultant problems in articulation and sound production can make the patient's speech difficult to understand if not totally incomprehensible. Speech therapy in these cases is usually extremely difficult and requires an extended period of treatment. Residual speech defects can be a major hurdle in so-

cial and vocational rehabilitation and occasionally a total loss of vocal communication persists.

Various types of communications devices exist, ranging from simple communication boards (Fig. 1–10) to complex electronic equipment that can be operated manually and artificially produces a human voice. This permits the patient a wider latitude of communication and the possibility of "speaking" to someone who may not be looking directly at him.

## COGNITIVE DISORDERS

### Intellectual Capacity

The patient's thought processes may be severely impaired in the period after coma. Frequently, intelligence tests show a marked drop from the pre-trauma performance level, with the impairment often most pronounced in the nonverbal portions of the test. Results for the verbal sections sometimes remain close to normal in those patients who do not have specific language disorders. A full battery of neuropsychological tests characteristically shows a wide scattering, with retention of certain functions contrasting with marked diminution in others. This differentiates the brain trauma victim from the congenitally impaired.

A majority of patients will improve fairly rapidly over a number of months. In most instances they regain at least the appearance of satisfactory intellectual function, although in some cases marked intellectual impairment will persist in spite of relatively satisfactory results on psychological tests. However, some patients are able to develop a superficial facade that masks profound thought disorders with severely impaired judgment and deficiencies in critical thinking that can prevent satisfactory social reintegration, even though no other handicaps are present. Others having had similar injury and length of coma will regain their premorbid status.

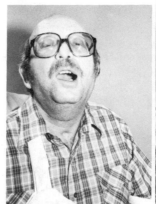 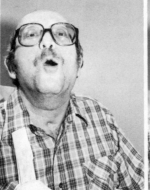 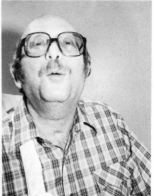

**Figure 27–4.** Note the effect of spasiticity on facial expression during vocalization.

## MEMORY DISTURBANCES

Mnestic disorders merit special consideration because of their severity and frequency following head injury.[1, 2, 4, 6, 8, 10] Immediately following coma, amnesia can be total, combined with disorientation for time and place, as well as loss of fixation memory. Orientation to place is usually the first to return, although it may not return for several months. Disorientation in time is usually more persistent.

Psychological memory tests (Wechsler) can be utilized. However, it is perhaps more clinically relevant to question the patient regarding events of his past life and his memory of major social and political events, as well as to evaluate his ability to perform basic learned skills. Memories of the patient's past life return slowly; this return can be helped with family photographs, personal anecdotes, and stories of specific significant life events recounted by members of the family. Frequently the patient remains confused regarding the temporal sequence of these events. It is important that the psychologist and the family work as a team in aiding the patient to reconstruct his past. It is common to have a period of permanent amnesia involving the events leading up to the accident. Such retrograde amnesia can include the events of several weeks or even months. Generally the patient regains memories of his past life fairly readily, but in some cases a loss of basic learned material persists, as though everything the person had ever learned was erased.

Therapy for the relearning process involves techniques that will assist the patient in remembering what he had previously learned until he is able to develop independent recall without cues and coaching. This process can be complicated by a short attention span and difficulty in recall of middle and long-term memory. The eventual outcome of vocational rehabilitation can easily depend on the patient's success in overcoming this problem.

## BEHAVIOR DISORDERS

One of the most common behavior changes seen following head trauma is a surprising degree of regression, with patients returning to a child-like state of dependency. They may adopt a totally infantile pattern, seeking signs of affection, playing with toys, and insisting on help in performing simple acts that they are physically capable of carrying out independently. The entire rehabilitation team together with the family must work to overcome this.

A total change of character is not unusual. This can take the form of a frontal lobe type syndrome in which a previously conservative individual becomes garrulous and expansive, losing critical awareness and control of himself and behaving without concern for the effect of his behavior on other people, failing to observe the usual social customs. It is less common to see development of neuroses such as obsessional behavior or true manic states, although depression is not uncommon. Some patients show a tendency to violence, either directed at the family or persons in general, or manifest other personality changes that seem to be exaggerations of premorbid tendencies. Individuals can develop a true psychotic state or permanent dementia.

Probably the most frequent post-traumatic behavior change is apathy and a general slowing down of activity, both mental and physical. In spite of great encouragement by family and therapists, many of these patients show a total loss of interest in anything that does not directly concern them and a loss of motivation in carrying out even the routine activities of daily living. Their morning toilet and dressing can take two or three times as long as it ordinarily had taken them prior to the accident. As a result of the multiple injuries and complex cognitive and mental sequelae, many of these patients are unable to reintegrate into a life that has become too rapid for them. They have difficulty in resuming prior friendships and relationships and tend to adopt an isolated life situation on the fringes of a society from which they feel rejected. This adds severe socioeconomic consequences to their loss of confidence and anxiety.

## SEIZURE DISORDERS

Contrary to general opinion, epileptic seizures are not common following head injury, whether the wound is closed or open. When seizures do occur, anticonvulsant medication must be administered with the usual guidelines and precautions. The systematic prophylactic use of anticonvulsant medication does not seem justified even in patients who have isolated electroencephalographic abnormalities unless these abnormalities are exceptionally marked or highly suggestive of seizure activity.

# HEAD INJURY IN CHILDREN

Classically, the prognosis for recovery from severe head injury in children is better than in adults. Sequelae are significantly less frequent, although there is again a variable relationship between length of coma and severity of residual effects. All of the same types of lesions that are seen in the adult can be seen in children. However, the greatest number of difficulties arise because of behavior problems and learning difficulties.

Behavior problems are the rule and usually take the form of a change in character; the child becomes unstable and impulsive, with frequent anger and aggressive acting-out. At times more severe problems occur that involve episodes of fugue, irrational behavior, and a tendency to become antisocial or delinquent. Learning difficulties and scholastic problems must be anticipated, frequently resulting in one or two years' loss in class level. It is important to carefully evaluate the child's academic ability and provide for an intermediate period of special classes or coaching before attempting to return the child to his normal class level in order to avoid the additional trauma of scholastic failure. Occasionally one sees a child who, with great difficulty, is able to recover his previous scholastic level but then is unable to acquire new skills and knowledge. The prognosis in these cases unfortunately is quite poor.

## OVERALL PROGNOSIS

The outlook following severe head injury remains somber. Most statistics show from 50 to 70 per cent of head-injured patients returning to some type of activity but most often at a lower level than prior to accident. The handicap is much more often the result of problems in mentation than motor dysfunction, although these at times can be totally disabling themselves, as can a severe communication disorder. Many attempts have been made to categorize the sequelae of head injury, but no classification has really been satisfactory because of the complexity and interrelationship of a multiplicity of factors.

The most frequent handicap is the loss of initiative and motivation coupled with a general slowing or bladypsyche that can be described as "intellectual viscosity."

The severity of the prognosis mandates a prolonged period of intensive rehabilitation carried out by a multidisciplinary team.

## REFERENCES

1. Brooks, D. N.: Long and short-term memory in head injury patients. Cortex 11:329, 1975.
2. Brooks, D. N.: Wechsler memory scale performance and its relationship to brain damage after severe head injury. J. Neurol. Neurosurg. Psychiatr. 39:593, 1976.
3. Cohadon F., Hubert L. M. and Richer E.: La réadaptation des traumatisés crâniens légers dans la prévention des séquelles subjectives. Bordeaux Méd. 5:1021, 1972.
4. Ducarne B.: Troubles neuropsychologiques des traumatisés crâniens ayant subi un coma plus ou moins prolongé, Psychol. Franç. 21:59, 1976.
5. Gilchrist E. and Wilkinson M.: Some factors determining prognosis in young people with severe head injuries. Arch. Neurol., 36:335, 1979.
6. Held J. P., Mazeau M. and Rodineau J.: Les troubles de la motilité et du langage chez les traumatisés crâniens. Ann. Méd. Phys., 18:337, 1975.
7. Jennett B.: Assessment of the severity of head injury. J. Neurol. Neurosurg. Psychiatr. 39:647, 1976.
8. Mandleberg, I. A.: Cognitive recovery after severe head injury. J. Neurol. Psychol., 38:1121, 1975; 39:1001, 1976.
9. Mazaux J. M.: Les aphasies traumatiques. Thèse Méd., Bordeaux, 1977.
10. Mazeau M., Ducarne B. and Held J. P., Devenir neuropsychologique à long terme des traumatisés crâniens sévères. Congrès IRMA, 1978.
11. Payen B.: Les paraostéoarthropathies chez l'hémiplégique. Thèse Méd., Paris, 1978.
12. Rhoades M. E., Garland D. E., Orthopedic prognosis of brain-injured patients. Clin. Orthop. 131:104, 1978.
13. Vigouroux R. P., Baurand C., Choux M. and Guillermain R.: Etat actuel des aspects séquellaires graves dans les traumatismes crâniens de l'adulte. Neurochirurgie 18: suppl. 2, 1 (1972).
14. Weber R., Normand J.: La rééducation des complications neurologiques graves des traumatismes cérébraux. Ann. Méd. Phys., 13:67, 1970.

# 28

# Sex

*by Ruth K. Westheimer, Ed.D.*

The health care professional has an obligation to become familiar with the important psychological changes that a person is subjected to when hospitalized for any length of time.

Separation from home, partner, and daily routine and the "shock" of undergoing occasionally dehumanizing procedures may bring about negative feelings. The individual may experience anxiety upon being reduced to the role of patient, in which almost every respect of life is controlled by other people, and having to expose intimate life details to strangers.

These factors, with the person's impaired physical condition, can bring about a loss of libido, which in itself is anxiety provoking.

Human beings are born with a libido and they die with a libido. When health professionals understand this concept and incorporate it into their dealings with patients, they will have made significant progress toward achieving a healthy attitude about sexuality for all people.

## THE OLDER PERSON AND SEX

In our western civilization, particularly in the United States, the tendency to worship the young, the beautiful, and the able-bodied can lead to a denial of sexual interest and feelings among people not in these categories. It also can lead to a negative self-concept in many who feel that they do not live up to the "ideal image" of sexual achievement as portrayed in the mass media. This applies particularly to western civilization because in some nonwestern societies studied by anthropologists and sociologists older members of the family are

530

highly respected and revered. They increase in status in the community as they age and have a special position in the family and community until they die.

Not so with us. Older women and men often identify with and adapt to the kind of stereotyped image they think they "ought" to present, namely, that of a person who is no longer sexually useful, no longer interested in sexual activity. For the menopausal woman who goes through "the change," who has passed the childbearing years, this kind of attitude becomes a part of a vicious circle. If she refrains from being sexually active, the physiological phenomena of aging may occur faster. Atrophy of the vaginal mucosa may occur, accompanied by diminished vaginal lubrication, which may cause dyspareunia. Accompanying these changes, which are most likely to be accentuated in the sexually inactive postmenopausal woman, is an actual shrinkage in size of the vaginal barrel. Loss of elasticity in tissues is one manifestation of aging in general and is observed in many parts of the body. Vasomotor instability ("hot flashes") and atrophic changes in the breasts and skin also may occur.

Older men who ask the physician repeated questions about the prostate and make complaints of vague abdominal pain are often attempting to relieve their anxiety by drawing attention to that part of the body. When the physician or health professional initiates a discussion on sex by making specific questions about erection, ejaculation, morning erection, nocturnal emissions (wet dreams), and masturbation, it becomes possible for the patient's anxiety to be relieved. It is important to convey that worthwhile sexual activity does not *only* consist of a firm erection and vigorous orgasm on every occasion. Most importantly, sexual expression is influenced by a positive concept of personal sexuality and self-esteem.

## QUALITIES OF THE COUNSELOR

To be an effective counselor, there are three basic ingredients a person must have: knowledge, ability to establish rapport, and the counselor's comfort with sexual matters. I would like to coin a new term, *sexual literacy*. Since the physician and the health professional in general already possess (so we hope) the skills of counseling, we just have to add the specific knowledge about physiology, recent research findings, and information from the field of human sexuality including anatomy, physiology, and psychosexual therapy.

What is the responsibility of the health professional in sex counseling of the elderly in general and of the elderly who have minor physical impairments in particular? Which approach should be taken and which questions addressed to open communication between the caregiver and the patient in this area?

In order to provide a basis for improving the quality of the patient's sexual activity, a sympathetic, nonjudgmental approach is needed. It is not enough to ask, "How is your sex life?" One has to ask specifically, "How has the health problem we talked about (for example, the minor cardiovascular situation or arthritis) affected your sexual functioning?" And one must *wait* for a response. This sort of counseling on the intimate aspects of life and love *cannot* be done in a hurry—the patient must realize that you the practioner *really want* to know—that this is not just a routine perfunctory question.

## THE COUNSELING APPROACH

Here are some examples of open-ended questions: "How have you managed to deal with the sexual part of your life to date? How does your spouse (partner, friend) feel about your disability? Has your desire for sexual activity, foreplay, orgasm, and resolution been affected by this? (If yes, describe the situation.) When did you first notice difficulty in your sexual functioning? Did you ever talk to a health professional about this? How do you feel about talking about this issue now? Would you like me to suggest some ideas that might provide some improvement or enrichment in your sexual functioning—maybe some suggestions specifically that have helped others in your particular condition?"

## COUNSELING ON MASTURBATION

It is important for the counselor to be aware of the taboos and preconceived notions in our society relating to self-stimulation. It is difficult for most people to talk about masturbation in general and about their own masturbatory activities in particular. We have to listen carefully in order to detect whether the patient feels guilty, ashamed, or disgusted about masturbation or if previous education and psychological influences have made it possible for the patient to engage in any masturbatory activity at all.

Once the subject has been approached and tactfully discussed, further clarifying questions can be asked: "Do you masturbate to orgasm? Do you have difficulties reaching an orgasm when you masturbate? Do you use fantasies when you masturbate? How do you feel about masturbating?"

For those older women and men who do masturbate, either because there is no partner available or for any other reason, it is important to alleviate their anxiety about this activity and give reassurance and permission that this is a perfectly acceptable form of sexual activity. Sometimes it is useful to suggest using fantasies, audiovisual aids, or vibrators. Vibrators seem to be more help for women wanting to achieve sexual release—orgasm—than for men. When suggesting use of a vibrator it is important to add that for many women the direct touch of the vibrator on the clitoris is not enjoyable, but rather circular motions around the clitoral area are. For some women an object or dilator or an additional vibrator inserted into the vagina is pleasurable and also keeps the vagina in "good health," delaying atrophy at the same rate that would be possible if the vagina were used for sexual intercourse. This is particularly important for the woman who has no partner for sexual activity. Another suggestion is to use a lubricant inside the vagina and around the clitoral area to prevent chafing and to enhance sexual feeling.

## COUNSELING ON SHARED SEXUAL ACTIVITY

On the subject of shared sexual activity, the counselor might ask: "How frequently do you and your partner engage in sexual activity? Do you tell your partner what pleases you most sexually? Do you engage in mutual masturbation? Has your disability had any influence on your talking about sexual activity with your partner?"

What is needed is education on *sexual enrichment*—and most important—the *giving of permission* . . . for sexual feelings to be accepted and welcomed.

We know that with age, caressing and touching become far more satisfying as reassurances of sensory adequacy than orgasm, because the sense of touch (especially in the fingertips and other highly sensitive areas) is attenuated. For this reason, oral as well as manual sexual stimulation is of profound gratification to the elderly. Similarly, perfumes as well as pheromones may tend to enhance sexual excitation through the olfactory pathways.

Most men need manual stimulation to achieve an erection at some time in their later years; erection is no longer psychogenic, emanating as a reflex from the brain on the thought of sex or sight of a desirable sexual partner. This concept too has to be taught and counseled about.

The health professional must know about the medications and other substances, including alcohol, used by the patient because they may affect his sexual functioning.

With the postmenopausal woman, the same careful listening and counseling procedure ought to be used. For women, counseling must include the information that increased dryness of the vagina and thinning and tendency to bleed of the vulvar and vaginal mucosa are likely to occur. Painful intercourse often results in the avoiding of any sexual activity. Some discussion with patients also ought to include reference to the changes in the breast that may occur with aging.

Often women feel that a partner's inability to attain or maintain an erection means that they are no longer attractive, that it is their failure. Intensive counseling is needed in this situation.

Minor physical impairments such as cardiovascular problems, arthritis, multiple sclerosis, extreme obesity, or any such disease are likely to affect the sexual functioning of the older man or the woman. Sometimes people will use the presence of illness or symptoms of an illness as a means of avoiding unwanted sexual activity or will use the existence of illness in a manipulative fashion to obtain something they want sexually.

## CHRONIC ILLNESS AND SEXUAL FUNCTION

In order to know the extent of the effects of chronic illness on sexual function, one must know something about the patient's previous sexual history.

### OSTOMY PATIENTS

Patients undergoing the three types of ostomy surgery (ileostomy, colostomy, ileal conduit) need further counseling as to their sexual functioning after recovery. For example, when impotence results from such an operation, it is important to counsel the men that touching, hugging, and kissing are still-available modalities of sensual expres-

sion; in addition, he certainly can help his partner achieve as many orgasms as she wishes either manually or orally (if that is in their repertoire) or by adding a vibrator to their sexual activity. Sometimes the ability to ejaculate is lost while the ability to have erections is still present, and sometimes retrograde ejaculation occurs. (In this condition seminal fluid is propelled posteriorly into the bladder rather than anteriorly through the distal urethra.) Some patients are distressed by this and to others it is of little concern.

Less data are available about women who have had ostomies. Suffice it to say, counseling is imperative—especially so if a man or a woman commences a new relationship. The patient must tell the new partner about the conditon—*long before* engaging in actual sexual activity. In these, like in many other situations, peer counseling with people who have undergone similar operations or have similar disabilities is very helpful.

### STROKE PATIENTS

There are not much data available on sexual activity and patients who have had strokes. Ford and Orfirer[1] reported on 105 stroke patients less than 60 years old and noted that 60 per cent of this group did not experience loss of libido following cerebrovascular accident. Counseling *must* include the partner because often it is the partner's concern that brings about decreased sexual activity.

Others also studying patients under the age of 60, noted that decreased libido after a stroke is more common in right-sided paralysis than in left-sided paralysis, a fact substantiated by a more recent study. Several researchers have found that diminishing of libido after stroke is common if the dominant hemisphere is damaged, but not common if the stroke affects only the nondominant hemisphere. In addition, they reported that patterns of sexual activity before the stroke are excellent predictors of sexual activity following occurrence of the stroke.

I would like to suggest that the counselor-health practitioner proceed with caution. If the patient is not interested in sexual activity, the counselor should not press the issue. On the other hand, for those interested, he should suggest specific positions and sexual aids. Some examples: (1) the couple could try to engage in sexual activity in a side-by-side position, with the stroke victim positioned in such a way that the "healthy" side is uppermost; (2) mutual masturbation, (3) oral-genital stimulation; (4) use of a vibrator; or (5) a female-superior position.

### ARTHRITIC PATIENTS

For the arthritic patient, when mechanical limitations on coital positions are present, some recommendations in terms of sexual activity are timing sexual activity to the "best" time of the day and taking a bath together before sexual activity to take advantage of heat applied to the affected joints. A renewed learning of sexual pleasuring has to occur. For example, for some, rear-entry position or a lateral position might be suggested.

## CARDIOVASCULAR PATIENTS

For the patient with cardiovascular impairment the following guidelines could be helpful.

If the patient has enjoyed sexual activity before the illness, it can be enjoyed afterward. I, however, believe that we can educate and counsel about good sexual functioning at any time even if previously the patient's sex life was not so rewarding to him or her. The question on the minds of patients whether sex life is over for them stems in part from the mass media, movies, and literature, which show us situations in which the person with a heart condition suddenly dies in the arms of a loved one. Many people believe that any sexual activity puts too great a strain on the damaged heart. Counseling is also important for the spouse of the patient who might feel guilty about wanting sexual activity and unsure if there are any risks involved. This ought to take place in the hospital before the patient is discharged so that feelings of depression, anger and guilt can be aired and dispelled.

In order to give adequate advice, the counselor must know about the previous sexual patterns of the patient. It is important to have a private talk with the patient because it is unlikely that certain types of historical material will be discussed as openly with the partner present.

While climbing stairs and walking, the heart beats from 107 to 130 times a minute. In comparison, the heart averages 117 beats a minute during sexual intercourse. When there is no pain, no shortness of breath, or tiredness when climbing stairs or doing some form of equal exercise, the heart can usually deal with the amount of energy required for sexual activity.

We have learned from the observations of Masters and Johnson[2] in the laboratory setting that the following changes occur during the *four phases* of sexual activity. Phase I: Arousal—the skin becomes flushed, breathing and pulse rate gradually increase, blood pressure is mildly elevated. Phase II: Plateau—a leveling of these signs. Phase III: Orgasm—the heart works hardest here; pulse rate may reach 150 beats per minute and blood pressure may reach 160/90. This phase lasts 15 to 20 seconds, and the energy used is similar to what it takes to climb a flight of stairs or take a brisk walk. Phase IV: Resolution—the body returns to a resting heart rate and blood pressure within a matter of seconds. Angina or palpitations occur most frequently in this phase.

The time sexual energy lasts is important. For the majority of people, it is relatively short. The average middle-aged person having sexual intercourse with the same partner twice a week has a total time from arousal to resolution of 10 to 16 minutes. During this time maximum stress on the heart lasts only 4 to 6 minutes.

Masturbation might be a first step in working slowly toward maximum sexual activity because the patient can control the amount of stimulation and is not pressured by time or ability to please the partner. Also, manual stimulation can provide the partner with sexual satisfaction until sexual relations are resumed, and sexual foreplay in a relaxed atmosphere allows a gradual increase in heart rate and blood pressure.

In terms of positions, it is important to counsel that no major changes in sex positions should be tried if this makes either partner anxious. However, the person who has had the heart attack should avoid positions that keep weight balanced on the arms for a long period of time. Anxiety and muscle fatigue can cause more work for the heart. Sometimes the partner who has not had the heart attack assumes the top position and the more active role; however, there is little research to support the theory that the passive partner uses less energy. For some people the side-by-side position, either toward each other, or with one behind the other, or sitting facing each other, is indicated. Oral-genital sexual activity, if both partners accept it, places no additional strain on the heart. Anal intercourse stimulates the rectal muscles and mucus lining and may lead to irregularities of heart rhythm. If acceptable to the partners, use of this position should be cleared with the physician before it is engaged in.

In good sexual counseling, these patients are instructed not to engage in sexual activity when angry, under stress, or tired because at these times the heart already beats faster and sex would be an additional source of stress. Another point worth mentioning is to engage in sexual activity in pleasant surroundings—the temperature ought not to be too hot or too cold. The patient should avoid very hot or cold baths because these affect the circulation by opening or closing the blood vessels respectively. A good rule is to be rested before sexual activity. Early afternoons after a nap or morning hours may be best, but it is important to change habits only if this does not cause anxiety and stress. It is important not to follow a heavy meal or an evening cocktail with sex. The circulatory system needs to help digest the food, and alcohol tends to change the amount of blood the heart pumps each minute. It is best to postpone sexual activity at least three hours or more after eating a heavy meal and drinking alcohol. Taking medication such as propranolol (Inderal) and nitroglycerin before engaging in sexual activity *must* be discussed with the physician. Women with a heart condition are advised against taking birth control pills or estrogen (for menopausal symptoms). The woman with a heart condition who wishes to begin a pregnancy must of course discuss this with her physician.

Kaplan[3] in her recent book also mentions that libido may be diminished with cardiac disease, coronary artery disease, postcoronary syndrome, and hypertension. The excitement phase may be diminished because of anxiety about sudden death and use of antihypertensive drugs. Kaplan writes that vascular disorders do not affect orgasm. In terms of pathogenic mechanism, vascular disorders disrupt erection in the male. The effect of local circulatory problems has not been studied in women because they seem far less disabled by disorders of the genital blood vessels.

## SEXUAL DYSFUNCTIONS IN DIABETICS

Diabetes mellitus is frequently associated with impotence in men. The earliest manifestation may be a mild to moderate decrease in firmness of the erection. It is important to determine whether or not the distress of erectile difficulties is primarily psychogenic or whether it is caused by an organic process apart from the disease itself.

One must consider other psychogenic stresses of life, such as depression and anxiety as well. Men with impotence problems, even if they are diabetic, respond just as well to psychosexual therapy as healthy men. When the impotence is an early symptom of diabetes, careful attention to an appropriate diet and the use of prescribed medication will frequently be effective.

If the erectile difficulties are more in the psychological realm, for example, caused by anxieties concerning sexual performance, the treatment modality of psychosexual therapy can be very helpful. Such methods might include discussion of the specific health problem, reduction of anxiety by use of fantasy material, and instruction in less demanding positions for sexual activity. Even at times when there may be no possibility of reversal of the problem, the spouse or sexual partner of the diabetic man should be included in the counseling. It must be made clear to her that the man's difficulty is not caused by his finding her less attractive, or by homosexual tendencies, and it is not because the man has another sexual partner. Open discussion with the partner about the disease and its complications is very important. The fact must also be stressed that, even without a firm erection, sexual pleasure and ejaculation can be satisfying. Sexual intimacy should be encouraged.

Research data on sexual dysfunction in diabetic women is sparse. There are many studies describing reproductive problems of women with diabetes, but only recently have researchers delved into this area. It seems that women with diabetes are more often nonorgasmic than women without this disease, even when they have had no problems in this area before the onset of the disease. Some reported a noticeable lessening of the intensity of orgasm a few years after the diagnosis of diabetes was made and also reported the need for longer periods of direct sexual stimulation, either in masturbatory or coital activity. Vaginal lubrication is not significantly altered in most diabetic women with sexual dysfunctions. It is important to rule out the possibility of infections. Dyspareunia, if associated with diabetes, may be due to poor vaginal lubrication, atrophic (estrogen-deficient) vaginitis, and other causes.

Again, whenever possible, counseling ought to be conducted together with the partner, and combined with the appropriate medication for treatment of the sexual problem.

## POSTMASTECTOMY PATIENTS

Sometimes physicians "forget" that patients continue to have sexual needs and sexual feelings, or they assume that patients are no longer interested in sexual activity. When breast cancer is discovered, a woman's first concern is for her survival. At the same time, she is apt to be deeply troubled by the fear of mutilation, by anxiety about her husband's or sexual partner's reaction, and by the fact that in our culture the breast is generally regarded as a symbol of femininity and attractiveness. Often the breast serves as a source of sexual arousal for the man as well as for the woman herself.

The surgical removal of one or both breasts may create psychological and psychosocial problems. One of the more serious concerns of the patient is how others will respond, and this is especially crucial in terms of intimate behavior. A woman may fear not only rejection in the form of aversion or denial but also rejection in the form of pity. Her reaction to mastectomy depends on her concept of her own femininity and sexuality.

Often women undergoing the procedure do not know, before the operation, whether they will have a simple breast biopsy performed or will undergo more extensive surgery. In this situation, the importance of skill and sensitivity of the counselor and the information provided cannot be overemphasized.

Suggestions for postoperative rehabilitation ought to include specific instructions in terms of sexual activity. When the topic is discussed in a matter-of-fact manner with the counselor or health care team, the implication is that sexual activity will quite naturally, continue. Frequently women report that they would have liked a discussion on the topic, either before surgery or during their hospitalization, but thought it was inappropriate because the health care professional did not broach the subject.

An equally crucial aspect is that of initiating sexual activity. Often women who regularly have initiated sexual activity before their mastectomy operation find that after the operation they tend to wait for their partner to initiate sex, for fear of rejection. In such cases it is imperative to set aside time for an open, honest discussion with a sensitive, skilled counselor. Some experts suggest that the male partner view the operation site and actually assist in changing the dressing during the hospital stay. Of course, touching, hugging, kissing, and reassurance are an integral part of such demonstrations of love and the promise of continued satisfying sexual activity.

## HELPING THE CHRONICALLY INSTITUTIONALIZED PATIENT

For the chronically institutionalized patient some of the issues just discussed are of greatest importance. Health care professionals, especially nurses and orderlies who are in daily contact with the patient, must be trained to accept the patient's sexuality. The patient's sexual interest and desire must be respected. An awareness of how to deal with the exposure of parts of a patient's body, which before hospitalization or institutionalization occurred in private, is essential. In addition, patients' masturbatory activities and their need for sexual intimacy and discussion about sexuality, have to be clarified with the staff.

One way to accomplish this is in seminars and discussion groups led by experienced sex educators and counselors. It is advisable to make clear at the beginning of such seminars that *no* personal questions will be asked of the participants. Once this pressure is removed, it is possible for participants to teach and learn from each other. Using tact and humor, this writer has effectively made use of puppets to instruct seminar participants in how to deal with this sensitive subject matter.

Institutions must begin to provide appropriate opportunities for sexual expression of their clientele and, above all, must make arrangements for possibilities of privacy, including, if possible, setting aside "dating rooms," comfortably furnished and with a clear "Do not disturb" sign at the door.

## CONCLUSION

The need for companionship at all ages, for touching and stroking, is certainly there to be cultivated, cherished, and even augmented by proper education. Education is particularly crucial because older people who have strong sexual desires often feel guilty and ashamed.

Since they have adopted the dominant values of contemporary society, i.e., that sexuality is only for the "young and beautiful," I believe that through education and counseling about sexual feelings the negative effects of these attitudes can be overcome.

Skills of promoting discussion, listening in a sympathetic, nonjudgmental way, and offering knowledgeable advice are important ingredients in sexual counseling. For example, one should convey the message that the pleasure of sexuality, the intimacy of the sex act, and the sharing of closeness and caressing have meaning in themselves and do not have to result in orgasm as the end product. One evening or during the day the partners could just caress. The next evening or day they might engage in touching the genitalia. On the third encounter they may be having sexual intercourse. The importance of a nonpressured situation should be emphasized.

For disabled people, helpers might be trained to actually facilitate sexual encounters between partners, including, when necessary, positioning the participants in a manageable manner and even, if required, assisting the partners during sexual activity.

Sexuality is much more than just a penis in a vagina. Sexuality is a total feeling and can have numerous expressions. It is important for the health professional to legitimatize sexual pleasure and to discuss openly and frankly, with tact, humor, and "sexual literacy" all aspects of the patient's sexual capabilities and limitations and if necessary to teach better sexual functioning.

## REFERENCES

1. Ford, A. B., and Orfirer, A. P.: Sexual behavior and the chronically ill patient. Med. Aspects Hum. Sexuality, 1:51–61, 1967.
2. Masters, W. H., and Johnson, V.: Human Sexual Inadequacy. Boston, Little, Brown & Co., 1970.
3. Kaplan, H. S.: The New Sex Therapy. New York, Brunner/Mazel Co., 1974.

# 29

# From Rehabilitation to Independent Living

by Nancy A. Brooks, M.A.

Acknowledgement: Consumer advocates Barney and Cathy Hoss reviewed an earlier draft of this work and made valuable suggestions for which the writer is grateful.

What happens to disabled people after they leave rehabilitation facilities and cease their outpatient training? Do they find general acceptance, adequate services, and opportunities to participate in conventional life styles? Or are they more often restricted to undesirable living conditions and isolated from their able-bodied neighbors?

Even limited answers to these questions are not yet available because disabled people living in the community have only recently become subjects of public and professional interest. But as long as the ultimate goal of rehabilitation is to return patients to their communities, professionals should consider these issues. Public attitudes, environmental barriers, and economic constraints are powerful social variables that can greatly influence whether disabled individuals will be able to utilize what they have learned in rehabilitation. As important as it is, rehabilitation is only a beginning in the process of community integration.

During rehabilitation patients begin to learn what it means to be a disabled person at the same time they are learning how to manage their new physical attributes. The rehabilitation process communicates expectations for the disabled individual through professional-client relationships, daily routine, and physical environments in the treatment setting. As disabled individuals respond to these stimuli, they begin to adopt a new social pattern: *the disabled person role*. Social habits learned here will be transferred to the community when patients leave the therapeutic setting for the larger social context. Therefore, professionals who are aware of the social ramifications of rehabilitation can direct the disabled person role into patterns that are suitable to current social conditions.

Giving attention to the social context of disability is especially relevant now, for an important social movement is changing expectations for disabled individuals. Well-publicized modifications in laws, architectural standards, and educational procedures have been achieved by the disability movement of the 1970's and have signaled a break with traditional assumptions about disability. Although general acceptance of these new assumptions has been slow, the ideals of the movement have challenged the rehabilitation team to prepare clients for more active roles in their communities. One derivative of these changes, the independent living movement, has particular significance for rehabilitation practices.

The goals of the independent living movement foresee disabled persons taking responsibility and exercising initiative as they assume community roles that are as normal as possible. Any tendency for rehabilitation processes to encourage dependency rather than assertiveness is disputed by the independent living ideology. Even the most severely disabled are assumed capable of responding to rehabilitation training and taking a legitimate place in the mainstream. Achieving these independent living goals requires special awareness from both clients and professionals because all members of the team need to know not only which self-care skills are required for normal functioning but also which social skills will help disabled people participate fully in the everyday world.

The purpose of this chapter is to further the goals of independent living by reviewing social expectations for disabled people and suggesting how rehabilitation professionals can help clients develop social skills appropriate to the disabled person role. Specifically, this chapter will utilize a sociological perspective in surveying attitudes toward the disabled, issues affecting intimate relationships with the disabled, and community resources to help disabled persons build independent lifestyles. Disability will be viewed here as a characteristic extending beyond physical impairment to include life style and self-concept.

In doing my own teaching and research in the sociology of disability, I have found that physical impairment is an encompassing social attribute that affects the total life experience. In fact, my interest in the area began while I was experiencing my own adjustment to the disabled role following a diagnosis of multiple sclerosis. While I was learning to cope with restricted strength and mobility, I also learned about social and environmental barriers that set my experience apart from the life styles of my peers. Participating in patient groups and disability advocacy projects taught me that my experiences were shared by many others. As a sociologist, I drew hypotheses from these observations and investigated them systematically in research. I will use illustrations from my own experiences when they are appropriate to this chapter in keeping with the sociological tradition of relating individual histories to broader social processes. Otherwise, I will draw from professional literature to explain major social conditions affecting disabled people who attempt to live independently in the community.

## THE MARGINAL SOCIAL ROLE

Although disabled individuals often establish accepted places for themselves in the community, disabled people as a group still face imposing social and environmental barriers. Rehabilitation clients have a justifiable concern about their re-entry into the community, for society is not congenial to people who see, hear, or move in unusual ways. Despite recent advances in legal and educational areas, the predominant response to the disabled is still stigmatization expressed through social and physical means.

## ATTITUDES TOWARD DISABILITY

Repeated investigation of attitudes expressed by able-bodied people indicates that to them the disabled trigger feelings of fear, awkwardness, and concern about contagion. Rejection of the disabled is similar to the negative attitudes directed toward other minority groups; both produce stereotypes and discriminatory behavior.

Face-to-face interactions between able-bodied and disabled people are likely to reveal these negative feelings. Subtle nonverbal cues express discomfort and tension. Comer and Piliavin have found that the able-bodied may fidget, lose eye contact, talk too loudly, keep a substantial distance from the disabled person, and generally attempt to avoid sustained interaction.[1] In these situations the disability becomes the focal point and the individual characteristics of the disabled person are ignored. Assistive devices may also become insurmountable obstacles to effective communication if the able-bodied person pointedly stares at the device or refuses to discuss anything else. My students who have simulated disabilities in public settings report that they are often treated as if they were either invisible or were sideshow freaks. Some students have become so anxious about the responses they received from strangers that they were unable to complete the four-hour simulation. Systematic research substantiates these observations and justifies disabled individuals' complaints about their public reception. Whatever the reason, the typical response to people with disabling conditions is to show pity or dislike.

These shared attitudes both reflect and influence social conditions. Since able-bodied people tend to feel uncomfortable around the disabled, attempts to integrate the disabled into workplaces, churches, and restaurants are gradual at best. Then, because the two groups have few opportunities for interaction, stereotyped ideas about disability are reinforced. A vicious circle results. However, there is hope for breaking this pattern. Yuker finds that public acceptance of disability varies with the disabled person's capacity to fill social roles.[2] When impairments require only minimal assistance and do not interfere with the fulfillment of major social roles such as work or childrearing, public attitudes are more accepting than when impairments obstruct usual role performance and interfere with social interaction. These findings affirm the significance of rehabilitation.

Yet the potential of rehabilitation can be undermined if service professionals also hold negative attitudes. For example, if professionals assume that a physical impairment is likely to be associated with a mental or emotional disability, they may be falling into the tendency described by Beatrice Wright to "spread" stigmatized characteristics.[3] Such a tendency could lead professionals to temper their expectations for client accomplishment, prepare less demanding programs, and thereby create self-fulfilling prophecies. The underlying assumptions that professionals hold are no doubt as important to rehabilitation outcome as patient motivation.

The accumulated effect of these evaluations of disability is to categorize the disabled as different and inferior. Efforts to integrate disabled individuals into the community and to establish independent living service programs must overcome inclinations to reinforce isolation and dependency. Social service agencies in particular have been attacked by advocates in the disability movement on the grounds that professional helpers have long used service provision as means for controlling disabled individuals' life styles and preventing clients from experiencing the dignity of risk. Once one becomes a client, dependent upon others who make decisions and provide services, one may find it difficult to graduate into responsible adult roles. We all have our dependency needs, and if services support those tendencies without assisting the full transition expected by the community, the disabled role may always contain elements of the sick patient role.

A further association between attitudes and rehabilitation services has been observed in the link between impairment and socioeconomic status. Acquiring a disability may lead to changed social standing if income levels or occupations or both are affected. In Western societies occupation and income are major sources of identification. Disrupting those indicators of social status may produce stress for both clients and their family members who had created relationships under earlier circumstances. Rehabilitation and service systems have great opportunity to exercise social control at this point. Acting upon underlying attitudes toward disability and their clients' social characteristics, professionals may direct rehabilitation programs and economic benefit applications in ways that will alter clients' social status or communicate the expectation that the client will always be dependent.

Rehabilitation professionals also reveal their own evaluation of disabled clients by managing differently those patients who do not demonstrate the desired "motivation." It is possible that staff may not respond objectively to the spinal cord–injured patient who enters rehabilitation with no observable legal source of income to support his expensive habits. Such a person may not appear to be a proper rehabilitation candidate. Certainly clients are not powerless, yet cases like this may elicit direct attempts to alter the disabled person's life style. How long clients remain in rehabilitation, what transitional supports are developed, and which economic benefits are sought are all instruments of social control through which professionals can express their attitudes toward disabled individuals.

## SELF-CONCEPT OF THE DISABLED

Attitudes and social systems that disparage people with disability may not only affect social status but may also cause the disabled to internalize stigma and devalue themselves. According to social-psychological principles, humans form self-concepts by incorporating the reactions received from other people. The resulting image that we carry in our mind's eye of who we are and what we are worth is not the same as a body image, which may also be affected by an acquired disability. Instead, the self-concept answers the question, "Who am I?" and is constantly being re-formed as we apply others' responses to ourselves. When disabled people constantly encounter social and physical barriers that exclude them from ordinary experiences, they may gradually come to believe they deserve such disrespect. Also, negative attitudes held by the patient prior to disablement may stimulate self-debasement.

The work I have done with my colleague Ronald Matson on the self-concepts of people with multiple sclerosis has found that MS people do have somewhat more negative self-concepts than able-bodied subjects.[4] However, our subjects also reported having a range of supporting resources. It is apparent that people with disabling conditions can develop coping strategies to bolster self-esteem and assist in confronting barriers and exercising self-determination. Rehabilitation can contribute to the development of positive self-concepts by teaching skills that give clients a sense of control over life. Trieschmann has found that perceived sense of control is associated with adjustment to spinal cord injury and can be influenced by rehabilitation processes.[5] When disabled individuals acquire the capacity for managing rigorous social and physical environments, they are likely to construct more positive self-concepts.

But answering the question, "Who am I?" may be difficult when stigmatization interferes with intimate relationships, the relationships having the greatest impact upon self-concepts. Since people who hold negative attitudes about disability are unlikely to participate in close relationships with disabled people, the reserve of potential friends and sexual partners is reduced. Even family members may respond to the disability by withdrawing from the disabled member. Maintaining the intimacy that is crucial to self-esteem becomes a major challenge for both the disabled and their "significant others."

## EFFECTS OF DISABILITY UPON INTIMATE RELATIONSHIPS

### THE FAMILY

When a family member becomes disabled, the entire group is subjected to the social-psychological stress of that experience. Families undergo an adjustment process as they respond to changing roles and functions. As shared activities become too difficult because of architectural and social barriers and family friends sever relationships, the family absorbs some of the stigma associated with disability. Medical and rehabilitation expenses added to home modifications and the purchase of expensive devices create economic strains. As a result of these costs and perhaps the loss of income from the disabled individual, the entire family may encounter downward social mobility.

In addition to change in social position, the family experiences change within itself. Previously established patterns in which family members played breadwinner, homemaker, or child roles may be rearranged. If the mother had been an active, decision-making family member around whom other roles were centered, her disability may cause others to alter their functions. If family relationships were already unstable, disability can be an overwhelming trauma. Whether these changes are temporary or permanent, they are likely to affect how individuals deal with each other even to the extent that rehabilitation outcome may be affected.

Not enough research has been done on the families of disabled adults to permit generalizations about factors influencing their adjustment. There are only preliminary observations to suggest that families may disintegrate, be strengthened, or simply cope, although the variables associated with those differences have not been identified. However, some family responses to disabled adult members can be described.

First, the family is subject to prevailing social evaluations of disability and may hold negative attitudes that interpose between established family relationships. Having a spouse or sibling become disabled does not necessarily reform discriminatory attitudes. Family members may express fear, awkwardness, or pity toward the disabled individual, and these feelings may be counterproductive to family adjustment.

Second, the family has an immediate concern about the dependency of a disabled member because its division of labor may be threatened. Will he or she be able to carry on as a producer, consumer, or other active member of the unit? This issue of dependency is increased by social pressures to support disabled individuals. "In sickness and in health" is a social requirement that may distress family members who do not want the caretaker role. Although some individuals may reject this obligation and seek divorce or institutionalization as an escape, other family members may welcome the new dependency as a means to gain power. The previously all-suffering wife may thrive on the caretaker role if she perceives an opportunity to gain control over the husband, the family finances, and the family decisions. Likewise, the disabled person can become a sickroom tyrant. Because the family is a social unit, its response to disability affects its own structure and functions as well as the disabled individual's adjustment.

For this reason, Lindenberg suggests that rehabilitation should include the family.[6] She reports that family support has been found to benefit rehabilitation outcome and that family involvement can be encouraged through educational and counseling activities. Although families may hold negative attitudes and encourage dependency, information and guidance from professionals can facilitate adjustment.

Giving information to the entire family about the disabling condition, the therapies, and alternative resources for the return home will alleviate one of the family's basic problems in this situation: *role ambiguity*. Since the family's understanding of the disability may be incomplete, family members have unclear expectations for the disabled individual. Zahn has shown that disabilities which are most obvious and stable produce the least difficulty for the family,[7] yet the social-psychological uncertainties of dealing intimately with a disabled individual still causes considerable stress. The family is pressed to deal with characteristics that are undesirable, little understood, and perhaps likely to change unpredictably. Nevertheless, families can adapt their structures to accommodate both family and individual needs.

Several family types may emerge as patterned responses to the issue of role ambiguity. If the family makes no place for the disabled individual, continuing its previous routine without regard to that person's needs, it may be termed a *rejecting family*. Although its behavior is not as extreme as that of the family that separates itself by divorce or "warehousing" the disabled in an institution, the rejecting family still responds to the ambiguous disabling characteristic through withdrawal. The opposite type, the *sacrificing family*, responds to the disabled member by placing the individual in the center of all family routines. Here the family responds to ambiguity by overemphasizing the disabled person's need for support. A *third family type* adapts its social structure by normalizing the experiences of the disabled person as much as possible without sacrificing other members. Traditional family roles may be modified during the normalizing process in order to keep the individual in the family while retaining basic family functions. Former homemakers may become breadwinners and young children may be given substantial family responsibilities while the disabled father assumes childrearing and home management obligations. The normalizing theme of this family type is also demonstrated as other family members neither withdraw from nor overprotect the disabled individual. These three family types illustrate the extreme forms that intimate relationships may take in response to disability. Maintaining intimate relationships calls for flexibility and communication skills in order to overcome the physical, psychological, and social barriers associated with disability.

## SEXUALITY

Sexual bonds create the ultimate intimate relationships, but this level of intimacy may be difficult for disabled individuals to achieve, even if they had sexual partners prior to the disability. As members of a stigmatized minority, the disabled often have been designated as either totally nonsexual or sexually perverse (see Chapter 28). Physically disabled people have been categorized with the aging and the mentally retarded as undesirable sexual types. Since these groups do not measure up to cultural standards of attractiveness, social mechanisms have isolated them from sexual contexts. None of these groups is likely to be depicted in sexually evocative advertisements or in the entertainment media. Resorts, singles' bars, beaches, and other areas where sexual encounters are expected to take place have been off limits to these groups. Many of those locations contain architectural as well as social barriers.

These sexual deterrents represent collective inclinations to maintain social distance from people who are considered different and objectionable. If the able-bodied were to accept the masculinity and femininity of disabled individuals, then intimate relationships might follow and norms would be disturbed. Furthermore, until recently there has been little information about sexuality and disability that could dispel these negative associations. Now sex research is expanding to include disabled persons and there is literature available, such as Comfort's work,[8] to reinforce counseling of disabled individuals and their partners.

Rehabilitation professionals can participate in making information available to explain the sexual implications of disability. In doing so, professionals communicate permission to accept disabled individuals as total human beings rather than as containers of impairments. The sexuality of disabled individuals should be viewed as a human characteristic that is not qualitatively different for able-bodied and disabled individuals but that may benefit from open attention or counseling or both.

## WOMEN AND DISABILITY

The situation of disabled women illustrates the impact of physical impairment upon sexuality, the family, and intimate relationships in general. To be female and disabled is to be faced with double problems of dependency and role ambiguity, for disabled women encounter singular difficulties in playing roles of sexual partner, spouse, and parent. These difficulties are magnified by lack of research and support systems.

In fact, sex research on disabled women lags far behind systematic investigation of disabled males. The working assumption has been that since women could take a passive role in sexual matters, their problems were minimal. However, disabled women not only require information about nontraditional sex acts that are suitable to their impairments, they also require counseling regarding the complications of contraception and pregnancy. What are the side effects of using birth control pills if one is paralyzed and in a wheelchair? What factors should be included in the decision to have children? What community resources are available for disabled women who need to escape overprotective home environments? These issues should be addressed during rehabilitation.

Disabled women have been stereotyped by family expectations and rehabilitation services, which have tended to direct disabled women toward home-bound domestic roles rather than toward employment. Yet after disabled women have been consigned to the domestic scene, they have not received preparation or assistance in mothering, a major facet of their lives. In the present state of assistive equipment and information, childrearing can be unnecessarily challenging to disabled mothers. Special equipment for handling infants and small children should be made available and childrearing courses should be prepared. Of course, this is not to say that the father, able-bodied or disabled, will not participate in child care, but is only a reminder that this traditional aspect of the female role has not been fully supported by rehabilitation practices.

It is likely that being female and disabled brings greater dependency to intimate relationships because of the overlay of traditional dependency expected from women in general. Those who have close relationships with disabled women may be tempted to overprotect and isolate. Through the process of rehabilitation and counseling, professionals can guide both male and female clients toward more satisfactory intimate relationships and also facilitate greater accomplishment in other social realms.

## THE TRANSITIONAL ROLE

Most disabled people are coping in a marginal social position, neither fully segregated nor fully integrated, but conventional social participation is now becoming somewhat less difficult because the disabled person role is gradually changing. Although underlying attitudinal issues have not been resolved, new possibilities have been introduced by the disability movement. Efforts to achieve architectural modifications and independent living services have brought specific improvements. However, balancing recently achieved opportunities with the traditional constraints of disability results in a virtual juggling act. While the media may occasionally extoll the virtues of a remarkable success, a "Billie Jean King in a wheelchair," most disabled people are still coping with an uncomfortable and unclear social position.

Rehabilitation professionals have the opportunity to influence the direction of this transitional social role. The social attitudes that form the basis of discrimination and unclear expectations can be molded, for attitudes are learned and subject to change. Given the medical mandate to educate the public, providing information about disabling conditions is a suitable role for professionals. By participating in public education, professionals can improve awareness of rehabilitation technology and training and also inform the community about possibilities for successful social functioning by the disabled. A more effective means for improving attitudes, however, is to combine instruction with opportunities to meet disabled people. Encouraging rehabilitation clients to participate in community programs will benefit both clients and the public. Professionals themselves may also benefit from attitude awareness programs such as disability simulations. Assuming a substantial impairment and negotiating the realities of public settings will show professionals what clients will encounter after discharge. My experience in directing simulations shows that even well-informed, sensitive nondisabled people acquire considerable insight from adopting a disfiguring or awkward impairment. Participation in disability-related experiences outside the rehabilitation setting reminds professionals that physical and social skills acquired during rehabilitation may not always be easily transferable to community living.

## MANAGING LIFE WITH A DISABILITY

According to Erving Goffman, author of the classic work, *Stigma: The Management of Spoiled Identity*, coping with the world of able-bodied people is a major feature of the disabled person role.[9] Uncertain face-to-face communication and confrontations with forbidding environments oblige disabled people to adopt the specialized role imposed by social values. Becoming a disabled person means learning how to manage marginality by guiding inter-

action and information-sharing into expected forms. "Good adjustment" as it is defined by the able-bodied is demonstrated when disabled people resign themselves to an inaccessible world and cause minimal difficulties for others. Above all, adjustment means not pushing acceptance too far. Goffman's view is that underlying prejudices demand that the disabled conform to existing conditions, no matter how restricting they may be.

## THE ADJUSTMENT TO COMMUNITY LIVING

These ideas are provocative, for they explain the pattern of isolation and dependency still characteristic of the disabled social role. However, the process of social adjustment to disability is little understood and requires more research. Although it is apparent that stigmatization blocks full social participation of disabled persons, there is enough observed variation in the adjustment of disabled individuals to warrant investigation of intervening variables. Knowing which factors direct the disabled to acquiesce and which stimulate resistance to social constraints would benefit those who re-enter the community. Simplistically, it appears that three variables affect the adjustment process. First, at the physical level, disabled people who learn techniques for mobility and self-care acquire resources for self-determination in their environments. Second, at the personal level, developing positive self-concepts gives disabled individuals the strength to confront their restrictions. Last, at the social level, learning appropriate new social skills and modifying old social patterns extends opportunities to participate in a range of social roles beyond the disability designation. If disabled people are to move beyond acceptance of a stigmatized social role, they require a full arsenal of tools and techniques for facing the challenges of being disabled in a healthist society.

Presently there are few support systems for those who leave rehabilitation to enter the community. Cogswell has observed that paraplegics make their adjustment to the community through a process of self-socialization.[10] Since there are few professionals available to guide the re-entry period, rehabilitation clients learn alone how to establish social relationships in their families, peer groups, and neighborhoods. Cogswell also suggests an adjustment model that describes the elements of learning to live with disability.[11] First, disabled people must abandon the former able-bodied role. Next, they must identify with the new role. Third, they are likely to overemphasize the new role before finally integrating new and old roles. This model is not rigid; disabled individuals will not pass through clear-cut stages in the given order. The elements of the Cogswell model are useful for showing that adjustment to disability is similar to other major life changes such as marriage, divorce, or occupational shifts. Demystifying the process of learning how to be a disabled person who lives in the community will demonstrate the strength of social forces that impose particular life styles upon social categories. Therapists who focus on the tragedy of disability overlook the broader human experience.

Managing this adjustment process calls for social competency on the part of disabled individuals. Being able to locate and utilize service systems, to establish and to maintain social ties, and otherwise to accommodate to the social constraints of disability requires a repertoire combining everyday politeness, assertiveness, and socially appropriate responses to stress. Such basic social competencies become especially important because of attitudinal barriers and the complications of disability, such as the need to acquire help from other people. Because disabled people require assistance from others at the same time that they need independence, communication skills are pressed to obtain the necessary help without submitting to dependency.

The issue of acquiring help from others is a typical source of social tension for the disabled, which can be understood through sociological analysis. People who must frequently receive help experience an imbalance in the ordinary exchange of benefits and services. The give-and-take of everyday life usually results in both giving and receiving, so that obligations are evenly distributed. There are numerous social sanctions available to apply against those who do not reciprocate in these exchanges, ranging from gossip to legal measures. However, social arrangements also provide accommodations for those who lack the resources or ability to repay an obligation. These accommodations usually create a subservient position for the recipient. We all know the experience of "being in debt" as the result of a favor we could not return. Sociologically, this is a position disabled people must frequently take toward those who give them assistance.

When I was adapting to the consequences of multiple sclerosis, I experienced the dissatisfaction of always having to be the person who said, "Thank you." After finding that other disabled people had similar feelings, I conducted an investigation of the techniques disabled people employ as they receive help.[12] The results indicated that the respondents preferred to avoid receiving help because they found that balancing needs for both assistance and dignity produced considerable stress. However, respondents also described strategies for obtaining and managing help that cause them to feel less subordinate. Many subjects reported that they prefer to initiate and direct the helping process in order to remain in control and obtain the most efficient and least hazardous assistance. Some respondents also perceived receiving help as an opportunity to meet other people or to achieve some personal advantage. Disabled people are not above manipulating their helpers to obtain secondary benefits.

Rehabilitation professionals can ease the potential imbalance of receiving help by teaching newly disabled people how to manage assistance. By demonstrating how disabled people can obtain necessary help and direct their helpers in the safest and most effective techniques, professionals can provide some sense of control over a stressful situation. Furthermore, staff can practice awareness of their own tendencies to provide help in ways that express either paternalistic or egalitarian relationships. Helping is one of the most distinctive means of communicating attitudes toward disability.

## ADAPTING THE LIFE STYLE

Just as interaction patterns reveal collective perceptions of disability, access to appropriate housing, transportation, and supporting services indicates general social placement of disabled persons. Like it or not, we live in a stratified society that symbolizes social value in material goods and life styles. Highly visible indicators such as housing and style of recreation communicate to others our location on the ranking system and also demonstrate the extent of our resources. When disabled people are relegated to inadequate living conditions, both social and physical segregation results. Practical requests for removal of barriers in effect demand equal access to social opportunities. When rehabilitation clients request respectable housing and transportation which is as independent as possible, they indicate a typical desire to be assimilated in their communities. Therefore, members of the rehabilitation team should keep in mind the social implications as well as the functional effects of placing their clients in the community.

Housing, for example, is more than shelter. A house or apartment symbolizes the resident's social standing and contributes to his or her self-concept. Also, there are specific features that make housing more suitable for the everyday functions of disabled people. A home should allow the resident to enter and leave safely and with minimal assistance. Within the home, there should be adequate space for moving about and making use of kitchen, bathroom, living room, and bedroom. Safety and security are also valid concerns for disabled residents, who may want to add fire alarms and police alerts.

If these components are available, usual home-related activities of eating, dressing, and toilet functions should be accomplished much faster and more easily than when basic features are inadequate. There are many devices and modifications available for home improvement, but the features just mentioned provide the basic foundation for appropriate housing. Furthermore, the living arrangement will be most suitable when the disabled individual can interact with other people and can also have privacy. The living environment is especially important to disabled people because they may not be able to leave their homes as often as able-bodied people do and are highly dependent upon their immediate surroundings to satisfy many needs and prevent environmental deprivation. In this regard, the location of housing is important since an isolated setting diminishes opportunities for social contact. For example, an apartment that opens onto a busy pedestrian area may provide stimulation for the person who lacks transportation.

Housing can contribute meaningfully to the physical and social well-being of disabled people who live in the community. Combining accessible design with reinforcing services such as attendant care or home chore assistance has characterized numerous independent living residential programs. Several disabled individuals have been introduced to community-based living through small group homes, cooperative apartment complexes, and accessible, low-income housing projects, a trend very well described by Laurie.[13] One long-standing illustration of comprehensive housing programs is the Fokus program in Sweden. Beginning in 1964 with the goal of integrating severely disabled people into the community, the Fokus Society developed integrated apartment complexes that provided advanced design and 24-hour assistance to severely disabled residents.[14] The program has been successful in expanding the productivity of participants and demonstrating a substantially lower cost than nursing home or institutional care would have produced. The plan has now been incorporated, with modifications, into other Swedish services.

Although accessible housing is a necessary component of community interaction, it is not a sufficient answer to the problems of dependency and isolation. America is a mobile society, and for disabled people to participate actively in a full range of social roles, they must be able to move from home to workplace to recreation and so forth. Having access to transportation gives disabled people the chance to experience ordinary life styles that tend to make use of many aspects of a community's physical environment. To require disabled people to remain in their homes is to continue the tradition of institutionalization on a smaller scale.

Some major obstacles to accessible transportation have been overcome by engineering advances. Hand controls for automobiles, lifts for vans and buses, and sidecars attached to motorcycles have given many disabled individuals the opportunity to expand the range and speed of their mobility and thereby increase chances for self-determination. Another major obstacle, community resistance to providing accessible public transportation, was challenged by Federal transportation regulations implementing Section 504 of the Rehabilitation Act of 1973. In keeping with the civil rights intent of the law, transportation regulations require that communities make public systems, such as bus and subway systems, accessible to people using wheelchairs. Although these regulations are highly controversial, the Transbus has been designed and introduced to city streets, and many communities have also developed specialized transportation systems that give door-to-door service by appointment. Both forms have legitimate applications and contribute to social integration. However, organized transportation programs, whether public or private, have run afoul of high energy costs and fiscal conservatism. At the time of this writing, public transportation for the disabled has a questionable future. No doubt disability advocacy groups will argue the merit of giving public support to potential taxpayers who are attempting to live independently.

Personal care assistance is another element of an independent life style that is especially relevant to severely disabled people. Having assistance with the activities of daily living may make the difference between spending many hours per day managing one's own dressing and hygiene and using the much more efficient assistance of an attendant, making time for employment, education, or social interaction. This is an interesting arrangement in which the disabled person accepts a limited amount of dependence while trying to accomplish independence in other areas. It is hoped that the disabled person will be able to maintain control over the attendant and not become susceptible to a medical model in which the caretaker determines what is to be done. The independent living movement specifically calls for consumer management over attendants and encourages disabled individuals to hire, manage, and pay for their own personal care.

Again, economic matters impede the fulfillment of these aims, for attendant care is expensive and usually requires financial reinforcement from public sources. Without this reinforcement, assistance can place an excessive drain on the disabled person's finances or may not be possible at all. Like public transportation, however, current public sources for attendant care are threatened by economic uncertainty.

Adding personal care to a normalized life style is also problematic because the attendant–disabled person arrangement is a new social relationship as it is defined by the independent living movement. Is it possible for a severely disabled person to manage such a relationship without causing abuses on both sides? There is little cultural support in the

United States for an occupation so close to the servant role, raising questions about the selection of people who would be attendants. Since I am interested in this relationship from a sociological perspective, when I interviewed the president of the Swedish militant organization for the disabled I inquired what types of people his group favored as attendants. He reported that students and housewives generally did well but that nurses were undoubtedly "too bossy." Apparently, people trained to give custodial care in the medical system may have difficulty adjusting to the independent living model. Despite this observation, it is quite probable that rehabilitation personnel, including nurses, could contribute to the effective use of personal assistance by training disabled clients in the management of personal attendants.

A more traditional contribution of professionals to independent living has been their role in developing and prescribing assistive devices. Certainly the many prosthetic and orthotic devices now available have greatly contributed to quality of life for disabled persons. Without these mechanical aids, many important social functions would be impossible.

Seen from the sociological perspective, devices are cultural artifacts that conform to pragmatic norms in the United States. Our culture encourages us to construct mechanisms that will solve our problems. But functional aids are also subject to evaluation within specific social settings. Although the usefulness of a given device may be acknowledged by a disabled person, the device may not be utilized if its appearance does not reinforce the public image the individual wishes to convey. Devices that appear excessively therapeutic may not be utilized as frequently as those that are unobtrusive. If devices carry only minimal symbolic association with the sick role, they are more comfortable to manage socially. Being a "bionic person" is not generally a desirable role.

What designers can do to ease these issues of social acceptability is to facilitate choice-making by the disabled individuals who will use the devices. Making alternatives available and giving clients adequate information about their prosthetic and orthotic aids will increase the likelihood that individuals will find devices to suit their life style. Disabled individuals who incorporate devices into their adapted life styles often become active consumers as they locate catalogs, specialists, and other disabled people to help them make choices about assistive aids. This consumer involvement often extends to the design and construction of original devices. Active involvement by the people who will use devices not only creates a better match between the function and the social environment, it may also lower the cost of purchasing expensive components that will not be put to use.

## ECONOMICS: THE BOTTOM LINE

The costs of being a disabled person go far beyond the expense of devices. People who require specialized transportation, new or modified housing, customized clothing, unusual diets or easy-to-prepare convenience foods, and/or costly personal assistance in addition to medical care and prescriptions are likely to experience decline in their standard of living. A further cost of disability is the restriction of choice. Many expensive items have no alternative and yet may be necessary to life or functioning. Also, disabled people may not be able to do comparison shopping because of limited strength and mobility. For many disabled people, quality of life diminishes as they confront the economic constraints of disability.

Fortunately, many benefit programs exist to alleviate these pressures. Both public and private programs contribute to the disabled population's standard of living through veteran's benefits, workman's compensation, Social Security programs, blindness agencies, charitable groups, and voluntary organizations. There is no doubt that these programs give essential aid to disabled persons and demonstrate public commitment to a vulnerable population. However, inequities and contradictory intentions are expressed through these economic benefits. While families of disabled children, totally dependent adults, and blind individuals receive an extra tax deduction, a working disabled adult gets no deduction or other substantial support for disability-related expenses. Even disabled veterans receive generous benefits for impairments that are not service related. But the "Catch 22" of receiving benefits emerges when disabled people who wish to become more independent try to utilize the benefit system and find that many programs have been constructed as disincentives rather than as ladders to achievement. Especially in the Social Security programs (SSDI, SSI, and Medicaid), eligibility for benefits has often been determined by very low ceilings of personal income. Furthermore, benefits generally have not been adequate to meet the high costs of disability. If disabled individuals attempt to overcome this low status position by working, they may lose all benefits even though personal income does not meet the costs of special transportation, devices, and perhaps attendant care. Too often benefit systems do not function as supports for people who could be productive.

Bowe calls for a radical transition from this dependency model to an investment model, arguing that rehabilitation has demonstrated its effectiveness in preparing the disabled to be independent and productive.[15] Disabled persons do have a good record as stable, capable community members. Now there is an opportunity to expand upon that record through the use of recent advances in rehabilitation training methods, rehabilitation engineering accomplishments, and the awakened interest of the disabled population itself. Rehabilitation professionals have the responsibility to publicize the value of their field and to convince policymakers that disabled persons need not be a drain on the economy if appropriate support systems can be put in place.

Even though strong arguments can be made for reducing dependency and isolation, stiff resistance must be overcome. Managing disability still requires both utilization of support systems and accommodation to a marginal social role.

## COMMUNITY RESOURCES

Supporting services have recently become more available in the community. Self-help groups, independent living referral centers, and disability advocate groups can now assist disabled persons as they seek active roles in the community. Since disabled individuals are similar to immigrants who have minimal skills and resources for coping with a strange environment, they may very well benefit from the experience of others who have made an earlier voyage or who have valuable skills and information to assist adaptation.

The independent living movement has made many practical contributions to the community living experience. Based on the premise that disabled individuals will be able to reach their full potential more readily when they live among able-bodied people, utilize community service systems, and exercise self-determination, independent living programs have stimulated the development of community resources to accommodate a variety of life styles. Most large communities contain independent living programs, and many smaller areas provide selected aspects of the independent living design. This design proposes that each community should contain its own arrangement for independent living and that at least some of the following elements should be available in each community: (1) community-based accessible housing, (2) referral centers for housing and services, (3) accessible transportation, (4) personal care aide services, and (5) independent living training. Although consumer management of these elements is a major goal, professional providers are also expected to develop and manage independent living programs in response to community needs.

The experience of constructing or participating in independent living programs has demonstrated that many disabled persons are capable of substantial independence. One aspect of the independent living philosophy includes the formation of self-help groups through which experienced persons

can act as role models and educators for those who are making the transition to community participation. By sharing problems and solutions, disabled individuals not only attack the real issues of independence, they also practice social skills that they can apply to relationships with able-bodied persons. Furthermore, self-help groups provide an opportunity to ventilate the stress of playing the disabled role in an able-bodied society.

Another consequence of the independent living movement has been the integration of community-wide services. Enlightened policymakers have begun to include disabled citizens in community programs. Many mental health organizations, housing facilities, and adult education services are becoming prepared to accommodate disabled persons. This trend has shown that returning rehabilitation clients to the community requires only an extension of existing services, not an entirely new system. Such integrated services not only reinforce the aims of full social participation for the disabled, they are likely to be less expensive than separate programs.

However, integration of disabled individuals into existing programs raises issues of program adequacy and consumer management. If disabled people are not adequately involved and their interests are not included in service delivery, the independent living philosophy will have been compromised. To counter the possibility that disabled people may be either overlooked or swallowed by community systems, there is a federal law that supports the rights of disabled persons. Channels now exist for this newly recognized minority group to demand civil rights in their communities, and civil rights often translate as equal opportunity to utilize public services. Although the full legal process of defining the Rehabilitation Act of 1973 through judicial decisions has not yet been completed, the law has established complaint systems through the Office of Civil Rights and can be used to achieve equal access to the community. Even the fiscal conservatism of the 1980s will not be able to still the assertion that disabled persons have the right to equal opportunity.

Rehabilitation staff members can prepare their clients to expect support from their communities and inform them about the range of existing services. (See suggested resources listed at the end of this chapter.) However, clients should also be prepared to be their own advocates in locating and utilizing their community services. Since independent living demands consumer initiative and responsibility, professionals should emphasize client choice and management within the rehabilitation setting. Any tendencies toward dependency should not be reinforced by the organization's needs for efficiency or authority. If clients learn that others will make decisions for them during rehabilitation, they may practice the same acquiescence when they are discharged.

The rehabilitation staff members should attend to their own personal characteristics that support dependency and should also teach appropriate social skills to clients. Sessions on interpersonal communication and assertiveness will be directly applicable to locating, managing, and evaluating community-based services. Experienced role models who have conquered community living should participate in group training while clients are still in the rehabilitation program. People who have "been there" can offer invaluable insight to those who are cautious about their debut into conventional society.

On the lighter side, another community resource that has strong potential for independent living is recreation. Going far beyond wheelchair basketball games, the concept of community-based recreation includes participation in the arts, skiing and other winter sports, tennis, and horseback riding. Besides the obvious benefit to health to be derived from most recreational activities, this form of community participation may accomplish several other social functions.

First, by adding a very conventional element to the disabled person's life style, recreation removes some obstacles to social interaction. Person-to-person conversations about recreational activities will produce more positive images about the disabled individual. Although not many disabled individuals will be able to share discussions about running shoes, an exchange of tips about fishing equipment or citizen's band radio may lead to more lasting exchanges.

Second, recreational activities are clear evidence of the ordinary life styles that many disabled people can accomplish. What better evidence of shared human capacities than to see people in wheelchairs exercising on the city bike paths or attending a country music concert? By going public with their individual leisure interests, disabled people may be able to alleviate some of the strangeness attached to their impairments.

Third, visible participation of disabled individuals in recreational and artistic facilities reinforces in the public mind the concept behind constructing accessible environments. If the accessible museum is seen in use, able-bodied people will have a better understanding of its purpose.

Community groups will be likely referrals to appropriate recreational activities. Local advocacy groups often compile listings of recreational facilities and organize groups that share particular interests. Recreation has long been tied to therapeutic purposes, both physical and psychological. Taking part in physical or creative activities produces feelings of fitness and self-worth, certainly valuable results for disabled individuals who may not have many opportunities to attain them.

Another dimension of the human experience that is also a community resource for personal reinforcement is religious participation. Serving both as a powerful interpretive framework for understanding the disability and also as a link to shared community experiences, religious organizations may supply crucial support to disabled persons. Long-standing architectural barriers are beginning to be modified in many religious gathering places, and some thinkers such as Harold Wilke have purposefully reached out to extend supportive religious functions to the disabled.[16] Participating in religious activities symbolizes acceptance into the human community and can be an important step for both able-bodied and disabled persons. However, congregations are likely to express prevailing social attitudes as well as religious explanations of impairment. If the particular doctrine presents impairment as a sign of sin or as a badge of suffering, the individual who has an impairment may encounter extreme, stereotyped receptions from the congregation. Nevertheless, individual spiritual needs should be recognized by professionals, and directories of accessible worship places should be available to clients who wish to utilize those community resources.

Professionals who act as liaisons to community resources transmit the message that disabled individuals have choices available to them as they establish themselves in their communities. There is no single avenue to community integration, only a series of alternatives that must be sought out, selected, and utilized. For this reason, the professional who is capable of walking the narrow line between assisting and controlling clients is making a significant contribution to future independence. Although more support systems are available to disabled people who are now living independently, consumers require self-control and social competency in order to achieve the delicate balance of receiving services and living independently. Professionals who understand both the opportunities and the strains of playing the disabled person role will prepare clients more effectively for community living.

## THE NEED FOR ADVOCACY

If the rehabilitation team can communicate to clients that the disabled person role requires active participation in response to a challenging environment, then clients will be better prepared to move from rehabilitation to independent living. Professionals can transmit this expectation through professional-client relationships that are educational as well as therapeutic, rehabilitation programs that include follow-up services, and community involvement that informs both able-bodied and disabled persons about the potential of disabled individuals. In short, the rehabilitation team can act consciously as the liaison to community living.

Because independent living is an extension of the rehabilitation process, professionals have a legitimate obligation to be advocacy role models to clients. Like other citizens, disabled individuals may not understand the significance of interest group activity, let alone comprehend the relevant issues to be confronted. Awareness of the disabled role may develop slowly among some clients, so professionals should provide important reading materials and group experiences. Magazines that describe life styles available to disabled consumers and excursions to accessible community functions will demonstrate the feasibility of living independently. But appreciation of the need to overcome barriers may only emerge with experience. Therefore, rehabilitation processes should include opportunities to achieve "the dignity of risk," one of the normalization principles that teaches disabled persons how to manage themselves when they fail. As they confront the realities of community living, the disabled will learn that there are many obstacles to be surmounted. From that understanding, disabled clients will recognize the importance of advocacy to bringing necessary changes.

To be successful advocacy role models, professionals should remain informed about legislation and public appropriations that affect community service systems and be prepared to speak out for the interests of clients who will be requiring assistance as they seek a better quality of life. State legislation concerning the zoning of group homes, for example, may be very susceptible to attention from professional interest groups. Expressing opinion about accessibility, transportation, and public acceptance will not only affect the outcome of policy formation but will also communicate the legitimacy of being disabled and further reinforce the rehabilitation process.

## THE AGE OF LIMITS

The test of the next decade will be to extend the achievements of the 1970s in easing social and economic pressures on people who have disabilities. New economic challenges test the endurance of advocates who seek more accessible housing, transportation, and personal care services. If these reinforcements are forthcoming, they will relieve pressures upon disabled people and their families who otherwise will be constrained by seriously inhospitable conditions.

The independent living movement can become a viable model for other vulnerable populations. The comprehensive provision of support services to people who have received appropriate training is a system that can be applied to the aging, the mentally retarded, and the mentally ill. Certainly the demographic predictions indicate that the aging population will increase in number as medical science continues to sustain the lives of individuals who might have otherwise died. Evidence already shows that providing services to such groups in the community is less expensive economically and more effective socially than retaining these populations in institutions. Rehabilitation and independent living services can only experience greater demand in the future.

On a more humanistic level, participation in the independent living movement is an opportunity for professionals to demonstrate that individuals can exercise control over social roles. In challenging rigid social stereotypes and teaching disabled individuals important social skills, professionals defy social categorization based on physical characteristics. The disabled person role, like other social expectations, is a product of collective assumptions. If both nondisabled and disabled persons come to understand that physical impairment need not determine entire life outcomes, then disability can become an incidental feature rather than an overwhelming characteristic. Just as feminist, black power, and senior citizen activist groups have argued convincingly that anatomy is not destiny, disabled individuals and their advocates can rebel against social and economic pressures that would keep disabled people dependent and vulnerable.

## SUGGESTED RESOURCES

**Publications**
*Accent on Living.* $4.50 Quarterly.
Cheever Publishing, Inc.
P.O. Box 700
Gillum Rd and High Dr
Bloomington, IL 61701

Bruck, Lilly
*Access: The Guide to a Better Life for Disabled Americans, 1978.*
Random House
20 E 50th St
New York, NY 10022

*Disabled U.S.A.* Free.
The President's Committee on Employment of the Handicapped
Washington, D.C. 20210

Frieden, Lex, Laurel Richards, Jean Cole, and David Bailey
*ILRU Sourcebook: A Technical Assistance Manual on Independent Living.* 1979. $19.95.
The Institute on Rehabilitation and Research
1333 Moursund
Houston, TX 77030

Goldenson, Robert M., editor in chief
*Disability and Rehabilitation Handbook.* 1978.
McGraw-Hill, Inc.
1221 Ave of the Americas
New York, NY 10020

Hale, Glorya, Editor
*The Sourcebook for the Disabled. An Illustrated Guide to Easier, More Independent Living for Physically Disabled People, Their Families and Friends.* 1979.
Paddington Press Ltd.
Distributed in U.S. by
Grosset & Dunlap
95 Madison Ave.
New York, NY 10010

Lifchez, Raymond et al.
*Getting There: A Guide to Accessibility for Your Facility.*
College of Environmental Design
University of California
Berkeley, CA

*Paraplegia News.* Monthly. $5.
5201 N 19th Ave, Suite 108
Phoenix, AZ 85015

*Rehabilitation Gazette.* $3.50 disabled, $6.00 non-disabled. Plus postage/handling 75¢.
4502 Maryland Ave
St. Louis, MO 63108

*Sports 'N Spokes.* $5.50. Bi-monthly.
5201 N. 19th Ave, Suite 108
Phoenix, AZ 85015

Task Force on the Concerns of Physically Disabled Women.
*Toward Intimacy: Family Planning and Sexuality Concerns of Physically Disabled Women,* 2nd ed. 1978.
Human Sciences Press
72 Fifth Avenue
New York, NY 10011

**Organizations**
American Coalition of Citizens with Disabilities
1346 Connecticut Ave, N.W., Room 308
Washington, D.C. 20006

Barrier-Free Environments, Inc.
P.O. Box 53446
Fayetteville, NC 28305

Boston Self Help Center, Inc.
18 Williston Rd
Brookline, MA 02146

Disability Rights Center
1346 Connecticut Ave
Washington, D.C. 20036

Easter Seal Society
2023 W Ogden Ave
Chicago, IL 60612

Handicapped Homemaker Research Center
University of Connecticut
Storrs, CT 06268

Self-Help Institute
Center for Urban Affairs
Northwestern University
2040 Sheridan Rd
Evanston, IL 60201

# REFERENCES

1. Comer, R. J., and Piliavin, J. A.: The effects of physical deviance upon face-to-face interaction: the other side. J. Pers. Soc. Psychol. 23 (1):33–39, 1972.
2. Yuker, H. E.: Attitudes of the general public toward handicapped individuals. Awareness Paper. Washington, D.C., White House Conference on Handicapped Individuals, 1977.
3. Wright, B. A.: Spread in adjustment to disability. *In* Stubbins, J. (ed.): The Social and Psychological Aspects of Disability. Baltimore, University Park Press, 1977, pp. 357–365.
4. Matson, R. R., and Brooks, N. A.: Adjusting to multiple sclerosis: an exploratory study. Soc. Sci. Med. 11:245–250, 1977.
5. Trieschmann, R. B.: Spinal Cord Injuries: Psychological, Social, and Vocational Adjustment. Elmsford, NY, Pergamon Press, 1980.
6. Lindenberg, R. E.: Work with families in rehabilitation. *In* Bolton, B., and Jacques, M. (eds.): The Rehabilitation Client. Baltimore, University Park Press, 1979, pp. 146–155.
7. Zahn, M. A.: Incapacity, impotence, and invisible impairment: their effects upon interpersonal relations. J. Health Soc. Behav. 14:115–123, 1973.
8. Comfort, A.: Sexual Consequences of Disability. Philadelphia, George F. Stickley Company, 1978.
9. Goffman, E.: Stigma: Notes on the Management of Spoiled Identity. Englewood Cliffs, NJ, Prentice-Hall, 1963.
10. Cogswell, B. E.: Self-socialization: readjustment of paraplegics in the community. J. Rehabil. 34 (3):11–13, 1968.
11. Cogswell, B. E.: Rehabilitation of the paraplegic: processes of socialization. Soc. Inq. 37 (winter): 11–26, 1967.
12. Brooks, N. A.: Receiving help: management strategies of the handicapped. J. Sociol. Soc. Welf. 5 (1):91–99, 1978.
13. Laurie, G.: Housing and Home Services for the Disabled: Guidelines and Experiences in Independent Living. New York, Harper and Row, 1977.
14. Brattgard, S. O.: Sweden: Fokus, a way of life for living. *In* Lancaster-Gaye, D. (ed.): Personal Relationships, the Handicapped and the Community: Some European Thoughts and Solutions. London, Routledge and Keegan-Paul, 1972, pp. 25–40.
15. Bowe, F.: Rehabilitating America: Toward Independence for Disabled and Elderly People. New York, Harper and Row, 1980.
16. Wilke, H. H.: Creating the Caring Congregation: Guidelines for Ministering with the Handicapped. Nashville, Abingdon, 1980.

# 30

# Insurance and Rehabilitation

*by Michael Mittelmann, M.D.*

## INTRODUCTION

The purpose of the chapter is to identify the basic principles involving insurance benefit payments for rehabilitation services. For several decades, rehabilitation professionals have spent considerable effort defining their specialty.[3] Parallel developments in the insurance industry initially saw payments being made for acute medical and surgical care but scant attention being paid to the rehabilitation needs of the patient. Private sector and federal programs present similarities and differences; they are subject to understanding and misunderstanding.

The discussion will be from the viewpoint of private sector insurance reimbursement. Rehabilitation under state and federal programs, Medicaid, Medicare, active military, and veterans programs is brought about through many steps beginning with legislation. Medicare is mentioned only in this chapter because private insurance companies and Blue Cross/Blue Shield administer this federal program under contract. Without using traditional contract language, in an era when strong efforts by the insurance industry are leaning in the direction of preparing understandable, easy-to-read material, we will briefly explore and analyze samples of various lines or types of insurance.

The training and education of insurance personnel in the field of rehabilitation is obviously very limited. A few elements may be found in the educational programs available through such organizations as the Health Insurance Association of America, the International Claim Association, the Insurance Institute of America, and home office training schools of insurance companies. Claim personnel have learned a considerable amount over the years because of contact with rehabilitation providers. Often the invitation has been extended to join weekly staff conferences involving individual patients (claimants) for whom the insurance representatives are responsible. An exchange of ideas often occurs, and the insurance benefits or the law can be explained by the insurance representative as needed.

A recent survey of insurance persons who are involved with medical and rehabilitation programs for their companies revealed that they serve in a number of national and local professional organizations or trade associations in which they interact with the rehabilitation community. Also, each company has executives who serve on boards of trustees of facilities and have responsibilities on executive committees of many national organizations and fund-raising groups such as the United Way. A number of insurance companies have rehabilitation consultants in medical and vocational specialties.

The hazard of any such text is that there would be a tendency to believe that once in print, the answer to the question or topic is forever engraved. In instances in which contracts exist, the final analysis must remain in the hands of insurance and legal experts, leaving the approach in this chapter simply as a guideline overview. Input from the medical community is indeed important when further explanation of the diagnosis or treatment is necessary, and particularly when new techniques or experimental procedures are utilized. Case illustrations are given in Tables 30–1 and 2 and a Glossary of Insurance Terms appears at the conclusion.

## GROUP HEALTH INSURANCE

This insurance, sometimes called Basic/Major Medical or Comprehensive Health Insurance, applies to persons who are members of a plan. Understanding the number of variations of coverages might resemble the challenge of solving the Rubik's cube. For the most part, a basic premise is that acute rehabilitation care is covered subject to conventional deductibles, coinsurance factors, and other contract specifications.

Not all contracts cover all care at every facility. As an illustration, one large group contract does not cover outpatient occupational therapy and does not cover confinement at skilled nursing facilities, but it does cover inpatient rehabilitation at a general hospital or rehabilitation center. Understanding the provisions of the contract in force is a necessity for the plan participant and the provider, particularly if questions develop. Almost-standard wording appears in most group contracts that limit coverage to charges incurred for rental of durable (not disposable) medical and surgical equipment. Administrative variations may recognize purchase when it is more economical or when the item prescribed by a physician is not available for rental. In any event, both the therapy and the supplies must be medically necessary for the treatment of injury or disease. Certain contracts extend benefits for repair of equipment when the purchase option has been used. Two cases are given in Table 30–1.

Cardiac rehabilitation programs, pain management programs, and other highly specialized rehabilitation programs are covered for patients who are getting medically necessary therapy. Coverage of sessions at health spas or follow-ups at Y's would not be allowable. Cost of exercise equipment, stationary bicycles, and weights would not be covered. There are parallels with the Medicare program, which excludes physical fitness equipment, self-help devices, and nonmedical items for environmental control. Costs of electric hospital beds, electric wheelchairs, and the like would be allowable if the medical condition warrants and there is an accompanying prescription by a physician.

In the future, we will recognize the efforts being made by group health carriers and policyholders to look closer at rehabilitation servies as many insurance and reinsurance companies have done for decades under automobile liability and workers' compensation contracts. This expanded involvement goes beyond conventional claims payment and accompanies the growing concern about quality medical management, cost accountability, and insurance affordability.

Although admittedly the number of instances are less than 10 per cent, one is always fearful of potential fraud or abuse. One policyholder's claim payment form contains a *warning*: "Any intentional false statement in this application or willful misrepresentation relative thereto is a violation of the law punishable by a fine of not more then $10,000 or imprisonment of not more than five years, or both. (18 U.S.C. 1001)." Another company's claim form, the Prescription Drug Record Form, states just above the patient's signature/date line: "I hereby certify the above drugs and medicines were necessary for the treatment of the illness/injury reported and were purchased by me for the individual named above." Bills, prescriptions, and other pertinent data are to be retained and made available to the insurer upon request.

## HEALTH MAINTENANCE ORGANIZATION SERVICES

Over 10 million persons in the United States receive care in health maintenance organizations (HMOs) or variants thereof. The presence or absence of short-term and long-term rehabilitation coverage under HMO contracts must be determined by the prepaid plan subscribers. Those who opt for this health care delivery approach and those who provide the services should be aware of the plan's special service provisions or limitations. They would be spelled out in what is sometimes called a service agreement. Necessary in-hospital and outpatient care for a member or an eligible family dependent would ordinarily be given in facilities approved by the HMO and by staff members of the HMO or affiliated physicians. Physical therapy or private duty nursing necessitates approval. The plan might set a yearly limit on physical therapy to 30 outpatient visits that would be paid by the HMO at 100 per cent (in other words, the members pay no fee, no deductible, and no coinsurance charge). At times members do pay up to 50 per cent of costs.

Coverage of occupational therapy, speech therapy, and hearing therapy is excluded by a great number of agreements. Coverage of audiology testing is frequently permissable for persons under age 18. Yet in others, physical therapy, occupational therapy, and speech therapy are provided under home health care services for homebound members. A limit on the number of home visits for services may accompany the requirement for a partial payment by the member for the actual charges.

Frequently HMOs do not pay for supplies, mainly orthopedic and prosthetic devices, artificial aids, hearing aids, eyeglasses, and other corrective appliances. There are HMOs that do have a prosthetic device benefit, using a separate clause in the

TABLE 30-1. CASE SYNOPSES

| TYPE OF INSURANCE | AGE/SEX | DIAGNOSIS | ITEM/MODIFICATION | | | EXPLANATION |
|---|---|---|---|---|---|---|
| Group health | 22/male | Quadriplegia, C-2 | Phrenic nerve stimulators (2); respirator; motorized, lift-hydraulic wheelchair | Included in hospital charges over $100,000 | Paid | Reasonable and necessary medical treatment; met contract definition (durable medical equipment) |
| | | | Environmental control unit with intercom speakers | $4900 | Not paid | Not medical equipment; excluded by contract |
| Group health | 25/female | Chronic neck muscle spasms | Medco-Sonlator with cabinet (used) | $ 800 | Not paid | Not reasonable and necessary for home use |
| Self-insurer with excess worker's compensation policy | 28/male | Paraplegia, T-12; ruptured diaphragm; multiple fractures, right femur, tibia | Standard wheelchair<br>Motor vehicle with hand controls<br>Home modifications | $ 400<br>$4000<br>$9400 | Paid | Policyholder paid up to first $50,000; insurance company not liable until entitlements exceed $50,000 |
| Homeowners | 33/male | Quadriplegia, C-5; status postcervical spine fusion | Molded cervical brace custom made from cast | $ 275 | Paid | Policy in force had medical payments limit of $1000 |
| Professional liability (malpractice) | 27/male | Popliteal artery injury; above-knee amputation | Above-knee prosthesis; standard wheelchair; roof repair on home that he could not accomplish himself | Over $1000 advance payments made to cover expenses incurred | Paid | Liability established in this case—clear responsibility; exposure sufficient to justify rehabilitation expense payments |

service agreement, enabling reimbursement for 80 per cent of the first $5000 and 100 per cent of the eligible expense beyond $5000. A $25,000 maximum may apply. A few HMOs help members obtain items at cost or arrange for temporary rentals but not purchase of crutches and canes. To show how precisely claims are analyzed, it is noted that prepaid plans will not provide for services or supplies covered by No-Fault automobile insurance or those that are governmental responsibility. Vocational rehabilitation more commonly falls under the employer's workers' compensation insurance coverage or the state-federal program; furthermore, the Health Maintenance Organization Act of 1973 does not require this supplemental service.

Office visits to a consultant physiatrist would normally be considered as a physician office visit if reasonable and necessary for the disease or injury. Again, an approval for the consultation is required. Physical therapy, occupational therapy, speech therapy, and physical medicine consultations in skilled nursing facilities would be considered for coverage in certain HMOs for 90 days per contract year.

## MISCELLANEOUS LINES OF INSURANCE

There are three types of policies whose primary purpose is well known, but there is little appreciation for the potential role of rehabilitation. These are self-insurance, homeowners, and professional liability (malpractice). A case synopsis for each situation is given in Table 30–1.

**Self-Insurance (With an Excess Workers' Compensation Policy).** Here the corporation assumes the liability for workers' compensation. It will handle the benefit payments until a limit is reached, and at that point the insurance (excess) carrier may become directly involved. Thus, a corporation's employee benefit or insurance department would pay until reaching a contractually specified amount, say $50,000, for the medical management and rehabilitation of an injured employee.

This is particularly important in the states of California, Florida, and Minnesota, in which there are mandated rehabilitation programs. Moreover, self-insurance is permissible in 47 states. Rehabilitation staff may find themselves communicating with persons who have such titles as company manager of workers' compensation, regional self-insurance manager, coordinator, or corporate medical director. At times, the self-insured corporation may contract with a private rehabilitation vendor of medical management and vocational rehabilitation services.

**Homeowners.** The policy covers the owner's premises, subject to numerous detailed provisions and exclusions. If a claim is made or suit is filed against an insured homeowner for bodily injury, an insurance carrier might be obligated to pay up to the limit of liability. The policy could have a provision for coverage of "Medical Payments to Others" (often called Coverage F), enabling payment for necessary medical expenses. Medical expenses means reasonable charges for medical services and prosthetic devices as well.

Rarely is a rehabilitation specialist aware of the frequently small dollar limit ($1000) on "Medical Payments To Others" coverage. Obviously, $1000 would barely pay for the care of a serious burn case or a victim of a major dog bite. Sometimes but not always other insurance, for instance, workers' compensation, protects the injured person. Finally, if liability is established or a settlement is made, the injured party may receive a sum of money that could be used for medical expenses.

**Professional Liability (Malpractice).** Customarily, a person undergoing rehabilitation because of a problem resulting from an alleged act of malpractice will be afforded what is necessary before or during the litigation process. The assumption is that the person (claimant) has other coverage or funding sources, perhaps group health or an individual health plan. Nonetheless, occasions arise in which an insurance carrier begins early payment if the liability is accepted prior to settlement or award. Table 30–1 summarizes the case in which a claimant underwent a below-knee amputation resulting from vascular embarrassment. The lower extremity prosthesis and related costs were paid promptly by the insurer of the surgeon because the liability was established. There was clear responsibility, and, furthermore, the exposure was sufficient to justify the medical and vocational rehabilitation expense payments.

## INDIVIDUAL HEALTH INSURANCE

By definition, this type of health, accident or disability policy would be sold to an individual person, not a group. Rehabilitation efforts beyond the basic hospital care may be initiated for a case by the insurer if the medical expense claim payments are expected to reach a level of, for example, $10,000, and if the financial reserves range in the vicinity of $75,000.

Candidate identification becomes an ongoing judgmental process in which the insurer's staff will consider the supplemental factors of anticipated duration of disability, as for example over one year, and also the length of the benefit period, which might extend over ten years. Appropriate early settlement of a case often proves to be of value and interest to the insured person.

Contract language will specify those covered medical expenses, as well as services and supplies that are medically necessary under broadly accepted medical standards. Charges for rental of durable medical and surgical equipment and artificial eyes, limbs, and nondental prostheses are allowed unless the benefit has been paid by other means such as under Medicare, workers' compensation, or No-Fault insurance plans. A case in which benefits were denied is explained in Table 30–2. The positive application of the concept of rehabilitation in this line of insurance is illustrated by the following case.

**Case 1.** A 30-year-old woman became disabled as a result of systemic lupus erythematosus. Her disability insurance policy provided a $500 monthly indemnity benefit after a 60-day waiting period. The benefit would have been payable for five years totaling $30,000. A rehabilitation benefit provision contained in the policy allowed $1500 for tuition, special books, and equipment. The $1500 was based on three months of total disability benefits. Because of inability to return to work as a medical secretary, she desired and the insurer approved payment for a course in the use of computers. Under the terms of the policy, the insurer had the option of denying rehabilitation if the rehabilitation effort did not lead toward returning the insured to her occupation. In this case, the specialized training in computers was not expected to lend itself to returning the insured to the work force as a medical secretary. It was felt that the individual was motivated and both she and the company would benefit from the special rehabilitation effort. As such, the rehabilitation benefit was extended beyond the policy terms in the amount of $5000 for completion of the computer course. The insured signed an agreement whereby if she should be unable to find employment, the insurer would continue to provide her with a monthly disability benefit. It was agreed that if she should remain totally disabled and unable to find employment for the duration of the five-year exposure during which time benefits would have been payable, the amount that was paid for the computer course, namely $5000, would be deducted from any remaining benefits that would be paid.

Although initially unable to find employment, she ultimately did find a new job. In summary, the total exposure for the insurer over five years would have been $30,000. In addition to the $5000 for the special education, 21 monthly indemnity payments were issued for the total amount of $10,500. The net savings to the insurance carrier amounted to $14,500: ($30,000–$15,500 = $14,500).

It is acknowledged that this case demonstrates that rehabilitation does apply in the handling of individual disability claims.

## MEDICARE

Generally, there is familiarity with this health insurance program under Title XVIII of the Social Security Act, which since its inception has helped to pay for rehabilitation care as well as for the rental or purchase of certain medically necessary items of durable medical equipment. Rehabilitation services for both inpatient and outpatient are standard benefits for which patients (beneficiaries) have coverage. In the early years of the program, the leadership of the rehabilitation community, particularly leading up to the changes in 1972, provided clarification but also emphasized the importance of the need for expansion of rehabilitation benefits. Efforts are continuing as of this writing, and an entire chapter would be required to detail the issues and how they are undergoing resolution. Coverage guides in Medicare outline what pertains to inpatient and outpatient multidisciplinary rehabilitation programs, in addition to pain centers, cardiac rehabilitation, and specific modalities (e.g., acupuncture), to name only a few.

It is truly mandatory for patients and providers to consult the regulations, coverage guides, and limitations that are bound in numerous handbooks and manuals, for example: Durable Medical Equipment Coverages and Limitations, March, 1981: 2100–2100.2 (Rev.), pages 2–38 through 2–42. Only a few comments will be offered to introduce this style of governmental insurance. A case is given in Table 30–2.

Publications make clear that coverage of the cost of hospital beds, pneumatic appliances, oxygen tents, wheelchairs, crutches, and many other items is subject to meeting a yearly deductible and payment of 80 per cent of the reasonable charges. Commercial catalogs often contain consumer information and sample certificates of medical necessity to be completed by the attending physician. Costs of repair of equipment in selected areas meet coverage criteria. Footwear would be excluded unless the orthopedic shoe is part of a leg brace. Medicare does not pay for supportive devices for the feet, eyeglasses or hearing aids, but under Part B (Medical Insurance) it will cover prosthetic devices that replace all or part of an internal body organ—leg, arm, back, and neck brace and artificial legs, arms and eyes.

In fiscal year 1982, the 16th year of Medicare, it was projected that $49 billion would be paid under Part A (Hospital) and Part B on behalf of 24 million beneficiaries. It is impossible to calculate the amount paid for equipment, since it is incorporated within a category called "Laboratory and Other." This group accounted for $673 million (8 per cent) of the total in 1979.[8]

Part A intermediaries and Part B carriers must make determinations that affect the payment or nonpayment to health providers of all specialties, suppliers, and beneficiaries. Controversies may ultimately have to be resolved by consultations, peer review, professional standards review organizations (PSROs), or in the established appeals and hearings mechanism or through adjudicative, litigation, and legislative processes. Fraud and abuse situations are being carefully and methodically

**TABLE 30–2. CASE SYNOPSES**

| TYPE OF INSURANCE | AGE/SEX | DIAGNOSIS | ITEM/MODIFICATION | | | EXPLANATION |
|---|---|---|---|---|---|---|
| Individual life and health | 9/female | Bilateral tibial torsion and femoral anteversion | External rotation hip orthoses with audio biofeedback attachments | $ 600 | Not paid | Supplies not medically necessary under broadly accepted medical standards; did not meet contract intent |
| Medicare (Part B) | 70/female | Quadriplegia, C-6 | Electric hospital bed | $ 850 | Paid | Covered if carrier's physician determines patient's condition was such that frequent change in body position was necessary; verified medical necessity |
| No-Fault | 50/male | Below-knee prosthesis, damaged in vehicle accident | Below-knee prosthesis, replacement | $ 1000 | Paid | Reasonable charge for necessary product |
| Workers' compensation | 45/male | Head injury, residuals | Motorized wheelchair | $ 1800 | Paid | Compensable items under state law; reasonable and necessary |
| | | | Accessories, repairs for standard and motorized wheelchairs | 500 | | |
| | | | Home modifications | 17,000 | | |
| | | | Motorized ceiling-mounted lift hoist | 2000 | | |
| | | | Electric bed | 1600 | | |
| | | | Air conditioning equipment | 1500 | | |
| | | | Home modifications | 2000 | Not paid | Not reasonable and necessary; considered home betterment |
| Workers' compensation reinsurance | 41/male | Paraplegia, T-12 | Standard wheelchair | $ 800 | Paid | Compensable items under state law; reasonable and necessary; Reinsurer reimburses primary carrier after contractual agreement is met |
| | | | Home modifications | 6700 | | |
| | | | Motor vehicle (trade-in) with hand controls | 1100 | | |
| General liability reinsurance | 29/male | Quadriplegia, C-6 | Standard and motorized wheelchairs | $ 1900 | Paid | Reinsurer reimburses primary carrier after contractual agreement is met |
| | | | Hospital bed | 820 | | |
| | | | Used, modified van; | 11,100 | | |
| | | | Home construction | 66,500 | | |

pursued in Medicare and other public programs, particularly in periods of tight monetary constraints. Fiscal intermediaries and carriers, in addition to the federal government, have a defined role to play in this activity.

## LONG-TERM DISABILITY INSURANCE

The intent of disability insurance is to pay a portion of wage loss benefits to disabled persons. Phillips reports that there are 20 million workers who are covered under short-term group accident and sickness policies.[5] There are over 11 million who have group long-term disability (LTD) insurance. This is in distinction to workers' compensation insurance for job-related accidents or illness. To handle this population, a large premium must be paid to offset the large payout, which can range from $1000 to $5000 per month in disability insurance benefit payments. The subject of cost control is of interest to the policyholder as insurance affordability becomes a key issue. Several large corporations have focused on the importance of verification of injury claims. There is an intensifying demand to spend appropriately what is perceived as limited financial resources for quality services.[3]

Rehabilitation provisions in disability policies might allow up to six times the monthy benefit for rehabilitation-related expenses. During a period of approved rehabilitation, the patient (claimant) may still be considered totally disabled and fully protected by the terms of the LTD contract. Payment reduction occurs if income is received from various sources, including Social Security disability benefits. Most would agree that early return to work with the original employer is one of the ideal goals in this specialized type of insurance just as it is in workers' compensation.

To be considered totally disabled in terms of the usual group LTD policy, a person must be unable, by reason of disease or accidental injury, to perform duties of the usual occupation. The requirement relates to the first 12 or 24 months of the disability. After that, the test changes to the inability to perform any reasonable occupation. A reasonable occupation in this sense means any gainful activity for which a person is or may reasonably become fitted by education, training, or experience.

A physiatrist could be called upon to act as a consultant or independent medical examiner. Carrier authorization is often permissible for any reasonable tests that are necessary to make a proper determination. For example, a patient manifesting lumbar radiculopathy associated with other residuals of lumbar laminectomy might require electromyography and nerve conduction velocity evaluation to support the clinical findings. The consultant would be asked in the final narrative report to de-

## TABLE 30–3. IMPAIRMENT RATINGS

**PHYSICAL**
(check one)
Patient is:
- [ ] (a) able to perform all usual activities (no limitations).
- [ ] (b) able to perform all usual activities except heavy physical exertion (very slight limitations).
- [ ] (c) able to perform all usual activities except excessive lifting, climbing, or bending (slight limitations).
- [ ] (d) able to perform all usual activities except moderate lifting, climbing, and bending (mild limitations).
- [ ] (e) able to perform only light activity such as walking, standing, and occasional lifting less than 25 lbs (moderate limitations).
- [ ] (f) able to perform only sedentary activities, primarily sitting (moderately severe limitations).
- [ ] (g) primarily house confined, able to perform very few activities (severe limitations).
- [ ] (h) completely incapacitated, is incapable of self-care (total limitations).

**MENTAL/NERVOUS**
(check one)
Patient:
- [ ] (a) has no mental/nervous impairment.
- [ ] (b) is able to function under stress and engage in interpersonal relations (no limitations).
- [ ] (c) is able to function in most stress situations and engage in most interpersonal relations (minimal limitations).
- [ ] (d) is able to function in some stress situations and engage in some interpersonal relations (mild limitations).
- [ ] (e) is able to engage in only limited stress situations and engage in only limited interpersonal relations (moderate limitations).
- [ ] (f) is unable to engage in any stress situations or engage in interpersonal relations (severe limitations).
- [ ] (g) has significant loss of psychological, physiological, personal, and social adjustment (total limitations).

termine the severity of the medical condition and to outline the patient's capabilities in relation to future employment. Table 30–3 permits the consultant to rate an individual's physical impairment and mental impairments or to add explanatory remarks or comments, if any. Accurate completion of the narrative report and the impairment rating assists the claim staff in further handling of the claim.

Certain carriers reimburse costs incurred by the patient, providing direct benefits such as prosthetic devices, automobile adaptations, or home modifications with the approval of the policyholder as a direct payment. On occasion, extracontractual arrangements for the purchase of ramps or architectural barrier removal at home can be made with the policyholder's approval.

## NO-FAULT AND AUTOMOBILE LIABILITY INSURANCE

No-Fault is the common term or form of automobile insurance, available in a number of states, in which an insurer pays benefits regardless of fault for medical expenses and economic losses incurred. The Michigan insurance law, for instance, Section 500.3107(a), specifies how reimbursement for rehabilitation and related devices would be covered: ". . . allowable expense consisting of all reasonable charges incurred for reasonably necessary products, services, and accommodations for an injured person's care, recovery, or rehabilitation." Under Connecticut General statutes, Chapter 690, No-Fault Motor Vehicle Insurance (Section 38-319) (B-1), " 'allowable expense' means reasonable charges . . . for reasonably needed products, services, and accommodations." Massachusetts General Law, Chapter 231, Section 34(a), states that personal injury protection provisions of a policy provides for payment for all reasonable expenses for necessary medical services. An unusual case is briefly abstracted in Table 30–2.

The implications for physicians and other health professionals are apparent. One should be sure when prescribing treatment that the records clearly support *why certain modalities or medications are used as well as the frequency and duration.* Documentation of the need for ancillary diagnostic studies including x-ray should not be disregarded. When certifying a medical impairment or disability, one should sign only when there is an explanation of "why" or "how long." If there is a temporary disability, it is recommended to try to project or estimate when return to work or other activities of daily life can be reasonably expected. Each disability day is important to industry and each day is important to the patient, who must be goal-oriented while receiving quality care. Insurance carriers expect, consistent with the law, that the treatment being provided is *reasonable and necessary* for the condition that has been diagnosed. Those who treat acute injury or alleged chronic residuals need to be aware of this because the vast majority of claims do not involve spinal cord injury, head injury, or traumatic amputations, but rather soft tissue injuries, including strains and sprains. What, we might ask, are the real clinical differences between musculoskeletal strains that occur during friendly Sunday afternoon neighborhood touch football games and those allegedly sustained by motorists during automobile collisions in which there is truly minimal vehicular damage?

How many people involved in an automobile accident or in the workers' compensation setting have been told by a physician to return to work on a Monday when the previous Thursday or Friday would have been equally appropriate? There has been much written and analyzed about the cost of each extra acute hospital day or each extra therapy session that might not be appropriate.

Payment under an automobile liability policy is predicated on the insured's legal liability. If there is no liability, nothing would be paid. However, in instances in which there is liability, a carrier may advance monies to the injured party for out-of-pocket expenses prior to final settlement. A case example is given in Table 30–2.

## WORKERS' COMPENSATION

In this system, the employer assumes the cost of occupational disability. Medical rehabilitation is provided in 50 states, even if it is unspecified in the law. For example, in California, where medical and vocational rehabilitation is mandated, a rehabilitation bureau has been established in the Division of Industrial Accidents, and rehabilitation programs are compulsory on the part of the employer or insurance carrier.

There are few comprehensive references that summarize the fundamental details in each state. One resource published annually by the United States Chamber of Commerce is the Analysis of Workers' Compensation Laws.[1] It contains in outline form many excellent charts, including one summarizing rehabilitation benefits in every state. A periodic update is made regarding the total financial effect on society: "Reporting in Social Security Bulletin, U.S. Department of Health and Human Services estimated that employers spent over $17 billion in 1978 to insure or self-insure their work injury risks. This was about $3 billion, or 20 per cent higher than the 1977 costs of Workers' Compensation. The previous year, 1976, the increase in cost was 27 per cent. The average cost per $100 of payroll jumped to $1.85 for 1978 compared with $1.73 for 1977. A substantial part of this growth can be attributed to inflation, but there has been a continued rise in statutory benefit amounts, amounts payable for medical care, and indemnity awards. Medical costs totaled $2.96 billion in 1978, while compensation benefits amounted to $6.78 billion—a total of $9.73 billion for about 70 per cent of all workers' compensation costs."

For comparison purposes, in 1978, Ætna Life and Casualty paid out, on behalf of workers' compensation policyholders, $332.7 million for medical and indemnity payments. By the end of 1980, however, $500.3 million was paid (for everything from strains and sprains to catastrophic spinal cord and head injury cases). The data pinpointing the totals going toward medical and vocational rehabilitation are unknown.

Rehabilitation equipment and environmental modifications are a component part of the total cost.[4] In another excellent reference, Ross reports that many states allow for replacement or repair of damaged equipment.[7] In a few, this includes eyeglasses, dentures, or hearing aids. Penalties may be imposed in certain jurisdictions if an employer fails, neglects, or refuses to provide such appliances and care. Certain Canadian provinces stipulate a clothing allowance because of wear on clothing caused by artifical limbs (e.g., $110/year/leg). The costs of electronic environmental control systems, home modifications, and vocational communication equipment (e.g., electric typewriter) are often reimbursed by the workers' compensation carrier or self-insurer for eligible employees, whereas this would not be the case under group health, individual health, or medicare plans.[4]

Employees working in shipyards or on some offshore oil rigs, for example, may have protection under Section 39 (c) (2) of the Longshoremen's and Harbor Workers' Compensation Act. The Secretary (of Labor) may at his discretion furnish such prosthetic appliances or other apparatus not normally covered but made necessary by an injury upon which an award has been made under this act to render a disabled employee fit to engage in a remunerative occupation.

Brief mention was made in an earlier section regarding the concept of self-insurance. Table 30–2 contains pertinent case summaries.

## REINSURANCE

Reinsurance is the process whereby, in exchange for part of the premium consideration, one company, called the reinsurer, assumes a part of the risk orginally accepted by another, the primary company. Reinsurance spreads the risk of loss among many companies so that in the event of a loss, financial conditions or stability of the participants will not be jeopardized. The reinsurance contract is between the primary insurer and the reinsurer. Cases are evaluated by rehabilitation experts within each reinsurance company. They review situations in which the primary company handled workers' compensation, general liability, long-term disability, and others.

Home modifications, work site adaptations, and certain items of durable medical equipment are compensable under state workers' compensation laws. They must be reasonable and necessary. Decisions are made by the primary carrier. A reinsurer then reimburses the primary carrier after contractual agreements have been met (Table 30–2). The demands of certain patients (claimants) may not be reasonable and necessary. A reinsurer has the right to agree or disagree, and a court ruling may decide the final outcome.

## DISCUSSION

The decade of the 1980s witnessed the International Year of Disabled Persons, 1981. This was brought about by the 1975 Declaration on the Rights of Disabled Persons (United Nations General Assembly).[6] It stated, "Disabled persons are entitled to the measures designed to enable them to become as self-reliant as possible. . . ." and ". . . disabled persons have the right to medical, psychological and functional treatment, including prosthetic and orthotic applicances. . . ." Hoehne commented in the Awareness Papers of the White House Conference on Handicapped Individuals, "Those who continue to contribute to the payment of the cost of those services are entitled to optimum efficiency and acceptable levels of cost effectiveness. The objective of promoting excellence in services to handicapped individuals is not in conflict with the objective of promoting cost effectiveness."[2] Most third party payers would support these views with the realization that each case is evaluated under the terms of a specific policy, contract, or entitlement.

Rehabilitation providers and other health care professionals commonly ask the question: "How does one manage to cope with the reimbursement system and the numerous variables?" Rehabilitation professionals could arrange for prompt telephone or written contact with the field office representing the insurance carrier. This serves to make the insurer aware of the need for a decision perhaps even before the bill is submitted. The patient or family or both are encouraged to pursue an inquiry because quite often they know the claim office location, the customer service representative, or the specific name of the person handling the claim. Correspondence should contain basic information (e.g., patient name, employer's name, Social Security number, policy number) to avoid the classic problem of mismatched or unidentifiable mail. Many facilities are now providing good information pertaining to the diagnosis, the prescription, the necessity, and the approximate cost. This greatly assists those who process the claim. It is as important to know early what is going to be paid as it is to know what might be denied so that alternative funding sources can be investigated. There may be occasions when the patient will want to seek the advice of legal counsel. Employer-policyholder awareness is improved by communication relative to the particular case—an invitation to visit the rehabilitation facility and to attend staff conferences or public forums, scientific publications and follow-up with the insurance company.

Legal and medical issues are interwoven with a wide variety of reimbursement mechanisms and policy provisions. Tables 30–1 and 2 contain 11 cases. In spite of the fact that dispositions and outcomes are given, the very complex aspects of how the ultimate resolution was determined, or for that matter the interpretation or the negotiation process, has not been addressed. We would deem it essential that rehabilitation providers and more importantly their patients become knowledgeable regarding the specific situations that arise. These generally are on a case-by-case basis, and conclusions may be reached that are different from those explained in this chapter. A keystone in rehabilitation is the inter- and multidisciplinary team; the most effective team includes not only the patient but also the fiscal third party payer. Each has something to learn from the other.

## REFERENCES

1. Analysis of Workers' Compensation Laws, Chamber of Commerce of United States, Washington, D.C. 1980, p. viii.
2. Hoehne, C. W.: Service delivery systems for handicapped individuals. The White House Conference on Handicapped Individuals—Awareness Papers. Washington, D.C. U. S. Government Printing Office 1:371, 232-034/6199 1977.
3. Mittelmann, M.: Rehabilitation issues from an insurer's viewpoint: past, present, future. Arch. Phys. Med. Rehabil. 61:587–591, 1980.
4. Mittelmann, M. and Settele, J.: Insurance reimbursement mechanisms for rehabilitation equipment and environmental modifications. Arch. Phys. Med. Rehabil. 63:279–283, 1982.
5. Phillips, W. R.: Current developments in group long-term disability insurance. CPCU Journal 33:163–167, 1980.
6. Rigdon, L. T.: Civil Rights. The White House Conference on Handicapped Individuals—Awareness Papers. Washington, D.C., U. S. Government Printing Office, 1:411, 232-034/6199, 1977.
7. Ross, E. M.: Workers' Compensation Rehabilitation Laws and Programs—An Analysis of the Member Jurisdictions of the International Association of Industrial Accident Boards and Commissions, October 1981.
8. Thirteenth Annual Report on Medicare—Fiscal Year, 1979, p. 3.

# A GLOSSARY OF INSURANCE TERMS

The definitions included in this chapter are for basic information and guidance. Just as there is difficulty in expressing complex medical terminology simply, so is there a problem with translating certain quasilegal contractual wording into explicit and readable format.

**Accident**—An event takes place without one's foresight or expectations; an undesigned, sudden, and unexpected event or occurrence.

**Accident insurance**—Replaces a substantial part of earned income lost through disability caused by accidental injury. May provide for payment of medical expenses occasioned by accidental injury and indemnity for death or loss of limbs or sight suffered through accident.

**Actuary**—A specialist trained in mathematics, statistics, and accounting responsible for rate, reserve, dividend calculations, and statistical studies.

**Adjuster**—An individual representing the insurance company in discussions leading to agreement about the amount of a loss and the company's liability.

**Agency**—Insurance sales office (over 30,000 in the United States).

**Agent**—One who solicits, negotiates, or effects contracts of insurance on behalf of the insurer.

**American Insurance Association**—An association of over 200 stock insurance companies writing casualty and surety lines.

**Allowable expense**—Terminology often seen in health care contracts. It means any necessary, reasonable, and customary item of medical or dental expense. A cost, part of which or all, that is covered by a plan.

**Application**—A form on which prospective insureds state facts requested by insurer and on the basis of which the insurer decides whether or not to accept the risk, modify the coverage offered, or decline the risk.

**Automobile insurance**—Involves, for example, two basic types of coverage: (1) liability insurance (coverage for losses caused by injuries to persons) and (2) insurance for physical damage related to the automobile itself.

**Benefit structure**—The types of coverages and levels of benefits for each account chosen by the policyholder under various lines of business.

**Beneficiary**—The person named (as in an insurance policy) to receive proceeds or benefits.

**Bodily injury liability insurance**—Protection against loss arising out of the liability imposed upon the insured by law for damages because of bodily injury, sickness, or disease substained by any person or persons (other than employees).

**Broker**—An insurance broker ordinarily is a solicitor of insurance who does not represent insurance companies in a capacity as agent but places orders for coverage with companies designated by the insured or with companies of his or her own choosing.

**Carrier**—An insurance company that "carries" the insurance.

**Casualty insurance**—That type of insurance primarily concerned with losses caused by injury to persons and legal liability imposed upon the insured for such injury or for damage to property of others.

**Claim**—As used in reference to insurance, claim may be a demand by an individual or corporation to recover under a policy of insurance for loss that may come within that policy.

**Claimant**—One that asserts a right or title. May be synonymous with patient, client, beneficiary, and so forth.

**Coverage**—Generally means the protection afforded by the policy to the insured. The type of coverage refers to the kind of plan and benefit provided by contract synonymous with "insurance."

**Claim analyst**—Reviews files and resolves complicated cases (e.g., referral to peer review).

**CLU**—A professional designation awarded by the American College of Life Underwriters signifying a Chartered Life Underwriter.

**Coinsurance**—A provision in an insurance policy requiring the insured to contribute a fair and just share of the total premium out of which losses are to be paid.

**Commissioner of Insurance**—The state official charged with the enforcement of laws pertaining to insurance. Sometimes called the Superintendent or Director.

**Comprehensive major medical insurance**—A type of major medical insurance.

**Contract**—A binding agreement between two or more parties for the doing or not doing of certain things. A contract of insurance is embodied in a written document usually called the policy.

**Contribution**—That part of the insurance premium paid by either the policyholder, or the insured, or both. The term "contributory" is used to describe a group insurance plan under which the insured shares in the cost of the plan with the policyholder.

**Coordination of benefits**—A method of integrating benefits payable under more than one group health insurance plan so that the insured's benefits from all sources do not exceed 100 per cent of the allowable medical expenses.

**CPCU**—The professional designation signifying a Chartered Property and Casualty Underwriter.

**Deductible**—The amount of covered expenses that must be incurred (or "cash paid") by the insured before benefits become payable by the insurer. Insurance is written on this basis at reduced rates.

**Direct writer**—An insurance that sells its policies through salaried employees or agents who represent it exclusively rather than through independent local agents or insurance brokers.

**Disability**—See Long Term Disability.

**Exclusions**—Specified conditions or circumstances for which the policy does not provide benefits.

**Experience rating**—The process of determining the premium rate for a group risk wholly or partially on the basis of that risk's experience.

**Exposure**—The physical elements of an object, or the personal characteristics of a person that, to the limit of liability provided by an insurance policy, make up the potential for loss under the contract.

**Field office**—A company office for the purpose of supervising business within a certain territory.

**Group contract**—A contract of health insurance made with an employer or other entity that covers a group of persons identified as individuals by reference to their relationship to the entity.

**Group insurance**—Broadly, any insurance plan by which a number of employees (and their dependents) are insured under a single policy issued to their employer with individual certificates given to each insured employee. The most commonly written lines are Hospital, Surgical, Medical Expenses, Major Medical, and Comprehensive Medical Expense plans.

**Health insurance**—Insurance against loss by sickness or accidental bodily injury.

**Health Insurance Association of America**—A voluntary association of over 300 U.S. and Canadian insurance companies. As with other trade associations its purpose is to develop a forum for members and act as a public service liaison, conduct research, and so forth.

**Indemnity**—The contractual relationship that exists when one party, for a consideration, agrees to reimburse another for loss caused by designated contingencies.

**Injury**—In group health insurance, refers to nonoccupational, accidental bodily injury occurring while insured.

**Insurance company**—An organization chartered under state or provincial laws to act as an insurer. Insurance is subject to formal regulation at the state and federal level.

**Insurance policy**—The entire written contract of insurance.

**Insurance**—Coverage by contract whereby one party undertakes to indemnify or guarantee another against a loss by a specified contingency or peril.

**Insurance Services Office (ISO)**—Formed in 1971 as a consolidation of several insurance industry service organizations performing advisory, actuarial, rating, statistical, and other research services.

**Insurer**—The party to the insurance contract who promises to pay losses or benefits. Any corporation primarily engaged in the business of furnishing insurance protection to the public.

**Limited policy**—A policy providing insurance against specified types of accidents or restricted in indemnity payments as contrasted with full coverage policies.

**Long-term disability (LTD)**—A group insurance coverage that provides disability or salary continuance benefits or both.

**Loss ratio**—Losses paid (claims payment and expenses) divided by the premium earned.

**Major medical plan**—A type of health insurance that provides benefits (e.g., hospital room and board) for most types of medical expenses subject to deductibles and limits.

**Medical expense insurance**—Coverage available in various forms against expenses incurred for medical treatment and care as a result of bodily injury or illness. Examples include major medical expense insurance, surgical expense insurance, and hospitalization insurance.

**Medical proof**—Documentation from a provider of services that supports the claim for cost of treatment of a disease or injury.

**Misrepresentation**—Willfully misleading with regard to information affecting the settling of a claim.

**Mutual company**—An insurance company whose management is directed by a board of directors elected by the policyholders.

**No-Fault automobile insurance**—Generally, an automobile insurance system whereby economic loss benefits are paid directly to injured individuals without regard to who is at fault in an accident. A name often given to this coverage is Personal Injury Protection (PIP).

**Noncontributory**—A term used to describe a group insurance plan under which the policyholder pays the entire cost.

**Policy**—The document in which is set forth the contract of insurance.

**Policyholder**—The individual, firm or other organization in whose name a policy is written.

**Premium**—The amount of payment required to continue the policy during its term.

**Processor**—An administrative employee who pays or denies claims based upon contractual language, administrative practices, and policy provisions.

**Reinsurance**—A method of sharing risks among several companies to protect against excessive loss.

**Risk**—The subject matter of insurance—either a person or an object such as a home, a car or a business, or the uncertainty of financial loss.

**Stock company**—An insurance company owned by stockholders who elect a board of directors to direct the company's management.

**Underwriter**—A technician trained in evaluating risks and determining rates and coverages for it. (Term derives from Lloyd's where each person willing to accept a portion of a risk wrote their name under the description of the risk after an evaluation).

**Underwriting**—The process of selecting risks and classifying them according to their degree of insurability so that the appropriate rates may be assigned. The process includes rejection of risks.

**Veterans benefits**—Benefits including disability and medical care available through the Veterans Administration.

**Workers' compensation**—Statutory disability and medical insurance for employees who suffer job-related diseases or injuries. Payments to dependents are made if the worker is killed in industry.

## GLOSSARY REFERENCES

Group Health Insurance I. New York, Health Insurance Association of America, 1976.

Osler, R. W., and Bickley, J. S.: Glossary of Insurance Terms. Santa Monica, Insurance Press, Inc., 1972.

Terms and Phrases Commonly Used in Property, Casualty & Life Insurance. The Hartford, (83102 Rev.)

Analysis of Workers' Compensation Laws. Washington, D.C., Chamber of Commerce of the United States, 1981.

Insurance Facts 1979. New York, Insurance Information Institute.

# 31

# Medicolegal Aspects

*by Lee S. Goldsmith, M.D., LL.B.,F.C.L.M.*

A recent trend has been to include in medical texts a chapter on the law. While the emphasis has too often been on problems associated with medical malpractice, that is not the case with the specialty of physiatry. In this specialty medical malpractice litigation is secondary. Of primary importance is legislation—that is, laws that affect the specialty enacted by the various state legislatures as well as by Congress. These laws have enabled the physiatrist to assist the patient in returning to a normal and fruitful existence.

The law may be divided into two categories. First is *statute law*, the law that is enacted by state legislatures and laws passed by the United States Congress, which become the law of the land. Second is what is called *common law*, the law that evolves on the basis of the decisions of judges in evaluating the cases they hear. Medical negligence law, or malpractice, as it is too commonly called, is generally based on the latter, while the various decisions to help the handicapped and prevent discrimination against them have evolved from the direct intervention of legislative bodies.

## MALPRACTICE

Though malpractice litigation is not as great a problem for physiatrists as it is for many members of the medical profession, no chapter relating to the law would be complete without some discussion of the subject. Malpractice refers only to professional negligence, and any professional is liable for malpractice. However, it is on physicians that most of the publicity has centered.

Malpractice, or professional negligence, refers to the requirement that the professional perform in accordance with expected standards and with the standards applicable at the time the care and treatment was rendered. The professional is expected to keep abreast of his field and is expected to avail himself of equipment and facilities available.

Standards of care were originally set down in an 1898 case, *Pike* v. *Honsinger*,[1] which stated in part:

A physician and surgeon, by taking charge of a case, impliedly represents that he possesses, and the law places upon him the duty of possessing, that reasonable degree of learning and skill that is ordinarily possessed by physicians and surgeons in the locality where he practices, and which is ordinarily regarded by those conversant with the employment as necessary to qualify him to engage in the business of practicing medicine and surgery. Upon consenting to treat a patient, it becomes his duty to use reasonable care and diligence in the exercise of his skill and the application of his learning to accomplish the purpose for which he was employed. He is under the further obligation to use his best judgment in exercising his skill and applying his knowledge. The law holds him liable for an injury to his patient resulting from want of the requisite knowledge and skill, or the omission to exercise reasonable skill, or the failure to use his best judgment. The rule in relation to learning and skill does not require the surgeon to possess that extraordinary learning and skill which belongs only to a few men of rare endowments, but such as is possessed by the average member of the medical profession in good standing. Still, he is bound to keep abreast of the times, and a departure from the approved methods in general use, if it injures the patient, will render him liable, however good his intentions may have been. The rule of reasonable care and diligence does not require the exercise of the highest possible degree of care, and to render a physician and surgeon liable, it is not enough that there

---

[1]*Pike* v. *Honsinger*, 155 N.Y. 201, 49 N.E. 760 (1898).

has been a less degree of care than some other medical man might have shown, or less than even he himself might have bestowed, but there must be a want of ordinary and reasonable care, leading to a bad result. This includes not only the diagnosis and treatment, but also the giving of proper instructions to his patient in relation to conduct, exercise and the use of an injured limb. The rule requiring him to use his best judgment does not hold him liable for a mere error of judgment, provided he does what he thinks is best after careful examination. His implied engagement with the patient does not guarantee a good result, but he promises by implication to use the skill and learning of the average physician, to exercise reasonable care, and to exert his best judgment in the effort to bring about a good result.

Though decided in 1898, *Pike* is still considered to be "good" law and forms the basis for the standards of care in every state in the United States. Physicians always question attorneys as to what is good practice and what are deviations from accepted practice. The answer is always changing—with the times, with the specialty, and with the advancement of medical knowledge. Twenty years ago there were no specialists in cardiac rehabilitation medicine, so there was no litigation involving this complex subspecialty of physiatry. Therefore, there could be no standard of care on which a judgment could be made and, of course, no errors for a specialist to make. However, as medicine has developed, malpractice litigation has increased. To the specialist there are two major concerns: first, how to prevent a malpractice suit and how to avoid becoming involved in such a suit, and second, how to recognize the areas that members of the speciality most often become involved with in litigation.

As just stated, the problems in the specialty of physiatry are far fewer than in most other specialties. However, as the specialty expands, so will the areas of liability.

## PROBLEM AREAS

EQUIPMENT MALFUNCTION. Any piece of equipment may malfunction, from the electromyographic equipment to a pair of parallel bars that suddenly break under the weight of a patient. The individual in immediate charge of the equipment or the institution maintaining it is ultimately responsible for that equipment.

INADEQUATE SUPERVISION. A too-common situation is the patient being trained to use crutches who falls and either reinjures himself or suffers an even greater injury. The fault is laid on the individual who planned the training and the individual who executed the training program with the patient.

CARDIAC REHABILITATION. In this category would be included the selection of patients for stress testing, the performance of the stress testing, the immediate follow-up of the patient who underwent the test, and the development of the rehabilitation program for the patient after completion of the test. As the patients are all at high risk to begin with, there will be a certain number of fatalities. When these fatalities occur, questions may be raised as to the manner in which the patient's case was managed. There has been a tendency to rely on standards set by various associations. Such standards are acceptable minimal criteria but must be modified for the given individual. Rote following of such standards is not a basis for a successful defense.

In this high-risk area of physiatry, documentation and communication are probably the best defenses. The physiatrist will not be the primary treating physician but will in all probability be acting in the capacity of a specialist doing a special test. Under these circumstances, the physiatrist must receive the necessary information prior to the performance of the test and must be willing to forego that test if the information is not present. Will the forwarding physician receive the information necessary for care of the patient and will he be capable of using that information? Will the patient be able to use the information and follow the plan that has been established? Is the plan sufficiently clear to be followed with minimal risk? The failure to answer these questions may raise the possibility of liability. However, if there is clear documentation in response to these questions, as well as to other relevant questions, the likelihood of a problem will diminish. The good attorney representing a patient—the attorney who prepares his case well—will always want to review the treating physician's records prior to the institution of a suit. When those records are clear and complete, the chances that a suit will be filed will diminish.

It is well accepted that the closer the relationship between a physician and a patient, the less likely that the patient will sue. Among those physiatrists working closely with a patient in long-term settings, this is probably true. However, this does not apply to the physiatrist working in the remote facility doing the stress testing. Under these circumstances there is little opportunity for communication with the patient and the family, and the opportunity to create such communication must be taken.

## INFORMED CONSENT

The subject of informed consent has received a great deal of publicity during the last 15 years, out of proportion to its legal importance. However, as with the concept of medical malpractice, it is not a new idea. The basic tenets of the theory were set forth by Justice Cardozo in 1914 in his decision on a case entitled *Schloendorff* v. *The Society of New York Hospital*:[2]

Every human being of adult years and sound mind has a right to determine what should be done with his own body; and a surgeon who performs an operation without the patient's consent, commits an assault for which he is liable in damages . . . This is true except in cases of emergency where the patient is unconscious and it is necessary to operate before consent can be obtained.

In the decisions that were rendered in the 1970s, emphasis was placed on the fact that the patient must be capable of giving informed consent—that is, the patient must have been given sufficient information so that the decision, when made, will be based on the facts in the particular case, the degree of risk, as well as the degree of potential benefit. Physicians have often answered with the argument that if they were required to give complete information, so much time would be spent with a particular patient that fewer patients would be seen and less care rendered. These represent opinions in the extreme. Giving information to a patient is required, but the detail necessary will vary with the patient, the patient's condition, and the procedure to be performed. The greater the risk associated with the procedure, the greater is the patient's right to have the information that he wants in order to make an informed decision.

1. A patient may expressly state that he does not wish any information concerning the procedure. If this is the case, that particular fact should be recorded in the patient's chart.

2. A patient may be too young or physically unable to give consent. Under these circumstances, the consent, except in the time of an emergency, should be obtained from someone who has the authority to give the consent for the patient.

3. A patient who comes into a doctor's office is impliedly consenting to a physical examination, and no special consent is necessary. However, if a special test is to be performed, a consent is necessary for that test. If a patient is to undergo a stress test, the patient should be informed of the risks, consequences, and potential benefits associated with that test.

A good method of proceeding is to have a notation placed in the patient's record that the consent was given, by whom it was given, and when on the particular day that it was given. (It is not necessary to itemize all the information that was given.) It is also good practice to have the patient sign a hospital consent form, with that form being co-signed by a physician and not by a nurse. That form may well be, under the proper circumstances, signed by a physiotherapist at the time it is signed by the patient.

Though the concept of informed consent is a requirement, and the patient has the right to have the information given, its real role is in the prevention of litigation. Obtaining the consent establishes communication, rapport, and friendship, all of which lessen the likelihood of litigation.

Many states have now enacted statutes relating to informed consent. New York statute is similar to many:

4. It shall be a defense to any action for medical malpractice based upon an alleged failure to obtain such an informed consent that:

(a) the risk not disclosed is too commonly known to warrant disclosure; or

(b) the patient assured the medical practitioner he would undergo the treatment, procedure or diagnosis regardless of the risk involved, or the patient assured the medical practitioner that he did not want to be informed of the matters to which he would be entitled to be informed; or

(c) consent by or on behalf of the patient was not reasonably possible; or

(d) the medical practitioner, after considering all of the attendant facts and circumstances, used reasonable discretion as to the manner and extent to which such alternatives or risk were disclosed to the patient because he reasonably believed that the manner and extent of such disclosure could reasonably be expected to adversely and substantially affect the patient's condition.[3]

Whatever the procedure in the individual physiatrist's state, the best method, both for the benefit of the patient and protection of the physiatrist's interests, is discussion with the patient followed by recording of the fact in the patient's record.

## MALPRACTICE AND ALLIED HEALTH CARE PROFESSIONAL

Few health care providers work in a professional vacuum, but in few health care professions are the interrelationships of the providers as closely intertwined as those of the physiatrist, physiotherapist, and physiotherapist assistant. While the professional duties of each may be clear, the interrelationships may lead to various potential liability problems that are not necessarily clear.

An individual who is self-employed and who is working alone with no other co-workers is responsible for the negligence of no one but himself. However, if that individual hires a second individual who is working as an employee, the first individual is responsible not only for his own acts but also for the acts of the employee, provided that those acts are performed in the course of the employment or can be stated to be part of the job description. As an example, consider the following: a physiatrist hires and pays a salary to a physiotherapist who works in the physiatrist's office three days each week. In addition, the physiotherapist works in his own office two days a week. The physiotherapist has taken out a malpractice insurance policy to cover any and all acts of negligence. The physiatrist has taken out a malpractice insurance policy to cover himself as well as any employees.

---

[2]*Schloendorff* v. *The Society of New York Hospital*, 211 N.Y. 125, 105 N.E. 92 (1914).

[3]New York State Public Health Law G2805–d.

If the physiotherapist was negligent on one of the days he was working in his own office, the physiatrist would have no responsibility. The physiotherapist's insurance carrier would come in and defend its insured. If the physiotherapist was to commit a negligent act while working for the physiatrist, the physiatrist's insurance carrier would be called in to defend and would have the primary responsibility for the defense. The fact that the physiotherapist had his own insurance would not release the physiatrist from the ultimate responsibility for the negligence.

If the physiatrist and the physiotherapist were working in separate offices and treatment information was passed on with prescriptions, the situations would be as follows:

1. If the physiatrist failed to properly evaluate the patient and ordered the wrong therapy, which the physiotherapist could not reasonably have known was wrong, the physiatrist would be responsible.

2. If the physiatrist failed to properly evaluate the patient and ordered the wrong therapy, which a reasonable physiotherapist should have known was wrong and should not have carried out, both would be responsible.

3. If the physiatrist provided the proper instructions but the physiotherapist carried them out improperly, the physiotherapist alone would be liable.

When a physiotherapist's assistant is brought into the situation, these analogies would prevail. The supervising employer is responsible for the acts of the employee. There is still another situation:

4. If the supervising employer knew, or had reason to believe, that the independent working physiotherapist might be negligent under a given set of circumstances, the physiatrist could be liable.

The law has expanded the concept of individual responsibility for the acts of others. While this has been emphasized within the hospital setting, it is being noted in the private setting as well.

### HOSPITAL-BASED PERSONNEL

When all personnel are employees of a hospital, it is not unusual for the physiatrist to have his own malpractice insurance policy; this is either paid for by the institution directly or the payment is reimbursed by the hospital. Under all circumstances the hospital is responsible for the acts of its employees, though the defense may be paid for by separate entities. That is, the physiatrist's insurance carrier would provide representation and pay the costs of any judgment, knowing that the hospital had already paid the premium. The same situation would prevail for the physiotherapist as well as the physiotherapist assistant.

Within the hospital setting the chains of command or responsibility are set forth in manuals and memoranda. Ultimately the chairman of the department has responsibility for any and all employees of that department and the hospital who are working within the area of his supervision.

## LEGISLATION

Legislation has proliferated during the last 20 years. Legislatures have acted both on the federal and state levels. The federal government has the power to enact any legislation as it relates to federal interests and affects federal funding. The states may supplement this legislation but cannot decrease what has been offered through federal legislation.

Federal legislation affects every area from education to vocational rehabilitation. A summary of existing legislation can be found in available federal publications.[4] However, those acts of primary interest to the physiatrist are cited in the following paragraphs.

### EDUCATION OF THE HANDICAPPED ACT

This act provides federal funding for educational programs relating to the handicapped. All states need not join the program, but those states that do must provide "all handicapped children with a free, appropriate education in the least restrictive setting."

The act is aimed at providing services in five basic areas. The first is in funding general grants for handicapped education that include funds for hospital and institutions and funds for physical therapy, audiology, speech therapy, occupational therapy, and counseling. The second is funds for preschoolers who are handicapped. The third is funds to develop regional resource centers. Fourth, regional resource centers are meant to provide assistance to educators in the development of the necessary programs. Fifth, funds are allocated for programs in teacher recruitment, research, and education.

Notwithstanding that legislation has been enacted and funds appropriated to obtain requisite results. It is quite possible that certain communities are not affording the proper education to handicapped children. In a 1972 case, *Mills* v. *Board of Education of the District of Columbia*,[5] an action was brought on behalf of seven students who claimed that they were not receiving the appropriate

---

[4]Summary of Existing Legislation Relation to The Handicapped. (Obtained from Superintendent of Documents, U.S. Government Printing Office, Washington, D.C. 20402, Publication No. E-80-22014.) Key Federal Regulations Affecting the Handicapped, Publication No. (OHDS) 80–22008.

[5]*Mills* v. *Board of Education of the District of Columbia*, 348 Federal Supp. 866 (1972).

public-supported education and were, indeed, being excluded from the District schools. These children, among whom were those who were emotionally disturbed, retarded, or hyperactive, had been excluded without being given their rights. As part of the defense, the District stated, referring to itself, "these defendants say that it is impossible to afford plaintiffs the relief they request unless:

(a) The Congress of the United States appropriates millions of dollars to improve special education services in the District of Columbia; or

(b) These defendants divert millions of dollars from funds already specifically appropriated for other educational services in order to improve special educational services. . . ."

The court rejected the arguments and basically stated that if additional funds were not available, the available funds would have to be equitably distributed so that no one particular class would suffer disproportionately.

This case involves circumstances that were present in the District of Columbia, but the situation could well be applicable to many other communities in which federal funding is used or in which there were marked inequalities.

## COMPREHENSIVE EMPLOYMENT AND TRAINING ACT

The Comprehensive Employment and Training Act (CETA) contains specific provisions relating to the handicapped. According to the act, a "handicapped individual" is one who "has a physical or mental disability which, for such individual, constitutes or results in a substantial handicap to employment." Though funding for this statute has been cut in recent years, it has provided an additional method of training for the handicapped as a method of entry into the job market. In communities where such programs continue, it is one of the areas into which handicapped individuals should be directed.

It should be noted that federal statutes operate through providing funds to the states and state agencies that control the distribution of those funds, or through specific federal agencies such as the Social Security Administration. Relatively complete summaries of federal legislation and regulations routinely appear in government publications.

## STATE ACTIVITIES

While basic funding may come from Congress, the various state legislatures can take steps to ease the lives of the handicapped without the infusion in many instances of large sums of money. The New York State legislature had presented to it, in 1981, various proposed acts that would have led to concrete assistance for the handicapped. A sample of such proposed legislation follows.

1. Many states now have enacted legislation providing special license plates for motor vehicles belonging to the handicapped. Such license plates, along with requirements for allocation of parking places in commercial lots, have facilitated parking and access to commercial enterprises. In addition, a suggestion was made for special license plates for vehicles owned by commercial organizations that specialize in the transportation of the handicapped. Such vehicles would not be ambulances, so that they would not be entitled to that specific designation. A special license plate would allow a van to park in a reserved parking place to facilitate easier access and allow transport of greater numbers of individuals.[6]

2. States have traditionally had complete control over establishments in which liquor is sold, either packaged or by the glass. New York State has also maintained the authority of prior approval before any reconstruction or new construction was permitted and required a fee at the time of filing. However, in 1981 it was proposed that this filing fee be waived when included in the plans of reconstruction or new construction was "an alteration to widen a doorway, construct an access ramp, refit a restroom or any other alteration designed to provide greater accessibility to physically disabled or handicapped persons."[7]

3. Considering that a handicapped individual has probably suffered a diminution in income, and also considering that the handicapped individual would want a modifcation made in his home to facilitate his movement in accordance with the specific disability, handicapped individuals faced a problem. If the home alterations contemplated were deemed by the tax assessor to improve the residence, the handicapped individual could face higher taxes. While the state does not control the manner in which local real estate taxes are collected or their amount, it can give the local authority the opportunity to waive such taxes if it desires. The exemption from the additional taxes would not be routinely given. The restrictions are clearly set forth to apply to: "(i) a blind or physically handicapped owner of the residence, or (ii) a blind or physically handicapped member of an owner's household, if such member resides in the property." The improvement, of course, must be of the type necessary to facilitate the activities of the blind or physically handicapped individual within the premises.[8]

4. A physically handicapped individual may well not be able to drive. However, a common experience of anyone is to be asked by commercial operations on occasion for some form of identification.

---

[6]State of New York S.1467–B A 1929–B (1981).
[7]State of New York S.1570 A 2104.
[8]State of New York S.1664–A A 2117–A.

The document most often requested is a driver's license. A bill has been proposed to enable the Commissioner of Motor Vehicles to issue a "nonoperating driver's license." Thus, nondriving individuals would have a valid and acceptable means of identification.[9]

5. A bill has been suggested to allow a blind individual a tax deduction for expenses relating to the obtaining, training, or maintaining of a guide dog. The theory is that the dog enables the individual to earn an income and without the dog no income would be earned. Therefore, the dog would be a valid business expense.[10]

6. In a step that could have wide-ranging significance, a bill was proposed for the creation of an office for a state advocate for the disabled within the executive department of the state government. The advocate would be directed to take the part of the disabled as an ombudsman when conditions so indicate, as well as to ensure that the disabled have their rights. A portion of the proposed legislation is:

. . . to advise and assist the governor, the legislature, and state agencies in the development of state policies designed to meet the needs of persons with disabilities;
. . . to stimulate community interest in the problems of persons with disabilities and to promote public awareness of resources available to persons with disabilities;
. . . to advise and assist political subdivisions of the state in the development of local programs for persons with disabilities;
. . . to serve as a clearinghouse for information relating to the needs of persons with disabilities;
. . . to conduct or cause to be conducted such studies of the needs of persons with disabilities as may be appropriate . . . .

In addition to this, provisions were to be made for the setting up of an advisory council that would be of assistance to the public advocate. The council would have representatives of providers as well as recipients of the services or the parents or natural guardians of recipients.[11]

If one considers the many federal statutes that have been enacted, with their provisions of benefits and the inherent requirement that the state act on those provisions, this proposed legislation would ensure that the state would be taking maximum advantage of the benefits available. It would furnish a central location for providers, as well as recipients, to contact to determine what is available to the particular individual, locality, or educational institution.

7. Handicapped individuals have always had difficulty voting—first, because many of the polling places may not be accessible to the individual, and second, because even if the polling place were accessible, the individual may not be able to get to the polling place. It was proposed that the election laws be amended to provide the permanently disabled with "absentee" ballots that would be mailed to the residence of the individual and could be returned by mail. Once a person was identified as a permanently disabled individual, the ballots would be mailed to him routinely.[12]

Federal legislation is constantly changing. During one session of a state legislature many bills are introduced, many having potential impact on the lives of the handicapped. A chapter on the law as it relates to the handicapped is therefore out of date by the time that it is written. Additional statutes will have been proposed and enacted in the interim. The reader is advised to check his particular state as to the available resources.

---

[9]State of New York S.1664–A A 4775–A.
[10]State of New York S.1664–A A 8664–A.

---

[11]State of New York (a) A 10707.
[12]State of New York (b) S.8836 A 11206.

# 32

# The Physiatrist, Physician to the Disabled

*by Asa P. Ruskin, M.D.*

The specialty of physical medicine and rehabilitation, or physiatry, is at the same time one of the oldest and one of the newer medical specialties. Physicians since antiquity have utilized physical modalities such as light, heat, cold, exercise, and hydrotherapy for medicinal purposes. In the late nineteenth and early twentieth centuries, electrotherapy, x-ray and radium therapy, added to the other physical modalities, developed into the specialty interest area then called physical therapy, and physician specialty groups and publications developed. During the formative phases, all of these modalities and techniques were directed primarily toward the treatment of acute medical conditions, as it must be admitted that society as a whole directed very little attention and support to care of the chronically ill and disabled.

It was the impetus of caring for the wounded veteran following World War I that began to turn medical interest toward the restoration of function and led simultaneously to development of the allied health professions of physical therapy and occupational therapy. The rapid training of masseurs and physical educators followed, as well as some specialized nurses needed for the treatment of the wounded. By far the greatest thrust to acceleration and development of the field of rehabilitation medicine followed on the heels of World War II, because it was not until the 1940s that the full capability of modern medicine resulted in the survival of vast numbers of war injured who would have perished in earlier combats.

The simple example of spinal cord injury should suffice to dramatize the point. Prior to the advent of antibiotics, a spinal cord–injured person had a life expectancy of less than six months; very little, if any, attention was given to rehabilitation. At the present time spinal cord injury in many cases hardly reduces the normal life expectancy, and returning the spinal cord–injured person to economic independence becomes vital, especially if one considers that daily civilian casualties cause over 10,000 such injuries annually, the vast majority in the under-30 age group.

Along with the increased survival of large numbers of persons suffering disabilities, both congenital and acquired, has arisen society's recognition of the needs and rights of these individuals to benefit from the medical and technological developments of our era so that they can achieve the highest possible productive capacity and quality of life.

The physiatrist is that physician who, after having completed his general medical training, has gone on to fulfill the full three-year residency training period in a specialized program accredited by the American Board of Physical Medicine and Rehabilitation that was first established by the Advisory Board for Medical Specialties in 1947. At the present time over 70 medical schools have departments of physical medicine and rehabilitation and over 2000 specialists have been certified as diplomates in this field. The physiatrist brings to bear on the problems of the disabled the entire panoply of medical knowledge, both diagnostic and therapeutic, encompassing not only a myriad of pharmaceutical advances but also the latest in electronic diagnostic and treatment modalities. The physiatrist is familiar with the interface between psychology and medicine that has given rise to behavior modification, biofeedback, and similar new areas of interest. The physiatrist also has in-depth knowledge of the capabilities of and techniques utilized by the various allied health professions and is able to prescribe specific intervention and coordinate the activities of various members of the rehabilitation team, which might include physical, occupational, and speech therapists, psychologists, social workers, rehabilitation nurse-clinicians, prosthetists, orthotists, biomedical engineers, and others as the need arises.

Physiatrists base their practice on six principles:

1. The evaluation and management of patients who have physical disabilities is an integral aspect of medical care.

2. Disability can often be prevented or reduced through appropriate medical management.

3. The goals of management include improvements in physical, social, psychologic, and vocational functioning, with or without change in the basic disease process. Such goals are a proper medical concern.

4. The restoration or maintenance of a patient's functional abilities frequently demands the efforts of many specialists, including nonmedical personnel and other specialized physicians as well as the physiatrist. It is the physiatrist who must coordinate this group in the best interests of each patient.

5. Family and community resources are often essential to the rehabilitative process, and the physiatrist must include them in his diagnostic and therapeutic efforts.

6. Planning for continuity of restorative care is a medical responsibility. Such care should be oriented toward reintegrating the patient into his social setting.

While the hospital-based physiatrist is primarily concerned with rehabilitation of the severely disabled person with conditions such as hemiplegia, paraplegia, amputation, severe arthritis, and the like, the physiatrist in a daily office practice or outpatient clinic is more concerned with treatment of that 70 per cent of the population that is disabled at some time in their lives with conditions ranging from low back ache, stiff neck, "pinched nerve," tennis elbow, and the vast assortment of aches and pains that the human body is heir to.

In all instances the physiatrist is a physician who recognizes that the patient is a complex human being in a complex world and who derives great satisfaction in restoring measures of self-sufficiency to his patients, recognizing that often the restoration of function is the only real and obtainable cure.

# Evolving Roles of Health Professionals in Care of the Disabled[1]

*by Asa P. Ruskin, M.D.*

A wide diversity of health professions now render care to the handicapped and disabled. The first major group is physicians; those in almost every medical specialty are concerned to some degree with the treatment and care of disabling conditions. Leaving aside psychiatry for purposes of this discussion, the field of physical medicine and rehabilitation, or physiatry, whose practitioners are known as physiatrists, is the only medical specialty that has made treatment and rehabilitation of the disabled its primary concern. An extensive list of allied health workers has evolved with the development of interest in the care and treatment of different aspects of disability and its rehabilitation. These include physical therapists, occupational therapists, speech pathologists, rehabilitation nurses, orthotists, prosthesists, bioengineers, and specialists in rehabilitation of the visually and hearing impaired. To this incomplete list must be added the entire gamut of health professionals who may be called upon for various aspects of rehabilitative care and services.

In order to understand how these myriad occupations interrelate and what direction future events might take, it is helpful to reflect on the history of their development.

Medical science, along with all of modern technology, has been evolving at such a fantastically rapid pace that it is extremely difficult for us to realize how much has occurred in the relatively brief moment of time that is represented by the lifetimes of our own fathers and grandfathers. The Archives of Physical Medicine and Rehabilitation can trace its roots directly to the *Journal of Electrotherapeutics* in the 1890s. Let us put this in context and consider what constituted the practice of medicine at that time. In Europe the great breakthroughs and discoveries of modern physiology were at their height. Pasteur in 1885 saved a boy with his new rabies vaccine, Claude Bernard in 1889 was describing his discoveries on the physiology of the internal organs. Lister's concepts of antisepsis, first mentioned in 1865, were beginning to take hold. Medicine in general was still at the threshold of the modern era and had not yet crossed into it. Chemotherapy with Paul Ehrlich's Salvarsan was yet to come in the 1900s; the germ theory of disease was still hotly debated, with the great pathologist Virchow arguing against the bacterial theories of Pasteur. Yellow fever was still being prevented by firing cannons to dispel the night air while no one thought that mosquitoes had anything to do with its spread. A growing number of surgeons were washing their hands prior to operating and many were rinsing them with antiseptic carbolic acid.

Modern medical education in the United States was in its infancy. While major universities with organized curricula had existed in Europe for some time, medical education here was primarily the province of proprietary schools established by a

[1]Lecture delivered to the New York Academy of Medicine, October 29, 1981, in the symposium "The Disabled in Society."

few physicians, which would hold courses for three or four months a year and give certificates after two such years to those who attended. The training was entirely by lecture, with little or no clinical experience provided, and the admission requirements were ability to read, write, and pay the tuition. These schools existed in the urban centers. The rural United States still depended largely on physicians trained by apprenticeship in the stable-boy-to-surgeon tradition. A few European-style medical schools existed, including Chicago (later to become Northwestern), Harvard, and New York Medical College of Columbia University. The present-day system of medical education did not have its real beginnings until the founding of Johns Hopkins University School of Medicine in 1893, which for the first time required a college degree as prerequisite for admission and providied a four-year curriculum, including laboratory and hospital teaching. Generalized reform of medical education did not occur until after the famous Flexner report of 1910.

Our electrotherapy ancestors of the 1890s represented one among many groups with different philosophies and modes of treatment based for the most part on unscientific and primitive concepts regarding the causes of diseases. It is interesting to note that the electrotherapists allied themselves frequently with homeopathic physicians, hydrotherapists, and other practitioners who espoused the use of natural means of treatment in opposition to the allopathic physicians, who had only recently given up bloodletting and concentrated on dangerous nonspecific medication with agents such as purgatives and mercurials. At least the natural methods caused less harm and sometimes lately I've been getting the feeling that reverberations and echos of that early dichotomy may still be heard on a quiet evening.

The *Journal of Electrotherapeutics*, which included x-ray, was replaced in 1902 by the *Journal of Advanced Therapeutics*. This had expanded to include coverage of 15 departments, including orthopedics, hydrotherapy, exercise, dietetics, psychotherapy, climatology, and phototherapy. The last of these came following the discovery of ultraviolet light and its medical utilization by Finsen in 1896.

Use of the term hydrotherapy in those days bore almost no resemblance to our present use of the term for whirlpool treatment and swimming pool exercises. Hydrotherapy then involved the taking of water internally or the application of wet compresses for many diseases. I mention in passing, however, one of the physicians interested in this field, Simon Baruch, who at age 22 was a Civil War battalion surgeon. His interest in hydrotherapy had an indirect effect on our profession, which will become apparent later in this discussion.

Those physicians who had expanded their interest from limited electrotherapeutics were now referred to as "physical therapists." There were frequent conflicts with nonphysician electrotherapy assistants, who, after gaining some experience in a physician's employ, would set up shop on their own. (At that time in history there were no licenses or regulations on who could declare himself to be a health practitioner, and Kickapoo Indian tonic was being widely sold.)

In 1887 the American Orthopedics Association was organized. This group differentiated itself from general surgeons by its use of mechanical devices. Within that specialty there were many who held that orthopedic surgeons should limit themselves to the use of braces and mechanical devices, avoiding operative surgery entirely. The orthopedic surgeons went through a period of continual conflict with the general surgeons, as well as considerable conflict with the instrument makers whose "descendants" were to become the orthotists and the prosthesists of today. It was not finally resolved until the First World War.

These early physicians, physiotherapeutists, concerned themselves with the use of these modalities as applied to the general practice of medicine. Rehabilitation as we know it today was not a consideration until the advent of World War I. Prior to United States entry into the war, it become apparent because of the many battlefield casualties that large numbers of American wounded could be anticipated, and a war preparedness committee was organized. Thus in 1917 things began to move very rapidly. An orthopedist, Dr. Joel Goldthwait, who directed the medical mechanical department of the Massachusetts General Hospital and who was a personal friend of Gen. Pershing, urged the creation of a special division of orthopedic surgery in the army. He also advocated the construction of specialized orthopedic surgery hospitals with the intention that they should deal with all physical reconstruction. This was the first important declaration of independence of orthopedic surgery. The move was strongly opposed by the general surgeons, and these specialized orthopedics hospitals were never constructed. Instead, in August 1917, the Surgeon General created a new division, the Division of Special Hospitals and Physical Reconstruction, which included general surgery, orthopedic surgery, head surgery, and neuropsychiatry. In this organizational structure the orthopedists supervised artificial limbs. The orthopedists already were associated with some trained orthopedic aides, prominent among them Mary McMillan, who was the chief aide to Dr. Goldthwait at the medical mechanical department of the Massachusetts General Hospital. It was under her direction that 800 women were given 30-day training courses in what was called "military massage." They constituted the first organized corps of reconstruction aides, which was later to form the nucleus of the group of physical therapy technicians. From there evolved the American Association of Physical Therapists.

During this hectic year of 1917, three months after creation of the Division of Special Hospitals, Dr. Frank Granger, President of the American Association of Electrotherapy and Radiology, as it was then called, was appointed to head the physiotherapy section of that division. Thus the physiotherapeutic physicians were established in the area of physical reconstruction, for which their skills and techniques had wide application. These war years saw evolution of several crossroads which were to have a significant effect on the future development of rehabilitation professions.

The army nursing corps refused to accept the responsibility of supervising and controlling the physical reconstruction aides. They considered these aides to be persons of lesser training and status, whose acceptance would have reduced the higher standards of nursing at that time. This is why the occupational designation physical reconstruction aide was set up and these individuals trained as a separate unit. Had this not occurred, physical therapy today might have been a branch of the nursing profession.

Another major crossroad resulted from the conflict over vocational rehabilitation. The Surgeon General wanted this established as part of a comprehensive reconstruction program, but this idea was opposed by a civilian federal board for vocational rehabilitation that had been established the year before, and also by the Red Cross Institute for Crippled and Disabled, which had been established prior to the war. As a result of a conference set up by the Secretary of War in January 1918, military and therefore medical control of vocational rehabilitation was limited to the immediate postinjury period and separated from general civilian vocational rehabilitation, which gained its independence at that time as a branch of the educational establishment rather than medicine.

In 1918 occupational therapists were added to the corps of reconstruction aides. Occupational therapists had existed in a psychiatric setting from the early 19th century, practising ergotherapy, or "work cure and moral treatment," and had organized as the National Association for the Promotion of Occupational Therapy in March 1917 under the direction of a nurse, a social worker, a psychiatrist, and an ex-patient. Their duties during the war as reconstruction aides were not clearly distinct from those of the physical reconstruction aides previously mentioned.

During the period between the wars, the rise of the majority of present-day medical specialties was seen. The physical therapy physicians continued to promote use of physical modalities in the treatment of general medical conditions and also were instrumental in developing training programs and accreditation measures for physical therapy technicians. During this period, the time of training for physical therapy technicians was lengthened from four months to a year, and a bachelor's degree in physical education became a requirement. Many of the schools of physical therapy, however, in the same way as the early medical schools, turned out inadequately prepared technicians. In 1934 the American Physical Therapy Association, which had developed from an organization created by 30 former military aides, asked the American Medical Association to take over the accreditation of physiotherapy schools and agreed that physical therapists would work on prescription and under the supervision of physicians. By 1936 the AMA Council on Medical Education and Hospitals had inspected 35 schools and published the "essentials of an acceptable school for physical therapy technicians."

Occupational therapists continued to progress primarily under medical leadership, with various physician presidents of the Occupational Therapy Association and training requirements that were increased to six months in 1924 and to nine months in 1932.

The tragedy of World War II, coming at a time of rapidly advancing medical technology, combined to create a situation in which, for the first time in history, vast numbers of war injured were able to survive their wounds. Largely through the efforts of an internist, Dr. Howard Rusk, who was appointed head of the US Air Force Convalescent Training Program, modern rehabilitation medicine took on a new impetus. In his efforts, both with the military and in his development of the first institute of rehabilitation medicine after the war, Howard Rusk was aided in no small measure by his personal friend, Bernard Baruch, son of the Civil War physician with an interest in hydrotherapy who had become an advisor to presidents.

By 1946 the term *physiatrist* was being used as a designation for a physician specializing in physical medicine, and in 1947 the Advisory Board for Medical Specialties and the American Medical Association established the American Board of Physical Medicine as the body conferring certification in that specialty and fully equal to all other medical and surgical specialties. In 1949 the board included the words "and Rehabilitation" in its title, thus recognizing that the physiatrist is as concerned with the rehabilitation of his patients as with the treatment of their medical problems. At the time of its recognition as a specialty, four accredited residencies in physical medicine existed, offering 12 positions. Growth of the specialty steadily accelerated since that time; by 1955, 258 physiatrists had been certified. I was personally given Certificate No. 594 in 1966; by 1971 the number had reached 960. Currently there are almost 2000 physiatrists certified as diplomates, of whom 377 were certified in the two years between 1977 and 1979. In 1980, 608 residency positions existed in 62 separate programs throughout the country, 43 per cent of which are filled by women. More than half of the residents are graduates of United States medical colleges.

The rapidly accelerating development of this specialty and the concomitant development of all the various rehabilitation-related allied health professions result not so much from the efforts of those in the individual professions themselves as from advances in medical technology. These developments have extended life span and suppressed acute diseases, vastly increasing the numbers of persons surviving with disability and chronic conditions. Development has also accelerated with the recognition by society that the care and treatment of these persons is an economic obligation and an economic necessity, as well as a moral one.

At the present time, a physician who wishes to enter the specialty of physiatry must, after completing four years of medical school, have some experience with general medicine and then a three-year residency program in one of the 62 approved academic programs. Following this intensive full-time training period, the physician may sit for Part 1, the written portion of his specialty board examination, and then, after an additional one- or two-year period of experience in the field, he may qualify to apply for the second, or oral, examination, which would convey certification.

Of the allied health professions, physical therapy requires that after high school the candidate take a four-year program leading to a bachelor's degree, of which two years are devoted exclusively to training in physical therapy itself. Many therapists take additional courses and do research leading to a master's degree after they have worked as therapists.

Occupational therapy likewise has evolved a four-year baccalaureate program. Both of these professions include in-hospital clinical practice as part of their training programs. Educational requirements for the other professions are too numerous and extensive to discuss at this time. Suffice it to say that there has been a general evolution toward expanding and upgrading educational requirements. However, simultaneous with this increase in education and training, new categories of allied health professional aides and assistants are developing. These individuals carry out the simpler tasks. The new categories provide opportunities for a greater number of individuals to enter the health care delivery professions, so as to better cope with the ever-expanding needs and expectations of our population.

Now, what of the future? We have seen that there has been a steady and progressive evolution from a group of physicians with an interest in the narrow application of a single therapeutic modality, electricity, to a wide area involving the treatment of all disabilities, regardless of cause. The specialty now is concerned with the relief of disabling pain, both acute and chronic. It treats patients of all ages, from the child with cerebral palsy and congenital deformity to the adult stroke victim. It is involved with almost every aspect of medicine that results in a decrease in a patient's function. Thus we have now subspecialty interest groups in cardiac rehabilitation, pulmonary rehabilitation, and kidney disease rehabilitation of patients on dialysis, and peripheral vascular disease clinics, prosthetic clinics, pain centers, rheumatic disease and arthritis centers, neuromuscular disease centers, and spinal cord injury centers. The specialty of physical medicine and rehabilitation is different from all other specialties because it is the only one that owes its individuality not to a disease or organ but to a philosophy. This was simply stated by Howard Rusk as being "the acceptance of a philosophy of responsibility that we in medicine are not finished with our patients when the fever is down and the stitches are out." It might seem from this that rehabilitation medicine is a simple thing and that all physicians could be automatically practitioners of rehabilitation medicine on accepting this concept. At one time it was quite common to hear it said that "rehabilitation is everybody's business." In answer to this, Krusen, one of the pioneers of modern physiatry, stated that "rehabilitation can only be the business of highly skilled workers who have made it their business. I agree that rehabilitation is everybody's interest."

It is only the physician with eight or more years of postgraduate training who has the knowledge and experience necessary to cull from all of the necessary areas of medicine—engineering, behavioral sciences, and the various allied health professional areas of expertise—those elements necessary to orchestrate the diagnosis and treatment of a specific disability in a given patient. It is clear to me that the role of the physiatrist will continue to evolve. The physiatrist will become the primary physician for chronic diseases, and in the light of the advancing numbers of patients subject to these conditions, we may anticipate elaboration of several subspecialties within this group. In like fashion, the various allied health professions, which have all increased the duration and scope of the training given in their respective schools, can be expected to undergo a redefinition of roles, with increasing responsibility and areas of interest.

It is important that all professional persons be able to function at a level commensurate with their ability and training, and that avenues for professional advancement and educational opportunities be accessible to all who wish to pursue them. It is, of course, essential that there be adequate regulations and safeguards to ensure that the degree of responsibility and autonomy of each practitioner is truly commensurate with the level of training and experience required for the specific tasks undertaken.

## REFERENCES

1. Lyons, A. S. and Petrucelli, R. J.: Medicine an Illustrated History. Harry N. Abrams, Inc., New York, 1978.
2. Bettmann, O. L.: A Pictorial History of Medicine. Charles C Thomas, Inc., Springfield, Ill., 1956.
3. Gritzer, G.: Division of labor in medicine: the case of rehabilitation. Doctoral thesis, New York University, Dept. of Sociology, 1978.
4. Ruskin, A. P.: Rehabilitation, the client, the physiatrist, and the team. In Murray, R. and Kijek, J. C. (eds): Current Perspectives in Rehabilitation Nursing. C. V. Mosby Co., St. Louis, 1979.
5. Ruskin, A. P.: Physiatry, past, present and future. NY State J. Med. August 1976.

# INDEX

Dear Colleague:
We invite your help to keep

# CURRENT THERAPY IN PHYSIATRY: Physical and Rehabilitation Medicine

in tune with your needs.

Use the postcard below to tell us what topics and features you especially liked or found particularly useful in this edition. We'd also appreciate your suggestions for future editions—what subjects you would like added or deleted. Thank you for your help.

ASA P. RUSKIN, M.D.

**P.S.** Need extra copies of **CURRENT THERAPY IN PHYSIATRY: Physical and Rehabilitation Medicine** for the hospital, office or friends? Please indicate how many copies on the postage paid order card below and we'll be glad to send them to you on 30-day approval.

**Available from your bookstore or the publisher**

Medical Editor　　CURRENT THERAPY IN PHYSIATRY: Physical and Rehabilitation Medicine

Comments: _____

_____

_____

_____

_____

_____

Name _____

Address _____

City _____ State _____ ZIP _____

Use this postcard to order additional copies of **CURRENT THERAPY IN PHYSIATRY**

**YES!** Please send me _____ copies of
**Ruskin: CURRENT THERAPY IN PHYSIATRY: Physical and Rehabilitation Medicine**
**About \$67.50 • Over 600 pages • Over 380 illustrations • Order #7853-X**

Bill me plus postage & handling. If not completely satisfied, I may return the book with the invoice within 30 days at no further obligation.

☐ Charge my credit card (Save postage & handling)
　☐ VISA
　☐ MASTERCARD
　　Credit card # ▢▢▢▢▢▢▢▢▢▢▢▢▢▢▢▢
　　Exp. Date ▢▢—▢▢　　Interbank # ▢▢▢▢

Signature _____

*Add sales tax where applicable*

☐ Send me future editions of **CURRENT THERAPY IN PHYSIATRY: Physical and Rehabilitation Medicine** as available.

Name _____

Address _____

City _____ State _____ Zip _____

Prices are US only and subject to change.
883　MO5269

TRANS
2
ACCT
9
ACT
TAX CODE
TERMS
SHIP
PRI
MSG

**BUSINESS REPLY MAIL**

FIRST CLASS   PERMIT NO. 101   PHILADELPHIA, PA

postage will be paid by addressee

# W.B. SAUNDERS COMPANY

west washington square
philadelphia, PA 19105

**BUSINESS REPLY MAIL**

FIRST CLASS   PERMIT NO. 101   PHILADELPHIA, PA

postage will be paid by addressee

# W.B. SAUNDERS COMPANY

west washington square
philadelphia, PA 19105